Complications of Cancer Therapy: Best Practices in Prevention and Management

Kanika Sood Sharma • Raajit Chanana
Gaurav Sood
Editors

Complications of Cancer Therapy: Best Practices in Prevention and Management

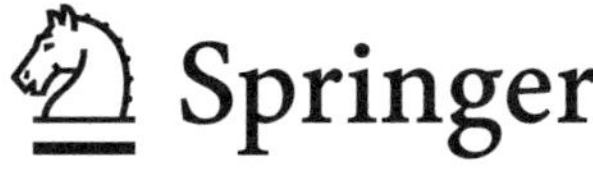

Editors
Kanika Sood Sharma
Department of Radiation Oncology
Dharamshila Narayana Superspeciality Hospital
New Delhi, India

Raajit Chanana
Department of Medical Oncology
Dharamshila Narayana Superspecialty Hospital
New Delhi, India

Gaurav Sood
Department of Liver and GI Surgery
BLK Super Speciality Hospital
New Delhi, India

ISBN 978-981-99-0986-5 ISBN 978-981-99-0984-1 (eBook)
https://doi.org/10.1007/978-981-99-0984-1

This Springer imprint is published by the registered company Springer Nature Singapore Pte Ltd.
The registered company address is: 152 Beach Road, #21-01/04 Gateway East, Singapore 189721, Singapore

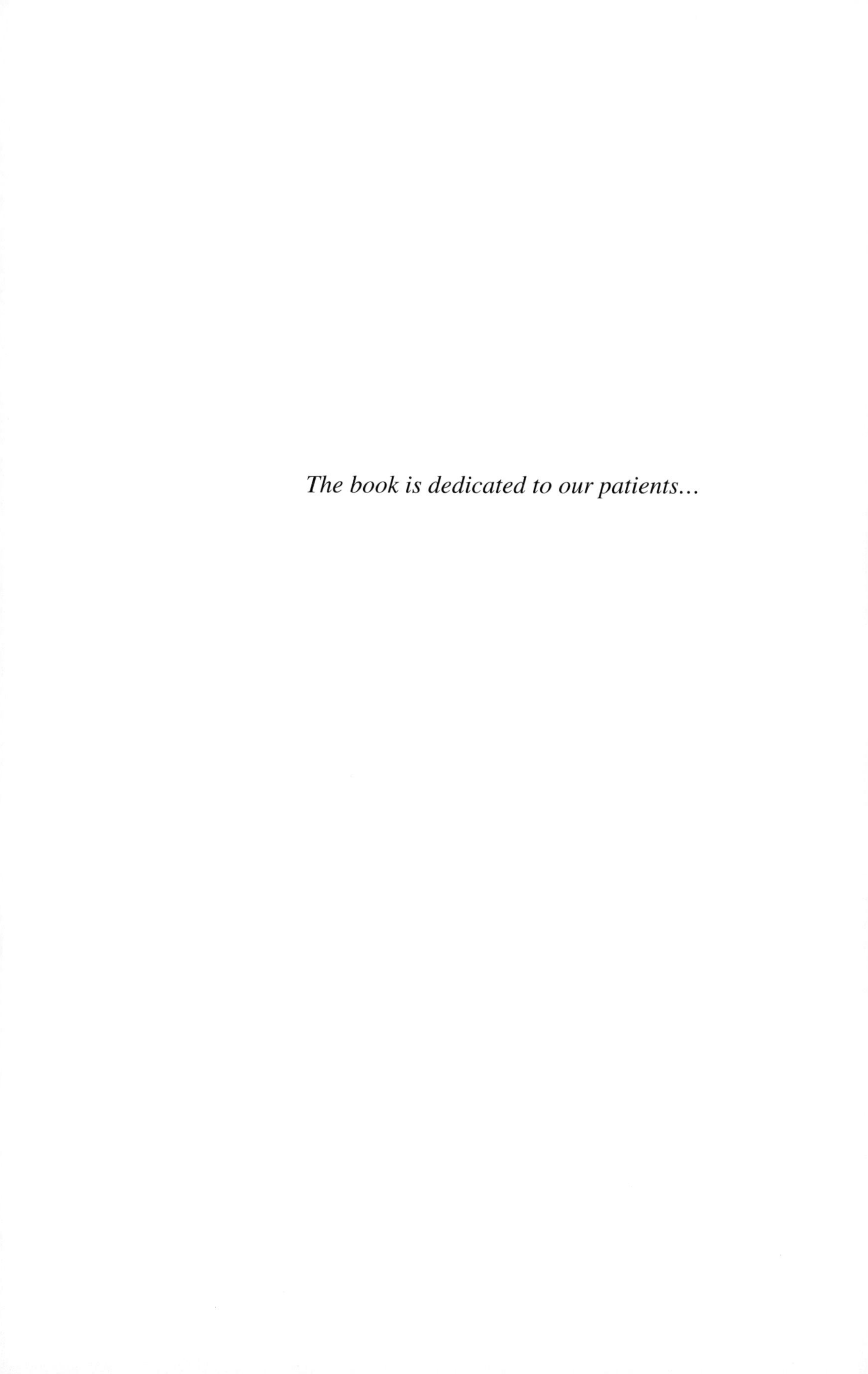

The book is dedicated to our patients…

Preface

Introduction

Cancer is one of the leading causes of mortality and morbidity worldwide. In India, majority of cancer patients present in advanced stage of disease which requires multi-modality treatment for management. There has been an increase in the medical care related to complications of this disease in last decade. The word "Complications" classically is defined as a medical problem that occurs during a disease, or after a procedure or treatment. It may be a direct outcome of the disease and its treatment or may be unrelated to it. These medical problems are unwanted, undesirable, unexpected/expected and above all unintended.

Some complications are referred to as accompaniments of treatment which fall in the category of expected side effects. The occurrence of these cannot be avoided but the intensity may be reduced by precautionary measures.

At the present era, financial toxicities which is described as the harmful effect of high cost of treatment on person's quality of life also comprise an important aspect of cancer treatment. Compared to a decade ago, patients with cancer are receiving expensive molecules and the list is growing. Inpatient hospitalizations, due to treatment complications have been the major drivers of the costs of cancer care. When compared with individuals without a cancer, cancer survivors have higher expenditure, even years after diagnosis. Early recognition and management of adverse events of cancer treatments are essential for optimal cancer care.

Types of Complications

Almost all effective medications have the potential to produce toxicity or side effects, either at therapeutic dose or at levels that exceed the therapeutic doses. All the modalities of cancer treatment (surgery, radiation, chemotherapy/immunotherapy/targetted therapy) can cause complications. By virtue of onset the complications may be acute which appear over a period of days, chronic or late which appears over a period of months or years after completion of cancer treatment. Direct complications may be an untoward effect of the malignancy where the invasion of the tumour can cause mechanical compression of the structure adjacent to it. Whereas indirect complications include systemic manifestations of the disease or related to the treatment sequelae. Some complications are attributed to specific procedures or technique. Cancer treatment entails multi-modality treatment which exposes the patients to array of procedures which interact to compound the side effects.

One such example is chemotherapy-induced neutropenia which can be aggravated/amplified with the usage of concurrent chemotherapy along with radiation therapy. Similar interaction of different treatment modalities is seen in aggravation of pneumonitis in patients receiving taxanes and thoracic radiation.

Incidence of Complications

Treatment-related side effects in routine care are common, continue throughout routine clinical care. The incidence of complications is understated due to underreporting by the patients as well as clinicians. Most patients consider side effects as a part and parcel of the cancer treatment and do not seek consultation for the same. There is also a disparity in the incidence of complications reported by physician and the patient which is evident many studies reporting treatment-related toxicities.

Acute chemotherapy toxicity can have negative effects for the patients and the health economy. Incidence of Grade III/IV acute toxicities have been reported in 35.6% of patients. The rate of hospital admission due to toxicity and go up to 13%. Nausea and fatigue are the most common side effects, along with diarrhoea and constipation. The highest hospitalization is required due to sepsis, pneumonia and acute kidney injury. A study has reported 7.5% deaths are related to chemotherapy.

Acute effects begin within 1 or 2 weeks after starting RT and often are inflammatory or reflect the depopulation of rapidly growing epithelial cells. There is usually a direct relationship between the radiation dose and volume to normal tissue and risk of toxicity. Type and incidence of complications depend on the site of cancer and modality of treatment employed.

Late side effects in adult cancer survivors and childhood cancer survivors will vary depending on the type of cancer and type of treatment. Late effects of RT often reflect fibrosis, vascular injury or gradual changes in slowly dividing tissues. Residual DNA damage may rarely cause delayed carcinogenesis. Fatigue (15–90%) and mental health issues (80%) are common long-term side effects associated with cancer treatment. Common late side effects of breast cancer treatment include lymphoedema, cardiotoxicity, fatigue, neuropathy, cognitive dysfunction, premature menopause and infertility, bone and musculoskeletal issues. Long-term side effects for colorectal cancer survivors include bowel, bladder, sexual dysfunction, complications related to ostomy, neuropathy and mental issues. Common side effects in Head and Neck cancer survivors include musculoskeletal and neuromuscular dysfunction, upper gastrointestinal dysfunction, lymphoedema, sleep apnoea, speech defects, oral health issues and mental health issues. Common long-term effects of prostate cancer include urinary, sexual or bowel dysfunction and mental issues.

Predictive Indicators

Some indictors can predict the higher incidence of certain complications and can forewarn the clinician. There are many factors which dictate the incidence of complications, and these include the pre-existing medical condition, nutritional status, social support and socio-economic status. Severity of the side effects may vary depending on the health and nutritional status of individual. The manifestation of toxicity depends on both cellular characteristics and affected organ's anatomy and physiology. Predictive indicators can be broadly classified as-patient related, tumour related and treatment related.

Pharmacogenomics or a patient's genetic composition strongly influences how chemotherapeutic agents are absorbed, metabolized and excreted by the body.

Disease site and number of chemotherapy agents are important factors which decide the likelihood of toxicity. These factors need to be accounted during formulation of the treatment care plan.

Future Considerations

With improved screening and treatment, the number of cancer survivors are expected to increase. These side effects often have significant impact on survivor's quality of life, morbidity and overall mortality. It is essential to identify both the immediate and late side effects of treatment to plan treatment management more comprehensively. Technological advancements in external-beam RT delivery, including intensity-modulated RT (IMRT), stereotactic RT (stereotactic RT and stereotactic body RT), image-guided brachytherapy and proton therapy have decreased RT toxicity by dramatically improving the ability to deliver RT that maximizes tumour dose and minimizes organ dose. The adoption of the best practices with incorporation of the preventive measures can reduce the incidence or the severity of complications. Planned health-education for patients with cancer can help us provide effective and evidence-based care to cancer patients.

New Delhi, India — Kanika Sood Sharma
New Delhi, India — Raajit Chanana
New Delhi, India — Gaurav Sood

Acknowledgement

Without the experience and support of our peers this book would not exist. We acknowledge the contribution of all the authors who have prepared the manuscript after exhaustive research and have shared their personal cases and experience.

We are indebted to our parents, spouse (Dr Prerna—wife of Dr Raajit) for the constant support and motivation in the preparation of the manuscript. Our appreciation to our children for bearing with us, who surely will love to see their names here.

- Vedika and Zian (children of Dr Raajit)
- Gaurika and Aayansh (children of Dr Kanika and Dr Gaurav)

Special thanks to Mr Sanjeev Maggoo for the secretarial support and coordination with the authors. Our heartfelt gratitude to our colleagues Dr Aditi Tanwar, Dr Manisha Himthani, Dr Amita Prakash, Dr Himanshu Joshi and Dr Payal Bhalla for helping in the editorial process in different capacities.

We also take the opportunity to thank Springer for providing a platform to write on this less talked but a pertinent topic.

Contents

Part II Cancer Surgery Related Complications

Part I

Radiation and Chemotherapy Related Complications

Chemotherapy-Induced & Radiotherapy-Induced Thrombocytopenia

1

Sarita Rani Jaiswal and Mahak Agarwal

Abbreviations

CIT	Chemotherapy induced thrombocytopenia
RIT	Radiotherapy induced thrombocytopenia
RDI	Relative Dose Intensity
TPO	Thrombopoietin
TPO-RA	Thrombopoietin-receptor agonists

1.1 Introduction

Thrombocyte is one of three major cellular components of blood produced in the bone marrow. They not only help in coagulation or regulation of haemostasis, but they mediate between the vascular system, the immune system and hemostasis [1]. Following damage to there adherence of the activated platelets to the surface of the damaged vessel and with release of various factors which causes simulation of coagulation cascade is stimulated and ultimately clot formation [2, 3]. As the clot

S. R. Jaiswal (✉)
Cellular Therapy and Immunology, Manashi Chakrabarti Foundation, New Delhi, India

Department of Blood and Marrow Transplantation, Dharamshila Narayana Super-Speciality Hospital, New Delhi, India

M. Agarwal
Department of Blood and Marrow Transplantation, Dharamshila Narayana Super-Speciality Hospital, New Delhi, India

K. Sood Sharma et al. (eds.), *Complications of Cancer Therapy: Best Practices in Prevention and Management*, https://doi.org/10.1007/978-981-99-0984-1_1

grows, there is narrowing of the blood vessel which prevents blood loss. This process is called coagulation [3]. The platelet counts are in the range of 150,000 to 350,000 platelets per microliter [4]. Thrombocytopenia is a condition or a disorder in which the platelet count is decreased below the normal lower range. The formation of blood clots is impaired, hence body is unable to control bleeding. When the count gets below 10,000 platelets per microliter, bleeding can occur without trauma at any place including the brain [5]. CIT is a disorder that develops as an adverse effect of myelo-suppressive chemotherapy [6]. These chemotherapeutic drugs not only kill cancer cells, they can also damage the platelet-forming cells in the bone marrow leading to damage in the process of megakaryopoiesis [7]. Thrombopoietin (TPO) is a predominant cytokine which is responsible for regulation of platelet counts [8]. The severity of CIT or RIT depends on the type of chemotherapy, intensity of the used drugs and the duration of treatment. Fortunately, CIT can be managed with platelet transfusions, additional medications, such as thrombopoietin agonists [9].

1.2 Incidence

The incidence of CIT varies widely depending on the agent or the combination of agents employed. In a study by Rong Lu et al., the incidence of most commonly used regimens which result in thrombocytopenia were 92.3%, 89.7%, 89.7% and 69.7% with DHAP (dexamethasone, cytarabine, cisplatin), ICE (Ifosfamide, carboplatin, etoposide), GDP (gemcitabine, dexamethasone, cisplatin) and Gemox (gemcitabine, and oxaliplatin) respectively [10].

1.3 Pathophysiology of Chemotherapy-Induced Thrombocytopenia

1.3.1 Reduces Platelets Production

It's important to understand the mechanism of CIT, as how platelets are made (Fig. 1.1) and not all chemotherapeutic drugs cause thrombocytopenia through the same mechanism. Stem cells differentiate into cells committed to megakaryocyte differentiation known as megakaryocyte colony-forming cells (MK-CFCs). These cells stop their mitotic divisions and enter into a process of endomitosis, leading to polyploid precursor cells with multiple times the normal diploid DNA content, which matures into large megakaryocytes. Finally, platelets are produced from the shredding of mature megakaryocytes; either a portion of the megakaryocyte membrane buds off into the sinusoid of bone marrow to produce platelets or mature megakaryocyte extrude long cytoplasmic processes through endothelial cells and large strands of platelet material (proplatelets) are released into the circulation (Fig. 1.1). These proplatelets eventually becoming mature platelets, possibly

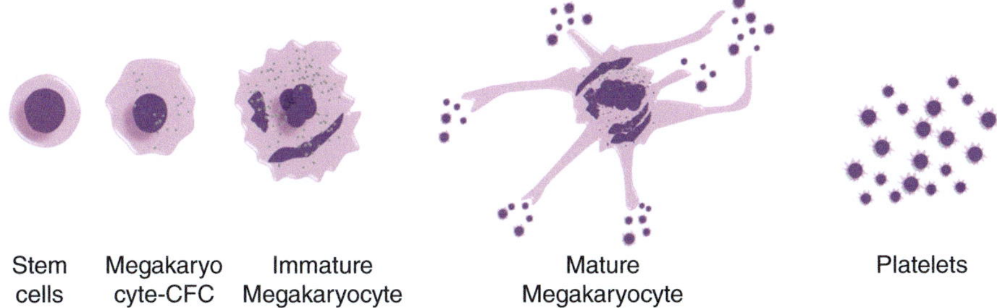

Fig. 1.1 Maturation of megakaryocyte and platelet production. Differentiation of stem cells led to megakaryocyte colony-forming cells (MK-CFCs) formation. MK-CFCs stop their mitotic divisions and enter into a process of endomitosis to form polyploid precursor immature megakaryocyte. These polyploid immature megakaryocyte precursor cells then mature into large mature megakaryocytes. Finally, platelets are produced from the shredding of mature megakaryocytes

through fragmentation in the lung. Different chemotherapy drugs have been seen to affect the megakaryocyte and platelet production pathway at different steps. Alkylating agents such as busulfan and carboplatin affect pluripotential stem cells. Cyclophosphamide spares hematopoietic stem cells because of their abundant levels of aldehyde dehydrogenase, but affects later megakaryocyte progenitors. The antibody-drug conjugate T-DM1 (trastuzumab [T] coupled to the microtubule toxin emtansine [DM1]) causes grade 3 or higher thrombocytopenia within one week in about 13% of patients by inhibiting megakaryocyte growth and differentiation. T-DM1 is internalized into megakaryocytes via the FcgRIIa receptor or by pinocytosis where it releases DM1, which inhibits megakaryocyte polyploidization and growth. Bortezomib, a proteosome inhibitor neither effect on stem cells nor megakaryocyte maturation but does inhibit NF-kB, which is a final regulator of platelet shedding. Hence a short duration of thrombocytopenia is observed.

1.3.2 Increases Platelets Destruction

Few of experimental chemotherapy agent like ABT-737 reduces the activity of the anti-apoptotic protein “Bcl-xL” and rapidly induces platelets to undergo apoptosis. After a single dose of ABT-737, platelets dropped to 30% of baseline by 2 h and re-turned to baseline after 72 h. This was not due to platelet activation. Rather, caspase-mediated apoptosis was induced with rapid appearance of phosphatidylserine on the platelet surface and clearance of these cells from the circulation by the reticuloendothelial system in the liver. The antibody-drug conjugates gemtuzumab ozogamicin (anti CD33) and inotuzumab ozogamicin (anti CD22) are both associated with acute thrombocytopenia (platelet counts dropping by 86% in 3–4 days in monkeys) and sinusoidal obliteration syndrome due to acute hepatic sequestration of platelets. Several data also show that etoposide also increases platelet apoptosis by reducing Bcl-x (L) activity. Finally, chemotherapy may accelerate platelet clearance by immune mechanisms [11]. The administration of single-agent fludarabine in lymphoma has been noted to produce an antiplatelet antibody-mediated ITP in up to 4.5% of patients. This ITP is commonly responsive to rituximab. ITP secondary to use of chemotherapy drugs have also been documented in certain circumstances. This leads to production of a drug-dependent antiplatelet antibody, causing platelet destruction, like by the drug oxaliplatin. However this effect is uncommon and needs yet to be proven.

1.4 Radiation Induced Thrombocytopenia (RIT)

Study by Chen F et al., demonstrated that radiation induced endothelial cell injury contributes to the slow recovery of platelets after radiation; it provides a deeper understanding into the pathogenesis of thrombocytopenia induced by radiation [12]. They also demonstrated that the supplementation of exogenous VEGF significantly promoted faster migration and platelet production of MKs toward the vascular niche and a rapid recovery of the platelet level in a radiation-induced thrombocytopenia (RIT) mouse model. Another study by Lambert MP. et al., shown that platelet factor-4 (PF4) is released by the damaged megakaryocytes locally, which leads to inhibition of platelet recovery [13]. Platelet factor 4 (PF4) is a negative autocrine in vivo regulator of megakaryopoiesis. Individuals with high level of PF4 may essentially be sensitive to develop thrombocytopenia whenever there is injury to the bone marrow. Blocking PF4 enhances platelet recovery while released PF4 from megakaryocytes limits the efficacy of TPO. This is possibly due to increased release of PF4 stimulated by TPO.

1.5 Guidelines for Platelet Transfusion

Initially, the recommended guideline for cut-off value of platelet transfusion was below 20,000/μL. Later, it was seen that there is an increased risk of bleeding, when the platelet count is less than 5000/μL and this risk of bleeding does not seem to change significantly between 10,000/μL and 100,000/μL [14]. It is also evident that platelet count of 7000/μL is necessary for the interaction with the endothelium. We follow the guidelines indicating platelet count less than 10,000/μL in our institution. However, it is important to check the platelet count manually as well, due to variability in platelet size following recovery from myelosuppression, resulting in falsely low platelet counts generated by standard cell counters (Table 1.1) [14].

Table 1.1 Triggers for platelet transfusion

Platelet concentration	Patient population
<5 × 10^9 cells/L	All patients who are even not bleeding and clinically stable
<10 × 10^9 cells/L	Patients with fever or post-hematopoietic cell transplantation or on chemotherapy
<20 × 10^9 cells/L	Patients receiving heparin; all outpatients or those who are to be discharged
<50 × 10^9 cells/L	Patients who are actively bleeding or who will undergo invasive procedure within the next 4 h
<100 × 10^9 cells/L	Neurosurgical patients
Any	Patients with dysfunctional platelet count (e.g., medication, disease-related, after bypass)

1.6 Evolution of Agents Directed at Thrombopoietin to Combat Thrombocytopenia

The clinically relevant TPO molecule development has occurred in 2 phases. (1) Recombinant TPO molecule (2) Recent TPO molecule. Amongst the recombinant TPO molecule, the PEG-rhMGDF is a non-glycosylated protein comprised of 153 amino acids coupled with polyethylene glycol and rhTPO is glycosylated TPO protein made in Chinese hamster ovary (Fig. 1.2). Both produced marked improvement on platelet counts and reduced the period of thrombocytopenia. The development of both was stopped in Europe and the USA due to rising titre of neutralising antibodies against PEG-rhMGDF, creating TPO deficiency and thrombocytopenia. However, rhTPO is continued in China and is licenced for CIT. Despite early failure, newer TPO molecules known as TPO-RA were developed with less side effect, like Romiplostin, eltrombopag, avatrombopag, heterombopag. TPO receptor (c-mpl) are found in all megakaryocytic cell lines, the CD34 leukemic cell lineKM1-2, and hepatocellular carcinoma cell line (Hep3B) and also on fetal liver cells and brain. The TPO receptor exists as an inactive dimer with proximal and distal HRD1 & HRD2 (hematopoetic receptor domain 1 and 2). Romiplostin and rhTPO bind to HRD2 where as other TPO-RA bind to transmembrane region of the receptor. Binding of TPO-RA to distal hematopoietic receptor domain 2 receptor domains (HRD2), or to the transmembrane region of the receptor, triggers a change in conformation of receptors and a number of signal transduction pathways, including activation of the JAK-STAT signalling pathway, which induce proliferation and differentiation of megakaryocytes. This leads to increase in platelet production (Fig. 1.3).

There are currently two approved molecules for treatment of thrombocytopenia targeting the TPO receptor. Eltrombopag was licenced in 2008 for thrombocytopenia due to chronic ITP. Romiplostim is a "peptibody" created by inserting 14 amino

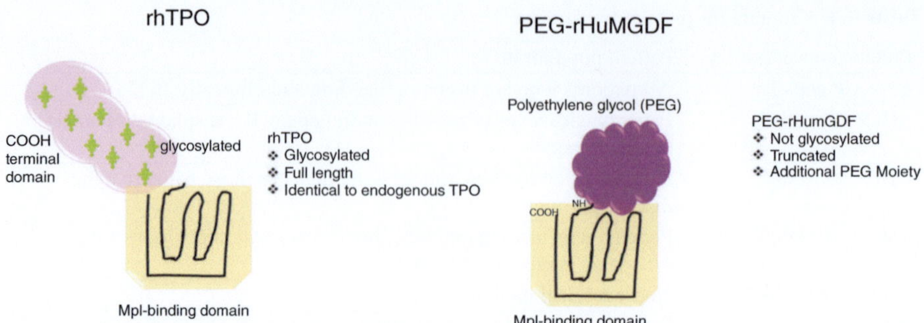

Fig. 1.2 Structure of chemotherapy drugs. Detailed composition of recombinant human thrombopoietin (rhTPO) and pegylated recombinant human megakaryocyte growth and development factor (PEG-rHuMGDF) drugs

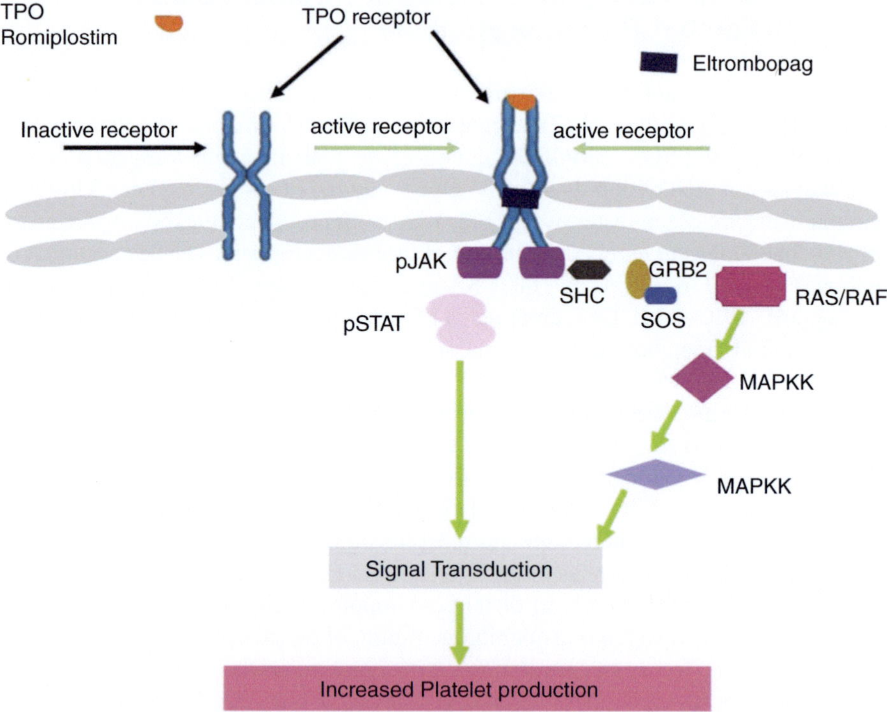

Fig. 1.3 Cellular mechanism action of Thrombopoietin Receptor Agonists (TPO-RA): Romiplostim and Eltrombopag are TPO agonists that bind to the TPO receptor and activate the JAK-STAT and MAPK signaling pathway, which induces the transcription of upstream genes of the platelet production. This leads to increased platelet production

acid peptides, approved in August 22, 2008 by FDA for long-term treatment for chronic ITP in adults who have not responded to other treatments. Along with rhTPO, the application of these molecules in CIT and RIT shall be discussed in the following sections.

1.7 Explore the Other Causes: Every Case of Thrombocytopenia in Chemotherapy Recipients are not due to Chemotherapy Alone

(a) Is there an associated immune thrombocytopenia or coagulopathy? Or is disease itself causing thrombocytopenia?
(b) Has the patient been introduced a newer medication recently? Has there been a recent infection or transfusion?
(c) Is there a chemotherapy- or disease-related thrombotic microangiopathy?
(d) Is the thrombocytopenia temporally related to radiation therapy?
(e) What dose and type of chemotherapy were given? Also what was the gap between the 2 cycles?

1.8 The Recent Recommended Approaches for CIT and RIT

There are many guidelines or algorithm available for treatment of thrombocytopenia. However, data is limited for treatment of the same condition induced by chemotherapy or radiotherapy (CIT and RIT). It depends on intent of the underlying treatment for a particular patient. Firstly, risk assessment for bleeding complications and the goal of treatment needs to be defined upfront (curative or palliative approach). Risk assessment is much emphasised when the patients are on anticoagulant therapy, or any other therapy related to the co-morbidity condition of the patient.

- For immediate recovery, platelet transfusion is necessary. Single donor platelets (SDP) are recommended compared to random donor platelets (RDP) for faster and sustained increment. This is more beneficial in patients of hematological malignancies undergoing chemotherapy or patients with severe aplastic anemia (SAA) who are in a state of bridge to transplantation.
- Rationalise the chemo regimen or dose of individual agent particularly those having more of myelosuppressive property
- Treat any other causes of thrombocytopenia: like rationalise the antibiotics if patient is on sepsis and receiving multiple antibiotics. For example, linezolid has been shown to cause myelosuppression, hence needs to be avoided [15].
- Look for coagulopathy judiciously and if any present, then treat them proactively. The data shows some tumors like adenocarcinoma of pancreas and gastric origin can cause chronic disseminated intravascular coagulation.

- To improve the haemostasis, various ant fibrinolytic agents like epsilon-aminocaproic acid (EACA) or Tranexamic acid (TXA) have been used. Tranexamic acid doses of 4–6 g per day in divided doses 6–8 h have been used in adults. However, these anti-fibrinolytic agents should be used cautiously as they increase the risk of thrombosis at the same time. National Comprehensive Cancer care Network (NCCN) recommend holding antifibrinolytics when endogenous platelet counts are >30 K/mcL and in patients with embolic strokes, active thromboembolism, and urinary tract bleeding [16].
- Recently, TPO-RA use is endorsed by NCCN, for the treatment of CIT. TPO, also known as c-Mpl ligand, is a relatively lineage-specific cytokine that stimulates megakaryocyte growth and maturation in vitro and is also a potent in vivo thrombopoietic growth factor which promotes megakaryocyte differentiation from hematopoietic stem cells and increases production of platelets.
- PF4 inhibition may have role in the condition which is associated with increased intra-marrow turnover of megakaryocytes such as RIT and CIT and also in ITP and MDS.

1.8.1 Treatment of Chemotherapy Induced Thrombocytopenia (CIT)

The clinical studies in the earlier days was done employing different cytokines, including IL-1, IL-3,IL-6, and IL-11, which showed their definite ability to stimulate platelet production either directly or indirectly in patients with CIT. However, its use is very limited because of side effects. Later the TPO molecules have shown clinical relevance. Following are few of the published data on use of these molecules in CIT.

1.8.2 Treatment with PEG-rhMGDF and rhTPO

In a major study by Basser et al. on 68 patients with advanced malignancy, who were treated with intravenous carboplatin 600 mg/m^2 and cyclophosphamide 1200 mg/m^2 and filgrastim 5 μg/kg/day in their first cycle [17]. In further cycles they received, additionally PEG-rhMGDF for 1, 3 or 7 days after chemotherapy. Patients showed a significantly higher platelet nadir with addition of study drug compared to cycle 1, (47.5 × 10^9/L vs. 36 × 10^9/L; $P = 0.003$). Not only the count but the duration days of grade 3 or 4 thrombocytopenia was also significantly shorter (0 vs. 3 days; $P = 0.004$) and no difference in the time of platelet recovery was observed. In another study done by Fanucchi et.al, PEG-rhMGDF was administration after treatment of lung cancer patients with carboplatin and paclitaxel for up to 16 days [18]. They found rise in platelet counts was statistically significant compared to placebo group. The median platelet count was 188 × 10^9/L *versus* 111 × 10^9/L ($p = 0.013$) in the study and placebo group respectively. Not only the number but duration of persistence was also increased from 7 days to 15 days ($P < 0.001$). The platelet count recovered to baseline in 14 days in the patients given PEG-rhMGDF, as compared with more than 21 days in those receiving placebo ($P < 0.001$). Neither the incidence of thrombosis was increased nor the survival affected. Another study by Moskowitz et al., in 2007 on 41 patients with Non-Hodgkin's lymphoma treated with ICE protocol has shown survival benefit from 21% to 31% ($p = 0.06$) after a median follow up of 8.6 years when they treated with PEG-rhMGDF [19].

Most important question is when to start, whether pre or post chemotherapy, with first or subsequent cycle and at what doses? A study at MD Anderson by Raj VS et al., in 2000 on 29 patients with gynaecologic cancer with rhTPO have shown a significantly reduced degree and duration of thrombocytopenia and enhanced platelet recovery after the administration of rhTPO days 2, 4, 6, and 8 after chemotherapy [20]. In patients who received the optimal biological dose of rhTPO (1.2 μg/kg of body weight) in cycle 2 (carboplatin plus rhTPO), the mean platelet count nadir was higher (44×10^9 cells/L and 20×10^9 cells/L; $P = 0.002$) and the duration of thrombocytopenia was shorter (days with a platelet count $<20 \times 10^9$ cells/L, 1 and 4 days [$P = 0.002$]. The need for platelet transfusion in this group was reduced from 75% of patients in cycle 1 to 25% of patients in cycle 2 ($P = 0.013$).

Although rhTPO is approved for CIT in China, and the numerous studies showed a definitive benefit in platelet count with the intervention compared to placebo, it is hard to assess from the published data as to whether any clinical endpoints such as relative dose intensity, remission rate, bleeding or any adverse events or survival were impacted.

1.8.3 Treatment of CIT with Newer TPO-RA

In a study performed at Memorial Sloan–Kettering Cancer Center from 2010–2012 on cancer patient, who already had persistent thrombocytopenia post chemotherapy were treated with 1–2 mg/kg of romiplostim weekly throughout the chemotherapy [21]. The platelet counts improved in all and 19/20 had platelet counts of 100×10^9/L or more. Three out of 20 patients developed deep vein thrombosis (DVT).

Another phase-II randomized prospective trial in solid tumour patients with CIT, conducted by Soff GA et al., in patients with mean platelet counts 62,000/μL for at least 4 weeks despite dose reduction or delay of chemotherapy [22]. In the randomization phase, 14 of 15 romiplostim-treated patients (93%) experienced correction of their platelet count within 3 weeks, compared with one of eight control patients (12.5%; $P < .001$). Including all romiplostim-treated patients ($N = 52$), the mean platelet count at 2 weeks of treatment was 141,000/μL compared to 57,000/μL in observation group. Forty-four patients who achieved platelet correction with romiplostim resumed chemotherapy with weekly romiplostim. Only 6.8% patient experienced recurrent reduction or delay of chemotherapy because of isolated CIT. They concluded that Romiplostim is effective in correcting CIT, and its maintenance prevents further delay in chemotherapy or any recurrence of CIT in most patients. Twenty-eight patients were continued on romiplostim for more than 6 months at a mean dose of 3.3 μg/kg. The incidence of venous thromboembolism (VTE) was

10.2% during the first year of romiplostim therapy with none discontinuing romiplostim.

In a report from four Boston cancer centers over 10 years, romiplostim had been utilized for CIT patients as a supportive care [23]. The patients who had a platelet count below 100×10^9/L for at least 3 weeks after their last chemotherapy treatment or a dose delay of longer than 1 week were enrolled. A total of 173 CIT patients (153 with solid tumors, 20 with lymphoma or myeloma) were treated. Approximately 90% received median of 4 cycles (range, 1–30) of chemotherapy on romiplostim. Amongst all the solid tumor patients, 71% had a platelet response, 79% avoided dose reductions/ delays of chemotherapy and 89% did not require platelet transfusion. The median baseline rise in the platelet count was statistically significant, $p = 0.001$ (116×10^9/L Vs 60×10^9/L ($P = 0.001$). The median weekly romiplostim dose was 3 mg/kg (interquartile range, 3–5 mg/kg). Patients who had extensive bone marrow involvement by tumor, prior pelvic radiotherapy or treated with temozolomide failed to show the response. Also response rate was lower in patients with aggressive lymphoma and myeloma. The incidence of adverse event like thrombosis was observed in 11% and bleeding rates 7.1%. In this study 2 different dosing algorithms were explored: (1) On days of chemotherapy administration (2) except on days of chemotherapy administration along with weekly doses. Patients on weekly dosing had a significantly higher median platelet count (143×10^9/L vs. 106×10^9/L; $P < 0.001$) and a higher rate of achieving a platelet response (81% vs. 63%; $P = 0.006$). Other clinical out-comes including the extent of chemotherapy RDI reduction and bleeding were better in patients receiving weekly treatment. The two ongoing trials of romiplostim in CIT are, NCT03937154 and NCT03362177.

In a randomized study (NCT00102726) on prophylaxis in 183 patients with CIT, receiving either placebo or eltrombopag with various doses 50 mg, 75 mg or 100 mg on days 2 through 11 for at least two 21-day chemotherapy cycles [24]. No toxicity was observed with eltrombopag, and it increased the platelet count in CIT compared to placebo group. Various other studies have documented the beneficial effects of eltrombopag and the maximum tolerated dose was capped at 100 mg due to the risk of thrombo-embolic events [3/183]. A larger randomised phase II study investigated eltrombopag 100 mg as prophylaxis for the prevention of CIT in patients receiving either gemcitabine alone (42 patients) or gemcitabine with carboplatin or cisplatin (32 patients) over six cycles of chemotherapy. The primary endpoint was the mean pre-treatment platelet count over six cycles of chemotherapy. The treatment was well tolerated with no increased risk of thrombosis (5/52 [9.6%] on eltrombopag and 2/23 [8.7%] on placebo) but was complicated by a 65% withdrawal rate. The geometric mean platelet count of the 48 eltrombopag–treated patients was 246×10^9/L compared with 193×10^9/L for the 23 placebo patients, but the difference did not attain statistical significance ($p = 0.103$). Patients receiving eltrombopag had a slightly lower rate of grade 3/4 thrombocytopenia (27/50 [54%] vs. 16/23 [70%]) and slightly higher nadir platelet counts than patients receiving placebo.

Zhu et al., carried out a real-world retrospective observational study in China, regarding the assessment of the response in lymphoma patients whose platelet counts dropped below 30 × 10^9/L and who were then treated with eltrombopag (n = 51), rhTPO (n = 50) or no platelet growth factor support (n = 52) [25]. The baseline platelet counts were 24 × 10^9/L in all three groups. After 10 days, the platelet count [median (standard division)] in those on eltrombopag and rhTPO was higher compared to placebo patients (131 × 10^9/L [71 × 10^9/L], 147 × 10^9/L [68 × 10^9/L], and 76 × 10^9/L [40 × 10^9/L] (in placebo group), respectively; $P < 0.001$). In this study the period [mean days (Standard deviation)] of thrombocytopenia (platelet counts <50 × 10^9/L) was 6.25 (2.61), 5.48 (2.62), and 8.33 (3.98) days, respectively ($P = 0.036$). The days [mean days (standard deviation)] required for recovery of platelet counts to more than 50 × 10^9/L was 6.33 (2.31), 5.44 (2.57), and 8.32 (2.53) days, respectively in eltrombopag, rhTPO and placebo groups ($P = 0.001$). Patients receiving eltrombopag or rhTPO were less likely to have grade 2/3 bleeding (5.9% and 4.0%) compared with untreated patients (11.5%). Many other studies are currently ongoing.

1.8.4 Other Drugs in the Pipeline

Avatrombopag has been studied in patients with CIT with solid organ malignancies but failed to show any benefit. Several CIT studies are ongoing with Avatrmbopag. Another molecule under study is Hetrombopag for which ongoing study is: NCT03976882: A Randomized, Double-blind, Placebo-controlled Multi-centre Study with an Open-label Extension to Evaluate the Efficacy and Safety of Hetrombopag for the Treatment of Chemotherapy-induced Thrombocytopenia in subjects with malignancy.

1.9 Conclusions

Thrombocytopenia is a common hematological complication developing following chemotherapy and radiotherapy in patients with malignancies, both hematological as well as non-hematological. This is one of known risk factor for bleeding and a serious obstacle to maintenance of dose intensity of chemotherapy regimens, compromising the therapeutic effect and ultimately the overall response. Oncologists should focus on addressing risk factors for thrombocytopenia, both in terms of preventing severe bleeding complications as well as maintain unhindered cancer-directed therapy. Platelet transfusion remains the cornerstone for acute management of thrombocytopenia in cancer. Novel agents like TPO-RA have shown beneficial effect in both CIT and RIT. In addition, whether a TPO plus anti-PF4 strategy can be developed to improve the outcomes in RIT remains to be seen.

Acknowledgement I am grateful to Dr. Suparno Chakrabarti for reviewing the manuscript.

Disclosures Nothing to disclose.

Authorship Contribution SRJ wrote the manuscript. MA contributed in reproduction of the figures and in referencing.

1. CIT frequently complicates cancer treatment causing delays in chemotherapy treatment, dose reductions, and discontinuation, ultimately compromising the outcomes.
2. Single donor platelet (SDP) transfusion is most effective way to prevent the acute complications due to thrombocytopenia.
3. Romiplostim (TPO-RA) is effective for the management of CIT in patients with solid tumors, as demonstrated by early recovery of platelet counts and low rates of chemotherapy dose reductions, treatment delays, bleeding, and platelet transfusions.
4. Romiplostim weekly dosing resulted in improved outcomes as compared with more intermittent intracycle dosing.
5. Romiplostim was generally ineffective in patients with BM invasion by tumour, prior pelvic irradiation or on temozolomide.
6. VTE is one of important side effect related to use of TPO-RA which should be looked for once patient is on continuous exposure.
7. Clinical development of rhTPO and PEG-rhMGDF has stopped in 2000 due to the development of neutralizing antibodies to PEG-rhMGDF.
8. The rhTPO is widely used to treat CIT in China and is unavailable elsewhere.
9. Eltrombopag is also approved and its dose is capped to 100 mg once daily for CIT and RIT.
10. The Clinical practice guidelines need to be followed for specific clinical circumstances with full understanding of overall condition of individual patient.

References

1. Koupenova M, Clancy L, Corkrey HA, Freedman JE. Circulating platelets as mediators of immunity, inflammation, and thrombosis. Circ Res. 2018;122(2):337–51.
2. Ghoshal K, Bhattacharyya M. Overview of platelet physiology: its hemostatic and nonhemostatic role in disease pathogenesis. ScientificWorldJournal. 2014;2014:781857.
3. Jurk K, Kehrel BE. Platelets: physiology and biochemistry. Semin Thromb Hemost. 2005;31(4):381–92.
4. Tranum BL, Haut A. Thrombocytosis: platelet kinetics in neoplasia. J Lab Clin Med. 1974;84(5):615–9.
5. Jinna S, Khandhar PB. Thrombocytopenia. Treasure Island: StatPearls; 2022.
6. Epstein RS, Weerasinghe RK, Parrish AS, Krenitsky J, Sanborn RE, Salimi T. Real-world burden of chemotherapy-induced myelosuppression in patients with small cell lung cancer: a retrospective analysis of electronic medical data from community cancer care providers. J Med Econ. 2022;25(1):108–18.
7. Zeuner A, Signore M, Martinetti D, Bartucci M, Peschle C, De Maria R. Chemotherapy-induced thrombocytopenia derives from the selective death of megakaryocyte progenitors and can be rescued by stem cell factor. Cancer Res. 2007;67(10):4767–73.
8. de Graaf CA, Metcalf D. Thrombopoietin and hematopoietic stem cells. Cell Cycle. 2011;10(10):1582–9.
9. Zhang X, Chuai Y, Nie W, Wang A, Dai G. Thrombopoietin receptor agonists for prevention and treatment of chemotherapy-induced thrombocytopenia in patients with solid tumours. Cochrane Database Syst Rev. 2017;11:CD012035.
10. Lu R, Lin Q, Chen S, Ye X. Chemotherapy-induced thrombocytopenia and platelet transfusion in patients with diffuse large B-cell lymphoma. Transl Cancer Res. 2020;9(3):1640–51.
11. Kuter DJ. Treatment of chemotherapy-induced thrombocytopenia in patients with non-hematologic malignancies. Haematologica. 2022;107(6):1243–63.

12. Chen F, Shen M, Zeng D, Wang C, Wang S, Chen S, et al. Effect of radiation-induced endothelial cell injury on platelet regeneration by megakaryocytes. J Radiat Res. 2017;58(4):456–63.
13. Lambert MP, Xiao L, Nguyen Y, Kowalska MA, Poncz M. The role of platelet factor 4 in radiation-induced thrombocytopenia. Int J Radiat Oncol Biol Phys. 2011;80(5):1533–40.
14. Szczepiorkowski ZM, Dunbar NM. Transfusion guidelines: when to transfuse. Hematology Am Soc Hematol Educ Program. 2013;2013:638–44.
15. Cossu AP, Musu M, Mura P, De Giudici LM, Finco G. Linezolid-induced thrombocytopenia in impaired renal function: is it time for a dose adjustment? A case report and review of literature. Eur J Clin Pharmacol. 2014;70(1):23–8.
16. Griffiths EA, Alwan LM, Bachiashvili K, Brown A, Cool R, Curtin P, et al. Considerations for use of hematopoietic growth factors in patients with cancer related to the COVID-19 pandemic. J Natl Compr Cancer Netw. 2020:1–4.
17. Basser RL, Underhill C, Davis I, Green MD, Cebon J, Zalcberg J, et al. Enhancement of platelet recovery after myelosuppressive chemotherapy by recombinant human megakaryocyte growth and development factor in patients with advanced cancer. J Clin Oncol. 2000;18(15):2852–61.
18. Fanucchi M, Glaspy J, Crawford J, Garst J, Figlin R, Sheridan W, et al. Effects of polyethylene glycol-conjugated recombinant human megakaryocyte growth and development factor on platelet counts after chemotherapy for lung cancer. N Engl J Med. 1997;336(6):404–9.
19. Moskowitz CH, Hamlin PA, Gabrilove J, Bertino JR, Portlock CS, Straus DJ, et al. Maintaining the dose intensity of ICE chemotherapy with a thrombopoietic agent, PEG-rHuMGDF, may confer a survival advantage in relapsed and refractory aggressive non-Hodgkin lymphoma. Ann Oncol. 2007;18(11):1842–50.
20. Vadhan-Raj S, Verschraegen CF, Bueso-Ramos C, Broxmeyer HE, Kudelka AP, Freedman RS, et al. Recombinant human thrombopoietin attenuates carboplatin-induced severe thrombocytopenia and the need for platelet transfusions in patients with gynecologic cancer. Ann Intern Med. 2000;132(5):364–8.
21. Parameswaran R, Lunning M, Mantha S, Devlin S, Hamilton A, Schwartz G, et al. Romiplostim for management of chemotherapy-induced thrombocytopenia. Support Care Cancer. 2014;22(5):1217–22.
22. Soff GA, Miao Y, Bendheim G, Batista J, Mones JV, Parameswaran R, et al. Romiplostim treatment of chemotherapy-induced thrombocytopenia. J Clin Oncol. 2019;37(31):2892–8.
23. Al-Samkari H, Soff GA. Clinical challenges and promising therapies for chemotherapy-induced thrombocytopenia. Expert Rev Hematol. 2021;14(5):437–48.
24. Kellum A, Jagiello-Gruszfeld A, Bondarenko IN, Patwardhan R, Messam C, Mostafa KY. A randomized, double-blind, placebo-controlled, dose ranging study to assess the efficacy and safety of eltrombopag in patients receiving carboplatin/paclitaxel for advanced solid tumors. Curr Med Res Opin. 2010;26(10):2339–46.
25. Zhu Q, Yang S, Zeng W, Li M, Guan Z, Zhou L, et al. A real-world observation of eltrombopag and recombinant human thrombopoietin (rhtpo) in lymphoma patients with chemotherapy induced thrombocytopenia. Front Oncol. 2021;11:701539.

Management of Radiation Proctitis

2

Vineeta Goel and Rachna Jain

2.1 What Is Radiation Proctitis?

Radiation proctitis is inflammation of the rectum that occurs as a result of acute damage to the rectum sustained from secondary to pelvic radiation therapy. Pelvic radiotherapy is an essential component of treatment for many pelvic malignancies—urological, gynaecological, and gastrointestinal malignancies (prostate, urinary bladder, cervix, uterus, and anus). During the course of pelvic radiotherapy, the rectum may be damaged, as it lies within the field of irradiation.

2.2 Types of Radiation Proctitis

Radiation proctitis can be classified as acute or chronic, depending upon the time duration of symptoms in relation to the treatment.

- Acute Radiation Proctitis - It occurs within six weeks of radiation therapy.
- Chronic Radiation Proctitis (CRP)—It may either occur as a sequel of acute radiation proctitis or may have a delayed inception (10-15 months to 30 years after radiation exposure) [1].

2.3 Incidence

Incidence of Acute Radiation Proctitis—The incidence of acute radiation proctitis is in the range from 8% to 13% when treated with brachytherapy alone and up to 21% when used in combination with other modalities [2].

V. Goel (✉) · R. Jain
Fortis Hospital, Shalimar Bagh, Delhi, India

K. Sood Sharma et al. (eds.), *Complications of Cancer Therapy: Best Practices in Prevention and Management*, https://doi.org/10.1007/978-981-99-0984-1_2

Incidence of Chronic Radiation Proctitis (CRP)—It is a relatively frequent late (after 3–6 months) side effect that affects 5–20% of cancer patients [3].

2.4 Risk Factors

Risk factors for radiation proctitis depends upon the volume of rectum irradiated, RT technique, total RT dose, and dose per fraction [4].

- Doses of radiation <45 Gy can cause lesser radiation proctitis.
- Doses between 45 and 70 Gy cause higher incidence of proctitis.
- Doses above 70 Gy causes significant injury to the surrounding area [5, 6].

Incidence of radiation proctitis is lesser with more conformal form of radiation techniques like IMRT, VMAT, IGRT as compared to 3 DCRT or conventional form of RT.

Factors which can increase the susceptibility to Radiation Proctitis [7, 8]:

- Coexisting vascular disease
- Connective tissue disease
- Inflammatory bowel disease
- Concomitant chemotherapy
- Smoking and alcohol
- Diabetes

2.5 Pathogenesis

Ionizing radiation can cause acute and chronic damage to normal rectum and colon. Proctitis manifests as vascular damage, mucosal ischaemia, thickening and ulceration. CRP occurs due to progressive epithelial atrophy and fibrosis associated with obliterative endarteritis, chronic mucosal ischemia, submucosal fibrosis, and new vessel formation, which leads to clinical symptoms [9] such as bleeding, ulcers, strictures and fistula formation. CRP is also termed as Radiation Associated Vascular Ectasias (RAVE) for cases where bleeding occurs from vascular ectasias, rather than ischemia and fibrosis [10].

2.6 Symptoms

Acute proctitis symptoms—diarrhea, mucus discharge, urgency, tenesmus, and uncommonly bleeding [7].

Chronic radiation proctitis—diarrhea, mucus discharge, urgency, tenesmus, and bleeding with potential iron-deficiency anemia that requires blood transfusions, obstructed defecation due to strictures with symptoms of constipation, rectal pain, urgency, and, rarely, fecal incontinence due to overflow [7].

2.7 Diagnosis

Diagnosis by endoscopy (colonoscopy or sigmoidoscopy) is important to exclude other causes of proctitis (inflammatory bowel disease, infectious colitis, ischemic colitis, diversion colitis, diverticular colitis) [11]. Figure 2.1 depicts the endoscopic findings.

There are three main forms of endoscopic findings in CRP:

- Inflammation predominant form (I-CRP)—edema, mucosal pallor, and ulcer
- Bleeding predominant form (B-CRP)—friability, spontaneous hemorrhage, and telangiectasia
- Mixed form—with features from both I-CRP and B-CRP [11].

Vienna Rectoscopy Score (VRS) is used for the endoscopic classification of CRP and is used to describe rectal mucosa [12]. The VRS divides the inner rectal mucosa into 12 mucosal areas.

Scoring of VRS: Each area is scored on the presence and grading of

- Telangiectasia (Grade 0–3)
- Congested mucosa (Grade 0–3)
- Ulceration (Grade 0–4)
- Stricture (Grade 0–4)
- Necrosis (Grade 0–1)

2.7.1 Role of Biopsies in Radiation Proctitis

When suspecting radiation proctitis, rectal biopsies are contraindicated as they may initiate chronic, poorly healing wounds and increase risk of rectal fistulas. Biopsy is justified only if a malignancy is suspected. Biopsies should be taken from the

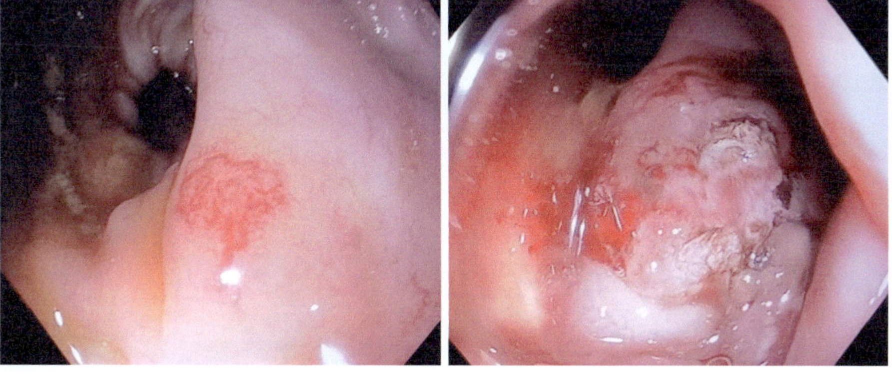

Fig. 2.1 Endoscopic features illustrating oedema, telangiectatic lesions and ulcers

posterior and lateral rectal walls. This helps to avoid the irradiated high-dose areas, which may cause complications. To summarize, biopsies should be avoided, as they do not contribute to the diagnosis.

2.8 Prevention

To prevent CRP, the high priority in RT is to exclude the rectum from the irradiation fields. Use of planning constraints is to reduce the irradiated rectal volume and decrease the risk of rectal toxicity [13]. The use of conformal radiation techniques like 3 DCRT,IMRT and IGRT can minimize the dose of radiation to the rectum while maximizing the dose to the target. When combining external radiation therapy and brachytherapy composite doses of external and brachytherapy to rectum should be evaluated.

Radiation proctitis depends upon the volume of rectum irradiated, RT technique, total RT dose, and dose per fraction [4]. Doses of radiation <45 Gy can cause lesser radiation proctitis. Doses between 45 and 70 Gy cause higher incidence of proctitis. Doses above 70 Gy causes significant injury to the surrounding area [5, 6].

2.9 Reirradiation Acceptable Doses

Re-irradiation is used in selected cases of primary rectal carcinomas with local relapse with pre-operative or post-operative radiation therapy done previously. Treatment was done with conventional fractionation 1.8–2 Gy per fraction upto a cumulative EQD2 (3) dose of 85–95 Gy [14].

2.10 Management

The management depends upon the type of radiation proctitis. Figure 2.2 depicts the management strategy for radiation proctitis.

2.10.1 Acute Proctitis

Medical management and supportive care includes hydration, antidiarrheals, anti-inflammatory drugs and steroid or 5-aminosalicylate enemas. Interruption of therapy is typically the definitive treatment.

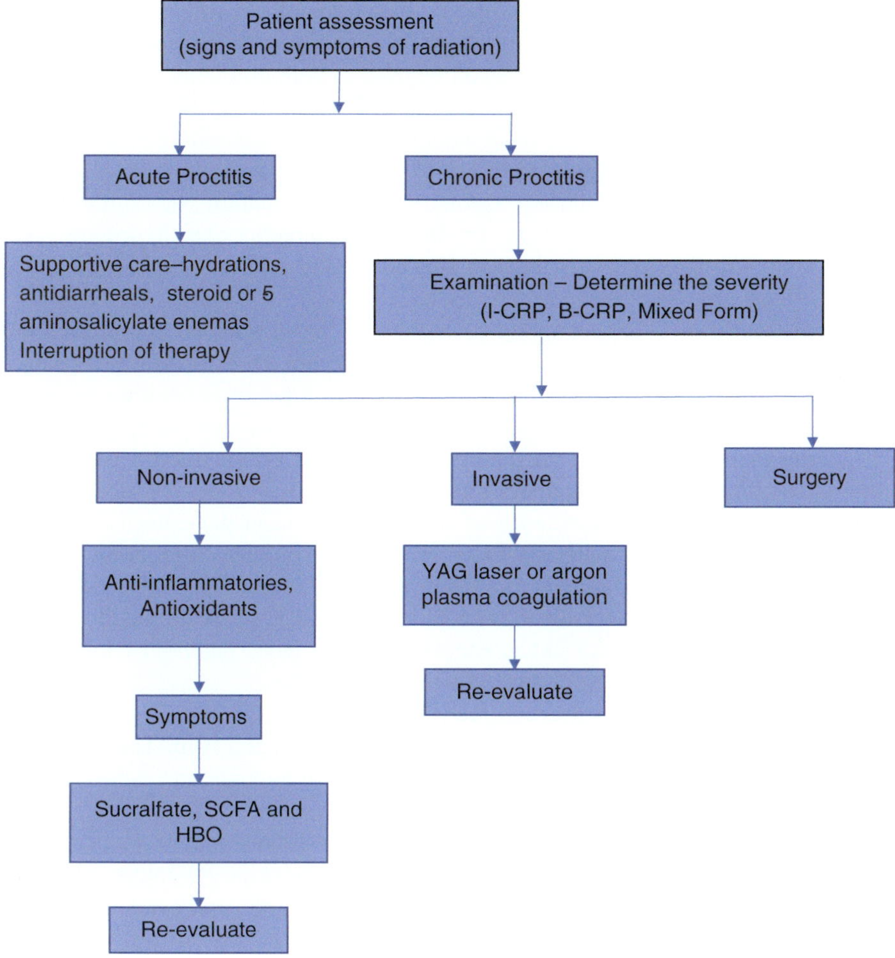

Fig. 2.2 Summarizes the management strategies for treatment of radiation proctitis

2.10.2 Chronic Proctitis

The management of chronic proctitis can be divided into:

1. **Non-invasive treatment** can be provided with the use of oral, rectal, or gaseous agents, which include anti-inflammatory agents, sucralfate, short-chain fatty acids, antioxidants and hyperbaric oxygen therapy.
   1.1 **Anti-Inflammatory Agents**—Agents such as sulfasalazine or 5-aminosalicylic acid (mesalamine) are usually first line treatments.

The mechanism of action of both nonsteroidal anti-inflammatory agents is through the inhibition of prostaglandin synthesis or free radical scavenging activity [15]. Mesalamine can be used as both oral tablet starting with a dose of 400 mg 2–3 times in a day for 1–2 weeks. In addition to oral mesalamine, one can also add rectal suppository of mesalamine which also provides good symptomatic relief.

Other anti-inflammatory agents used in combination with sulfasalazine or 5-aminosalicylic acid are prednisone, betamethasone, hydrocortisone, and metronidazole. Steroids can also be used to produce anti-inflammatory effects.

1.2 **Sucralfate**—It is a complex of highly sulphated sucrose and aluminium hydroxide which stimulate epithelial healing and the formation of a protective barrier. Rectal sucralfate (3 g) enema is superior in treating radiation proctitis as compared to anti-inflammatory regimens and can help in relieving symptoms in 75% of patients [16]. Rectal enema should be used as retention enema. One can even use a small disposable feeding tube inserted in rectum for local instillation of sucralfate enema suspension.

1.3 **Short chain fatty acids (SCFA)**—are the main oxidative fuel of the colonic mucosa and stimulate colonic mucosal proliferation [17]. SCFA also exerts a vasodilatory effect on the arteriole walls to improve blood flow [18]. Supplementation with SFCA enemas may accelerate healing by improving the hypoxic injury experienced by the colonocytes.

1.4 **Hyperbaric oxygen therapy (HBO)**—It involves the pathological process of ischemia that compromise blood flow to the rectal wall. The benefit of HBO is achieved through the decrease of tissue hypoxia, through its angiogenic and antibacterial effects [19].

1.5 **Antioxidants**—Cytoprotective effects of antioxidants help in reducing cellular oxidative stress, which is caused by radiation injury to intestinal tissue. Vitamin A along with other therapies help in significantly reducing rectal symptoms of CRP.

2. **Invasive** treatments include ablation, endoscopic coagulation and surgery

2.1 **Ablative Procedures**—Ablative techniques are reserved for the treatment of symptoms refractory to medical management and include formalin, endoscopic coagulation, and argon plasma coagulation. These techniques can be associated with complications that include bleeding, perforation, fistulas, and stenosis.

2.2 **Endoscopic Coagulation**—Endoscopic coagulation devices are effective for the control of radiation induced bleeding through coagulation of focal bleeding telangiectasias. It is done with either Argon Plasma Coagulation (APC) or YAG laser coagulation. Figure 2.3 depicts the endoscopic APC. They are based on the delivery of thermal coagulation and is done in patients suffering from significant radiation proctitis [20]. Single sessions help to improve symptoms, but generally 2–3 treatments are needed to achieve optimum results [21].

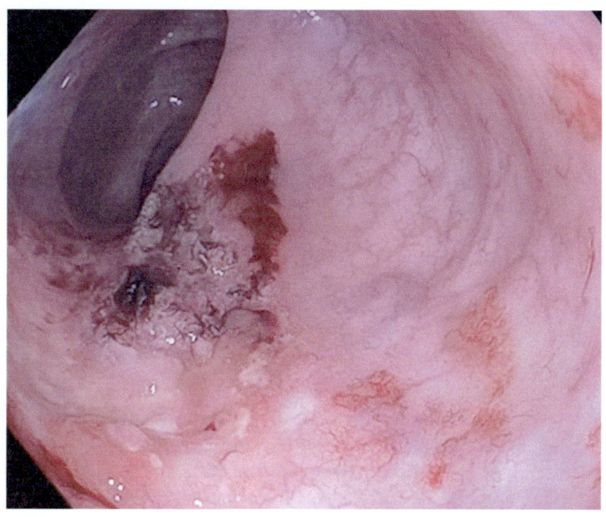

Fig. 2.3 Endoscopic features illustrating APC

2.3 **Surgery**—It is considered as the last option for patients with radiation proctitis. Less than 10% [22] of patients with CRP require surgery. In patients where surgery is done, it is directed at specific complications of radiation proctitis like perforation, intractable bleeding, fistulas, and strictures. Rarely faecal diversion with either a colostomy or ileostomy is done. Diverting the direction of stool decreases symptoms of tenesmus, pain, drainage, and infection. However, improvements in symptoms are unlikely to persist without additional interventions. Colostomy can also help to improve symptoms related to stricture and incontinence. Stool diversion colostomy allows rest to injured rectum. Many a times even fistulas and ulcers heal after diversion colostomy and then these colostomies can even be reversed.

References

1. Schultheiss TE, Lee WR, Hunt MA, et al. Late GI and GU complications in the treatment of prostate cancer. Int J Radiat Oncol Biol Phys. 1997;37(1):3.
2. Zeitlin SI, Sherman J, Raboy A, et al. High dose combination radiotherapy for the treatment of localized prostate cancer. J Urol. 1998;160(1):91.
3. Krol R, Smeenk RJ, van Lin EN, Yeoh EE, Hopman WP. Systematic review: anal and rectal changes after radiotherapy for prostate cancer. Int J Color Dis. 2014;29(3):273–83.
4. Talcott JA, Manola J, Clark JA, Kaplan I, Beard CJ, Mitchell SP, Chen RC, O'Leary MP, Kantoff PW, D'Amico AV. Time course and predictors of symptoms after primary prostate cancer therapy. J Clin Oncol. 2003;21(21):3979–86.
5. Coia LR, Myerson RJ, Tepper JE. Late effects of radiation therapy on the gastrointestinal tract. Int J Radiat Oncol Biol Phys. 1995;31:1213.
6. Beard CJ, Propert KJ, Rieker PP, et al. Complications after treatment with external-beam irradiation in early-stage prostate cancer patients: a prospective multiinstitutional outcomes study. J Clin Oncol. 1997;15:223.

7. Shadad AK, Sullivan FJ, Martin JD, Egan LJ. Gastrointestinal radiation injury: symptoms, risk factors and mechanisms. World J Gastroenterol. 2013;19(2):185–98.
8. Theis VS, Sripadam R, Ramani V, Lal S. Chronic radiation enteritis. Clin Oncol (R Coll Radiol). 2010;22(1):70–83.
9. Leiper K, Morris AI. Treatment of radiation proctitis. Clin Oncol (R Coll Radiol). 2007;19(9):724–9.
10. Mahmood S, Bollipo S, Steele S, et al. It's all the RAVE: time to give up on the "chronic radiation proctitis" misnomer. Gastroenterology. 2021;160:635.
11. Wu XR, Liu XL, Katz S, Shen B. Pathogenesis, diagnosis, and management of ulcerative proctitis, chronic radiation proctopathy, and diversion proctitis. Inflamm Bowel Dis. 2015;21(3):703–15.
12. Wachter S, Gerstner N, Goldner G, Potzi R, Wambersie A, Potter R. Endoscopic scoring of late rectal mucosal damage after conformal radiotherapy for prostatic carcinoma. Radiother Oncol. 2000;54(1):11–9.
13. Fonteyne V, De Neve W, Villeirs G, De Wagter C, De Meerleer G. Late radiotherapy-induced lower intestinal toxicity (RILIT) of intensity-modulated radiotherapy for prostate cancer: the need for adapting toxicity scales and the appearance of the sigmoid colon as co-responsible organ for lower intestinal toxicity. Radiother Oncol. 2007;84(2):156–63.
14. Mohiuddin M, Marks G, Marks J. Long-term results of reirradiation for patients with recurrent rectal carcinoma. Cancer. 2002;95(5):1144–50.
15. Shioyama Y, Tsuji H, Suefuji H, Sinoto M, Matsunobu A, Toyama S, Nakamura K, Kudo S. Particle radiotherapy for prostate cancer. Int J Urol. 2015;22(1):33–9.
16. Theodorescu D, Gillenwater J, Koutrouvelis P. Prostatourethral-rectal fistula after prostate brachytherapy. Cancer. 2000;89:2085–91.
17. Cook SI, Sellin JH. Review article: Short chain fatty acids in health and disease. Aliment. Pharmacol. Ther. 1998;12:499–507.
18. Pinkawa M. Spacer application for prostate cancer radiation therapy. Future Oncol. 2014;10(5):851–64.
19. Susil RC, McNutt TR, DeWeese TL, et al. Effects of prostate-rectum separation on rectal dose from external beam radiotherapy. Int J Radiat Oncol Biol Phys. 2010;76:1251–8.
20. Mendenhall WM, McKibben BT, Hoppe BS, Nichols RC, Henderson RH, Mendenhall NP. Management of radiation proctitis. Am J Clin Oncol. 2014;37(5):517–23.
21. Kuku S, Fragkos C, McCormack M, Forbes A. Radiation induced bowel injury: the impact of radiotherapy on survivorship after treatment for gynaecological cancers. Br J Cancer. 2013;109(6):1504–12.
22. Jao SW, Beart RW, Gunderson LL. Surgical treatment of radiation injuries of the colon and rectum. Am J Surg. 1986;151(2):272–7.

Radiation Enteritis in Patients Receiving Abdominal Radiation Therapy

3

Vineeta Goel, Deepak Kumar, Mansi Chaudhary, and Rachna Jain

3.1 Introduction

Radiation enteritis (RE) is a clinical syndrome which occurs due to radiation induced changes in small and large bowel. Bowel is inadvertently irradiated during radiation for abdomino pelvic cancers and can result in radiation enteritis with variable severity.

It was first reported in 1897 by David Walsh during radiation therapy to stomach during the era when Xray was discovered and came in use for cancer treatment [1]. It is an unavoidable side effects of radiation therapy and its development and progression depends upon dose, duration and individual sensitivity of the bowel to radiation therapy [2].

Radiation enteritis is defined as acute if it occurs during and within 3 months of radiation treatment and is called as chronic if it persists or occurs after 3 months of treatment [3].

Diagnosis of acute radiation enteritis is often clinical based on symptomatology of patients undergoing or recent history of radiation treatment. Acute RE is generally self-limiting and responds to symptomatic treatment. Chronic radiation enteritis is more worrisome as it can have direct impact on quality of life of patients especially for long term cancer survivors.

Both incidences and severity of radiation enteritis have significantly reduced with the use of newer technique of radiation therapy such as three dimensional radiation therapy (3DCRT), Image Guided Radiation Therapy (IGRT), Intensity Modulated Radiation Therapy radiation (IMRT) as compared to 2D RT and which were commonly used in past. Advances in diagnostic techniques also enable in detecting and diagnosing this entity at early time so that active management can be offered suitably.

V. Goel (✉) · D. Kumar · M. Chaudhary · R. Jain
Fortis Hospital, Shalimar Bagh, Delhi, India

K. Sood Sharma et al. (eds.), *Complications of Cancer Therapy: Best Practices in Prevention and Management*, https://doi.org/10.1007/978-981-99-0984-1_3

3.2 Pathophysiology

Radiation therapy causes direct or indirect damage of nuclear DNA of actively dividing cells which results in impairment of cell division and therefore death of dividing cells [4]. Inside intestinal mucosa, stem cells within intestinal crypts are mainly vulnerable to death because these are actively dividing and differentiating cells and their loss causes loss of mucosal integrity of cells [5–7].

Acute radiation injury also generates cascade of inflammatory process. This process causes a transient mucosal atrophy and lamina propria gets infiltered by plasma cells and polymorphonucleocytes.

Due to loss of stem cell in intestine, mucosal epithelial gets denuded which results in crypt ulceration and micro abscess formation at local site [8, 9]. These events leads to nutrients malabsorption, increase fluid loss and increase permeability to gut pathogen which in return further augments mucosal inflammation.

The mechanism of chronic radiation injury is still unclear. However, chronic radiation enteritis probably is caused due to end arteritis in the submucosa which results in tissue ischemia and necrosis, submucosal fibrosis and lymphatic dilatation [10]. These changes further progress to involve lamina propria and muscularis propria also. Probably it occurs due to imbalance of metalloproteinase enzyme which plays a major role in collagen deposition. Other than these TGF-B, and its effectors, connective tissue growth factor which causes fibrosis due to up regulation of Rho pathway [11, 12].

These pathological changes may result in vascular degeneration, telangiectatic vessel formation, mucosal ulcer, intestinal wall necrosis and serosa wall fibrosis which later on may result in fistula, adhesions, bleeding or life threating strictures [13].

Concurrent chemotherapy during radiation therapy further augments radiation enteritis due to increase damage of non-dividing cells [14].

3.2.1 Clinical Manifestations

Symptoms of acute radiation enteritis can appear after hours of radiation exposure or sometimes manifest from second to third week onward to attain peak in severity at last week of radiation therapy, which usually last for 5–6 weeks. Common symptoms of acute RE include nausea, vomiting, abdominal pain, diarrhoea with mucus or blood and loss of appetite. These symptoms are mostly low grade, self-limiting and resolve within few weeks of radiation treatment completion.

These symptoms may sometimes result in functional disorder such as malabsorption of fat, lactose or Vitamin B12 or bile salt as normally upper bowel tract is involved in absorption of these nutrients.

In some individuals symptoms may progress in severity such as intractable bowel pain, malena, severe enteritis or sepsis due to intrabdominal bacterial translocation through inflamed bowel loop.

Acute radiation effects may sometime translate into chronic injury and presents with chronic side effects. Chronic radiation enteritis may develop after 3 months to may be up to 30 year post radiation therapy. Incidences and prevalence of chronic radiation enteritis ranges from 10% to 20% [15, 16]. Symptoms manifests as chronic malabsorption, chronic abdominal pain, persistent weight loss, diarrhoea, gastrointestinal bleeding, stricture, fistula, obstruction and perforation. These symptoms usually have similar presentation as other intestinal pathologies such as inflammatory bowel disease, celiac disease, diverticular disease, infection or recurrent malignancy and so careful workup is needed to differentiate it as association with radiation therapy or a new entity.

3.2.2 Risk Factors for Radiation Enteritis

There are number of risk factors which plays a major role for development of radiation enteritis which can be classified as patient related and treatment related factors. Table 3.1 depicts the patient and treatment related risk factors for radiation enteritis.

Among these, patients factor such as low body mass index, co-morbid condition such as diabetes, hypertension, chronic vascular disease, pre-existing inflammatory bowel disease and smoking which increases possibility and severity of radiation enteritis. A previous history of abdominal surgery causes changes in anatomical configuration, adhesion and fibrosis of bowel leading to more chances of developing both acute and chronic radiation enteritis. Patients suffering from inflammatory bowel disease have relative contraindication of radiation therapy due to high risk of developing radiation side effects. Genetic factors may also seems predisposes to individual sensitivity to radiation, as some experience less severe side effects while some patients experiences severe side effects to identical course of radiation treatment [17].

Treatment related factors such as radiation dose received by bowel, fractionation, technique, and concurrent use of chemotherapy predisposes for development of both acute and chronic radiation enteritis.

Table 3.1 Risk factors for radiation enteritis

Patient related risk factors	Treatment related factors
Previous abdominal surgeries	Radiation technique
Diabetes Mellitus	Dose received by bowel-V15Gy and V45Gy
Hypertension	Fractionation
Smoking	Concurrent use of chemotherapy
Inflammatory bowel disease	
Chronic vascular diseases	

Total dose and volume of radiation received by bowel is an important determinants of radiation enteritis [18]. As an example for individual small bowel loop, volume receiving 15 Gy (V15) <120 cc has probability of developing <10% radiation enteritis. However, if entire volume of peritoneal cavity is considered then volume receiving 45 Gy (V45) < 195 cm^3 has <10% risk of developing radiation enteritis if delivered in conventional fractionation. Similarly, Volume received by individual small bowel loop to a dose of 50 Gy should be <5% for a <5% risk of late perforation or obstruction formation [19, 20].

Use of altered dose fractionation has been reported to be associated with higher risk of RE as compared to conventional fractionation [21, 22]. Radiation technique also plays a role as risk factor for radiation toxicity. Modern techniques of radiation treatment as IMRT, IGRT has reported to be less toxic for the bowel compared to 3DCRT for upper abdominal malignancy. Incidences of grade 3–4 upper GI toxicity as nausea decreased from 11% to 0% and diarrhoea from 18% to 3% with use of IMRT in pancreatic malignancy [23, 24]. Similarly, Standard field versus extended filed radiation therapy where patients receiving later technique experience more adverse effects (grade 3–4: 3.5% vs. 19%) compared to former [25].

Concurrent use of chemotherapy with radiation therapy augments increase bowel toxicity compared to radiation alone. A French study shown that acute toxicity rise from 2.2% with radiation alone to 13.5% with concurrent chemotherapy in rectal cancer [26].

3.2.3 Prevention

Incidences and severity of radiation enteritis can be prevented by embracing physical and medical strategies.

Physical strategies includes adoption of advance radiation techniques in upper abdominal malignancies. Radiation therapy in past was delivered based on anatomical bony landmark. Simple anterior posterior (AP-PA) radiation portal was used to treat the disease because of which lot of small bowel in treatment field. But Radiation therapy has evolved in past decade and now with the use of IGRT and IMRT we could limit the dose to the bowel as desired as per the standard dose constraints guidelines. IMRT has advantage of smaller field of radiation exposure, multiple beams arrangements and more conformal dose delivery which could maximize the normal tissue sparing by creating various shapes and steep dose gradients [27]. In addition small measures like prone or lateral positioning sometimes also helps in reducing bowel radiation doses. Another small strategy especially useful while irradiating pelvic malignancies is treatment in full bladder position. Full or distended urinary bladder helps in physically displacing bowel out of radiation field.

Sulfasalazine has proven benefit to inhibit eicosanoids, a causative agent for enteritis. It is also used to treat inflammatory bowel disease (IBD). A dose of 500 mg twice daily results significant decrease in rate of GI toxicity compared to placebo [28].

Statin and angiotensin converting enzyme (ACE) inhibitors has shown to decrease GI toxicity due to their anti-inflammatory, anti-thrombotic and anti-fibrotic properties which has been shown in *In vitro* studies [29].

Amifostine is a cytoprotective agent used to reduce xerostomia in head and neck cancer radiation therapy. Few studies has shown it is protective against radiation induced bowel toxicity but further research is needed to prove its true value [30].

Probiotics preparations have viable microorganism known as lactobacillus acidophilus plus bifidobacterium bifidum bacteria in large number which could alter the host's gut microflora. Few trials has shown probiotics improves in diarrhoea symptoms in radiation induced small bowel disease. A probiotic preparation known as VSL#3 has been tested and investigated with such property in randomised controlled trials. Further research is warranted to prove its actual benefits [31]. Patients are even encouraged to increase probiotic intake in their diet including consumption of yoghurt.

Vitamin E (tocopherol) and Pentoxifylline, a xanthine derivative, combination has shown to have antioxidant properties with reducing radiation induced fibrosis in pelvic malignancy [32] Hille et al. reported symptomatic improvement in chronic grade 1–2 enteritis in 71% patients receiving combination therapy compared to 33% in supportive group alone [33]. Further study is still needed to fully evaluate its effectiveness.

3.2.4 Diagnosis

Diagnosis of acute RE is generally clinical while there are few tests available for diagnosis of chronic RE.

A detail history and clinical examination is prerequisite to arrive at the diagnosis of acute radiation enteritis. A systemic algorithm should be followed for making the diagnosis and its effective management.

Contrast enhanced Computed Tomography (CT) has high sensitivity in detecting mucosal and serosa thickening of the bowel resulting due to inflammation or stricture. Additional finding which could be detected are bowel edema along with increased density of mesentery and it can also differentiate bowel adhesions [34].

Magnetic Resonance Enterography (MRE) uses MR with oral contrast and is highly sensitive in detecting small bowel edema/thickening (>3 mm), mural enhancement and dilatation or small bowel ileus in case of chronic enteritis [35].

However these investigations has its own limitations in detecting occult bleeding, ulceration or erosion for which endoscopy could be used as an adjunct for arriving at diagnosis.

Small bowel capsule endoscopy is very useful and informative tool to diagnose radiation enteritis. This may detect mucosal changes as edema, loss of villous structure, ulcer, stricture, bleeding or inflammatory changes. However, there are two major limitations of this procedure including risk of capsule retention during passage through gut and biopsy from gut to diagnose the histology is not be possible by this technique [36, 37]. To overcome such limitations, patency capsule test can be performed prior to capsule endoscopy to assess the patency of GI tract and can reassure to perform capsule endoscopy [38]. To enhance the visualisation of small bowel, double balloon enteroscopy is an useful diagnostic tool. It has an added advantage over capsule endoscopy and could also allow to procure biopsy from concerned area/bowel mucosa identified to be abnormal for tissue diagnosis.

3.2.5 Grading of RE

Radiation therapy Oncology Group (RTOG) describe to grade the severity of radiation enteritis [39].

3.2.5.1 Acute Toxicity

Grade 1: Increased frequency or change in quality of bowel habits not requiring medication/rectal discomfort not requiring analgesics.

Grade 2: Diarrhea requiring parasympatholytic drugs (e.g. Lomotil)/mucous discharge not necessitating sanitary pads/rectal or abdominal pain requiring analgesics.

Grade 3: Diarrhea requiring parenteral support/severe mucous or blood discharge necessitating sanitary pads/abdominal distention.

Grade 4: Acute or subacute obstruction, fistula or perforation; GI bleeding requiring transfusion; abdominal pain or tenesmus requiring tube decompression or bowel diversion.

3.2.5.2 Chronic Enteritis

Grade 1: Mild diarrhea; mild cramping; bowel movement 5 times daily; slight rectal discharge or bleeding.

Grade 2: Moderate diarrhea and colic; bowel movement more than 5 times daily; excessive rectal mucus or intermittent bleeding.

Grade 3: Obstruction or bleeding, requiring surgery.

Grade 4: Necrosis/perforation fistula.

3.2.6 Management

Low grade (grade I–II) acute RE is usually successfully managed symptomatically and conservatively. Majority of the patients report resolution of symptoms within few days of treatment interruption itself along with few symptomatic medications. This includes anti-diarrhoea medication, such as loperamide, 5HT3 blocker for nausea and vomiting and antacids. Dietary modification also play a vital role in resolving and preventing radiation induce diarrhoea. A diet which is lactose free diet, low fat and low residue diet which are generally recommended to consume during the course of treatment [40]. Patients presenting with abdominal cramps benefits from anti cholinergic, antispasmodic and analgesic agents.

Severe grade (Grade III–IV) of radiation enteritis need active and timely management. Proper investigation and imaging should be done prior to diagnosis as part of management. Patients with severe diarrhoea presents with dehydration and malabsorption. Diarrhoea should be managed with Oral Rehydration Solution (ORS), probiotics, anti-bacterial drugs and intravenous fluids along with supplements in cases of severe dehydration. Anticholinergic drugs are used to decrease the gut motility and antispasmodic with Opioid analgesic to decrease the abdominal pain.

The Somatostatin analogue octreotide is also used for managing severe diarrhoea due to both chemotherapy and radiation induced. A study has reported octreotide to be more effective in resolving diarrhoea compared to anticholinergic agents such as diphenoxylate hydrochloride plus atropine [41].

Trimacilone acetate, a potent steroid, administered intramuscularly has been studied to effectively preventing radiation enteritis for patient undergoing pelvic radiation therapy [42].

Mild cases of chronic enteritis is manged by low fibre diet, anticholinergic drug and stool softeners. Generally symptoms improves after their use within few days. Few cases may also require anticholinergic and opioid agonist to relieve the symptoms. High fibre diet helps in forming consistency of stool and manages patient with reduce rectal compliance.

Chronic watery diarrhoea due to bile acid malabsorption is managed with bile salt sequestering agents like cholestyramine [43]. However, the drug is not easily palatable and due to which majority discontinue it before the course. Alternative agents are Colestipol and Colesevelam which also binds to bile salts and is better tolerable but are expensive and not in general use [44].

Hyperbaric oxygen therapy (HBO) is an effective treatment modality for chronic bowel injury caused due to radiation. It decreases the tissue hypoxia and prevent from ischemic damage of bowel due to ionising radiation. Few study has also quoted its antibacterial property. This treatment is given for several week in an enclosed hyperbaric chamber [45]. However, results of recent hyperbaric oxygen therapy II (HOT2) trial did not support the benefit of HBO in chronic bowel injury secondary to radiation therapy [46]. Further studies are still needed to firmly establish its benefit.

3.2.6.1 Low Fiber Diet in Patients with Partial Bowel Obstruction

The human gut can't easily digest fiber which is a part of the plant based diet. Fibers also add bulk to stools. A high fiber diet (particularly rich in insoluble fibers) can worsen symptoms in patients with partial bowel obstruction. Insoluble fibers are found in rough parts of the plant based diet e.g. skins, grains and seed. Low fiber diet helps patients with partial bowel obstruction by reducing the risk of bowel obstruction caused by food and improves symptoms. The daily recommended amount of fiber is 38 g for men and 25 g for women, whereas a typical low fiber diet contains less than 10–15 g of fiber per day.

3.2.6.2 How to Modify Fiber Intake

1. Remove stalks, stems, seeds and skin from fruits and vegetables.
2. Cook and chop vegetables well as these are well tolerated.
3. Reduce tough, fibrous fruits and vegetables.
4. Avoid dried fruits, nuts and seeds.
5. Whole grain, high fiber breads and cereals need to be avoided.

3.2.6.3 General Dietary Tips for Patients with Partial Bowel Obstruction

1. Chew food well and eat slowly.
2. Have frequent small meals spread through the day (6–7 meals).
3. Cook foods well.
4. Cut food into small portions.
5. Read food labels carefully and avoid foods rich in fiber (more than 2 g fiber per serving).
6. Avoid tough or stringy foods.
7. If symptoms of bowel obstruction worsen, rest the bowel by taking fluids for short period to time to help settle the gut.
8. Aim to maintain a balanced diet.
9. If diet is very limited, take multivitamins/mineral supplements.
10. Plan to consume minimum 1.5L fluid per day

3.2.6.4 How to Get Back to Usual Foods After Relief in Partial Bowel Obstruction?

1. When patient starts feeling better, slowly add foods back into the diet.
2. Add new food 1 at a time, in small amounts. This helps to figure out which food is tolerated well.
3. If symptoms like diarrhea, gas, bloating or cramps occur when new food is added, avoid that food.

3.2.7 Surgical Management of Chronic RE

Surgical management of radiation enteritis may be needed in case of severe grade IV toxicity when presented with fistula, stricture or obstruction. Theses adverse complications are generally more common in patients who receive radiation therapy in post operative setting.

Conservative management of obstruction include bowel rest along by placing naso gastric tube with continuous aspiration along with Total Parenteral Nutrition (TPN).

However, if bowel obstruction is not relieved by conservative approach, then it is managed by surgical exploration. Surgical exploration is generally considered as the last resort. Surgery for radiation induced intestinal obstruction is generally very challenging and is associated with high morbidity and mortality. Main challenge in these surgeries is because large and multiple bowel segments are affected by radiation treatment and there is a lot of fibrosis in abdominal cavity.

Type and extent of surgery depends upon nature of affected bowel segments either single or multiple affected bowel segment and length of affected small bowel involved in pathogenesis. Surgical management includes adhesolysis, release of obstruction, strictureplasty or internal bypass if needed.

Strictureplasty conserve bowel length and also relieve obstruction caused due to stricture. However, Strictureplasty is not recommended in case of perforation, haemorrhage and fistula. However, post operative complication as anastomotic leak can be up to 30% and among them 40–60% may require further laparotomy for its correction. Such major surgery result in gut shortening, malabsorption and risk of adherence, stricture and fibrosis [47]. To reduce post operative complication anastomotic repair should be performed with non-irradiated bowel loop.

3.3 Conclusions

Radiation enteritis is a known and inevitable complication in patients receiving radiation therapy for upper abdominal malignancies. However, its severity can be predicted based on risk factors and could be prevented by adopting advance techniques as of radiation therapy. Proper and timely diagnosis is prerequisite to decrease its severity and effective management.

References

1. Walsh D. Deep tissue traumatism from roentgen ray exposure. Br Med J. 1897;2:272–3.
2. Kountouras J, Zavos C. Recent advances in the management of radiation colitis. World J Gastroenterol. 2008;14(48):7289–301.
3. Stacey R, Green JT. Radiation-induced small bowel disease: latest developments and clinical guidance. Ther Adv Chronic Dis. 2014;5(1):15–29.
4. Bismar MM, Sinicrope FA. Radiation enteritis. Curr Gastro Enterol Rep. 2002;4:361–5.
5. Hall EJ. Radiobiology for the radiologist. Philadelphia: Lippin-Cott Williams & Wilkins; 2000.
6. McGovern D. Radiation and other physiochemical injury. In: Weinstein WHC, Bosch J, editors. Clinical gastroenterology and hepatology. Philadelphia: Elsevier Mosby; 2005.
7. MacNaughton WK. Review article: new insights into the pathogenesis of radiation-induced intestinal dysfunction. Aliment Pharmacol Ther. 2000;14:523–8.
8. Rodier JF. Radiation enteropathy—incidence, aetiology, risk factors, pathology and symptoms. Tumori. 1995;81:122–5.
9. Pia de la Maza M, Gotteland M, Ramirez C, et al. Acute nutritional and intestinal changes after pelvic radiation. J Am Coll Nutr. 2001;20:637–42.
10. Yarnold J, Brotons MC. Pathogenetic mechanisms in radiation fibrosis. Radiother Oncol. 2010;97:149–61.
11. Strup-Perrot C, Mathe D, Linard C, et al. Global gene expression profiles reveal an increase in mRNA levels of collagens, MMPs, and TIMPs in late radiation enteritis. Am J Physiol Gastrointest Liver Physiol. 2004;287:G875–85.
12. Bourgier C, Haydont V, Milliat F, et al. Inhibition of Rho kinase modulates radiation induced fibrogenic phenotype in intestinal smooth muscle cells through alteration of the cyto-skeleton and connective tissue growth factor expression. Gut. 2005;54:336–43.
13. Oya M, Yao T, Tsuneyoshi M. Chronic irradiation enteritis: its correlation with the elapsed time interval and morphological changes. Hum Pathol. 1996;27:774–81.

14. Pawlik TM, Keyomarsi K. Role of cell cycle in mediating sensitivity to radio-therapy. Int J Radiat Oncol Biol Phys. 2004;59:928–42.
15. Andreyev HJ, Davidson SE, Gillespie C, Allum WH, Swarbrick E, British Society of Gastroenterology; Association of Colo-Proctology of Great Britain and Ireland; Association of Upper Gastrointestinal Surgeons; Faculty of Clinical Oncology Section of the Royal College of Radiologists. Practice guidance on the management of acute and chronic gastrointestinal problems arising as a result of treatment for cancer. Gut. 2012;61:179–92.
16. Birgisson H, Påhlman L, Gunnarsson U, Glimelius B. Late gastrointestinal disorders after rectal cancer surgery with and without preoperative radiation therapy. Br J Surg. 2008;95:206–13.
17. West CM, Barnett GC. Genetics and genomics of radiotherapy toxicity: towards prediction. Genome Med. 2011;3:52.
18. Letschert JG, Lebesque JV, de Boer RW, et al. Dose-volume correlation in radiation-related late small-bowel complications: a clinical study. Radiother Oncol. 1990;18:307–20.
19. Robertson JM, Lockman D, Yan D, et al. The dose-volume relationship of small bowel irradiation and acute grade 3 diarrhea during chemoradiotherapy for rectal cancer. Int J Radiat Oncol Biol Phys. 2008;70:413–8.
20. Roeske JC, Bonta D, Mell LK, et al. A dosimetric analysis of acute gastrointestinal toxicity in women receiving intensity modulated whole-pelvic radiation therapy. Radiother Oncol. 2003;69:201–7.
21. Varghese C, Rangad F, Jose CC, Raveendran P, Subhashini J, Ramadas K, et al. Hyperfractionation in advanced carcinoma of the uterine cervix: a preliminary report. Int J Radiat Oncol Biol Phys. 1992;23:393–6.
22. MacLeod C, Bernshaw D, Leung S, Narayan K, Firth I. Accelerated hyperfractionated radiotherapy for locally advanced cervix cancer. Int J Radiat Oncol Biol Phys. 1999;44:519–24.
23. Abelson JA, Murphy JD, Minn AY, Chung M, Fisher GA, Ford JM, Kunz P, Norton JA, Visser BC, Poultsides GA, et al. Intensity-modulated radiotherapy for pancreatic adenocarcinoma. Int J Radiat Oncol Biol Phys. 2012;82(4):e595–601.
24. Milano MT, Chmura SJ, Garofalo MC, Rash C, Roeske JC, Connell PP, Kwon OH, Jani AB, Heimann R. Intensity-modulated radiotherapy in treatment of pancreatic and bile duct malignancies: toxicity and clinical outcome. Int J Radiat Oncol Biol Phys. 2004;59(2):445–53.
25. Du XL, Sheng XG, Jiang T, Yu H, Yan YF, Gao R, Lu CH, Li QS. Intensity-modulated radiation therapy versus para-aortic field radiotherapy to treat para-aortic lymph node metastasis in cervical cancer: prospective study. Croat Med J. 2010;51(3):229–36.
26. Gerard JP, Conroy T, Bonnetain F, et al. Preoperative radio-therapy with or without concurrent fluorouracil and leucovorin in T3-4 rectal cancers: results of FFCD 9203. J Clin Oncol. 2006;24:4620–5.
27. Mundt A, Roeske J, Lujan A. Intensity-modulated radiation therapy in gynecologic malignancies. Med Dosim. 2002;27:131–6.
28. Kiliç D, Egehan İ, Ozenirler S, Dursun A. Double-blinded, randomized, placebo-controlled study to evaluate the effectiveness of sulphasalazine in preventing acute gastrointestinal complications due to radiotherapy. Radiother Oncol. 2000;57:125–9.
29. Gaugler M, Vereycken-Holler V, Squiban C, Vandamme M, Vozenin-Brotons M, Benderitter M. Pravastatin limits endothelial activation after irradiation and decreases the resulting inflammatory and thrombotic responses. Radiation Res. 2005;163(5):479–87.
30. Leonard C, Shapiro H, Henkenberns PL, Cornish P, Dahl K. Amifostine used as a normal tissue protectant in patients receiving pelvic radiotherapy. Int J Radiat Oncol Biol Phys. 2005;63:S448.
31. Chitapanarux I, Chitapanarux T, Traisathit P, Kudumpee S, Tharavichitkul E, Lorvidhaya V. Randomized controlled trial of live lactobacillus acidophilus plus bifidobacterium bifidum in prophylaxis of diarrhea during radiotherapy in cervical cancer patients. Radiat Oncol. 2010;5:31.
32. Gothard L, Cornes P, Brooker S, Earl J, Glees J, Hall E, Peckitt C, Tait D, Yarnold J. Phase II study of vitamin E and pentoxifylline in patients with late side effects of pelvic radiotherapy. Radiother Oncol. 2005;75(3):334–41.

33. Hille A, Christiansen H, Pradier O, Hermann RM, Siekmeyer B, Weiss E, Hilgers R, Hess CF, Schmidberger H. Effect of pentoxifylline and tocopherol on radiation proctitis/enteritis. Strahlenther Onkol. 2005;181(9):606–14.
34. Xiao J, Li Q. Multi-slice spiral CT evaluation of chronic radiation colitis and rectitis. Exp Ther Med. 2020;20(4):3033–40.
35. Algin O, Turkbey B, Ozmen E, Algin E. Magnetic resonance enterography findings of chronic radiation enteritis. Cancer Imaging. 2011;11(1):189–94. https://doi.org/10.1102/1470-7330.2011.0026.
36. Yamashina T, Takada R, Uedo N, et al. Prospective small bowel mucosal assessment immediately after chemoradiotherapy of unresectable locally advanced pancreatic cancer using capsule endoscopy: a case series. Ann Gastroenterol. 2016;29:386–8.
37. Nakamura M, Hirooka Y, Watanabe O, et al. Three cases with active bleeding from radiation enteritis that were diagnosed with video capsule endoscopy without retention. Nagoya J Med Sci. 2014;76(3–4):369–74.
38. Assadsangabi A, Blakeborough A, Drew K, et al. Small bowel patency assessment using the patency device and a novel targeted (limited radiation) computed tomography-based protocol. J Gastroenterol Hepatol. 2015;30:984–9.
39. Cox JD, Stetz J, Pajak TF. Toxicity criteria of the Radiation Therapy Oncology Group (RTOG) and the European Organization for Research and Treatment of Cancer (EORTC). Int J Radiat Oncol Biol Phys. 1995;31(5):1341–6.
40. Bye A, Kaasa S, Ose T, Sundfør K, Tropé C. The influence of low fat, low lactose diet on diarrhoea during pelvic radiotherapy. Clin Nutr. 1992;11:147–53.
41. Yavuz M, Yavuz A, Aydin F, Can G, Kavgaci H. The efficacy of octreotide in the therapy of acute radiation-induced diarrhea: a randomized controlled study. Int J Radiat Oncol Biol Phys. 2002;54:195–202.
42. Cetin E, Ozturk AS, Orhun H, Ulger S. Role of triamcinolone in radiation enteritis management. World J Gastroenterol. 2014;20:4341–4.
43. Kurien M, Thurgar E, Davies A, et al. Challenging current views on bile acid diarrhoea and malabsorption. Frontline Gastroenterol. 2018;9:92–7.
44. Wedlake L, Thomas K, Lalji A, Anagnostopoulos C, Andreyev H. Effectiveness and tolerability of colesevelam hydrochloride for bile-acid malabsorption in patients with cancer: a retrospective chart review and patient questionnaire. Clin Therapeut. 2009;31:2549–58.
45. Bennett M, Feldmeier J, Hampson N, Smee R, Milross C. Hyperbaric oxygen therapy for late radiation tissue injury. Cochrane Database Syst Rev. 2012;5:CD005005.
46. Glover M, Smerdon GR, Andreyev HJ, et al. Hyperbaric oxygen for patients with chronic bowel dysfunction after pelvic radiotherapy (HOT2): a randomised, double-blind, sham-controlled phase 3 trial. Lancet Oncol. 2016;17(2):224–33.
47. Galland RB, Spencer J. Surgical management of radiation enteritis. Surgery. 1986;99(2):133–9.

Radiation Induced Liver Disease in Patients Receiving Radiation for Hepatobilliary Cancer

4

Suman Mallik and Monidipa Mondal

4.1 Introduction

Radiation induced liver disease (RILD) is one of the important dose dependant serious complication of radiation of liver. Mean dose of liver when goes beyond 30–35 Gy there is higher chance of RILD. Case JT first described radiation induced liver injury long back 1924 [1]. Availability of modern radiotherapy techniques and better understanding of pathophysiology of radiation induced liver disease allows us to offer safer mode of radiotherapy and lesser chances of RILD. Evidences of conformal radiotherapy, radio-embolization and high dose focal radiotherapy has shown that it is safe to irradiate small volume of liver with high dose of radiotherapy saving at least 700 cm^3 volume of liver. V effective is another well correlated indicator of radiation dose and radiation related liver disease.

RILDs are classified in two groups Classic RILD and Non classic RILD. Anicteric hepatomegaly, ascites and elevated alkaline phosphatase (two times) are features of classic RILD. Classic RILD usually occurs 2 weeks to 3 months of radiotherapy [2].

On the other hand non-classic RILD occurs between 1 week to 3 months after therapy. It is characterized by fivefold increase in hepatic transaminases and declining of liver functions. Classic symptoms of classic RILD are absent in non-classic RILD.

The RTOG 84-05 study evaluated escalation of dose from 27 to 33 Gy at 1.5 Gy twice daily fractionation. Patients who received more than 33 Gy to whole liver, 10% of them had developed classic RILD. Diagnosis of classic RILD is done by clinical presentation and laboratory finding. MRI, SPECT (single photon emission computer tomography) and CT scan show certain feature suggestive of RILD. Treatment of RILD is primarily symptomatic and it is treated similarly as non RILD patients.

S. Mallik (✉) · M. Mondal
Narayana Superspeciality Hospital, Howrah, West Bengal, India

K. Sood Sharma et al. (eds.), *Complications of Cancer Therapy: Best Practices in Prevention and Management*, https://doi.org/10.1007/978-981-99-0984-1_4

4.2 Description, Listing of Complications Encountered with Incidence Rates

4.2.1 Pathophysiology

Liver biopsy after radiation induced liver damage and radiological evidences suggest venoocclusion, retrograde sinusoidal congestion and subsequent parenchymal atrophy are the causative factors of RILD. Activation of hepatic stellate cells are considered as an early event of RILD process. They are responsible for regeneration of hepatocytes, secretion of lipoproteins and growth factors [3]. Venoocclusive nature is correlated with decreased hepatic arterial perfusion and portovenous perfusion on multiparametric MRI. Classic RILD is divided in to 4 stages acute radiation hepatitis, pre hepatic fibrosis, hepatic fibrosis and cirrhosis. Acute radiation hepatitis occurs usually within 1 month of radiotherapy. Liver fibrotic and cirrhotic stage radiation induced liver disease occurs typically after 6 to 12 months. Radiation causes release of TNF-alpha due to apoptosis of sinusoidal apoptotic cell. It activates coagulation cascade and cause deposition of fibrin in central vein and thrombosis (Fig. 4.1) [4]. Kupffer cells secretes TGF-beta which enhances radiation induced hepatocyte apoptosis. Kupffer cells secrete Galactin-3, activate qHSCs through JNK and p38 MAPK pathways. It promotes qHSCs proliferation and differentiation into myofibroblastic hepatic stellate cells. It promotes protein deposition in the extracellular matrix and results in liver fibrosis and RILD [4].

Actual mechanism of non-classic RILD is less understood compared to RILD. Non-classical RILD occurs in patients with underlying liver disease where there is significant hepatocyte loss and dysfunction in addition to the veno-occlusive process. It involves loss of regenerating hepatocytes and reactivation of hepatitis.

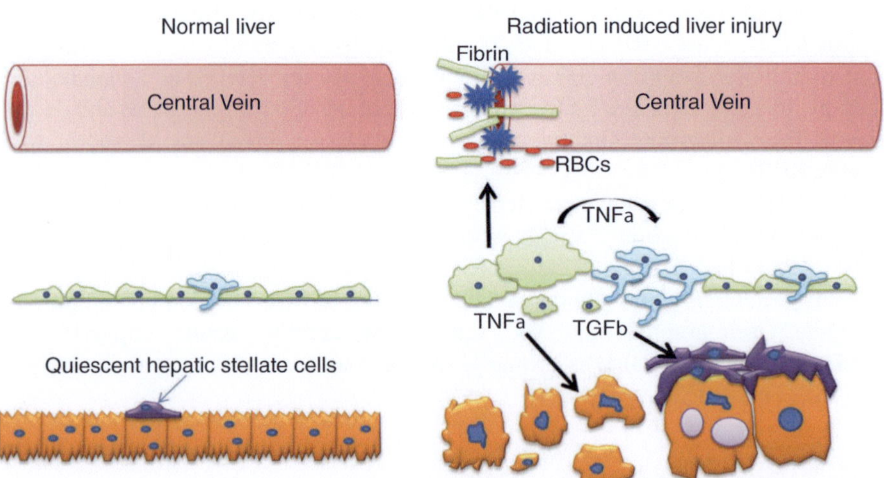

Fig. 4.1 Pathophysiology of RILD. (Adopted from Kim J, Jung Y. Radiation-induced liver disease: current understanding and future perspectives. Exp Mol Med;49(7):e359)

Therefore, they present with jaundice, markedly elevated bilirubin and serum transaminase (5 times greater than the laboratory reference range) or increase in 2 or more points of Child-Pugh Score (CP score). The severity of non- classic RILD can also be determined by ALBI (Table 4.1).

4.2.2 Timing of Manifestation of RILD

RILD typically occurs 4–8 weeks after completion of RT but has been described in the literature as early as 2 weeks and as late as 7 months after radiation. The signs and symptoms of classic RILD may appear as early as 2 weeks but may occur upto 6 month of radiation treatment, whereas in non-classic form symptoms appear within 3 months of radiation treatment [5].

4.2.3 Imaging Finding

Computed tomography (CT) scan RILD is seen as well demarcated area of hypoattenuation on plain CT and hyper attenuation on contrast-enhanced CT, as compared to surrounding normal liver with a sharp demarcation line [straight-border" sign] along the trajectory of the radiation beam, which is non anatomical in distribution. Straight border sign is seen commonly with non-conformal radiotherapy. Dynamic contrast enhanced CT shows 3 types of pattern according to Kimura at al [6]. **Type 1**, hyperdensity in all enhanced phases, which is observed in otherwise normal irradiated liver; **Type 2**, hypodensity in the arterial and portal venous phases; and **Type 3**, isodensity in all enhanced phases. MRI shows region of hypointensity on T1-weighted images, hyperintensity on T2-weighted images, slight hyperintensity on diffusion-weighted imaging (DWI), and low apparent diffusion coefficient (ADC). Functional imaging with single photon emission computed tomography (SPECT) is a more reliable option.

4.2.4 Other Investigations

Ascitic fluid cytology in RILD shows features of transudate with serum ascites-albumin gradient (SAAG) > 1.1.

Table 4.1 Clinical presentation of classic RILD and non classic RILD

Clinical presentation of classic RILD	Clinical presentation of non classic RILD
1. Anicteric hepatomegaly	1. Elevation of Transaminases (five times)
2. Ascites	2. Increase two or more points of Child Pugh score
3. Elevation of alkaline phosphatase. (two times)	3. Absence of classic features. Commonly presenting with elevation of bilirubin with low albumin

4.2.5 Incidence

Among the patients receiving hepatic radiation of 30–35 Gy, ~6–66% of patients present significant RILD [1]. The wide range of incidence reflects that the probability of RILD depends on multiple factors-volume of liver irradiated, dose per fraction and techniques of radiotherapy used, baseline liver function (CP score), underlying liver disease (chronic hepatitis B, hepatitis C infection, hepatic cirrhosis). The tolerance of partial liver volume irradiation is higher as liver parenchyma has parallel arranged functional unit. Incidence is higher with hypofractionated, accelerated radiotherapy. The incidence of RILD is significantly low (5–25%) with stereotactic radiotherapy in patients with low CP score. Patients with primary hepatobiliary malignancies have a lower tolerance to liver radiation than the patients with liver metastases. Along with these factors, portal vein thrombosis, concurrent use of systemic therapy, prior hepatic surgery, transarterial chemo-embolisation (TACE), transarterial radioembolization (TARE) increases the risk of RILD. Incidence of RILD is decreasing because of our better knowledge of liver tolerance, use of highly conformal radiotherapy techniques (IMRT, SBRT) with image guidance. Following table (Table 4.2) shows incidence of liver toxicities with SBRT.

4.2.6 For Common Complications

4.2.6.1 Predictors

Pre-existing liver disease like cirrhosis, non alcoholic steatohepatitis are one of the risk factors of RILD. Patients with good baseline liver function do well compared with poor liver function patient. Child Pugh A patients tolerates radiation better compared group B or C patient due to better hepatic reserve. Previous hepatic surgery and subsequent inadequate hepatic regeneration and cytotoxic chemotherapy are also associated with poor tolerance. For healthy liver 32 Gy in 2 Gy fractionation can cause 5% risk of classic RILD on other hand for cirrhotic liver 28 Gy in 2 Gy fractionation can produce classic RILD in 5% of patients [18].

A review by Emami et al. in 1990 suggests tolerance dose for one third, two third and whole liver are 50 Gy, 35 Gy and 30 Gy respectively to produce 5% chance of RILD at 5 years [19]. Validity of V30 data for classic and non-classic RILD is limited and mostly evaluated in HCC patients. It is useful in segregating high risk with low risk patients.

NTCP modelling and understanding of concept of effective volume estimation (Veff) from University of Michigan allowed more focal dose escalation with lesser incidence of RILD [20]. Two studies of SBRT was published from Princess Margaret Hospital in the year 2008 and 2009. One SBRT in HCC and intrahepatic cholangiocarcinoma [median dose prescription of 36 Gy (range 24 Gy to 54 Gy) and other one was SBRT in hepatic metastasis(range 28–60 Gy in 6 fractions). Despite similar median doses to liver 17% of HCC or intrahepatic cholangiocarcinoma patients experienced progression from Child-Pugh A to Child-Pugh B within 3 months

Table 4.2 Studies of SBRT liver with incidence of RILD

Study, year [reference], type of study	Sample size	Dose fractionation	Follow up (median)	Toxicities	Local control
Méndez Romero et al. 2006 [7] phase I–II	17 liver mets, 8 HCC	10–12.5 Gy × 3# or 5 Gy × 5#	12.9 months	4 RILD ≥ grade 3, one grade 5 (HCC patient with CP B)	82% at 2 years
Tse et al. 2008 [8] phase I	41, HCC/ IHC	9–10 Gy × 6#	17.6 months	10 (8 HCC, 2 IHC) grade 3 liver enzyme, 3 (2 HCC, 1 IHC) grade 3 hyperbilirubinemia, no grade 4–5, No RILD	65% at 1 year
Jung et al. 2013 [9] retrospective	92, HCC	10–20 Gy × 3–4#	25.7 months	11 grade 2, 6 grade 3 or higher RILD	92.1% at 3 years
Cardenes et al. 2010 [10], phase I	17, HCC	12 Gy × 3# 16 Gy × 3# (CP A) or 8 Gy × 5# (CP B)	24 months	2 grade 3 liver toxicity in patients with CP B at 42 Gy/3#	100% at 1 year
Jang et al. 2019 [11], phase II	65, HCC	15–20 Gy × 3#	41 months	3% ≥ Grade 3 liver toxicity, 1 RILD	95% at 3 years
Durand-Labrunie et al. 2020 [12], phase II	43, HCC	15 Gy × 3#	4 years	31% grade 3 acute adverse event, 19% abnormality in LFT	98% at 18 months
Takeda et al. 2016 [13], phase II	90, HCC	35–40 Gy/5#	41.7 months	11% ≥ Grade 3 toxicity	96% at 3 years
Goodman et al. 2016 [14]	81, liver mets	32–60 Gy/3–5#	2.25 years	4.9% ≥ Grade 3 liver toxicity	91% at 4 years
Mc Partlin et al. 2017 [15], phase I and II	51, liver mets	22.7–62.1 Gy/6#	2.3 years	3% Grade 3 toxicity, Acute grade III thrombocytopenia in 2 patients, no RILD	49.8% at 1 year, 26% at 4 years
Mendez Romero et al. 2017 [16], Retrospective	40, liver mets	37.5 Gy/3# 50.25 Gy/3#	2.2 years	7.5% ≥ Grade3 toxicity 3 cases of grade 3 elevation of liver enzymes	66% at 3 years 81% at 3 years
Scorsetti et al. 2018 [17] phase II	61, liver mets	25 Gy × 3#	6.1 years	No RILD	78% at 5 years

HCC hepatocellular carcinoma, *IHC* intrahepatic cholangiocarcinoma, *CP* child pugh

compared to very low incident with liver metastasis (95% confidence interval 0–5.3%) [8, 21].

For patients with Hepatitis B infection Lyman NTCP parameters for classic and non classic RILD have been calculated and those are $n = 0.26$, $m = 0.4$ and TD50 50 Gy [22]. In liver SBRT it is recommended to save 700 mL of healthy liver tissue where maximum dose allowed 15 Gy in 3 fractions [$\alpha/\beta = 3$]. This volume concept has been extrapolated from "critical volume" of hepatectomy series [23].

4.2.6.2 Early Warning Signs and Diagnostic Workup

There are several factors which are associated with higher chance of RILD. Mullikin T C et al. after evaluating 102 patients [51 with primary liver tumour and 51 with metastasis] concluded pre radiotherapy liver stiffness (LS) >3.0 kPa[hazard ratio [HR] 4.9; 95% confidence interval [CI], 1.6–14; $P = 0.004$], body mass index, clinical cirrhosis, CP score, albumin, presence of primary liver tumour and mean liver dose are significantly associated with higher post RT RILD. LS > 3.0 and mean liver dose were significantly associated with RILD in multivariate analysis [24]. Pre radiotherapy liver stiffness is measured by magnetic resonance elastography. Global liver function can be defined using 99mTc sulphur colloid SPECT. Normal liver sequester 80% of this isotope. In cirrhosis and parenchymal liver disease there is significant reduction of functional liver volume (<43%) [25–27].

Pre radiotherapy assessment of functional liver volume and subsequent treatment decision is associated with very low incidence of grade 3 hepatic toxicity [28].

Indocyanine green (ICG) also helps in differentiating cirrhotic liver with non-cirrhotic liver. In cirrhotic liver Indocyanine green dye shows rapid clearance and disappearance in contrary to metabolic liver disease where it is retained. Normally a liver retain 4–10% of ICG after 15 min and most cirrhotic patients shows value more than mentioned. Increase in ICGR15 value after radiotherapy is associated with higher risk of RILD [29, 30].

Liver specific gadolinium based contrast agent gadoxetate disodium (Evoist) is taken up by hepatocytes based on liver perfusion. It is correlated with ICGR15 retention. It also helps in measuring functional liver with improved spatial resolution of MRI images [31–35]. Studies have shown very low incidence of RILD or non classical RILD in modern era of radiotherapy. SBRT produces transient hypodensity on CT scan that appears within months after treatment and then resolves [22]. Elevated pre-RT LS measured by MRE was associated with an increased risk of developing RILD. In the context of a known hepatic malignancy or metastasis, increased LS likely demonstrate a liver compromised by fibrosis with reduced hepatic reserve.

4.2.7 Management of Complications Evidence of Same Including Guidelines/Algorithm/Summary Illustration

Once classic or non-classic RILD sets in, there is no specific curative management apart from standard supportive care. That includes diuretics, fluid balance, electrolytes balance, paracentesis as required and steroids to reduce hepatic congestion. Use of anticoagulants, trombolytics and tissue plasminogen activator have shown some benefit in relieving hepatic vein thrombosis. Post radiotherapy MRI changes are an indication of early radiation induced liver injury. Those patient may be picked early to start low molecular weight heparin, pentoxiphylline and urdeoxycholic acid for prevention of severe symptoms. Hedgehog inhibitors and CXCR4 inhibitors are under evaluation for radiation induced liver injury. Candidates who are considered for SBRT liver as bridge to transplant, liver transplant is curative in those patient in case of radiation induced liver injury [36–39]. Use of radioprotectors like amifostine have been evaluated to prevent RILD but it lacks strong evidence to be considered as routine for liver directed radiotherapy in modern era [40, 41].

4.2.8 Tips and Tricks to Prevent Complications

Radiation induced liver disease is best prevented than cured. It is dependent on baseline liver function, body mass index, clinical cirrhosis, CP score, albumin, presence of primary liver tumour, radiation dose, radiation volume and dose fractionation. Following evidence based approach is followed with reasonable safe outcome in Princess Margaret Hospital, Toronto, Ontario [42, 43] (Table 4.3).

Proton beam therapy is advantageous in patients with higher risk of developing non-classic RILD such as those with cirrhosis or CP score 2 because proton beam

Table 4.3 Evidence based dose fractionation and DVH protocol in primary and metastatic liver tumour to limit toxicity

Target	Dose
Palliative whole liver irradiation	Liver metastases: 30 Gy, in 2 Gy per fraction, 21 Gy in seven fractions
	Primary liver cancers: 28 Gy, in 2 Gy per fraction, 21 Gy in seven fractions
Therapeutic partial liver RT (standard fractionation)	Liver Metastasis: <32 Gy in 2-Gy fractions for liver metastases.
	Primary liver cancer: Mean normal liver dose (liver minus gross tumor volume) < 28 Gy in 2-Gy fractions for primary liver cancer
Nonuniform liver recommendations (SBRT, three to six fractions)	Metastasis: <15 Gy in three fractions <20 Gy in six fractions
	Primary liver cancer Mean normal liver dose (liver minus gross tumor volume) < 13 Gy in three fractions <18 Gy in six fractions
Critical volume model-based	700 mL of normal liver receives # 15 Gy in three to five fractions

therapy can significantly reduce functional liver irradiation by sharp fall of isodose due to Bragg peak effect with good local control [44–46].

Patients with primary liver cancers have a higher chance of having non classic RILD after external beam radiation [2, 47–49].

4.3 Conclusion

Radiation induced liver disease is rare in modern radiotherapy era. It is best prevented than cured by careful pre radiotherapy workup for indication of radiation and assessment of functional reserve of liver parenchyma. Liver is a parallel structure. It is associated with regeneration of functional unit by compensatory hypertrophy after liver directed local therapy. Treatments of active hepatitis B or C are also important to prevent radiation induced liver toxicity. High precision radiotherapy including particle beam therapy, better understanding of functional volume of liver by modern imaging techniques and refined indications of focal RT has decreased incidence of radiation induced liver toxicity.

Ten Key Points

1. Incidence of RILD is low in modern radiotherapy era.
2. RILD can be classified in classic and non-classic RILD.
3. Anicteric hepatomegaly, ascites and elevated alkaline phosphatase (two times) are features of classic RILD.
4. Non classic RILD characterized by fivefold increase in hepatic transaminases and declining of liver functions.
5. Veno-occlusion, retrograde sinusoidal congestion and subsequent parenchymal atrophy are the causative factors of RILD.
6. Pre-existing liver disease like cirrhosis, non alcoholic steatohepatitis, CP score B, previous hepatic surgery, TACE and subsequent inadequate hepatic regeneration and cytotoxic chemotherapy are associated with poor tolerance.
7. Liver functional volume can be defined using 99mTc sulphur colloid SPECT, Indocyanine green and also with liver specific gadolinium contrast agent gadoxetate disodium (Evoist) based MRI perfusion study.
8. Critical volume of liver 700 cm^3 should receive less than 15 Gy mean dose in 3–5 fractions radiotherapy (SBRT) to minimize the risk of RILD.
9. There is no specific curative management apart from standard supportive care in RILD.
10. Patients with primary liver cancer with compromised liver function should be dealt cautiously using modern radiation techniques including particle beam therapy.

References

1. Case JT. The occurrence of hepatic lesions in patients treated by intensive deep roentgen irradiation. Am J Roentgenol. 1924;12:27.
2. Lawrence TS, Robertson JM, Anscher MS, Jirtle RL, Ensminger WD, Fajardo LF. Hepatic toxicity resulting from cancer treatment. Int J Radiat Oncol Biol Phys. 1995;31(5):1237–48.
3. Benson R, Madan R, Kilambi R, Chander S. Radiation induced liver disease: a clinical update. J Egypt Natl Canc Inst. 2016;28(1):7–11.
4. Kim J, Jung Y. Radiation-induced liver disease: current understanding and future perspectives. Exp Mol Med. 2017;49(7):e359.
5. Toesca DAS, Ibragimov B, Koong AJ, Xing L, Koong AC, Chang DT. Strategies for prediction and mitigation of radiation-induced liver toxicity. J Radiat Res. 2018;59(suppl_1):i40–9.
6. Kimura T, Takahashi S, Takahashi I, Nishibuchi I, Doi Y, Kenjo M, et al. The time course of dynamic computed tomographic appearance of radiation injury to the cirrhotic liver following stereotactic body radiation therapy for hepatocellular carcinoma. PLoS One. 2015;10(6):e0125231.
7. Mendez Romero A, Wunderink W, Hussain SM, De Pooter JA, Heijmen BJ, Nowak PC, et al. Stereotactic body radiation therapy for primary and metastatic liver tumors: a single institution phase i–ii study. Acta Oncol. 2006;45(7):831–7.
8. Tse RV, Hawkins M, Lockwood G, Kim JJ, Cummings B, Knox J, et al. Phase I study of individualized stereotactic body radiotherapy for hepatocellular carcinoma and intrahepatic cholangiocarcinoma. J Clin Oncol. 2008;26(4):657–64.
9. Jung J, Yoon SM, Kim SY, Cho B, Park JH, Kim SS, et al. Radiation-induced liver disease after stereotactic body radiotherapy for small hepatocellular carcinoma: clinical and dose-volumetric parameters. Radiat Oncol. 2013;8:249.
10. Cardenes HR, Price TR, Perkins SM, Maluccio M, Kwo P, Breen TE, et al. Phase I feasibility trial of stereotactic body radiation therapy for primary hepatocellular carcinoma. Clin Transl Oncol. 2010;12(3):218–25.
11. Jang WI, Bae SH, Kim MS, Han CJ, Park SC, Kim SB, et al. A phase 2 multicenter study of stereotactic body radiotherapy for hepatocellular carcinoma: safety and efficacy. Cancer. 2020;126(2):363–72.
12. Durand-Labrunie J, Baumann AS, Ayav A, Laurent V, Boleslawski E, Cattan S, et al. Curative irradiation treatment of hepatocellular carcinoma: a multicenter phase 2 trial. Int J Radiat Oncol Biol Phys. 2020;107(1):116–25.
13. Takeda A, Sanuki N, Tsurugai Y, Iwabuchi S, Matsunaga K, Ebinuma H, et al. Phase 2 study of stereotactic body radiotherapy and optional transarterial chemoembolization for solitary hepatocellular carcinoma not amenable to resection and radiofrequency ablation. Cancer. 2016;122(13):2041–9.
14. Goodman BD, Mannina EM, Althouse SK, Maluccio MA, Cardenes HR. Long-term safety and efficacy of stereotactic body radiation therapy for hepatic oligometastases. Pract Radiat Oncol. 2016;6(2):86–95.
15. McPartlin A, Swaminath A, Wang R, Pintilie M, Brierley J, Kim J, et al. Long-term outcomes of phase 1 and 2 studies of SBRT for hepatic colorectal metastases. Int J Radiat Oncol Biol Phys. 2017;99(2):388–95.
16. Mendez Romero A, Keskin-Cambay F, van Os RM, Nuyttens JJ, Heijmen BJM, JNM IJ, et al. Institutional experience in the treatment of colorectal liver metastases with stereotactic body radiation therapy. Rep Pract Oncol Radiother. 2017;22(2):126–31.
17. Scorsetti M, Comito T, Clerici E, Franzese C, Tozzi A, Iftode C, et al. Phase II trial on SBRT for unresectable liver metastases: long-term outcome and prognostic factors of survival after 5 years of follow-up. Radiat Oncol. 2018;13(1):234.
18. Dawson LA, Normolle D, Balter JM, McGinn CJ, Lawrence TS, Ten Haken RK. Analysis of radiation-induced liver disease using the Lyman NTCP model. Int J Radiat Oncol Biol Phys. 2002;53(4):810–21.

19. Emami B, Lyman J, Brown A, Coia L, Goitein M, Munzenrider JE, et al. Tolerance of normal tissue to therapeutic irradiation. Int J Radiat Oncol Biol Phys. 1991;21(1):109–22.
20. Kutcher GJ, Burman C. Calculation of complication probability factors for non-uniform normal tissue irradiation: the effective volume method. Int J Radiat Oncol Biol Phys. 1989;16(6):1623–30.
21. Lee MT, Kim JJ, Dinniwell R, Brierley J, Lockwood G, Wong R, et al. Phase I study of individualized stereotactic body radiotherapy of liver metastases. J Clin Oncol. 2009;27(10):1585–91.
22. Cheng JC, Wu JK, Lee PC, Liu HS, Jian JJ, Lin YM, et al. Biologic susceptibility of hepatocellular carcinoma patients treated with radiotherapy to radiation-induced liver disease. Int J Radiat Oncol Biol Phys. 2004;60(5):1502–9.
23. Schefter TE, Kavanagh BD, Timmerman RD, Cardenes HR, Baron A, Gaspar LE. A phase I trial of stereotactic body radiation therapy (SBRT) for liver metastases. Int J Radiat Oncol Biol Phys. 2005;62(5):1371–8.
24. Mullikin TC, Pepin KM, Evans JE, Venkatesh SK, Ehman RL, Merrell KW, et al. Evaluation of pretreatment magnetic resonance elastography for the prediction of radiation-induced liver disease. Adv Radiat Oncol. 2021;6(6):100793.
25. Koay EJ, Owen D, Das P. Radiation-induced liver disease and modern radiotherapy. Semin Radiat Oncol. 2018;28(4):321–31.
26. Hoefs JC, Wang F, Kanel G, Braunstein P. The liver-spleen scan as a quantitative liver function test: correlation with liver severity at peritoneoscopy. Hepatology. 1995;22(4 Pt 1):1113–21.
27. Rimola A, Soto R, Bory F, Arroyo V, Piera C, Rodes J. Reticuloendothelial system phagocytic activity in cirrhosis and its relation to bacterial infections and prognosis. Hepatology. 1984;4(1):53–8.
28. Kirichenko A, Gayou O, Parda D, Kudithipudi V, Tom K, Khan A, et al. Stereotactic body radiotherapy (SBRT) with or without surgery for primary and metastatic liver tumors. HPB. 2016;18(1):88–97.
29. Suresh K, Owen D, Bazzi L, Jackson W, Ten Haken RK, Cuneo K, et al. Using indocyanine green extraction to predict liver function after stereotactic body radiation therapy for hepatocellular carcinoma. Int J Radiat Oncol Biol Phys. 2018;100(1):131–7.
30. Yoon HI, Koom WS, Lee IJ, Jeong K, Chung Y, Kim JK, et al. The significance of ICG-R15 in predicting hepatic toxicity in patients receiving radiotherapy for hepatocellular carcinoma. Liver Int. 2012;32(7):1165–71.
31. Asayama Y, Nishie A, Ishigami K, Ushijima Y, Takayama Y, Okamoto D, et al. Histogram analysis of noncancerous liver parenchyma on gadoxetic acid-enhanced MRI: predictive value for liver function and pathology. Abdom Radiol. 2016;41(9):1751–7.
32. Richter C, Seco J, Hong TS, Duda DG, Bortfeld T. Radiation-induced changes in hepatocyte-specific Gd-EOB-DTPA enhanced MRI: potential mechanism. Med Hypotheses. 2014;83(4):477–81.
33. Richter C, Andronesi OC, Borra RJH, Voigt F, Lock S, Duda DG, et al. Inter-patient variations of radiation-induced normal-tissue changes in Gd-EOB-DTPA-enhanced hepatic MRI scans during fractionated proton therapy. Clin Transl Radiat Oncol. 2019;18:113–9.
34. Besa C, Bane O, Jajamovich G, Marchione J, Taouli B. 3D T1 relaxometry pre and post gadoxetic acid injection for the assessment of liver cirrhosis and liver function. Magn Reson Imaging. 2015;33(9):1075–82.
35. Van Beers BE, Pastor CM, Hussain HK. Primovist, Eovist: what to expect? J Hepatol. 2012;57(2):421–9.
36. Bearman SI, Lee JL, Baron AE, McDonald GB. Treatment of hepatic venocclusive disease with recombinant human tissue plasminogen activator and heparin in 42 marrow transplant patients. Blood. 1997;89(5):1501–6.
37. Richardson PG, Elias AD, Krishnan A, Wheeler C, Nath R, Hoppensteadt D, et al. Treatment of severe veno-occlusive disease with defibrotide: compassionate use results in response without significant toxicity in a high-risk population. Blood. 1998;92(3):737–44.

38. Richardson PG, Ho VT, Giralt S, Arai S, Mineishi S, Cutler C, et al. Safety and efficacy of defibrotide for the treatment of severe hepatic veno-occlusive disease. Ther Adv Hematol. 2012;3(4):253–65.
39. Richardson PG, Riches ML, Kernan NA, Brochstein JA, Mineishi S, Termuhlen AM, et al. Phase 3 trial of defibrotide for the treatment of severe veno-occlusive disease and multi-organ failure. Blood. 2016;127(13):1656–65.
40. Symon Z, Levi M, Ensminger WD, Smith DE, Lawrence TS. Selective radioprotection of hepatocytes by systemic and portal vein infusions of amifostine in a rat liver tumor model. Int J Radiat Oncol Biol Phys. 2001;50(2):473–8.
41. Feng M, Smith DE, Normolle DP, Knol JA, Pan CC, Ben-Josef E, et al. A phase I clinical and pharmacology study using amifostine as a radioprotector in dose-escalated whole liver radiation therapy. Int J Radiat Oncol Biol Phys. 2012;83(5):1441–7.
42. Dawson LA, Biersack M, Lockwood G, Eisbruch A, Lawrence TS, Ten Haken RK. Use of principal component analysis to evaluate the partial organ tolerance of normal tissues to radiation. Int J Radiat Oncol Biol Phys. 2005;62(3):829–37.
43. Pan CC, Kavanagh BD, Dawson LA, Li XA, Das SK, Miften M, et al. Radiation-associated liver injury. Int J Radiat Oncol Biol Phys. 2010;76(3 Suppl):S94–100.
44. Wang X, Krishnan S, Zhang X, Dong L, Briere T, Crane CH, et al. Proton radiotherapy for liver tumors: dosimetric advantages over photon plans. Med Dosim. 2008;33(4):259–67.
45. Petersen JB, Lassen Y, Hansen AT, Muren LP, Grau C, Hoyer M. Normal liver tissue sparing by intensity-modulated proton stereotactic body radiotherapy for solitary liver tumours. Acta Oncol. 2011;50(6):823–8.
46. Fukumitsu N, Sugahara S, Nakayama H, Fukuda K, Mizumoto M, Abei M, et al. A prospective study of hypofractionated proton beam therapy for patients with hepatocellular carcinoma. Int J Radiat Oncol Biol Phys. 2009;74(3):831–6.
47. Lawrence TS, Ten Haken RK, Kessler ML, Robertson JM, Lyman JT, Lavigne ML, et al. The use of 3-D dose volume analysis to predict radiation hepatitis. Int J Radiat Oncol Biol Phys. 1992;23(4):781–8.
48. Kawashima M, Furuse J, Nishio T, Konishi M, Ishii H, Kinoshita T, et al. Phase II study of radiotherapy employing proton beam for hepatocellular carcinoma. J Clin Oncol. 2005;23(9):1839–46.
49. Mizumoto M, Okumura T, Hashimoto T, Fukuda K, Oshiro Y, Fukumitsu N, et al. Proton beam therapy for hepatocellular carcinoma: a comparison of three treatment protocols. Int J Radiat Oncol Biol Phys. 2011;81(4):1039–45.

Managing Hyperemesis in the Era of Concurrent and Sequential Chemo-radiation

5

Rakesh Kumar Sharma, Ankur Bahl, and Sapna Singla

5.1 Introduction

Nausea and vomiting induced by cancer treatment (CINV) is one of the most feared adverse events amongst cancer patients leading to detrimental quality of life. It is experienced by approximately 60–80% of oncology patients when unattended [1]. Even after adequate prophylaxis, 30–40% of the patients suffer from CINV [2]. In the Indian setting, following chemotherapy, 51% and 69.5% of patients experience vomiting and nausea respectively [3].

In addition, CINV if left untreated can lead to dehydration, metabolic derangements, poor self-care, functional debility, depleted nutritional status, anorexia, poor performance status, changes in mental status, esophageal tears, wound dehiscence, and delay in administration of further chemotherapy [4]. With appropriate measures, CINV can be tackled in up to 80% of patients undergoing chemotherapy [5, 6].

5.2 Risk Factors

Various factors determine the likelihood and severity of nausea and vomiting following anticancer treatment (chemotherapy and/or radiotherapy). Patient's related factors include female sex and younger age. In addition, individuals with excessive expectations of nausea and vomiting prior to treatment are more prone to develop the same. Conversely, high amount of alcohol consumption lowers the risk of

R. K. Sharma · A. Bahl (✉)
Department of Medical Oncology, Fortis Memorial Research Institute, Gurugram, Haryana, India

S. Singla
Department of Anesthesia, Artemis Hospital, Gurugram, Haryana, India

K. Sood Sharma et al. (eds.), *Complications of Cancer Therapy: Best Practices in Prevention and Management*, https://doi.org/10.1007/978-981-99-0984-1_5

development of CINV. Chemotherapy related factors determining the risk of development of CINV include intrinsic emetogenicity, dosage, combination chemotherapy regimen, schedule and route of administration of which, intrinsic emetogenicity is the most important factor to consider to formulate an antiemetic prophylactic regimen. Factors pertaining to radiotherapy include the dosage, schedule and area of the body being irradiated [4, 7].

Various emetic syndromes associated with CINV should also be considered while formulating an antiemetic prophylaxis regimen, of which acute CINV is of the utmost importance, first described with cisplatin [4]. Based on cisplatin model, CINV is classified as acute if the onset is within 24 h of administration and delayed if it occurs beyond 24 h. An ideal prophylactic strategy should encompass both the acute and delayed CINV components.

Due to the availability of robust prophylactic measures, anticipatory emetic syndrome which is a conditioned emetic response to previous chemotherapy has markedly declined [4].

Chemotherapeutic agents are further classified based on emetogenicity potential. This classification was proposed by Hesketh & Grunberg and chemotherapeutic agents were divided into four groups comprising of highly, moderately, low and minimally emetogenic [4].

5.3 Types of Antiemetic Drugs

Various class of anti-emetic drugs used in oncology are described in Table 5.1.

Table 5.1 Anti-emetic drugs

Class	Drugs
5-HT3 receptor Antagonists	Ondansetron, granisetron, dolasetron, palonosetron
NK-1 Receptor Antagonist	Aprepitant, fosaprepitant, rolapitant, netupitant
Steroids	Dexamethasone
Antipsychotics	Haloperidol, alprazolam, lorazepam, olanzapine
Phenothiazines	Prochlorperazine
Benzamides	Metoclopramide
Cannabinoids	Dronabinol
Miscellaneous	Ginger Acupuncture Behavioral therapy

5.4 Antiemetic Prophylaxis Strategy

The most important consideration for formulating a prophylactic strategy is intrinsic emetogenicity of the chemotherapeutic agent. Ideal strategy for chemotherapy combination regimens is determined by the emetogenicity level contributed by the most emetic chemotherapeutic agent of the regimen followed by the contribution of other agents [8–10]. Based on intrinsic emetogenicity anti-emetic prophylaxis are recommended by various guidelines are summarised in Tables 5.2 and 5.3.

Patients being treated with concurrent chemoradiation should receive prophylaxis based on emetogenic risk level of chemotherapeutic agent unless RT emetic risk exceeds emetic risk of chemotherapeutic agent used [10].

Table 5.2 Anti-emetic prophylaxis for chemotherapy [8–10]

	Prophylactic strategy	
Risk	Acute	Delayed
High	Four drug combination comprising of NK1 antagonist, 5-HT3 antagonist, dexamethasone and olanzapine (Day-1)	Olanzapine ± dexamethasone (Day 2 to 4)
Moderate	Combination of 5-HT3 antagonist, dexamethasone ± olanzapine (Day-1)	Dexamethasone (Day 2 to 3)
Low	5-HT_3 antagonist or dexamethasone	None
Minimal	No prophylaxis needed	

Table 5.3 Anti-emetic prophylaxis approach for radiation therapy (RT) [8–10]

Emetogenic risk	Prophylaxis	Duration
High	Dexamethasone with 5-HT_3 antagonist	On the day of RT and next day if no RT planned for that day
Moderate	5-HT_3 antagonist ± dexamethasone	Before each dose
Low	Usually not needed	
Minimal	Usually not needed	

5.5 Breakthrough Nausea and Vomiting

Patients developing breakthrough nausea and vomiting despite prophylaxis need re-evaluation of emetogenic risk, other illnesses and concomitant medications. Drugs of different class if not used previously can be added (olanzapine, NK1 receptor antagonist, lorazepam or alprazolam, a dopamine receptor antagonist, dronabinol, or nabilone) [10].

5.6 Conclusion

Nausea and vomiting secondary to anti-neoplastic therapy and radiotherapy is one of the most common adverse event encountered in oncology practise that leads to significant deterioration in quality of life and hampers the delivery to cancer treatment. With adequate formulation of prophylactic strategy it can be prevented in majority of patients.

Ten Key Points

1. Nausea and vomiting are one of the most common adverse events encountered in oncology practice.
2. It affects 60–80% of oncology patients.
3. Hesketh classified chemotherapy into four groups based on emetic risk.
4. With the availability of appropriate prophylaxis, the incidence of anticipatory vomiting is on declining trend.
5. Antiemetic prophylaxis is recommended for the patients who will receive emetogenic anticancer agents.
6. Prophylactic strategy should encompass both acute and delayed phase.
7. Four drug olanzapine regimen is preferred for patients at highly emetogenic chemotherapy, especially cisplatin containing regimens.
8. Patients possessing high risk factors for nausea & vomiting should be considered for three drug anti-emetic prophylaxis even with moderately emetogenic chemotherapy.
9. Radiation induced nausea and vomiting is managed in a similar risk based strategy as used in CINV management.
10. Breakthrough nausea & vomiting is managed with agents not used in first line setting.

References

1. De Boer-Dennert M, De Wit R, Schmitz PIM, Djontono J, Beurden VV, Stoter G, et al. Patient perceptions of the side-effects of chemotherapy: the influence of 5HT3 antagonists. Br J Cancer. 1997;76(8):1055–61.

2. Roila F, Herrstedt J, Aapro M, Gralla RJ, Einhorn LH, Ballatori E, et al. Guideline update for MASCC and ESMO in the prevention of chemotherapy- and radiotherapy-induced nausea and vomiting: results of the Perugia consensus conference. Ann Oncol Off J Eur Soc Med Oncol. 2010;21(Suppl 5):v232–43.
3. Baburaj G, Abraham A, George L, Shetty V, Thempalangad R, Rajesh K, et al. A study on utilization and evaluation of antiemetics in chemotherapy-induced nausea and vomiting. Indian J Med Paediatr Oncol. 2017;38(3):334–9.
4. Hesketh PJ. Chemotherapy-induced nausea and vomiting. N Engl J Med. 2009;358(23):2482–94.
5. Chepsy C, Philip BG. An evidence practice gap in antiemetic prescription with chemotherapy. J Pharm Care. 2014;2:22–6.
6. Jordan K, Schaffrath J, Jahn F, Mueller-Tidow C, Jordan B. Neuropharmacology and management of chemotherapy-induced nausea and vomiting in patients with breast cancer. Breast Care. 2014;9(4):246–53.
7. Herrstedt J. Antiemetics: an update and the MASCC guidelines applied in clinical practice. Nat Clin Pract Oncol. 2008;5(1):32–43.
8. Roila F, Molassiotis A, Herrstedt J, Aapro M, Gralla RJ, Bruera E, et al. MASCC and ESMO guideline update for the prevention of chemotherapy- and radiotherapy-induced nausea and vomiting and of nausea and vomiting in advanced cancer patients. Ann Oncol. 2016;27:v119–33.
9. Razvi Y, Chan S, McFarlane T, McKenzie E, Zaki P, DeAngelis C, et al. ASCO, NCCN, MASCC/ESMO: a comparison of antiemetic guidelines for the treatment of chemotherapy-induced nausea and vomiting in adult patients. Support Care Cancer. 2019;27(1):87–95.
10. Hesketh PJ, Kris MG, Basch E, Bohlke K, Barbour SY, Clark-Snow RA, et al. Antiemetics: ASCO guideline update. J Clin Oncol. 2020;38(24):2782–97.

Complications of Intravesical Therapy for Early Bladder Tumors

6

Milap Shah and Puneet Ahluwalia

6.1 Introduction

The entire spectrum of intravesical agents available for the treatment of early bladder tumors can be divided into four categories: (1) intravesical immunotherapy (2) intravesical chemotherapy (3) combination therapy (4) newer agents. Each agents has benefits and risk profile of its own, however none of them are free of adverse events (AE). The complications of intravesical therapy can be classified into (1) Local symptoms—those occurring due to direct effects on the bladder (2) Systemic symptoms—those occurring due to systemic absorption of the drug. Local symptoms are in most cases unavoidable and mild which can be managed symptomatically. Systemic symptoms can be mild or sometimes even life threatening which can be controlled and prevented through proper selection criteria, standard administration protocol and early diagnosis of signs and symptoms.

6.2 Risk Factors [1]

The commonly attributed risk factors responsible for drug related toxicity are:

1. Transurethral resection done recently-it is not an absolute contraindication, however systemic absorption might be more if administered immediately after TURBT.
2. Visible hematuria-should be considered as a contraindication for immediate administration of intravesical agent

M. Shah
Department of Urologic Oncology, Max Institute of Cancer Care, New Delhi, India

P. Ahluwalia (✉)
Max Hospital, Delhi, India

K. Sood Sharma et al. (eds.), *Complications of Cancer Therapy: Best Practices in Prevention and Management*, https://doi.org/10.1007/978-981-99-0984-1_6

3. Traumatic catheterization
4. Active urinary tract infection (UTI)—urine culture should be done to document the absence of infection before administration of intravesical agent.
5. Impaired healing due to previous pelvic radiation, steroids, diabetes, immunocompromised states.

6.3 Intravesical Immunotherapy

6.3.1 BCG (Bacillus Calmette-Guérin)

Intravesical BCG was introduced as an intravesical treatment for urothelial cancer of the bladder a quarter of a century ago by Morales et al. [2]. Numerous strains of BCG are available, including TICE®, Connaught and RIVM. No differences between them strains in (1) their ability to prevent or delay progression, (2) clinical efficacy and (3) side effects was noted in a meta-analysis [3]. There is Level I evidence that as compared to intravesical chemotherapy, intravesical BCG treatment is associated with more side effects. However, serious events are observed in less than 5% cases [4]. Contrary to the existing notion, it has been clearly proven that addition of maintenance phase does not increase the BCG related toxicity as compared to induction phase alone. However, the interruption of treatment was more during the first year of intravesical BCG course [5, 6].

6.3.2 BCG Related Adverse Events

6.3.2.1 Local/Minor symptoms

Usually after the third dose of intravesical instillation, the most common side effects are dysuria and increased frequency of micturition due to inflammatory response and lymphokine release [7]. Low grade fever, malaise and flu-like symptoms also occur but are mild and self-limiting in nature. The severity of these symptoms help to differentiate between symptoms due to local inflammatory response and BCG systemic sepsis. Urine and blood cultures are necessary to rule out bacterial urinary tract infection with sepsis. Visible hematuria also occurs in a small cohort of patients after second or third instillation. Incidence rate is 1% to 30% [8, 9]. Though hematuria resolves by itself, further instillations should be withheld till urine is clear. In case of persistent hematuria, hemorrhagic cystitis and recurrence of tumor should be ruled out [9].

6.3.2.2 Systemic/Major Adverse Reactions

Significant adverse events are uncommon and more than 95% of patients who receive BCG tolerate the treatment well.

Fever

Lamm et al. concluded that high grade fever of more than 103F was the most common severe adverse event (2.9%) amongst the cohort of 2400 patients who received intravesical BCG [8]. As per the recent European Association of Urology (EAU) guidelines, if high grade fever persists for more than 48 h then there should be permanent discontinuation of BCG instillations and prompt treatment with more than two antimicrobial agents should be started while diagnostic evaluation is conducted [4].

Symptomatic Prostatitis and Epididymo-Orchitis

Although these are rare side effects, occurring in less than 1% of patients, the actual incidence is probably much higher [8]. As per study conducted by Mukamel et al., 40% of patients who underwent prostate biopsy after intravesical BCG instillations had granulomatous prostatitis [10]. Symptoms are rarely present, but urine culture should be performed and quinolones should be started. If no response is observed then isoniazid (INH) (300 mg/day) and rifampicin (600 mg/day) for 3 months should be given and further instillations should be withheld. Serum prostate specific antigen values might also be raised in such cases due to induration. Hence some urologists start INH and rifampicin therapy but biopsy is a more definitive to rule out prostate cancer [8]. Epididymo-orchitis is also rare. The approach in such cases is also similar to prostatitis patients. However, in case of refractory cases and abscess formation, orchiectomy may be required [4, 8].

BCG Sepsis

BCG sepsis is potentially the most fatal complication of intravesical BCG instillation. As per literature, the reported incidence rate is 0.4%, with 1 in 12,500 patients resulting in death due to fulminant sepsis post BCG instillation for non-muscle invasive bladder tumor (NMIBC) [8]. BCG sepsis results if instillation is performed in any of the cases as mentioned in contraindications below (Sect. 6.3.2.4). High grade fever and hemodynamic instability are common features. Disseminated intravascular coagulopathy (DIC), respiratory failure, jaundice and leukopenia occur at a later stage [1]. Blood and urine culture may be negative in such cases and hence treatment should be based on clinical judgement. In case of severe infection, high-dose quinolones or INH, rifampicin and ethambutol should be started daily for 6 months along with high-dose corticosteroids as long as symptoms persist. Empirical non-specific antibiotic treatment to cover Gram-negative bacteria and/or Enterococcus should also be given [4, 11].

Allergic Reactions

Arthritis or migratory arthralgia in 0.5% of cases and skin rash in 0.3% have been reported. These reactions are uncommon and they do not necessitate discontinuing BCG in patients with high risk tumors. Prophylactic INH and antihistamine control most symptoms [1, 4].

6.3.2.3 Rare Complications [1, 7, 12]

- Contracted bladder (<1%)
- Ureteral obstruction (0.3%)
- Immune complex glomerulonephritis
- Granulomatous hepatitis and pneumonitis
- Choroiditis and other ocular reactions
- Nephrogenic adenoma
- Cardiac toxicity
- Suppurative lymphadenitis
- Mycotic aneurysm
- Aortoduodenal fistula,
- Lupus vulgaris
- Musculoskeletal lesions
- Penile tuberculosis

6.3.2.4 Contraindication for Intravesical BCG instillation [4]

The absolute contraindications of BCG intravesical instillation are:

- During the first two weeks after TURB;
- In patients with visible haematuria;
- After traumatic catheterisation;
- In patients with symptomatic urinary tract infection.

6.3.3 Interferon α (INF α)

IFNs have immunomodulatory and anti-proliferative properties. Out of all IFNs, IFN-α is best studied as an intravesical agent. The best efficacy is noted at 50 million units as response is dose dependent. However, IFN-α is less effective than BCG as well as intravesical chemotherapy [13, 14]. Therefore, its role is only considered as salvage treatment in BCG refractory cases [15–17]. Side effects occur in less than 30% cases and are similar to those of BCG such as low grade fever, allergic reactions, malaise, flu-like symptoms and nausea. These are due to inflammatory response and lymphokine release [16, 18]. Visible hematuria and symptomatic cystitis is rare and self-limiting occurring in less than 10% cases [19]. Chronic adverse reactions include fatigue, weight loss and anemia. In a randomized, phase 2 study using BCG with IFN 2-α O'Donnell et al. reported systemic adverse events in 5.3% of patients [15]. The majority of cases (4.1%) were infectious or inflammatory.

6.3.4 Mycobacterium Phlei Cell Wall-Nucleic Acid Complex (MCNA/Urocidin)

MCNA has a better safety profile as compared to intravesical BCG. As per literature, the side effects encountered due to MCNA are dysuria, hematuria, fatigue, pollakiuria and urgency. However, the side effects are mild in nature and does not necessitate the stoppage of therapy [20].

6.3.5 Intravesical Treatment with α-Emitter Bi-213-Anti-Epidermal Growth Factor Receptor-Monoclonal Antibody

Single shot of Bi-213- anti-EGFR-MAb intravesical instillation was studies in a pilot study of 5 patients who were BCG refractory. No side effects were noted in these patients. Hence, to evaluate the utilization of this agent in a larger population, a phase-I trial was planned [21].

6.4 Intravesical Chemotherapy

As per the recent EAU guidelines, there is strong recommendation to offer one immediate instillation of intravesical chemotherapy after transurethral resection of the bladder (TURB) in low risk group [4]. Intravesical chemotherapy has become an integral part of management of management of low risk tumors over the past few years. Due to higher molecular weight and lesser systemic absorption, these agents are better tolerated than intravesical BCG. Due to the same reasons they do not carry the small but real risk of BCG sepsis and death. The most commonly used drugs for this are MMC, valrubicin, epirubicin, doxorubicin and gemcitabine [1].

6.4.1 Mitomycin-C (MMC)

Side effects occur in 3–30% cases after MMC instillation. The most common side effects are chemical cystitis which present as irritative (increased frequency, urgency and nocturia) lower urinary tract symptoms (LUTS), dysuria, suprapubic pain and discomfort [22]. Contact dermatitis can also occur due to spillage or direct skin contact of the medication [23]. Other rare adverse events occurring in upto 4–12% cases include eczema-like desquamation of the skin (perineum, face, palms, chest and sole) [22]. Proper cleaning of hands and local parts can prevent this. Other rare complications include myelosuppression, bladder contracture, extravasation of MMC can cause peritonitis, pelvic pain, necrosis, fibrosis and ulceration [22, 24, 25].

6.4.2 Doxurubicin and Epirubicin

The incidence of side effects ranges from 13 to 56%. The side effects profile is similar to MMC with most common side effect being chemical cystitis. This also presents as dysuria, irritative LUTS and suprapubic pain [26]. Systemic side effects occur in less than 5% cases [26]. In comparison of epirubucin and doxorubicin, the incidence of local toxicity was 15.6% versus 36.7% respectively and cystitis was less common with epirubicin [26].

6.4.3 Valrubicin

Valrubicin is notable for being the only US Food and Drug Administration (FDA)-approved intravesical medication specifically for BCG-unresponsive CIS. Despite its FDA approval, this agent is infrequently used because of its unimpressive long-term results and poor tolerability. Significant local toxicity was noted with 90% of patients experiencing at least one adverse event and 3 patients halting the induction course midway because of severe bladder symptoms [27]. Furthermore, treatment with valrubicin is more irritative than most other agents with 86% of patients experiencing 1 or more local bladder symptom of either frequency, dysuria, and urinary urgency [28]. Because of the poor response rates and durability of response with significant local symptoms compared with other intravesical therapies, valrubicin is rarely used as a viable salvage option for patients [29].

6.4.4 Gemcitabine

Gemcitabine and the taxane class of chemotherapy have been the most widely studied intravesical cytotoxic agents in the salvage setting and have demonstrated moderate efficacy [1]. As per literature, gemcitabine has shown a high plasma clearance, indicating even if it is distributed to the systemic circulation after intravesical administration, it will be quickly eliminated, reducing the risk of systemic toxicity [30]. Adverse reactions include nausea, increased frequency of urination, fatigue, intermittent gross hematuria and skin reaction [31].

6.4.5 HIVEC (Hyperthermic Intravesical Instillation of Chemotherapy)

As per literature, several complications have been reported posted hyperthermia treatment (HT) which include hematuria (RR-1.28, CI-95%), UTI (0–23%), sepsis (0–23%), stricture (0–10%), allergic reaction, dysuria, frequency, urgency and incontinence. Grade III or higher adverse events have been reported in more than 10% cases across various clinical trials [32].

6.5 Photodynamic Therapy (PDT)

Various agents have been tried and tested for PDT in BCG-refractory cases such as 5-aminolevulinic acid (5-ALA), hexaminolevulinate (HAL) and Radachlorin. 5-ALA use has resulted in side effects including nausea, hypotension, tachycardia, and some skin sensitivity. These are resolved within 24 h but require intervention to maintain hemodynamic stability in some patients [33]. PDT with intravesical hexaminolevulinate (HAL) exhibited adverse events such as severe, irritative voiding complaints without any noted hemodynamic instability [34]. Radachlorin, a third photosensitizer has also been investigated in a prospective trial of 34 patients with high-risk NMIBC and BCG failure. This trial demonstrated that radachlorin was also safe without significant adverse events [35].

6.6 Combination Intravesical Therapy

6.6.1 Immunotherapy Combinations

BCG with IFN leads to local adverse toxicity during treatment but without effecting long- term quality of life. Patients who received BCG with IFN experience more toxicity, including systemic side effects, such as fever and malaise [36].

Quadruple immunotherapy (BCG, INF, IL-2, and G-CSF) can cause decline in age related immune response [37].

6.6.2 Chemotherapy Combinations

Gemcitabine and MMC regimen is generally well tolerated with most adverse events related to the MMC component or Gemcitabine induced nausea [38].

Gemcitabine and Docetaxel—Gemcitabine can induce nausea but neither Gemcitabine nor Docetaxel irritate the bladder [39]. Hence due to the relatively safer toxicity profile, this combination appears promising.

6.6.3 Adenovirus-Mediated Interferon-Based Gene Therapy

As per the results of phase I trial published in 2013, there were no dose limiting side effects of intravesical rAd-IFN-a/Syn3. The most common complaints reported by patients after completion of treatment were urgency, headache, fatigue, and nausea. LUTS was effectively managed with anticholinergic therapy [40].

6.7 Newer Intravesical Agents

6.7.1 Vicinium (VB4-845)

Vicinium is a protein consisting of fused epithelial cell adhesion molecule antibody to Pseudomonas exotoxin A, which inhibits protein synthesis. Publicly available data are limited but intravesical installation demonstrated promising tolerability and 3-month CR rates of up to 40% with no significant adverse events [41].

6.7.2 Fosciclopirox (CPX-POM)

Ciclopirox Prodrug (CPX-POM) is an investigational small-molecule, novel anti-cancer agent being developed for the treatment of NMIBC. Phase I trial was recently completed and the results published showed no significant dose- limiting adverse events [42].

6.7.3 Apaziquone

It is a newer agent having lesser systemic side effects due to short half- life, poor penetration through avascular tissue and bio-reductive nature. It is theoretically established that since it has a safe systemic side effect profile, it can be used intravesically [43, 44].

6.7.4 Macrophage Migration Inhibitory Factor (MIF)

MIF levels are elevated in many cancers, including bladder cancer, and MIF levels have been noted to increase during tumorigenesis in a mouse model of bladder cancer. In a dose response study on mice, no significant toxicity was noted. Plans for first-in-human use studies are under way [45].

6.8 Conclusion

BCG intravesical treatment is associated with more side effects compared to other intravesical agents. However, serious side effects are encountered in <5% of patients and can be treated effectively in almost all cases. Other intravesical agents used as a primary or salvage therapy have better side effect profile, but there are conflicting evidences in terms of progression, prevention of recurrence and survival as compared to BCG in treatment of non-muscle invasive bladder cancer Table 6.1.

Table 6.1 Common adverse reactions of commonly used intravesical agents [4, 39]

Agent	Common adverse events
BCG	Local—cystitis, hematuria, granulomatous prostatitis, epididymo-orchitis Systemic—Malaise, fever, arthralgia, BCG sepsis
IFN	Fever
IL-2	Fever
GM- CSF	Injection site reaction
Doxorubicin/ Epirubicin	Irritative voiding symptoms
MMC	Rash, Dysuria, Bone marrow suppression
Gemcitabine	Nausea
Docetaxel	Tolerated well

References

1. Koya MP, Simon MA, Soloway MS. Complications of intravesical therapy for urothelial cancer of the bladder. J Urol. 2006;175(6):2004–10.
2. Morales A, Eidinger D, Bruce AW. Intracavitary bacillus Calmette-Guerin in the treatment of superficial bladder tumors. J Urol. 1976;116(2):180–3.
3. Sylvester RJ, van der MA, Lamm DL. Intravesical bacillus Calmette-Guerin reduces the risk of progression in patients with superficial bladder cancer: a meta-analysis of the published results of randomized clinical trials. J Urol. 2002;168(5):1964–70.
4. Babjuk M, Burger M, Capoun O, Cohen D, Comperat EM, Dominguez Escrig JL, et al. European Association of Urology Guidelines on Non-muscle-invasive Bladder Cancer (Ta, T1, and Carcinoma in Situ). Eur Urol. 2022;81(1):75–94.
5. van der Meijden AP, Brausi M, Zambon V, Kirkels W, de Balincourt C, Sylvester R, et al. Intravesical instillation of epirubicin, bacillus Calmette-Guerin and bacillus Calmette-Guerin plus isoniazid for intermediate and high risk Ta, T1 papillary carcinoma of the bladder: a European Organization for Research and Treatment of Cancer genito-urinary group randomized phase III trial. J Urol. 2001;166(2):476–81.
6. Brausi M, Oddens J, Sylvester R, Bono A, van de Beek C, van Andel G, et al. Side effects of Bacillus Calmette-Guerin (BCG) in the treatment of intermediate- and high-risk Ta, T1 papillary carcinoma of the bladder: results of the EORTC genito-urinary cancers group randomised phase 3 study comparing one-third dose with full dose and 1 year with 3 years of maintenance BCG. Eur Urol. 2014;65(1):69–76.
7. Lamm DL. Complications of bacillus Calmette-Guerin immunotherapy. Urol Clin North Am. 1992;19(3):565–72.
8. Lamm DL, van der Meijden PM, Morales A, Brosman SA, Catalona WJ, Herr HW, et al. Incidence and treatment of complications of bacillus Calmette-Guerin intravesical therapy in superficial bladder cancer. J Urol. 1992;147(3):596–600.
9. Molina JM, Rabian C, D'Agay MF, Modai J. Hypersensitivity systemic reaction following intravesical bacillus Calmette-Guerin: successful treatment with steroids. J Urol. 1992;147(3):695–7.
10. Mukamel E, Konichezky M, Engelstein D, Cytron S, Abramovici A, Servadio C. Clinical and pathological findings in prostates following intravesical bacillus Calmette-Guerin instillations. J Urol. 1990;144(6):1399–400.
11. DeHaven JI, Traynellis C, Riggs DR, Ting E, Lamm DL. Antibiotic and steroid therapy of massive systemic bacillus Calmette-Guerin toxicity. J Urol. 1992;147(3):738–42.

12. Nieder AM, Sved PD, Stein JP, Skinner DG, Soloway MS. Cystoprostatectomy and orthotopic ileal neobladder reconstruction for management of bacille Calmette Guerin-induced bladder contractures. Urology. 2005;65(5):909–12.
13. Malmstrom PU. A randomized comparative dose-ranging study of interferon-alpha and mitomycin-C as an internal control in primary or recurrent superficial transitional cell carcinoma of the bladder. BJU Int. 2002;89(7):681–6.
14. Jimenez-Cruz JF, Vera-Donoso CD, Leiva O, Pamplona M, Rioja-Sanz LA, Martinez-Lasierra M, et al. Intravesical immunoprophylaxis in recurrent superficial bladder cancer (Stage T1): multicenter trial comparing bacille Calmette-Guerin and interferon-alpha. Urology. 1997;50(4):529–35.
15. O'Donnell MA, Lilli K, Leopold C, National Bacillus Calmette-Guerin/Interferon Phase 2 Investigator G. Interim results from a national multicenter phase II trial of combination bacillus Calmette-Guerin plus interferon alfa-2b for superficial bladder cancer. J Urol. 2004;172(3):888–93.
16. Torti FM, Shortliffe LD, Williams RD, Pitts WC, Kempson RL, Ross JC, et al. Alpha-interferon in superficial bladder cancer: a Northern California Oncology Group Study. J Clin Oncol. 1988;6(3):476–83.
17. Punnen SP, Chin JL, Jewett MA. Management of bacillus Calmette-Guerin (BCG) refractory superficial bladder cancer: results with intravesical BCG and Interferon combination therapy. Can J Urol. 2003;10(2):1790–5.
18. Belldegrun AS, Franklin JR, O'Donnell MA, Gomella LG, Klein E, Neri R, et al. Superficial bladder cancer: the role of interferon-alpha. J Urol. 1998;159(6):1793–801.
19. Sylvester RJ, van der Meijden AP, Witjes JA, Kurth K. Bacillus Calmette-Guerin versus chemotherapy for the intravesical treatment of patients with carcinoma in situ of the bladder: a meta-analysis of the published results of randomized clinical trials. J Urol. 2005;174(1):86–91. discussion-2
20. Morales A, Herr H, Steinberg G, Given R, Cohen Z, Amrhein J, et al. Efficacy and safety of MCNA in patients with nonmuscle invasive bladder cancer at high risk for recurrence and progression after failed treatment with bacillus Calmette-Guerin. J Urol. 2015;193(4):1135–43.
21. Autenrieth ME, Horn T, Kurtz F, Nguyen K, Morgenstern A, Bruchertseifer F, et al. [Intravesical radioimmunotherapy of carcinoma in situ of the urinary bladder after BCG failure]. Urologe A. 2017;56(1):40–3.
22. Eijsten A, Knonagel H, Hotz E, Brutsch HP, Hauri D. Reduced bladder capacity in patients receiving intravesical chemoprophylaxis with mitomycin C. Br J Urol. 1990;66(4):386–8.
23. de Groot AC, Conemans JM. Systemic allergic contact dermatitis from intravesical instillation of the antitumor antibiotic mitomycin C. Contact Dermatitis. 1991;24(3):201–9.
24. Nieuwenhuijzen JA, Bex A, Horenblas S. Unusual complication after immediate postoperative intravesical mitomycin C instillation. Eur Urol. 2003;43(6):711–2.
25. Zein TA, Friedberg N, Kim H. Bone marrow suppression after intravesical mitomycin C treatment. J Urol. 1986;136(2):459–60.
26. Thrasher JB, Crawford ED. Complications of intravesical chemotherapy. Urol Clin North Am. 1992;19(3):529–39.
27. Steinberg G, Bahnson R, Brosman S, Middleton R, Wajsman Z, Wehle M. Efficacy and safety of valrubicin for the treatment of bacillus Calmette-Guerin refractory carcinoma in situ of the bladder. The Valrubicin Study Group. J Urol. 2000;163(3):761–7.
28. Dinney CP, Greenberg RE, Steinberg GD. Intravesical valrubicin in patients with bladder carcinoma in situ and contraindication to or failure after bacillus Calmette-Guerin. Urol Oncol. 2013;31(8):1635–42.
29. Haas CR, McKiernan JM. Salvage therapy using bacillus Calmette-Guerin derivatives or single agent chemotherapy. Urol Clin North Am. 2020;47(1):47–54.
30. Shelley MD, Jones G, Cleves A, Wilt TJ, Mason MD, Kynaston HG. Intravesical gemcitabine therapy for non-muscle invasive bladder cancer (NMIBC): a systematic review. BJU Int. 2012;109(4):496–505.

31. Brooks NA, O'Donnell MA. Treatment options in non-muscle-invasive bladder cancer after BCG failure. Indian J Urol. 2015;31(4):312–9.
32. Sousa A, Pineiro I, Rodriguez S, Aparici V, Monserrat V, Neira P, et al. Recirculant hyperthermic IntraVEsical chemotherapy (HIVEC) in intermediate-high-risk non-muscle-invasive bladder cancer. Int J Hyperth. 2016;32(4):374–80.
33. Berger AP, Steiner H, Stenzl A, Akkad T, Bartsch G, Holtl L. Photodynamic therapy with intravesical instillation of 5-aminolevulinic acid for patients with recurrent superficial bladder cancer: a single-center study. Urology. 2003;61(2):338–41.
34. Bader MJ, Stepp H, Beyer W, Pongratz T, Sroka R, Kriegmair M, et al. Photodynamic therapy of bladder cancer—a phase I study using hexaminolevulinate (HAL). Urol Oncol. 2013;31(7):1178–83.
35. Lee JY, Diaz RR, Cho KS, Lim MS, Chung JS, Kim WT, et al. Efficacy and safety of photodynamic therapy for recurrent, high grade nonmuscle invasive bladder cancer refractory or intolerant to bacille Calmette-Guerin immunotherapy. J Urol. 2013;190(4):1192–9.
36. Nepple KG, Lightfoot AJ, Rosevear HM, O'Donnell MA, Lamm DL, Bladder Cancer Genitourinary Oncology Study G. Bacillus Calmette-Guerin with or without interferon alpha-2b and megadose versus recommended daily allowance vitamins during induction and maintenance intravesical treatment of nonmuscle invasive bladder cancer. J Urol. 2010;184(5):1915–9.
37. Hurez V, Padron AS, Svatek RS, Curiel TJ. Considerations for successful cancer immunotherapy in aged hosts. Clin Exp Immunol. 2017;187(1):53–63.
38. Cockerill PA, Knoedler JJ, Frank I, Tarrell R, Karnes RJ. Intravesical gemcitabine in combination with mitomycin C as salvage treatment in recurrent non-muscle-invasive bladder cancer. BJU Int. 2016;117(3):456–62.
39. Brooks NA, O'Donnell MA. Combination intravesical therapy. Urol Clin North Am. 2020;47(1):83–91.
40. Shore ND, Boorjian SA, Canter DJ, Ogan K, Karsh LI, Downs TM, et al. Intravesical rAd-IFNalpha/Syn3 for patients with high-grade, bacillus Calmette-Guerin-refractory or relapsed non-muscle-invasive bladder cancer: a phase II randomized study. J Clin Oncol. 2017;35(30):3410–6.
41. Bree KK, Brooks NA, Kamat AM. Current therapy and emerging intravesical agents to treat non-muscle invasive bladder cancer. Hematol Oncol Clin North Am. 2021;35(3):513–29.
42. Weir SJ, Wood R, Schorno K, Brinker AE, Ramamoorthy P, Heppert K, et al. Preclinical pharmacokinetics of Fosciclopirox, a novel treatment of urothelial cancers, in rats and dogs. J Pharmacol Exp Ther. 2019;370(2):148–59.
43. Loadman PM, Phillips RM, Lim LE, Bibby MC. Pharmacological properties of a new aziridinylbenzoquinone, RH1 (2,5-diaziridinyl-3-(hydroxymethyl)-6-methyl-1,4-benzoquinone), in mice. Biochem Pharmacol. 2000;59(7):831–7.
44. Li D, Gan Y, Wientjes MG, Badalament RA, Au JL. Distribution of DT-diaphorase and reduced nicotinamide adenine dinucleotide phosphate: cytochrome p450 oxidoreductase in bladder tissues and tumors. J Urol. 2001;166(6):2500–5.
45. Meyer-Siegler KL, Leifheit EC, Vera PL. Inhibition of macrophage migration inhibitory factor decreases proliferation and cytokine expression in bladder cancer cells. BMC Cancer. 2004;4:34.

7 Predictors and Treatment of Platinum Induced Nephrotoxicity

Yasir Rizvi

7.1 Introduction

The platinum-based drugs cisplatin, carboplatin and oxaliplatin are widely used in the treatment of various malignancies. Nephrotoxicity due to these platinum based drugs is an important factor limiting the therapeutic usefulness of these compounds. Drug-induced nephrotoxicity may affect any component of the nephron structure such as the glomerulus, tubules, and renal microvasculature [1]. Renal toxicity impedes effective cancer therapy and can impact the quality of life of cancer patients. This chapter is intended as a guide for recognition of risk factors that may predispose to nephrotoxicity due to platinum based agents and its early diagnosis and treatment.

7.2 Incidence of Nephrotoxicity

Cisplatin is commonly used in the treatment of many solid-organ cancers, including those of the head, neck, lung, testis, ovary, and breast. Cisplatin is a strong cellular toxin and nephrotoxicity of cisplatin has been recognized since its introduction over 25 years ago [2]. The kidney accumulates cisplatin by peritubular uptake and concentration of the drug achieved in the renal cortex is several folds greater than other organs [3]. High peak plasma free platinum concentrations are associated with an increased risk of AKI [4]. Vasoconstriction in the kidney microvasculature [5] and release of proinflammatory cytokines [6] also add to renal injury. Cisplatin use can lead to various manifestations of renal involvement as outlined in Table 7.1.

Y. Rizvi (✉)
Department of Nephrology, VMMC and Safdarjung Hospital, New Delhi, India

Department of Nephrology, Dharamshila Narayana Superspeciality Hospital, New Delhi, India

K. Sood Sharma et al. (eds.), *Complications of Cancer Therapy: Best Practices in Prevention and Management*, https://doi.org/10.1007/978-981-99-0984-1_7

Table 7.1 Renal manifestations of cisplatin treatment [2]

• Acute kidney injury (20–30%)
• Hypomagnesemia (40–100%)
• Fanconi-like syndrome
• Distal renal tubular acidosis
• Hypocalcemia
• Renal concentrating defect
• Hyperuricemia
• Transient proteinuria
• Thrombotic microangiopathy
• Erythropoietin deficiency

7.3 Clinical Presentation

The most important clinical manifestation of cisplatin nephrotoxicity is kidney injury, which may be acute or chronic. Other kidney manifestations have been described, including electrolyte disturbances, thrombotic microangiopathy, and anemia (due to decreased erythropoietin production) as summarised in Table 7.1.

Acute kidney injury (AKI) from cisplatin exposure typically manifests with a slow rise in serum creatinine after five to seven days of therapy. The timing of AKI may be earlier (within three to five days of therapy) in patients with comorbid risk factors, such as pre-existing chronic kidney disease (CKD), older age, or concomitant use of nephrotoxic drugs.

Most patients experience a mild to moderate increase in serum creatinine (i.e., 1.5 to 2.9 times baseline), while some may progress to more severe AKI (serum creatinine >3.0 times baseline) or require renal replacement therapy. These patients generally have azotemia in the setting of bland urinalysis and minimal proteinuria. The urine output in these patients is generally preserved which is consistent with the induction of a concentrating defect in tubules.

Severe AKI is usually uncommon in the absence of pre-existing CKD and/or other comorbid risk factors as mentioned above. Although renal function improves in most patients, a subgroup of patients may develop permanent renal impairment [1].

Tubulointerstitial injury is a predominant finding on pathologic examination of human kidneys affected by cisplatin toxicity. Both proximal and distal tubules are affected, and in patients with AKI, there may be acute tubular necrosis.

7.4 Electrolyte Disturbances

Hypomagnesemia is common and may be present in 42–100% of patients depending on total cisplatin dose and length of exposure. Hypomagnesemia and renal magnesium wasting may persist for up to 6 years after initial dose [1].

Renal salt wasting syndrome has been reported in up to 10% of patients, manifesting as hyponatremia and severe orthostatic hypotension in the setting of high urinary sodium concentration. Patients typically present with polyuria, hypovolemia, and hyponatremia. This syndrome may present 2–4 months after initiation of cisplatin therapy [4].

Fanconi-like syndrome: Cisplatin-mediated nephrotoxicity is accompanied by the development of a Fanconi-like syndrome, with increased urinary excretion of glucose and amino acids in the urine.

Syndrome of in-appropriate antidiuretic hormone secretion (SIADH) has been documented in patients receiving vigorous hydration [5] but is less common now as cisplatin-associated nausea is treated with new-generation antiemetics, diminishing the stimulus for antidiuretic hormone secretion.

Thrombotic microangiopathy: Rare cases have been reported in patients who were also receiving bleomycin or gemcitabine with cisplatin [7].

Anemia—Cisplatin is frequently associated with anemia that is disproportionate to its myelosuppressive effect on the other blood cell lines. Animal and human studies suggest that cisplatin leads to a deficiency of erythropoietin due to its tubular toxicity.

Among the new platinum agents, the third generation mainly represented by oxaliplatin, is a recent agent that has been reported to have fewer adverse effects and has relevant safety in patients with pre-existing renal impairment [8]. However, there are case reports of oxaliplatin therapy leading to acute intravascular hemolysis and AKI [7].

7.5 Risk Factors

The main predisposing factors for nephrotoxicity due to platinum based drugs have been outlined in Table 7.2.

Due to increasing incidence of Chronic Kidney Disease in India, many patients being diagnosed with cancer may have varying degree of pre-existing renal dysfunction and present a clinical challenge for chemotherapy.

Table 7.2 Risk factors for cisplatin nephrotoxicity [2, 9]

- Older age
- Female sex
- Dose
- Frequency
- Cumulative dose
- Hypoalbuminemia
- Pre-existing renal disease due to any cause
- Concomitant use of other drugs with potential nephrotoxicity
  - Aminoglycosides like amikacin, gentamicin
  - Amphotericin-B
  - NSAID
  - ACE inhibitors/ARB

7.6 How to Monitor Patients During Chemotherapy

Patients on Platinum based chemotherapy should be regularly monitored for any evidence of renal toxicity. The monitoring comprises of the following:

A. **Clinical:**
   1. Maintain adequate hydration during chemotherapy
   2. Monitor blood pressure—avoid hypotension or hypertension
   3. Blood sugars should be well controlled for patients with pre-existing diabetes
   4. Monitor urine output
B. **Biochemical:** Blood tests may be regularly conducted as clinically indicated:
   1. Kidney function test: Blood urea, serum creatinine especially to monitor the trend of creatinine
   2. Electrolytes: Serum Sodium, Potassium, Calcium, Phosphate, Magnesium
   3. Acid base analysis: ABG or serum bicarbonate levels
   4. Urine routine and microscopy to assess for proteinuria

The frequency of monitoring may vary depending upon the clinical scenario and institutional practice. In patients with risk factors for cisplatin nephrotoxicity, more frequent monitoring (i.e., daily for the first few days after cisplatin administration) may be advisable.

7.7 Precautions

Prevention of kidney injury is a point of focus for patients undergoing cisplatin therapy. Aggressive Short-duration, low-volume hydration; dose adjustment for pre-existing renal impairments; magnesium supplementation; avoidance of other potential nephrotoxins, and, when appropriate, use of lower doses of cisplatin may help in reducing the incidence of nephrotoxicity. Although a number of pharmacologic agents have been evaluated to decrease nephrotoxicity, none has an established role.

7.8 Management

Management of nephrotoxicity due to platinum based chemotherapeutic agents depends on the degree of renal involvement.

7.9 Patients with Acute Kidney Injury

The general approach to the management of acute kidney injury (AKI) after cisplatin administration is the same as that for other causes of AKI. Cisplatin discontinuation is appropriate in patients who develop AKI, particularly those with moderate to severe AKI (increase in serum creatinine to >2.0 times baseline). If the inclusion of cisplatin in the treatment regimen is considered to be life-saving or life extending, retreatment with cisplatin may be considered after recovery from AKI.

Management issues in AKI

1. Volume status—avoid dehydration / fluid overload
2. Correct Dyselectrolytemia
3. Maintain Acid Base balance
4. Intravenous antibiotic dosing to be adjusted as per eGFR
5. Rule out other causes of kidney injury like UTI, Obstructive uropathy
6. Avoid other drugs with potential nephrotoxicity
7. Hemodialysis indications:
   - Advanced uraemia
   - Resistant hyperkalemia
   - Resistant Metabolic acidosis
   - Fluid overload
   - Uraemic encephalopathy

7.10 Patients with Electrolyte Disturbances

In general, patients with electrolyte disturbances after cisplatin administration are treated with appropriate supplementation. Discontinuation of cisplatin is not required in this setting, especially if the patient's cancer is being effectively treated with cisplatin or treatment with cisplatin is potentially life-saving or life-extending. However, discontinuation of cisplatin may be necessary if the patient has concurrent AKI or if the electrolyte disturbances are difficult to manage even with aggressive supplementation.

7.11 Fanconi-Like Syndrome

Patients who develop proximal tubular dysfunction (Fanconi-like syndrome) after cisplatin administration should be managed with oral or intravenous (IV) supplementation depending upon the severity of the deficiency. Patients with evidence of a renal tubular acidosis should receive alkali therapy (e.g., sodium bicarbonate, sodium citrate, potassium citrate) to correct their metabolic acidosis.

7.12 Salt Wasting

Patients with renal salt wasting following cisplatin should be acutely treated with IV saline to correct volume depletion and hyponatremia if present. Salt tablets can be administered once the patient is volume repleted and should be dose titrated to symptoms and blood pressure to avoid symptomatic hypotension and hypovolemic hyponatremia.

Take Home Points

- Nephrotoxicity due to platinum based chemotherapeutic drugs is an important factor limiting the therapeutic usefulness of these compounds.
- Clinicians should be aware regarding the risk factors that may contribute to enhanced nephrotoxicity of these drugs.
- Patients on platinum based chemotherapy should have a baseline renal assessment done before initiating therapy to detect any pre-existing renal disease.
- The patient should be regularly monitored during therapy for any evidence of renal toxicity.
- Platinum based drugs can lead to varied presentation of renal toxicity such as AKI, dyselectrolytemia, Salt wasting and Fanconi like syndrome.
- Early recognition and prompt therapy can prevent patient from developing advanced renal toxicity.
- Most of the patients developing AKI due to platinum based therapy recover after stopping the drug. *However* some patients may have persistent renal dysfunction.
- Concomitant use of other potentially nephrotoxic drugs should be avoided during platinum based chemotherapy wherever clinically feasible.

References

1. https://www.asn-online.org/education/distancelearning/curricula/onco/Chapter11.pdf. Last accessed on 28 May 2022.
2. Miller RP, Tadagavadi RK, Ramesh G, Reeves WB. Mechanisms of cisplatin nephrotoxicity. Toxins (Basel). 2010;2(11):2490–518.
3. Hayati F, et al. Prevention of cisplatin nephrotoxicity. J Nephropharmacol. 2015;5:57–60.
4. Reece PA, Stafford I, Russell J, et al. Creatinine clearance as a predictor of ultrafilterable platinum disposition in cancer patients treated with cisplatin: relationship between peak ultrafilterable platinum plasma levels and nephrotoxicity. J Clin Oncol. 1987;5:304.
5. Luke DR, Vadiei K, Lopez-Berestein G. Role of vascular congestion in cisplatin-induced acute renal failure in the rat. Nephrol Dial Transplant. 1992;7:1.
6. Ramesh G, Reeves WB. p38 MAP kinase inhibition ameliorates cisplatin nephrotoxicity in mice. Am J Physiol Renal Physiol. 2005;289:F166.
7. Jain A, Dubashi B, Parameswaran S, Ganesh RN. Oxaliplatin induced acute tubular necrosis. Indian J Cancer. 2015;52(3):363–4.
8. Labaye J, Sarret D, Duvic C, Hérody M, Didelot F, Nédélec G, Noël LH. Renal toxicity of oxaliplatin. Nephrol Dial Transplant. 2005;20:1275–6.
9. Perazella MA, Portilla D, Safar M. Cisplatin nephrotoxicity. UpToDate. Last accessed on 1 June 2024.

8 Radiation Cystitis After Pelvic Radiation in Survivors of Pelvic Malignancies

Swarupa Mitra, David Simson, and Soumitra Barik

8.1 Introduction

Radiation cystitis is a very common complication of pelvic radiotherapy. Incidence of radiation cystitis varies between 23% and 80% [1] Radiation cystitis may present commonly as dysuria, frequency, urgency, and haematuria. Haemorrhagic cystitis in the form of intractable haemorrhage is not an uncommon late complication seen in urology clinics.

Newer advancements in radiation technologies like Intensity modulated radiotherapy (IMRT) and Image Guided radiotherapy (IGRT) are promising, as they allow reduction in margins of the planning target volume (PTV), which significantly reduces the genitourinary toxicity as compared to conventional radiotherapy. The total delivered radiation dose to the genitourinary tract explains the differences in radiation toxicities between different radiation modalities. The bladder is an organ that is sensitive to small increments of radiation dose [2].

8.2 Epidemiology

The incidence of radiation cystitis reported is varied in different studies. This is because of the marked differences seen in collection of data, variations in dosimetry, size of radiation fields, and techniques of radiotherapy used. Nevertheless, acute

S. Mitra (✉)
Department of Radiation Oncology, Rajiv Gandhi Cancer Institute and Research Centre, New Delhi, India

Radiation Oncology, Fortis Memorial Research Institute. FMRI, Gurgaon, India

D. Simson · S. Barik
Department of Radiation Oncology, Rajiv Gandhi Cancer Institute and Research Centre, New Delhi, India

K. Sood Sharma et al. (eds.), *Complications of Cancer Therapy: Best Practices in Prevention and Management*, https://doi.org/10.1007/978-981-99-0984-1_8

radiation cystitis is generally seen in 50% of patients receiving pelvic radiation therapy for cancers of prostate or of cervical cancer as published in most studies. The mean duration for developing radiation cystitis is 31.8 months after treatment. Incidence of severe haematuria ranges from 5% to 8% and can develop up to 14 years following radiotherapy treatment. But the actuarial risk of developing haematuria is 5.8% at 5 years and 9.6% at 20 years. Males are more likely to develop radiation cystitis than females [3, 4].

With the introduction of Intensity-modulated radiotherapy (IMRT), a technique that can deliver higher doses to the target area while minimizing dose to the surrounding organs, namely, bladder and rectum, this number is decreasing. IMRT is being offered extensively for the treatment of various pelvic cancers because the complication rates with IMRT is lower than that with the traditional conventional or 3-dimensional (3D) conformal beam therapy, although not all studies show a significant difference.

The rates of genitourinary toxicity with IMRT compared with those with 3D conformal radiotherapy is as follows.

Grade 2: IMRT, 17–36%; 3D conformal radiotherapy, 42–60%
Grade 3: IMRT, 0.3–0.5%; 3D conformal radiotherapy, 1–2%

8.3 Etiology and Pathophysiology

The pathophysiology of radiation cystitis is not well understood. Multiple mechanisms of damage to the bladder with radiation have been suggested as described in Table 8.1.

Radiation causes cell death in 2 ways—Indirect and Direct.

INDIRECT—With Radiation therapy the energy from ionizing radiation is transferred to the molecules of the tumor cells and surrounding exposed tissues. Radiation interacts with intracellular water generating free radicals that interfere with synthesis of DNA, resulting in cell death. Rapidly dividing cells are most susceptible to

Table 8.1 The proposed pathophysiology of radiation cystitis

Site of the bladder	Proposed mechanism of radiation damage
Urothelium	Nuclear irregularity Cellular oedema Increased cytoplasmic elements Disruption of tight junctions & polysaccharide layer
Vasculature	Vascular endothelial cell oedema Endothelial cell proliferation Perivascular fibrosis
Detrusor Muscle	Smooth muscle oedema Replacement of smooth muscle with fibroblasts Increased collagen deposition Vascular ischaemia of bladder wall

radiation injury. Cells are most sensitive to radiation during the M and G2 phases of the cell cycle.

DIRECT—Radiation causes direct cell death by mitotic arrest, point mutations in deoxyribonucleic acid (DNA), and damage to the cell membrane.

It also causes changes in the blood vessels with subendothelial proliferation, oedema, and medial thickening, thus depleting blood supply to the irradiated tissue. Subsequent collagen deposition results in severe scarring and further obliteration of the lumen of the blood-vessels and may also obstruct revascularisation. As a result, tissue hypoxia and necrosis set in leading to mucosal ischemia and epithelial damage. Concomitant use of chemotherapeutic agents works synergistically to further increase the radiation induced damages.

In the case of urinary bladder, the subepithelial tissues are exposed to the alkalinity of the urine which in turn causes submucosal fibrosis. Vascular endothelial cell oedema manifests at 3 months and endothelial cell proliferation after 6 months. Vascular ischaemia, oedema, and cellular destruction replace the bladder smooth muscle fibres with fibroblasts and lead to increased collagen deposition and subsequent decreases in bladder compliance and capacity.

Radiation Cystitis can be described as Early and Late.

Early Radiation Cystitis—This is usually self-limiting and responds to conservative symptomatic therapy or observation.

These are those changes that appear within 12 months after radiation treatment. This includes submucosal inflammation and fibrosis, perineural inflammation, surface ulceration, and epithelial atypia (e.g., nuclear pleomorphism, hyperchromatism, granular cytoplasm).

Late Radiation Cystitis— This commonly presents with hematuria, ranging from mild to life-threatening.

These changes are seen after more than 12 months of treatment. They are essentially fibrovascular changes, with luminal occlusion, vascular ectasia, and necrosis of vessel walls. Cells with epithelial damage manifest cytoplasmic vacuolization and epithelial proliferation.

Clinical symptoms result from these pathological changes [5].

1. Pain and discomfort—Due to the formation of ulcers, radiation neuritis, and post radiation fibrosis.
2. Voiding Dysfunctions—Due to ischemia and fibrosis causing loss of bladder muscle fibres.
3. Abnormal Neural Stimulation—Due to ischemia causing denervation super sensitivity.

The rate of long-term complications depends on 3 factors:

1. Volume and area of bladder affected—The trigone is more symptomatic than the dome of the bladder.
2. Dose rate—Dose rates <0.8 Gy/h decreases risk of cystitis and daily fraction size >2 Gy/fraction increase risk.

3. Total dose—Toxicity increases when the total dose to bladder exceeds 60 Gy. Conformal radiation techniques allow higher doses to be delivered to the tumour while maintaining lower total dose delivered to the bladder.

8.4 Clinical Presentation

Bladder toxicities due to radiation can be divided into acute and late toxicities.

Acute toxicities generally occur during or within 3–6 months of radiation and late toxicities occur after 6 months of radiotherapy. Symptoms that occur between 3 and 6 months after radiotherapy are also termed subacute toxicity [6].

Acute symptoms usually consist of pain or burning sensation while urination, increased frequency and urgency, a sensation of incomplete bladder emptying, suprapubic pain or discomfort. Bladder spasms in men can present with referred pain in the glans penis. The reported incidence of acute radiation cystitis varies between 23% and 80% for patients receiving pelvic radiotherapy for various tumors [1, 7–11]. The wide variation in incidence is caused by actual variation in tumor type, dose-volume factor. These symptoms are usually subjective and not severe, hence may not be reported by the patient and physicians. Acute symptoms usually subside within several weeks of completion of radiotherapy.

Late bladder toxicities usually appear between several months to several years after completion of radiotherapy with a median time of approximately 13–20 months. The vast majority of late complications occur within 2–3 years of radiotherapy. Bladder injury may appear due to "global injury" when a major portion of the bladder is irradiated, or "focal injury" when a small portion of the bladder is irradiated. Late symptoms arising out of global injury are dysuria, frequency, urgency, reduced bladder capacity, reduced flow, incontinence, and cystitis. Focal injury may later manifest as hematuria, obstruction due to clot formation, ulceration, necrosis, and fistula formation [12]. Overall late toxicities occur in less than 10% of patients with bladder, prostate, or cervical cancer [1].

8.5 Grading of Bladder Toxicities

Several scoring systems have been used to describe acute and late bladder toxicities. National Cancer Institute (NCI) Common Terminology Criteria for Adverse Events (CTCAE) proposed a grading system depending upon the level of intervention required for therapy (Table 8.2) [13]. CTCAE grading does not differentiate between acute and late toxicities. Similarly, the Radiotherapy Oncology Group (RTOG) and the European Organisation for Research and Treatment of Cancer (EORTC) (Table 8.3) have proposed a grading system for acute and late genitourinary toxicities [14]. LENT-SOMA scale (Late Effects of Normal Tissues-Subjective, Objective, Management, and Analytic system) considers subjective and objective endpoints separately [15]. Although it is comprehensive, it is most commonly used in clinical studies.

Table 8.2 Common Terminology Criteria for Adverse Events (CTCAE) v5.0

Complication	Grade 1	Grade 2	Grade 3	Grade 4	Grade 5
Haematuria	Asymptomatic; clinical or diagnostic observations only; intervention not indicated	Symptomatic; urinary catheter or bladder irrigation indicated; limiting instrumental ADL	Gross haematuria; transfusion, IV medications, or hospitalization indicated; elective invasive intervention indicated; limiting self-care ADL	Life-threatening consequences; urgent invasive intervention indicated	Death
Cystitis noninfective	Microscopic haematuria; minimal increase in frequency, urgency, dysuria, or nocturia; new onset of incontinence	Moderate haematuria; moderate increase in frequency, urgency, dysuria, nocturia or incontinence; urinary catheter placement or bladder irrigation indicated; limiting instrumental ADL	Gross haematuria; transfusion, IV medications, or hospitalization indicated; elective invasive intervention indicated	Life-threatening consequences; urgent invasive intervention indicated	Death
Urinary fistula	–	Symptomatic, invasive intervention not indicated	Invasive intervention indicated	Life-threatening consequences; urgent invasive intervention indicated	Death
Urinary tract obstruction	Asymptomatic; clinical or diagnostic observations only; intervention not indicated	Symptomatic but no hydronephrosis, sepsis, or renal dysfunction; urethral dilation, urinary or suprapubic catheter indicated	Altered organ function (e.g., hydronephrosis or renal dysfunction); invasive intervention indicated	Life-threatening consequences; urgent intervention indicated	Death

Table 8.3 Radiation Therapy Oncology Group (RTOG)/European Organisation for Research and Treatment of Cancer (EORTC) morbidity scoring criteria for genitourinary toxicities.

Toxicity/complication	Grade1	Grade 2	Grade 3	Grade 4	Grade 5
Acute	Frequency of urination or nocturia twice pre-treatment habit/dysuria, urgency not requiring medication	Frequency of urination or nocturia that is less frequent than every hour. Dysuria, urgency, bladder spasm requiring local anaesthetic (e.g., Pyridium)	Frequency with urgency and nocturia hourly or more frequently/ dysuria, pelvis pain or bladder spasm requiring regular, frequent narcotic/gross haematuria with/ without clot passage	Haematuria requiring transfusion/acute bladder obstruction not secondary to clot passage, ulceration, or necrosis	Death
Late	Slight epithelial atrophy; minor telangiectasia (microscopic haematuria)	Moderate frequency; generalized telangiectasia; intermittent macroscopic haematuria	Severe frequency and dysuria; severe telangiectasia (often with petechiae). Frequent haematuria; reduction in bladder capacity (<150 cm^3)	Necrosis/Contracted bladder (capacity <100 cm^3). Severe haemorrhagic cystitis	Death

8.6 Dosimetric Correlation with Radiation Cystitis

8.6.1 Bladder Cancer

Patients treated with a dose 60–66 Gy to the whole bladder resulted in late grade 3 or more toxicity 0–42% [16, 17]. Patients treated with a hypofractionated dose of 52.5–57.5 Gy had grade 3 or more late toxicities in 4–18% [18, 19]. With partial bladder irradiation up to a dose of 67.5 Gy, the grade 3 or higher late toxicities was seen in 1–23% of patients [18, 20, 21].

8.6.2 Prostate Cancer

Bladder neck and prostatic urethra remain adjacent to treatment volume in prostate cancer. The majority of studies did not find any correlation between dose and genitourinary toxicity in prostate cancer. As the bladder is a highly distensible organ and interfraction and intrafraction filling uncertainties remain during the treatment course, it is difficult to arrive at a conclusive dose-volume relationship. In a multi-institutional trial of 669 prostate cancer patients, there was no difference in genitourinary toxicities in patients treated with 68Gy and 78 Gy. Grade 3 or more toxicities were seen in 13% and 12% in high dose and low dose arms respectively [22]. Patients treated with hypofractionated RT to a dose of 60 Gy in 20 fractions (3 Gy per fraction) in the CHHiP Trial, 5 year cumulative RTOG grade 2 or worse bladder toxicities was 11.7% [23].

8.6.3 Cervical Cancer

Locally advanced carcinoma of cervix treated with a higher EBRT dose (>60 Gy) results in unacceptable toxicities and poor outcomes. Hence EBRT is combined with brachytherapy for treatment [24]. Total combined dose with EBRT and brachytherapy to the region close to the brachytherapy applicator approximates 70–90 Gy [7]. In a study of 141 patients with follow up of 39 months, patients treated with bladder dose to D2cc of </= 95 Gy, 13% of patients had grade 1–4 late toxicities compared to 17% of patients who received a dose of >95 Gy to D2cc of the bladder. The difference in toxicities was not significant indicating the threshold for focal dose is not clear from available data [25–27]. Patients with locally advanced carcinoma cervix treated with EBRT (40–50 Gy) with concurrent chemotherapy followed by MRI based image-guided adaptive brachytherapy (IGABT) in EMBRACE I studies resulted in 5 year cumulative grade 3 or worse genitourinary toxicities was 6.8% [28].

8.7 Dose Volume Histogram (DVH) Analysis

The urinary bladder is a highly distensible organ. Its volume continuously changes with filling. Also, the bladder can move with positioning, bowel filling, and respiration. So, the dose-volume histogram obtained from a single planning CT may not represent the true dose distribution during treatment. With treatment to the whole pelvis, a static simulation 3D CT scan is not likely to represent the true bladder position during several weeks of therapy. Determining a true bladder DVH has not been possible. DVH obtained from planning CT at best can correlate with true dose distribution (Fig. 8.1) [7].

In the absence of robust data, clinicians can use dose limits listed in the conventional fractionation arm of the Radiation Therapy Oncology Group (RTOG) 0415 study of prostate cancer, which included a solid bladder constraint of—

- no more than 15% of the volume to receive a dose >80 Gy,
- no more than 25% of the volume to receive a dose >75 Gy,
- no more than 35% of the volume to receive a dose >70 Gy, and
- no more than 50% of the volume to receive a dose >65 Gy [29].

For hypofractionated RT, one can use dose constraints as per CHHip Trial Protocol,

- no more than 5% of the bladder volume to receive a dose >60 Gy,
- no more than 25% of the volume to receive a dose >48.6 Gy,
- no more than 50% of the volume to receive a dose >40.8 Gy.

For bladder cancer, there is no published robust data to guide dose-volume constraints. Restricting whole bladder or partial-bladder doses to 64–65 Gy in 36 daily fractions or 40–42 twice-daily fractions produce a level of late bladder complications equivalent to Radiation Therapy Oncology Group Grade 3 toxicity in <6%.

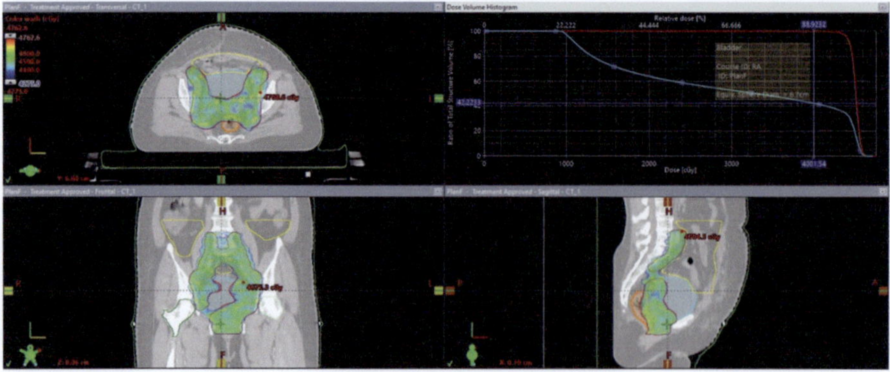

Fig. 8.1 Dose colour wash and Dose volume histogram (DVH) in locally advanced carcinoma cervix treated with volumetric arc therapy

In gynaecological malignancies, limiting EBRT doe to 40–50 Gy rarely results in any long-term sequelae. The addition of brachytherapy increases the dose to the bladder. In cervical cancer, the upper dose limit for brachytherapy has not yet been clearly defined.

8.8 Clinical Predictor or Risk Factor for Bladder Toxicities

Patients who underwent surgeries like TURBT, prostatectomy, or hysterectomy have a higher risk of developing bladder toxicities [30, 31]. Patients undergoing concurrent chemotherapy increase the risk of chronic hemorrhagic cystitis, incontinence, contractions, vesicoureteral reflux, and urothelial malignancies [32]. High dose per fraction have resulted in increased toxicities in some studies [33]. Increase in age is also associated with an increase in genitourinary toxicities after radiotherapy.

8.9 Management

As previously discussed, hematuria is one of the manifestations of radiation cystitis. However, hematuria in a patient who received pelvic radiation may not always be due to radiation cystitis. Any common causes for hematuria, such as urinary tract infection or renal stones should be excluded in the beginning [34]. Sometimes, the reddish discoloration of urine may not be due to blood, but instead, it could be due to certain drugs like phenazopyridine or iron supplements. Therefore, a good history and clinical examination are of utmost importance.

At the same time, a doctor should be vigilant when the hemoglobin drops persistently in a patient who has received pelvic radiation. One of the reasons could be radiation cystitis causing microscopic hematuria. Hence, a high level of suspicion should be there in those patients who received considerable radiation doses to the urinary bladder.

In a patient who presented with profuse bleeding, the initial management should be resuscitation [35]. Blood and colloidal infusions should be given to manage hypovolemic shock. At the same time, continuous or intermittent bladder irrigation should be started. A three-way catheter is used for this purpose. One end of it is used to instill irrigation fluid, the second is the output catheter through which urine and irrigation fluid comes out, and through the third port, the balloon is inflated. This catheter is wide bore enough to manually evacuate blood clots. The bladder irrigation should continue until the urine is clear. Most patients respond to this treatment. However, if the patient does not have severe symptoms and is stable, it is best to proceed with the diagnostic tests given below.

8.10 Diagnostic Tests

Apart from the routine blood work that includes a complete hemogram, kidney function test, and coagulation profile, an ultrasonographic evaluation of the kidneys, ureters, and bladder is essential to rule out other causes of hematuria. In addition, a contrast-enhanced MRI or CT scan may be helpful to know the cancer status or the primary organ. Sometimes, hematuria could be due to the direct invasion of the locally recurrent cancer.

At the same time, the patient may require a cystoscopy evaluation. Cystoscopy could be both diagnostic and therapeutic. The bladder mucosa will look white and frosted with telangiectasias and occasional sharp-edged ulcers on cystoscopy evaluation (Fig. 8.2) [36]. In severe cases, necrosis and fistula formation are seen. Moreover, the radiation oncologist should always correlate the cystoscopy findings to the dosimetric parameters when such cystoscopic findings are observed. Usually, a biopsy from the ulcer is avoided when the cystoscopic findings strongly suggest radiation cystitis. However, in cases where a bladder in invasion or growth is suspected, a biopsy is a must.

Apart from the diagnostic importance of cystoscopy, this procedure can be used to evacuate blood clots. After evacuating the blood clots, the doctor can see the bleeding points that can be fulgurated (discussed later in this chapter).

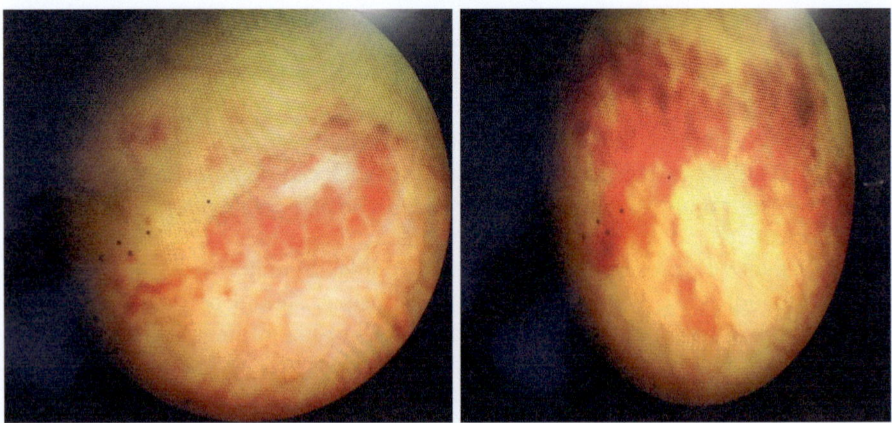

Fig. 8.2 Radiation cystitis

8.11 Treatment of Grade 1 and 2 Radiation Cystitis

Most symptoms of early grade radiation cystitis patients are self-limiting. Mild bleeding can be controlled using oral agents such as tranexamic acid or ethamsylate. An overactive bladder can be tackled using solifenacin or mirabegron [37].

Cranberry juice and extracts have long been used to reduce the severity of radiation-induced cystitis with mixed results. In a randomized double-blinded trial conducted among prostate cancer patients receiving external beam radiotherapy, one arm received cranberry extract capsules, and the other was given a placebo. There was a trend towards reduced acute cystitis in those on the experimental arm (65% vs. 90%, $p = 0.058$) [38]. However, its long-term effects are not reported. On the other hand, Campell et al. and Cowan et al. did similar studies with no difference in outcomes [39, 40].

Conjugated estrogens have been tried with promising results in managing radiation cystitis. It acts by decreasing the fragility of the microvasculature of bladder mucosa. In a small case series done by Lieu et al., 80% of the patients had an excellent response to therapy. Other agents used to treat hemorrhagic cystitis include sodium pentosan polysulphate, corticosteroids, and pentoxifylline tocopherol [41]. All interventions mentioned above constitute a low level of evidence. Hence, the routine use of these agents outside of a clinical trial is not advised.

8.12 Treatment of Grade 3 and 4 Radiation Cystitis

In grade 3 and 4 cystitis, after the initial resuscitation of the patient, a cystoscopic evaluation of blood clots and bladder irrigations is done.

In refractory cases of hemorrhagic cystitis, cystoscopic fulguration is beneficial. Ravi et al. used Yttrium-Aluminum-Garnet (YAG) laser to fulgurate. 93% of the patients responded with just one therapy session, and 97% had a complete response with one or multiple sessions [42]. Other small case series and reports used Argon Plasma Coagulation (APC) during cystoscopy with 100% response with just one application [43].Another option is Potassium Titanyl Phosphate (KTP) laser. Zhu et al. and Talab et al. used KTP with varying results. The advantage of the KTP laser is that it can selectively target the vasculature while sparing the overlying mucosa. This can prevent fibrosis and scarring. However, there is considerable risk vesical perforation, especially while performing multiple laser sessions on a heavily radiated urinary bladder.

8.12.1 Intravesical Therapy

Two intravesical agents, Alum and Formalin, have been tested in several small and large series.

After diluting, formalin, an organic compound (aldehyde), is instilled into the bladder for 15 to 30 min. The procedure must be done under spinal or general anesthesia. The response to formalin therapy is up to 90%. One of the contraindications for formalin therapy is vesicoureteral reflux. However, this procedure causes many irreversible side effects, including bladder contracture, ureteral stricture, and fistula formation. Even death has been reported as a complication of formalin therapy [44].

Another agent, alum (aluminum ammonium or potassium sulfate), is used as intravesical therapy. The advantage is that it does not require anesthesia. However, it is contraindicated in patients with renal failure because alum is absorbed systemically, and it cannot be excreted in patients with renal failure, causing toxicity [45]. The response rates were 78% and 100% in two older series.

Other less commonly used agents in intravesical therapy are sliver nitrate and prostaglandin [46]. Due to the unacceptable toxicities, especially of formalin and alum, these agents are not routinely used in current clinical practice.

Two agents, hyaluronic acid and chondroitin sulfate have been studied to prevent acute and chronic cystitis [47]. These agents are instilled into the bladder during external beam radiotherapy or brachytherapy to avoid acute and chronic cystitis. But, the results of these studies are mixed.

8.12.2 Hyperbaric Oxygen Therapy

In this technique, the patient will be subjected to pure oxygen at 2 to 3 times the atmospheric pressure at sea level (2 to 3 atmos). The biological rationale behind using this therapy is that it allows better oxygen diffusion into tissues, stimulates neovascularization, and promotes fibroblast proliferation [48]. Therefore, it decreases radiation-induced changes in bladder mucosa.

Even though the protocols differ in different centers, the patient usually undergoes daily treatment lasting 60 to 90 min for 6 to 8 weeks [49]. As the patient has to lie or sit in a pressurized cabin, this treatment is unsuitable for claustrophobics. Side effects include barotrauma to the eyes and ears, and retinal vasoconstriction. Nevertheless, these complications are now rare after refining and mastering the technique.

Apart from a randomized trial comparing intravesical therapy with hyaluronic acid and hyperbaric oxygen therapy, which showed comparable results, there are no other significant studies [50]. However, many prospective and retrospective studies consistently showed an excellent response rate of approximately 80% [51]. The response rate is better when there is minimal delay between the onset of bleeding and the start of therapy.

8.12.3 Systemic Therapy

Intravenous injections of recombinant factor VII, 30 microgram/kg daily, for 10 days stopped bleeding in a case of refractory radiation-induced hemorrhagic cystitis [52, 53]. Another agent that has been tried systemically is WF10, with some benefits. However, both these agents are not used in current clinical practice due to the low level of evidence.

8.12.4 Arterial Embolization

This technique comes in handy when other conservative measures fail. This procedure is generally done in the cath lab, where an interventional radiologist sub-selectively targets the branches of the anterior division of the internal iliac artery. Embolization is usually performed using polyvinyl alcohol particles or tris-acryl gelatin microspheres [54].The major complication of this technique is gluteal pain in cases of internal artery embolization. In a case series of 20 patients with intractable hematuria, 3 cases were of radiation-induced hemorrhagic cystitis; arterial embolization showed a 100% response at a median follow-up of 16 months [55].

8.13 Surgery

The surgical option comes as the last resort if all other options fail. Sometimes, internal iliac artery ligation or cystectomy and urinary diversion need to be done to save the patient's life [56]. Another alternative to cystectomy is percutaneous nephrostomy in frail patients. After performing the procedure, the bleeding gradually stopped within a week in one case report.

8.14 Conclusion

Radiotherapy is an integral part of comprehensive cancer management. Most patients with Cancers of the Cervix, Prostate, Rectum and other pelvic malignancies, receive external beam Radiotherapy as a part of their curative treatment. Radiation Cystitis is a predictable outcome, intensity of which depends on the total and fractionated doses of radiotherapy, the volume of normal organs exposed, the radiation technique used, patient related factors like chronic medical conditions, and other associated treatment. With use of conformal and targeted radiation methods, there is a significant reduction in the radiation cystitis incidence with safer delivery of treatment to patients with pelvic malignancies.

References

1. Marks LB, Carroll PR, Dugan TC, Anscher MS. The response of the urinary bladder, urethra, and ureter to radiation and chemotherapy. Int J Radiat Oncol Biol Phys. 1995;31(5):1257–80.
2. Sveistrup J, Rosenschöld PM, Deasy JO, Oh JH, Pommer T, Petersen PM, Engelholm SA. Improvement in toxicity in high risk prostate cancer patients treated with image-guided intensity-modulated radiotherapy compared to 3D conformal radiotherapy without daily image guidance. Radiat Oncol. 2014;9(1):44.
3. Crew JP, Jephcott CR, Reynard JM. Radiation-induced haemorrhagic cystitis. Eur Urol. 2001;40:111–23.
4. Denton AS, Clarke NW, Maher EJ. Non-surgical interventions for late radiation cystitis in patients who have received radical radiotherapy to the pelvis. Cochrane Database Syst Rev. 2002;3:CD001773.
5. Browne C, Davis NF, Mac Craith E, Lennon GM, Mulvin DW, Quinlan DM, Mc Vey GP, Galvin DJ. A narrative review on the pathophysiology and management for radiation cystitis. Adv Urol. 2015;2015:346812. https://doi.org/10.1155/2015/346812.
6. Marks LB, Carroll PR, Dugan TC, Anscher MS. The response of the urinary bladder, urethra, and ureter to radiation and chemotherapy. Int J Radiat Oncol Biol Phys. 1995;31(5):1257–80. https://doi.org/10.1016/0360-3016(94)00431-J.
7. Amdur RJ, Parsons JT, Fitzgerald LT, Million RR. Adenocarcinoma of the prostate treated with external-beam radiation therapy: 5-year minimum follow-up. Radiother Oncol. 1990;18(3):235–46. https://doi.org/10.1016/0167-8140(90)90059-6.
8. Pilepich MV, Krall JM, Sause WT, Johnson RJ, Russ HH, Hanks GE, Perez CA, Zinninger M, Martz KL, Gardner P. Correlation of radiotherapeutic parameters and treatment related morbidity in carcinoma of the prostate—analysis of RTOG study 75-06. Int J Radiat Oncol Biol Phys. 1987;13(3):351–7. https://doi.org/10.1016/0360-3016(87)90008-3.
9. Quilty PM, Duncan W, Kerr GR. Results of a randomised study to evaluate influence of dose on morbidity in radiotherapy for bladder cancer. Clin Radiol. 1985;36(6):615–8. https://doi.org/10.1016/s0009-9260(85)80246-4.
10. Sack H, Nosbuesch H, Stuetzer H. Radiotherapy of prostate carcinoma: results of treatment and complications. Radiother Oncol. 1987;10(1):7–15. https://doi.org/10.1016/s0167-8140(87)80064-6.
11. Shipley WU, Rose MA, Perrone TL, Mannix CM, Heney NM, Prout GR Jr. Full-dose irradiation for patients with invasive bladder carcinoma: clinical and histological factors prognostic of improved survival. J Urol. 1985;134(4):679–83. https://doi.org/10.1016/s0022-5347(17)47381-2.
12. Viswanathan AN, Yorke ED, Marks LB, Eifel PJ, Shipley WU. Radiation dose-volume effects of the urinary bladder. Int J Radiat Oncol Biol Phys. 2010;76(3 Suppl):S116–22. https://doi.org/10.1016/j.ijrobp.2009.02.090.
13. Common Terminology Criteria for Adverse Events (CTCAE) [Internet]. National Cancer Institute, Cancer Therapy Evaluation Program; c2020 [cited 1 July 2020]. Available online: https://ctep.cancer.gov/protocolDevelopment/electronic_applications/ctc.htm#ctc_500.
14. Cox JD, Stetz J, Pajak TF. Toxicity criteria of the Radiation Therapy Oncology Group (RTOG) and the European Organization for Research and Treatment of Cancer (EORTC). Int J Radiat Oncol Biol Phys. 1995;31(5):1341–6. https://doi.org/10.1016/0360-3016(95)00060-C.
15. LENT SOMA scales for all anatomic sites. Int J Radiat Oncol Biol Phys. 1995;31(5):1049–91. https://doi.org/10.1016/0360-3016(95)90159-0.
16. Rödel C, Grabenbauer GG, Kühn R, Papadopoulos T, Dunst J, Meyer M, Schrott KM, Sauer R. Combined-modality treatment and selective organ preservation in invasive bladder cancer: long-term results. J Clin Oncol. 2002;20(14):3061–71. https://doi.org/10.1200/JCO.2002.11.027.
17. Mameghan H, Fisher RJ, Watt WH, Meagher MJ, Rosen IM, Mameghan J, et al. The management of invasive transitional cell carcinoma of the bladder. Results of definitive and preopera-

tive radiation therapy in 390 patients treated at the Prince of Wales Hospital, Sydney, Australia. Cancer. 1992 Jun 1;69(11):2771–8. https://doi.org/10.1002/1097-0142(19920601)69:11<2771::aid-cncr2820691124>3.0.co;2-d.

18. Cowan RA, McBain CA, Ryder WD, Wylie JP, Logue JP, Turner SL, Van der Voet J, Collins CD, Khoo VS, Read GR. Radiotherapy for muscle-invasive carcinoma of the bladder: results of a randomized trial comparing conventional whole bladder with dose-escalated partial bladder radiotherapy. Int J Radiat Oncol Biol Phys. 2004;59(1):197–207. https://doi.org/10.1016/j.ijrobp.2003.10.018.
19. Duncan W, Quilty PM. The results of a series of 963 patients with transitional cell carcinoma of the urinary bladder primarily treated by radical megavoltage X-ray therapy. Radiother Oncol. 1986;7(4):299–310. https://doi.org/10.1016/s0167-8140(86)80059-7.
20. Yavuz AA, Yavuz MN, Ozgur GK, Colak F, Ozyavuz R, Cimsitoglu E, Ilis E. Accelerated superfractionated radiotherapy with concomitant boost for invasive bladder cancer. Int J Radiat Oncol Biol Phys. 2003;56(3):734–45. https://doi.org/10.1016/s0360-3016(03)00111-1.
21. Efstathiou JA, Bae K, Shipley WU, Kaufman DS, Hagan MP, Heney NM, Sandler HM. Late pelvic toxicity after bladder-sparing therapy in patients with invasive bladder cancer: RTOG 89-03, 95-06, 97-06, 99-06. J Clin Oncol. 2009;27(25):4055–61. https://doi.org/10.1200/JCO.2008.19.5776. Epub 2009 Jul 27
22. Al-Mamgani A, van Putten WL, Heemsbergen WD, van Leenders GJ, Slot A, Dielwart MF, Incrocci L, et al. Update of Dutch multicenter dose-escalation trial of radiotherapy for localized prostate cancer. Int J Radiat Oncol Biol Phys. 2008;72(4):980–8. https://doi.org/10.1016/j.ijrobp.2008.02.073. Epub 2008 May 19
23. Dearnaley D, Syndikus I, Mossop H, Khoo V, Birtle A, Bloomfield D, et al. Conventional versus hypofractionated high-dose intensity-modulated radiotherapy for prostate cancer: 5-year outcomes of the randomised, non-inferiority, phase 3 CHHiP trial. Lancet Oncol. 2016;17(8):1047–60. https://doi.org/10.1016/S1470-2045(16)30102-4. Epub 2016 Jun 20. Erratum in: Lancet Oncol. 2016;17(8):e321
24. Logsdon MD, Eifel PJ. Figo IIIB squamous cell carcinoma of the cervix: an analysis of prognostic factors emphasizing the balance between external beam and intracavitary radiation therapy. Int J Radiat Oncol Biol Phys. 1999;43(4):763–75. https://doi.org/10.1016/s0360-3016(98)00482-9.
25. Pötter R, Haie-Meder C, Van Limbergen E, Barillot I, De Brabandere M, Dimopoulos J, et al. GEC ESTRO Working Group. Recommendations from gynaecological (GYN) GEC ESTRO working group (II): concepts and terms in 3D image-based treatment planning in cervix cancer brachytherapy-3D dose volume parameters and aspects of 3D image-based anatomy, radiation physics, radiobiology. Radiother Oncol. 2006;78(1):67–77. https://doi.org/10.1016/j.radonc.2005.11.014. Epub 2006 Jan 5
26. Georg P, Lang S, Dimopoulos JC, Dörr W, Sturdza AE, Berger D, et al. Dose-volume histogram parameters and late side effects in magnetic resonance image-guided adaptive cervical cancer brachytherapy. Int J Radiat Oncol Biol Phys. 2011;79(2):356–62. https://doi.org/10.1016/j.ijrobp.2009.11.002. Epub 2010 Apr 10
27. Kirisits C, Pötter R, Lang S, Dimopoulos J, Wachter-Gerstner N, Georg D. Dose and volume parameters for MRI-based treatment planning in intracavitary brachytherapy for cervical cancer. Int J Radiat Oncol Biol Phys. 2005;62(3):901–11. https://doi.org/10.1016/j.ijrobp.2005.02.040.
28. Pötter R, Tanderup K, Schmid MP, Jürgenliemk-Schulz I, Haie-Meder C, Fokdal LU, et al. EMBRACE Collaborative Group. MRI-guided adaptive brachytherapy in locally advanced cervical cancer (EMBRACE-I): a multicentre prospective cohort study. Lancet Oncol. 2021;22(4):538–47. https://doi.org/10.1016/S1470-2045(20)30753-1.
29. Lee WR, Dignam JJ, Amin MB, Bruner DW, Low D, Swanson GP, et al. Randomized phase III noninferiority study comparing two radiotherapy fractionation schedules in patients with low-risk prostate cancer. J Clin Oncol. 2016;34(20):2325–32. https://doi.org/10.1200/JCO.2016.67.0448. Epub 2016 Apr 4

30. Chen GD, Lin LY, Wang PH, Lee HS. Urinary tract dysfunction after radical hysterectomy for cervical cancer. Gynecol Oncol. 2002;85(2):292–7. https://doi.org/10.1006/gyno.2002.6614.
31. Green N, Treible D, Wallack H. Prostate cancer: post-irradiation incontinence. J Urol. 1990 Aug;144(2 Pt 1):307–9. https://doi.org/10.1016/s0022-5347(17)39438-7.
32. Levine LA, Richie JP. Urological complications of cyclophosphamide. J Urol. 1989;141(5):1063–9. https://doi.org/10.1016/s0022-5347(17)41173-6.
33. Lindholt J, Hansen PT. Prostatic carcinoma: complications of megavoltage radiation therapy. Br J Urol. 1986;58(1):52–4. https://doi.org/10.1111/j.1464-410x.1986.tb05427.x.
34. Mallick S, Madan R, Julka PK, Rath GK. Radiation induced cystitis and proctitis—prediction, assessment and management. Asian Pac J Cancer Prev. 2015;16(14):5589–94.
35. Smit SG, Heyns CF. Management of radiation cystitis. Nat Rev Urol. 2010;7(4):206–14.
36. Liem X, Saad F, Delouya G. A practical approach to the management of radiation-induced hemorrhagic cystitis. Drugs. 2015;75(13):1471–82.
37. Jaszczyński J, Kojs Z, Stelmach A, Wohadło Ł, Łuczyńska E, Heinze S, et al. Post-irradiation bladder syndrome after radiotherapy of malignant neoplasm of small pelvis organs: an observational, non-interventional clinical study assessing VESIcare®/solifenacin treatment results. Med Sci Monit. 2016;22:2691–8.
38. Hamilton K, Bennett NC, Purdie G, Herst PM. Standardized cranberry capsules for radiation cystitis in prostate cancer patients in New Zealand: a randomized double blinded, placebo controlled pilot study. Support Care Cancer. 2015;23(1):95–102.
39. Campbell G, Pickles T, D'Yachkova Y. A randomised trial of cranberry versus apple juice in the management of urinary symptoms during external beam radiation therapy for prostate cancer. Clin Oncol (R Coll Radiol). 2003;15(6):322–8.
40. Cowan CC, Hutchison C, Cole T, Barry SJ, Paul J, Reed NS, et al. A randomised double-blind placebo-controlled trial to determine the effect of cranberry juice on decreasing the incidence of urinary symptoms and urinary tract infections in patients undergoing radiotherapy for cancer of the bladder or cervix. Clin Oncol (R Coll Radiol). 2012;24(2):e31–8.
41. Delanian S, Chatel C, Porcher R, Depondt J, Lefaix JL. Complete restoration of refractory mandibular osteoradionecrosis by prolonged treatment with a pentoxifylline-tocopherol-clodronate combination (PENTOCLO): a phase II trial. Int J Radiat Oncol Biol Phys. 2011;80(3):832–9.
42. Ravi R. Endoscopic neodymium: YAG laser treatment of radiation-induced hemorrhagic cystitis. Lasers Surg Med. 1994;14(1):83–7.
43. Suzuki S, Chino A, Fukui I, Hayashi T, Kozuka T, Suganuma T, et al. Successful use of endoscopic argon plasma coagulation for hemorrhagic radiation cystitis: a case report. Jpn J Clin Oncol. 2014;44(7):692–5.
44. Dewan AK, Mohan GM, Ravi R. Intravesical formalin for hemorrhagic cystitis following irradiation of cancer of the cervix. Int J Gynaecol Obstet. 1993;42(2):131–5.
45. Seear MD, Dimmick JE, Rogers PC. Acute aluminum toxicity after continuous intravesical alum irrigation for hemorrhagic cystitis. Urology. 1990;36(4):353–4.
46. Rigaud J, Hetet JF, Bouchot O. Management of radiation cystitis. Prog Urol. 2004;14(4):568–72.
47. Hazewinkel MH, Stalpers LJ, Dijkgraaf MG, Roovers JP. Prophylactic vesical instillations with 0.2% chondroitin sulfate may reduce symptoms of acute radiation cystitis in patients undergoing radiotherapy for gynecological malignancies. Int Urogynecol J. 2011;22(6):725–30.
48. Pasquier D, Hoelscher T, Schmutz J, Dische S, Mathieu D, Baumann M, et al. Hyperbaric oxygen therapy in the treatment of radio-induced lesions in normal tissues: a literature review. Radiother Oncol. 2004;72(1):1–13.
49. Corman JM, McClure D, Pritchett R, Kozlowski P, Hampson NB. Treatment of radiation induced hemorrhagic cystitis with hyperbaric oxygen. J Urol. 2003;169(6):2200–2.
50. Shao Y, Lu GL, Shen ZJ. Comparison of intravesical hyaluronic acid instillation and hyperbaric oxygen in the treatment of radiation-induced hemorrhagic cystitis. BJU Int. 2012;109(5):691–4.
51. Oscarsson N, Arnell P, Lodding P, Ricksten SE, Seeman-Lodding H. Hyperbaric oxygen treatment in radiation-induced cystitis and proctitis: a prospective cohort study on patient-perceived quality of recovery. Int J Radiat Oncol Biol Phys. 2013;87(4):670–5.

52. Connolly SS, D'Arcy FT, Corcoran MO. Recombinant activated factor VII to control life-threatening haemorrhagic radiation cystitis. Ir J Med Sci. 2010;179(3):431–3.
53. Geisler JP, Linnemeier GC, Manahan KJ. Recombinant factor VIIa to treat late radiation-induced hemorrhagic cystitis: a case report. J Reprod Med. 2008;53(5):360–2.
54. Loffroy R, Pottecher P, Cherblanc V, Favelier S, Estivalet L, Koutlidis N, et al. Rôle actuel de l'embolisation artérielle transcathéter dans le traitement des hémorragies vésicales et prostatiques. J Radiol Diagn Inter. 2014;95:1017–24.
55. Delgal A, Cercueil JP, Koutlidis N, Michel F, Kermarrec I, Mourey E, et al. Outcome of transcatheter arterial embolization for bladder and prostate hemorrhage. J Urol. 2010;183(5):1947–53.
56. Takeuchi T, Zaitsu M, Mikami K, Takeshima Y, Matsunaga T, Okamoto N, et al. A case of severe hemorrhagic cystitis caused by melphalan with successful bladder preservation by ligation of bilateral internal iliac arteries. Case Rep Med. 2010;2010:569138.

Pelvic Insufficiency Syndrome After Pelvic Radiation Encountered After Treatment of Gynaecological Malignancies

9

Sapna Nangia and Robin Khosa

9.1 Introduction

Radiation for gynecological cancers may result in insufficiency fractures of the sacrum and pelvic bones. These are most likely to occur in the background of osteoporosis and result from bone atrophy, secondary to radiation induced vascular injury. The latter results in absorption of lamellar bone and replacement by immaturely formed bone [1]. Occurring in a significant number of patients undergoing pelvic radiation, an average 14% [2], a high index of suspicion is advisable. A number of series have noted larger numbers. Femoral neck lesions may occur in 1.5% of patients undergoing radiation for cervical cancer [3].

Patients often present with complaints of low backache and symptoms may be mistaken for recurrent or metastatic lesions, intervertebral disc or osteoporosis related issues. Femoral head / neck lesions present as pain in the groin. As many as 40% patients suffering from pelvic insufficiency fractures (PIFs) may be asymptomatic, with bone lesions being identified only on routine imaging studies [2].

9.2 Causation

The most common site for pelvic insufficiency is the sacro-iliac joints followed by the sacrum, together accounting for nearly three quarters of all fractures. Fractures of the sacral ala may progress to involve sacral foramina [4]. The median number of sacral fractures has been noted to be 2 [4]. Other bony sites that may have insufficiency related injury include the pubis, lumbar vertebrae, iliac blade, acetabulum

S. Nangia (✉)
Apollo Proton Cancer Centre, Chennai, India

R. Khosa
Indraprastha Apollo Hospital, New Delhi, India

K. Sood Sharma et al. (eds.), *Complications of Cancer Therapy: Best Practices in Prevention and Management*, https://doi.org/10.1007/978-981-99-0984-1_9

and femoral heads. These sites correspond to weight bearing regions. Lesions that present as a single site fracture may progress to multiple sites in more than a quarter of patients [5].

In a systematic review comprising 21 studies and 3929 patients, Sapienza et al. noted that pelvic insufficiency occurred 7–19 months after radiotherapy [2]. The factors associated with a higher risk of this complication were noted to be older age, post menopausal status, osteoporosis, low body weight/body mass index and definitive treatment. The cut-off for weight has variously been defined as 49 kg and 55 kg. In addition, a higher radiotherapy dose, 50.4 Gy was noted to be significantly associated with the risk of PIF by Oh et al. [5]. Contradictory findings have been noted regarding the association of PIF with concurrent chemotherapy [5, 6]. Higher risk has been noted at age >50 years and also >70 years. Smoking, rheumatoid arthritis and multiparity have been noted to be additional risk factors [7].

9.3 Correlation with Radiation Technique and Dose

The risk of pelvic insufficiency fractures is the least with IMRT and the most with AP-PA pelvic radiation [2]. No differences have been observed between IMRT and 3DCRT by Vitzthum et al., hazard ratio 0.90; 95% (CI, 0.74–1.11) in patients with gynecological cancer [8]. The authors studied a cohort comprising 28,354 patients of the Surveillance, Epidemiology and End Results (SEER) data base, aged 65 patients or more, treated for gynecological, gastrointestinal and prostate cancers. They noted different pattern in prostate cancers i.e., patients undergoing IMRT had a smaller risk of fractures compared to 3DCRT. In addition they also noted that brachytherapy was associated with the least risk of PIF.

Ramlov et al. studied the dosimetric correlates associated with pelvic insufficiency fractures in 101 patients treated for locally advanced cervical cancer. The authors performed a detailed analysis of the correlation of D50% for sacrum and pelvic bones as well correlation of and noted that sacrum D50% during EBRT was significantly related to the risk of symptomatic PIF in women aged >50 years. The predicted risk of fractures in women aged >50 years was 22% at sacrum D50% of 35 Gy and 35% at 40 Gy. This has helped formulate dose constraints for the sacrum. The location of PIFs had no correlation with sites of high dose arising due to SIB to pelvic nodes [9].

Mir et al. [4] have postulated a nomogram for identifying the risk of sacral insufficiency fractures and based on age and V40Gy3. The entire sacrum, including sacral foramina surrounded by bone and excluding the coccyx was used for the dosimetric analysis. In this analysis too, there was no correlation with high dose regions arising from SIB to pelvic nodes.

The impact of constraints for the bone marrow on risk of PIFs will require prospective evaluation, but is likely to reduce the dose received by the iliac blade.

In an analysis of patients undergoing radiotherapy for anal cancer, a dose response relationship has been noted with cortical bone thinning in the femoral neck, a 2 cm^3 volume of the femoral neck receiving ≥40 Gy corresponding with 20% cortical thinning of the bone [10].

9.4 Evaluation

Plain X Rays: Lesions of the femoral head may present as destruction and subluxation of the femoral heads. Sclerosis of the acetabulum may be noted. Fractures lines and sclerosis may be recognised. However, X rays have poor sensitivity for PIFs.

Tc99m MDP scans: The most common finding is symmetric increased activity resulting in a typical H pattern in the sacrum, arising from injury in the SI joints and sacrum. Though multifocal abnormalities are typical, unilateral abnormalities may also occur. Scintigraphy abnormalities may also be noted in other bones i.e. pubis, iliac blades, femoral heads and the acetabulum [11].

9.4.1 CT Scan

Demonstration of fracture lines is best possible on CT scan imaging. Fracture lines in the sacrum are often vertical and bilateral, though horizontal fractures may also occur. Fractures may also be demonstrated in the ilium and pubis and may be associated with endosteal callus formation [12]. Sclerotic linear changes/diffuse osteolytic changes may be noted instead of fracture lines, Fig. 9.1a, b [13].

On magnetic resonance (MR) imaging the typical findings are diffuse low signal intensity on T 1 weighted imaging and diffuse high signal intensity on STIR images. Findings on MR imaging are often more widespread than on X ray imaging, demonstrate marrow edema and radiation osteitis and may often be accompanied by high signal intensity of adjacent muscles such as the piriformis, glutei, internal obdurator and iliac muscles on STIR images [12]. A coronal image improves identification of fractures and FS-T2w images have been considered the best for identification of marrow oedema and exclusion of metastases Fig. 9.2 [14].

9.4.2 FDG PET CT

Variable FDG uptake may be noted in PIF, due to underlying inflammation. In most patients mild and diffuse intake is noted, though intense and heterogenous uptake may be noted in some, the latter mimicking bone metastases. The uptake may persist even 6 months after diagnosis and may even be note to increase due to aggravation of the lesion due to weight bearing [15].

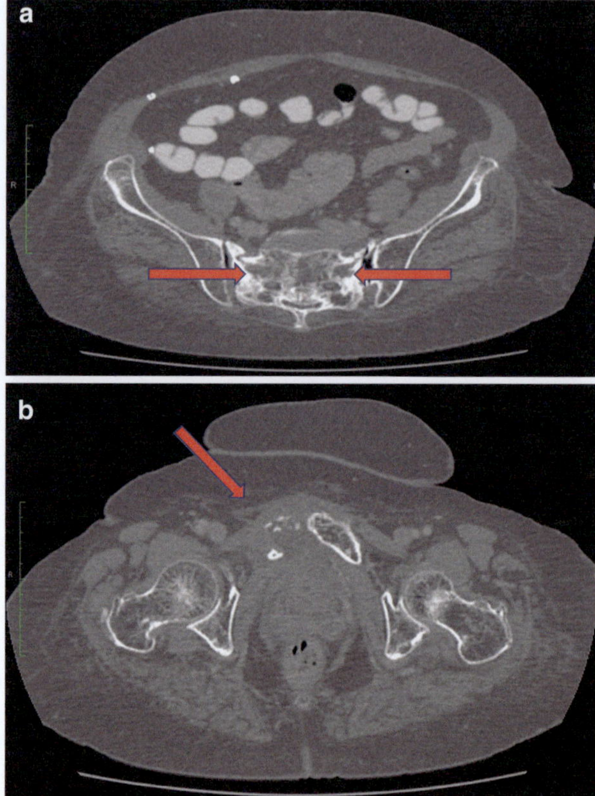

Fig. 9.1 (**a**) Pelvic CT scan, 1 year after radiation, showing osteolytic lesions in bilateral ala of sacrum suggestive of sacral insufficiency fracture. (**b**) Contrast enhanced CT scan images showing osteolysis of the right inferior pubic ramus with cortical thinning and irregularity with areas of lysis seen in the left inferior pubic ramus

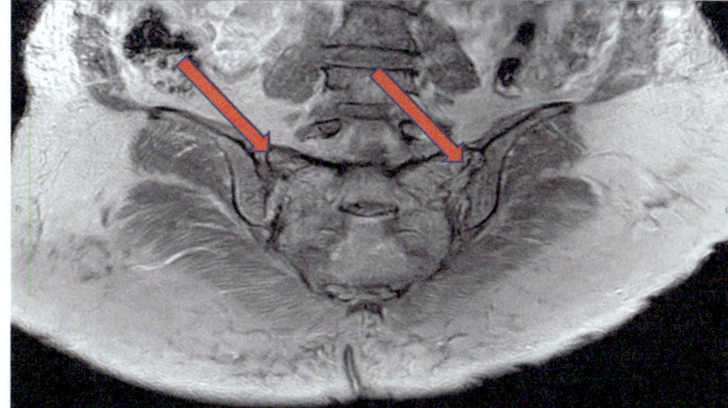

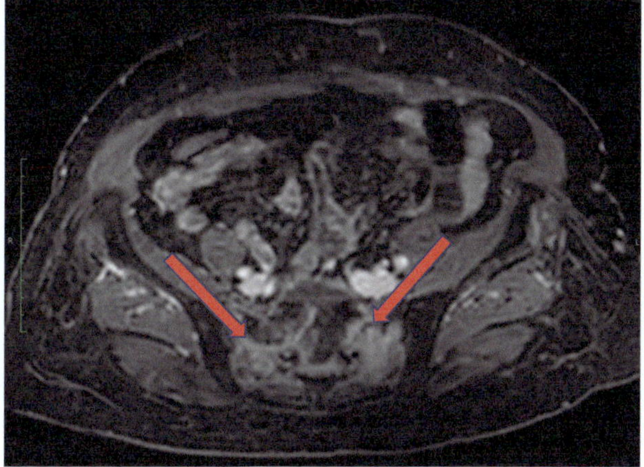

Fig. 9.2 Coronal and axial images of Magnetic resonance imaging showing diffuse altered signal intensity of the sacrum seen as heterogeneous signal on T1/T2W images with diffuse T2 fat sat hyperintensity representing edema. There are linear hyperintenses line seen through the bilateral ala of sacrum representing insufficiency fractures. Patchy enhancement is seen in the entire extent of the sacrum. The fracture line is also seen extending through the body of sacrum on the right side

9.5 Management

Deterioration in the bone health was noted almost universally in 132 eligible patients analysed from the 300 enrolled in the PARCER study [16]. Recognition of the problem of insufficiency and its high frequency is therefore important.

9.5.1 Prevention

Due attention to prescribing dose constraints to the sacrum and femoral heads during the radiation planning process is critical. In the authors' experience (unpublished), the D50% of the sacrum could be reduced from 44.8 Gy to 38.2 Gy in successive cohorts of patients treated without a dose constraint for the sacrum and following delineation of the sacrum and a constraint to decrease D50% sacrum to ≤35 Gy, respectively.

The dose prescription should also incorporate a constraint for the femoral head and neck aiming to achieve not >40 Gy to 2 cm^3 of femoral head and neck.

Pharmacologic preventive measures such as calcium and Vit D supplementation should be routinely prescribed to all post menopausal women undergoing pelvic radiotherapy.

9.5.2 Treatment of Established Pelvic Insufficiency Fractures

Patients present with low backache and occasionally pedal edema and conservative management with rest and NSAIDs is the preferred mode of treatment; some patients may require narcotic analgesics. Symptoms are more likely in patients with multiple sites of involvement [5]. Pain killers may be required for durations varying from 1 to 29 months, median 3 months.

Bone directed treatments such as calcium supplements and Vitamin D supplements are prescribed, though there is no study on their efficacy. Similarly hormone replacement therapy may be considered but has not been studied in this context. Though bisphosphonates have been used, there is concern regarding the impact of their anti angiogenic property on bone healing; further studies are advisable for their use in this indication [7].

Surgical treatment measures may include vertebroplasty and joint replacement.

Patients with lesions involving the femoral head present with pain in the groin and may be treated, as per severity by various methods that include non surgical measures like crutches and rest or surgical measures like internal fixation, with or without bone grafting, arthroplasty, insertion of prosthesis or total hip replacement [3].

9.6 Images

Figs. 9.1 and 9.2.

9.7 Conclusion

Bone changes in pelvic bones are wide spread after pelvic radiation and may lead to fractures in weight bearing bones. This significantly increases post treatment morbidity and also mortality. Prescription of a constraint for the sacrum femoral head and neck, helps to decrease the risk of this complication, Attention to bone health by calcium supplementation and Vitamin D supplementation of women undergoing pelvic radiation is advisable.

Ten Key Points

1. Pelvic insufficiency is widespread after pelvic radiation for gynaecological cancer. Nearly 40% patients are asymptomatic.

2. Pelvic insufficiency fractures occur mostly in postmenopausal women and are related to osteoporosis, low body weight and radiation dose received by the sacrum and femoral head and neck.
3. The most common site is the sacrum, followed by other weight bearing bones.
4. Patients present with low backache and occasionally pedal edema.
5. An X ray pelvis may miss pelvic insufficiency fractures.
6. An H sign is typically noted in the sacrum on radio nuclear bone scan. CT scans help identify the fracture line as well as sclerosis. MRI has the highest sensitivity and helps to identify radiation osteitis better as well distinguishes from metastatic lesions.
7. An important dose volume parameter is the Sacral D50% during EBRT. D50% 35 Gy reduces the fractures risk significantly compared to D50% 40 Gy, in post menopausal women.
8. An addition dose parameter is the femoral neck volume receiving 40 Gy, a volume higher than 2 cm^3 increasing the risk of bone loss.
9. Preventive strategies are calcium and vitamin D supplementation and dose constraints for the sacrum and femoral head, along with bone marrow constraints.
10. Treatment strategies include rest, NSAIDs, supports such as crutches and walkers and occasionally vertebroplasty and hip prosthesis and replacement.

References

1. Rafii M, Firooznia H, Golimbu C, Horner N. Radiation induced fractures of sacrum: CT diagnosis. J Comput Assist Tomogr. 1988;12(2):231–5.
2. Sapienza LG, Salcedo MP, Ning MS, Jhingran A, Klopp AH, Calsavara VF, et al. Pelvic insufficiency fractures after external beam radiation therapy for gynecologic cancers: a meta-analysis and meta-regression of 3929 patients. Int J Radiat Oncol Biol Phys. 2020;106(3):475–84.
3. Leabhart JW, Bonfiglio M. The treatment of irradiation fracture of the femoral neck. J Bone Jt Surg. 1961;43(7):1056
4. Mir R, Dragan AD, Mistry HB, Tsang YM, Padhani AR, Hoskin P. Sacral insufficiency fracture following pelvic radiotherapy in gynaecological malignancies: development of a predictive model. Clin Oncol (R Coll Radiol). 2021;33(3):e101–9.
5. Oh D, Huh SJ, Nam H, Park W, Han Y, Lim DH, et al. Pelvic insufficiency fracture after pelvic radiotherapy for cervical cancer: analysis of risk factors. Int J Radiat Oncol Biol Phys. 2008;70(4):1183–8.
6. Gondi V, Bentzen SM, Sklenar KL, Dunn EF, Petereit DG, Tannehill SP, et al. Severe late toxicities following concomitant chemoradiotherapy compared to radiotherapy alone in cervical cancer: an inter-era analysis. Int J Radiat Oncol Biol Phys. 2012;84(4):973–82.
7. Razavian N, Laucis A, Sun Y, Spratt DE, Owen D, Schonewolf C, et al. Radiation-induced insufficiency fractures after pelvic irradiation for gynecologic malignancies: a systematic review. Int J Radiat Oncol Biol Phys. 2020;108(3):620–34.
8. Vitzthum LK, Park H, Zakeri K, Heide ES, Nalawade V, Mundt AJ, et al. Risk of pelvic fracture with radiation therapy in older patients. Int J Radiat Oncol Biol Phys. 2020;106(3):485–92. https://doi.org/10.1016/j.ijrobp.2019.10.006.
9. Ramlov A, Pedersen EM, Røhl L, Worm E, Fokdal L, Lindegaard JC, et al. Risk factors for pelvic insufficiency fractures in locally advanced cervical cancer following intensity modulated radiation therapy. Int J Radiat Oncol Biol Phys. 2017;97(5):1032–9.

10. Okoukoni C, Randolph DM, McTyre ER, Kwok A, Weaver AA, Blackstock AW, et al. Early dose-dependent cortical thinning of the femoral neck in anal cancer patients treated with pelvic radiation therapy. Bone. 2017;94:84–9.
11. Abe H, Nakamura M, Takahashi S, Maruoka S, Ogawa Y, Sakamoto K. Radiation-induced insufficiency fractures of the pelvis: evaluation with 99mTc-methylene diphosphonate scintigraphy. AJR Am J Roentgenol. 1992;158(3):599–602.
12. Blomlie V, Rofstad EK, Talle K, Sundfør K, Winderen M, Lien HH. Incidence of radiation-induced insufficiency fractures of the female pelvis: evaluation with MR imaging. AJR Am J Roentgenol. 1996;167(5):1205–10.
13. Tokumaru S, Toita T, Oguchi M, Ohno T, Kato S, Niibe Y, et al. Insufficiency fractures after pelvic radiation therapy for uterine cervical cancer: an analysis of subjects in a prospective multi-institutional trial, and cooperative study of the Japan Radiation Oncology Group (JAROG) and Japanese Radiation Oncology Study Group (JROSG). Int J Radiat Oncol Biol Phys. 2012;84(2):e195–200.
14. Zhong X, Zhang L, Dong T, Mai H, Lu B, Huang L, et al. Clinical and MRI features of sacral insufficiency fractures after radiotherapy in patients with cervical cancer. BMC Womens Health. 2022;22(1):166. https://doi.org/10.1186/s12905-022-01758-2.
15. Oh D, Huh SJ, Lee SJ, Kwon JW. Variation in FDG uptake on PET in patients with radiation-induced pelvic insufficiency fractures: a review of 10 cases. Ann Nucl Med. 2009;23(6):511–6.
16. Chopade P, Chopra S, Jain J, Panda S, Patil A, Patil G, et al. Serial bone density changes in women undergoing pelvic (chemo) radiation: results from PARCER trial. Int J Radiat Oncol Biol Phys. 2022;114(3):463–71.

Radiation Induced Xerostomia in Patient Receiving Radical Radiation Therapy to the Face and Neck

10

Shyam Singh Bisht and Soumya Sarkar

Xerostomia is defined as dryness of mouth due to diminished function of salivary glands. It is one of the major complications of radiation therapy in head and neck cancers. The DAHANCA 6 and 7 trial reported acute and late severe xerostomia in 15% and 18% patients respectively receiving five weekly fractions of radiation therapy up to a total dose of 66–68 Gy [1]. Xerostomia also leads to long term side effects on oral health, taste, dental hygiene, voice quality and nutritional status of the patients.

10.1 The Salivary Apparatus

The parotid and the submandibular glands are the main salivary glands contributing to 80% of salivary flow, whereas the remaining is contributed by minor salivary glands present in oral cavity and pharynx [2]. Parotid gland secretions are serous and watery, whereas submandibular gland secretion contains mucins. Submandibular glands are responsible for saliva secretion in the unstimulated state and it contributes to the subjective sensation of moisture in the mouth [3]. The salivary gland hypofunction is due to the damage of salivary acinar cells resulting in change of the composition, volume and quality of the saliva produced. Despite having a slow turnover rate, the production and quality of saliva changes after radiation therapy over a period of time.

S. S. Bisht (✉) · S. Sarkar
Medanta Cancer Institute, Gurugram, Haryana, India

K. Sood Sharma et al. (eds.), *Complications of Cancer Therapy: Best Practices in Prevention and Management*, https://doi.org/10.1007/978-981-99-0984-1_10

10.2 Effect of Radiation Therapy on Salivary Function

Radiotherapy induced xerostomia has been strongly related to the radiation dose, fraction size, volume of irradiated tissue, fractionation schedule and type of ionizing radiation.

10.2.1 Dose Volume Relationship

A radiation dose of >52 Gy to the salivary glands leads to severe damage to the glands [4]. Head and neck cancer patients routinely receives a total dose of 60–70 Gy, thus predisposing the patients to chronic xerostomia. Study by Zhong-He Wang et al. [5] reported that there was shrinkage of salivary glands after radiotherapy, where the magnitude of volume reductions was associated with total mean dose delivered. Volume loss at mean doses >30 Gy to the glands was significantly more than at low doses. The average rate of volume loss of the glands has been observed to be higher in the first 3 weeks of radiotherapy compared to last 3 weeks of radiotherapy. Rapid decline in saliva outflow is seen in the first week of radiation and by the completion of radiation therapy saliva secretion virtually ceases. However, compensatory hypersecretion of the unirradiated salivary gland is seen after few months which lessens the degree of xerostomia to some extent but rarely compensates fully. It has also been shown that minimal gland function reduction occurs at <10 to 15 Gy mean dose. Gland function reduction gradually increases at radiation doses of 20 to 40 Gy, with a strong reduction of >75% at >40 Gy mean dose. Stimulated parotid salivary glands dose-volume models strongly corelated with both stimulated salivary function and quality-of life post radiation therapy [6]. It has been reported that post radiation stimulated salivary outflow decreases exponentially for each parotid gland at a rate of 4% per Gray of mean parotid dose [7].

10.2.2 Fractionation

The effects of fractionation size on xerostomia are conflicting. Continuous hyper fractionated accelerated radiotherapy (CHART) data showed that hypofractionation is protective for late effects [8]. But study in animal models showed reduction in acini cell number at 16 weeks after radiation therapy to be worse for CHART hyperfractionation than for conventional fractionation [9]. Thus, the effect of fractionation on xerostomia is still ambiguous.

10.2.3 Radiation Techniques

The parotid glands lie within the radiation portals of most of the head and neck malignancies. With conventional radiotherapy (CRT) techniques, often it becomes difficult to spare the parotid glands from receiving higher doses. With the advent of intensity modulated radiotherapy (IMRT), parotid sparing radiotherapy could be achieved to a greater extent. Pow et al. studied the effect of IMRT vs. CRT on salivary outflow and quality of life in patients with nasopharyngeal carcinoma patients. They showed that at 1 year post radiation therapy 83.3% patients the IMRT arm had recovered 25% of their pre-radiation stimulated parotid saliva flow compared to 9.3% in the CRT arm. Xerostomia related symptoms were significantly less common in the IMRT at 1 year post-radiotherapy [10]. In another trial by Kam et al., 60 patients with nasopharyngeal carcinoma received either conventional two-dimensional radiation therapy (2DRT) or IMRT. At 1 year post treatment, patients treated with IMRT had lower incidence of observer-rated severe xerostomia than patients with 2DRT (39.3% vs. 82.1%; $p = 0.01$). However, there was no significant difference between the two groups in patient reported outcome [11]. In the landmark PARSPORT trial, the incidence of xerostomia at 1 year was 74% vs. 39% in the conventional vs. the IMRT arms. At 1–2 years, significant recovery was seen in saliva secretion with IMRT compared to conventional radiotherapy, along with clinically significant improvements in dry-mouth-specific and global quality of life scores. At 2 years post treatment, grade 2 or worse xerostomia was 83% vs. 29% in conventional arm vs. IMRT arm respectively ($p < 0.0001$). There was no compromise in the locoregional control or overall survival [12]. This study taught the natural history of radiation induced xerostomia and established the role of IMRT in head and neck malignancies.

The pathogenesis of xerostomia also involves damage to the submandibular glands. Sparing of single submandibular gland by surgical transfer to the submental space before radiotherapy can prevent xerostomia. Submandibular glandulopexy in a trial has been reported as leading to significant reduction in xerostomia post radiation therapy [13]. But this method of submandibular gland sparing has its limitation as it cannot be used for all oral cavity and oropharyngeal tumors. It involves the risk of an operative procedure which might delay radiation therapy due to wound healing problems. Hence, this method was not widely applied. The effect of submandibular gland sparing by IMRT in prevention of xerostomia was studied by Saarilhati et al. In a subset of head and neck cancer patients receiving parotid sparing IMRT, the contralateral submandibular gland with low risk of recurrence was spared (mean dose <25 Gy). Patients with submandibular gland sparing IMRT had less grade two or grade three xerostomia and required less saliva substitutes in future. None of these patients had local recurrence in the vicinity of the spared glands during follow up. Although evidence regarding submandibular gland sparing radiotherapy is adding up, the safety and efficacy of submandibular gland sparing is extremely limited. Moreover, meaningful reduction of mean dose to submandibular gland has an increased risk of underdosing of level II lymph nodes which may compromise regional tumor control. At present, submandibular gland sparing radiotherapy should only be undertaken under a clinical trial setting.

The minor salivary glands, dispersed throughout the oral cavity are also an important source of mucins. The mean radiation dose to oral cavity in some studies has shown to be an independent predictor of xerostomia, although there are conflicting data.

Radiation also changes the chemical composition of the saliva. There is increase in sodium concentration in saliva post radiation. Saliva becomes highly viscous and pH changes towards acidity [14]. The concentrations of immunoproteins likely secretory immunoglobin A, lysozyme etc. are reported to increase, but with decreased salivary outflow it leads to a significant immunoprotein deficit. All these radiation induced changes leads to altered oral flora growth with more acidogenic and carcinogenic microorganisms than non-carcinogenic microorganisms.

10.3 Endpoints and Toxicity Scoring

Xerostomia can be defined subjectively according to the patient's symptoms. Objective criteria include measured salivary production at rest or stimulation and imaging endpoints. Salivary function is quantifiable. Grade 4 xerostomia is defined by the Late Effects Normal Tissue-Subjective, Objective, Management, Analytic (LENT-SOMA) scale as an objective reduction of >75% of baseline salivary function. Whole mouth salivary function is typically assessed by asking the subject to produce as much saliva as possible within a given period. This can be performed in an unstimulated (at rest) or stimulated manner (in response to a salivary stimulant). However, salivary function measurements are uncertain and variable, with standard deviations of 20–30%. Observer-based can be Common Terminology Criteria for Adverse Events, include the requirement for frequent drinks of water or diet alterations. Imaging endpoints include. Scintigraphy of parotid gland ejection fraction over a timed interval and dynamic magnetic resonance imaging sialography of ductal flow. To best define xerostomia, QUANTEC recommend that an observer-based system (e.g., the Common Terminology Criteria for Adverse Events) be supplemented by a validated QOL measurement device (e.g., the XQ (xerostomia questionnaire) or salivary measurements (e.g., whole mouth-stimulated measurements).

10.4 Management of Xerostomia

10.4.1 Radiation Therapy Planning

Parotid and submandibular salivary glands can be adequately delineated on contrast-enhanced computed tomography images. However, irradiated parotid glands typically shrink during radiation therapy, due to cell loss. On the basis of weekly computed tomography scans of 15 patients, studies have reported little change in the medial parotid gland position during radiation therapy and shrinking of the lateral edges on average, 1 mm/week during RT. Significant improvement in xerostomia rates has been established in a number of studies by using parotid sparing radiation therapy techniques. Sparing at least one parotid gland appears to eliminate xerostomia, and sparing at least one submandibular gland also appears to reduce xerostomia risk and increase stimulated and unstimulated salivary function. Blanco et al. demonstrated that sparing at least one parotid gland with mean dose <20 Gy minimized the incidence of grade 4 xerostomia. Limiting both parotids to a mean dose of <25 Gy resulted in minimal grade 4 xerostomia [5]. Deasy et al. supported similar dose constraints for parotid sparing radiotherapy along with submandibular gland sparing to modest mean doses of <35 Gy whenever oncologically safe [15].

10.5 Prevention of Radiation Induced Xerostomia

Amifostine has been used prophylactically as a radioprotector in patients with head and neck cancer. Amifostine and its active metabolite, WR-1065 is preferentially taken up by tissues such as salivary glands due to increased levels of alkaline phosphatase in normal tissues compared tumor cells. Inside the cells it prevents damage by acting as a free radical scavenger. The benefits of this drug were established in phase 3 randomised trial by Brizel et al. Patients with head and neck carcinoma were treated with Amifostine 200 mg/m^2 daily 15 to 30 min before radiation therapy. Patients received radiation once daily (1.8–2 Gy) to total doses of 50–70 Gy. Median saliva production was greater with Amifostine and had significant reduction of grade 2 acute and chronic xerostomia [16]. In spite of this trial the drug was not incorporated in clinical practice as it showed lack of benefit in patients treated with concurrent chemoradiation therapy. The dose limiting side effects like hypotension, vomiting and Steven Johnson syndrome were also a deterrent in its clinical application.

10.5.1 Treatment of Xerostomia

The general approach to treating patients with radiation induced xerostomia involves symptomatic management and prevention of oral complications. Symptomatic treatment includes increase in existing saliva flow, replacing saliva secretion, control of dental caries and treatment of infection. Maintaining orodental hygiene, avoidance of smoking, use of dentures can reduce xerostomia. Various over the counter products that can function as saliva substitutes have been developed specifically for patient with xerostomia. Different formulations like rinses, aerosols and chewing gums are available which promote salivary gland functions.

10.5.1.1 Salivary Substitutes

Artificial saliva provides temporary relief in some patients. Lubrication of oral mucosa with salivary substitutes provides symptomatic relief of dry mouth and also helps in swallowing function and maintaining oral hygiene. Increased water intake also helps in symptom alleviation of xerostomia.

10.5.1.2 Salivary Stimulants

Role of Pilocarpine has been investigated as a salivary stimulant for the treatment of radiation induced xerostomia. Pilocarpine is a parasympathomimetic agent that functions primarily as a muscarinic agonist with mild beta-adrenergic activity. It provides increased salivation and symptomatic relief to patients due to cholinergic stimulation of residual functional salivary gland tissue. Johnson et al. studied the role of pilocarpine hydrochloride for the treatment of radiation induced xerostomia and concluded that pilocarpine can improve symptoms associated with post-irradiation xerostomia, including oral dryness, discomfort, and difficulty in speaking and also reduce the need for comfort agents [17]. The recommended dose of pilocarpine is 5 mg three times a day. Strict patient selection is necessary for treatment with pilocarpine as it is contraindicated in patients with bronchospasm, congestive heart failure, chronic obstructive pulmonary disease, acute bronchial asthma and acute congestive glaucoma.

Cevimeline, an acetylcholine analogue selectively stimulates M3 muscarnic receptors in the salivary glands. It has a longer half life and sialagogic action than pilocarpine. Recent study shows that cevimeline at 30–45 mg thrice daily induced better unstimulated, but not stimulated, salivary production than placebo and relieved symptoms of xerostomia without any severe adverse effects [18].

10.5.1.3 Acupuncture

The role of acupuncture in the management of xerostomia has been evaluated in studies. Blom et al. showed that acupuncture treatment results in significant improvement in salivary flow rate in patients with xerostomia upto 6 months and additional acupuncture therapy can maintain this improvement upto 3 years [19]. Transcutaneous electrical nerve stimulation (TENS) is also being studied as a treatment option for radiation induced xerostomia.

10.5.1.4 Gene Therapy

Salivary glands are proven to be attractive target sites for multiple clinical gene transfer applications. Multiple studies in animal models have yielded proofs of concept for novel treatments using gene therapeutics for damaged salivary glands following radiation therapy. Further studies involving gene transfer may give a clinically applicable solutions for this condition in future.

10.6 Unanswered Questions

There are some unanswered questions which can be the topic of future research like the implication of submandibular glands or minor glands within the oral cavity sparing on xerostomia and quality of life, best quantitative threshold which corresponds to patient's quality of life, spatial sensitivity of different salivary glands to radiation, Dosimetric constraints of submandibular and minor salivary glands and use of adaptive radiotherapy to account of temporal change in parotids during radiation.

10.7 Conclusion

Xerostomia is an important acute and late sequelae of radiation therapy compromising the quality of life in head and neck cancer patients. Significant advances have been made in understanding the natural course of radiation induced xerostomia and its management. The best approach to manage xerostomia begins with proper clinical assessment of each patient, followed by salivary gland sparing radiation planning. To prevent severe xerostomia, attempts should be made to spare at least one parotid gland to a mean dose of <20 Gy or both glands to receive less than 25 Gy (mean dose). For complex, partial-volume RT patterns (IMRT), each parotid mean dose should be kept as low as possible, consistent with the desired clinical target volume coverage. A lower parotid mean dose usually results in better function. Submandibular gland sparing also significantly decreases the risk of xerostomia. With proper care post radiation therapy, maintaining oral hygiene, appropriate treatment with available pharmacological options and regular follow up salivary function recovery can take place to a varied extent. With the development in imaging biomarkers and understanding the recovery of salivary glands at cellular and molecular levels better prevention and treatment of radiation induced xerostomia will be possible.

References

1. Mortensen HR, Overgaard J, Specht L, et al. Prevalence and peak incidence of acute and late normal tissue morbidity in the DAHANCA 6&7 randomised trial with accelerated radiotherapy for head and neck cancer. Radiother Oncol. 2012;103(1):69–75. https://doi.org/10.1016/j.radonc.2012.01.002.
2. Ortholan C, Benezery K, Bensadoun RJ. Dose de tolérance à l'irradiation des tissus sains: les glandes salivaires [Normal tissue tolerance to external beam radiation therapy: salivary glands]. Cancer Radiother. 2010;14(4–5):290–4. https://doi.org/10.1016/j.canrad.2010.03.007.
3. Dirix P, Nuyts S. Evidence-based organ-sparing radiotherapy in head and neck cancer. Lancet Oncol. 2010;11(1):85–91. https://doi.org/10.1016/S1470-2045(09)70231-1.
4. Porter SR, Scully C, Hegarty AM. An update of the etiology and management of xerostomia. Oral Surg Oral Med Oral Pathol Oral Radiol Endod. 2004;97(1):28–46. https://doi.org/10.1016/j.tripleo.2003.07.010.
5. Wang ZH, Yan C, Zhang ZY, et al. Radiation-induced volume changes in parotid and submandibular glands in patients with head and neck cancer receiving postoperative radiotherapy: a longitudinal study. Laryngoscope. 2009;119(10):1966–74. https://doi.org/10.1002/lary.20601.
6. Blanco AI, Chao KS, El Naqa I, et al. Dose-volume modeling of salivary function in patients with head-and-neck cancer receiving radiotherapy. Int J Radiat Oncol Biol Phys. 2005;62(4):1055–69. https://doi.org/10.1016/j.ijrobp.2004.12.076.
7. Chao KS, Deasy JO, Markman J, et al. A prospective study of salivary function sparing in patients with head-and-neck cancers receiving intensity-modulated or three-dimensional radiation therapy: initial results. Int J Radiat Oncol Biol Phys. 2001;49(4):907–16. https://doi.org/10.1016/s0360-3016(00)01441-3.
8. Leslie MD, Dische S. Parotid gland function following accelerated and conventionally fractionated radiotherapy. Radiother Oncol. 1991;22(2):133–9. https://doi.org/10.1016/0167-8140(91)90009-6.

9. Price RE, Ang KK, Stephens LC, Peters LJ. Effects of continuous hyperfractionated accelerated and conventionally fractionated radiotherapy on the parotid and submandibular salivary glands of rhesus monkeys. Radiother Oncol. 1995;34(1):39–46. https://doi.org/10.1016/0167-8140(94)01491-k.
10. Pow EH, Kwong DL, McMillan AS, et al. Xerostomia and quality of life after intensity-modulated radiotherapy vs. conventional radiotherapy for early-stage nasopharyngeal carcinoma: initial report on a randomized controlled clinical trial. Int J Radiat Oncol Biol Phys. 2006;66(4):981–91. https://doi.org/10.1016/j.ijrobp.2006.06.013.
11. Kam MK, Leung SF, Zee B, et al. Prospective randomized study of intensity-modulated radiotherapy on salivary gland function in early-stage nasopharyngeal carcinoma patients. J Clin Oncol. 2007;25(31):4873–9. https://doi.org/10.1200/JCO.2007.11.5501.
12. Nutting CM, Morden JP, Harrington KJ, et al. Parotid-sparing intensity modulated versus conventional radiotherapy in head and neck cancer (PARSPORT): a phase 3 multicentre randomised controlled trial. Lancet Oncol. 2011;12(2):127–36. https://doi.org/10.1016/S1470-2045(10)70290-4.
13. Jha N, Seikaly H, McGaw T, Coulter L. Submandibular salivary gland transfer prevents radiation-induced xerostomia. Int J Radiat Oncol Biol Phys. 2000;46(1):7–11. https://doi.org/10.1016/s0360-3016(99)00460-5.
14. Ben-Aryeh H, Gutman D, Szargel R, Laufer D. Effects of irradiation on saliva in cancer patients. Int J Oral Surg. 1975;4(5):205–10. https://doi.org/10.1016/s0300-9785(75)80027-5.
15. Deasy JO, Moiseenko V, Marks L, Chao KS, Nam J, Eisbruch A. Radiotherapy dose-volume effects on salivary gland function. Int J Radiat Oncol Biol Phys. 2010;76(3 Suppl):S58–63. https://doi.org/10.1016/j.ijrobp.2009.06.090.
16. Brizel DM, Wasserman TH, Henke M, et al. Phase III randomized trial of amifostine as a radioprotector in head and neck cancer [published correction appears in J Clin Oncol. 2000;18(24):4110–1]. J Clin Oncol. 2000;18(19):3339–45. https://doi.org/10.1200/JCO.2000.18.19.3339.
17. Johnson JT, Ferretti GA, Nethery WJ, et al. Oral pilocarpine for post-irradiation xerostomia in patients with head and neck cancer. N Engl J Med. 1993;329(6):390–5. https://doi.org/10.1056/NEJM199308053290603.
18. Chambers MS, Posner M, Jones CU, et al. Cevimeline for the treatment of postirradiation xerostomia in patients with head and neck cancer. Int J Radiat Oncol Biol Phys. 2007;68(4):1102–9. https://doi.org/10.1016/j.ijrobp.2007.01.019.
19. Blom M, Lundeberg T. Long-term follow-up of patients treated with acupuncture for xerostomia and the influence of additional treatment. Oral Dis. 2000;6(1):15–24. https://doi.org/10.1111/j.1601-0825.2000.tb00316.x.

Osteoradionecrosis of the Mandible Post Radiation of Head and Neck Cancers 11

Pooja Nandwani Patel

11.1 Introduction

Osteoradionecrosis (ORN) is a relatively rare but morbid and costly complication of radiation therapy (RT). It is a condition with bone and mucosal breakdown after RT. As it's a morbid complication affecting cosmetic and functional outcomes [1], prophylactic and therapeutic measures should be taken for its prevention. There are various definitions of ORN but till date there is no accepted standard classification or grading. The most prevalent definition is a site of bone necrosis (death) in an irradiated field unrelated to tumor recurrence that fails to heal over 3 to 6 months period.

In today's era of advanced conformal radiation techniques, the incidence today (1–5%) has gone quite down compared to previous years incidence in 1990's (around 20%) [2]. There has been lot of focus on the predisposing factors related to ORN including patient variables—tobacco, alcohol, comorbidities, tumor location, stage and dental hygiene [3] and treatment variables—dental extraction [4] 2 weeks prior to radiation treatment, surgery [5, 6], chemotherapy and radiation treatment technique [7–9] used. Still till date the pathophysiogenesis for ORN remains unclear [10].

P. N. Patel (✉)
Department of Radiation Oncology, Sterling Hospitals, Sindhubhavan, Ahmedabad, Gujarat, India

K. Sood Sharma et al. (eds.), *Complications of Cancer Therapy: Best Practices in Prevention and Management*, https://doi.org/10.1007/978-981-99-0984-1_11

11.2 Description/Listing of Complications Encountered—With Incidence Rates

The first report on ORN of mandible after radiotherapy was published in 1922 by Regaud and later in 1926 Ewing termed it as radiation osteitis. ORN has also been termed as radiation osteomyelitis, radio-osteonecrosis, osteonecrosis, osteomyelitis of irradiated bone, radio-osteomyelitis and septic osteoradionecrosis. The pathogenesis includes sequence of events by radiation therapy including endarteritis, hypovascularity, hypocellularity in turn leading to tissue hypoxia and thereby causing tissue breakdown and nonhealing of wounds for a long period of time. There are various other theories and definitions proposed for ORN with none being till date as standard. Delanian proposed the possible mechanism as Fibroatrophic where there is early inflammation followed by fibrosis and remodeling resulting in terminal tissue necrosis with reactive oxygen species and TGF-b1 production. However with many studies still claim hypovascularity and hypocellularity as the histologic proof. Minipig study in 2012 showed at 4 h after a dose of 25 Gy in 1 fraction to the mandible, microvascular damage preceded the observation of bony destruction on histology [11]. An another study from Netherland in 2018 proved bone biopsies at the time of implant placement demonstrated less vascular density in the irradiated group and preferential obliteration of microvascular structures at doses >50 Gy [12]. Shuster et al. [13] proved ORN cases had no increased osteoclast activity indicating a destructive lytic process with ORN. Clinically bone in the radiation portal becomes devitalized and exposed for more than 3 months without any signs of healing in absence of recurrence. Mandible is the most common bone where ORN is seen as it is a very dense bone with less blood supply. Vascular cause for ORN is also supported clinically—ORN development in mandible is up to 6 times more likely than in the better vascularized maxilla. Amongst the various different staging systems available, Marx's staging system [14] is most commonly used (Table 11.1). ORN can develop during a wide range of time period after radiation therapy (from few months to several years) [15–17]. The incidence rates were as high as 20% in the 1990s [2] as reported in clinical trials (DAHANCA 7) but in today's modern era of conformal radiotherapy the incidence rates have been quite low (1–5%) [2, 7, 9, 17].

Table 11.1 Marx's classification of ORN

Stage	Description
I	Exposed alveolar bone without pathologic fracture, which responds to hyperbaric oxygen therapy
II	Disease does not respond to HBOT, and requires sequestrectomy and saucerization
III	Full thickness bone damage or pathologic fracture, usually requires complete resection and reconstruction with free tissue

11.3 Predictors/Risk Factors for the Mentioned Complication

There has been lot of focus on the predisposing factors related to ORN including patient variables—tobacco, alcohol, comorbidities, tumor location, stage and dental hygiene [3] and treatment variables—dental extraction [4] 2 weeks prior to radiation treatment, surgery [5, 6], chemotherapy and radiation treatment technique [7–9] used. Tobacco consumption leads to a complex sequaelae including infection, trauma, poor dental hygiene, impaired local wound healing, increasing surgical complications after head and neck surgery leading to cascade of events leading to ORN [2–6]. Alcohol along with tobacco can act as a strong irritant and thereby significantly contributing to breakdown of mucosa and exposure of bone. Presence of any comorbidities leads to compromised general condition affecting healing of local tissues and eventually increasing the risk of ORN. Tumor located in oral cavity with mandibular bone invasion as compared to oropharyngeal cases have more risk of ORN [15]. Owosho et al. from MSKCC [16] had higher ORN in advanced oropharyngeal cancers compared with oral cavity cancer (as high dose upto 70 Gy used in oropharyngeal tumors compared with adjuvant dosing of 60 Gy most often used in oral cavity). Risk is also pronounced with marginal bone resection [18]. Poor dental hygiene and periodontal disease again leads to vicious cycle of impaired wound healing, trauma thereby introducing bacteria to enter into the underlying demineralized bone and leading to chances of ORN. Review of literature shows no difference in rates of ORN for extractions done before or after Radiation therapy [19, 20] however preferably all loose, caries teeth should be removed before the start of Radiation therapy. Radiation therapy starting with less than 2 weeks of dental extractions or dental extractions in less than 1 year period time of radiation therapy completion leads to compromised wound healing and increasing the risk of ORN. Surgery done prior to radiation therapy affects vascularization and increasing the risk further. Even the addition of chemotherapy is related to increased risk of ORN. Higher doses of RT and nonconformal techniques leads to increased risk of ORN. Better conformal plans IMRT vs 3DCRT also decreases the risk of ORN [15].

11.4 Early Warning Signs and Diagnostic Work Up

The diagnosis of ORN starts with typical clinical presentation of exposed bone through overlying skin and mucosa often painless or along with pain and swelling. Often there may be non resolving painful mucosal ulcer, trismus, orocutaneous fistula with exposed bone seen, fetor oris with or without active infection. Clinically bone in the radiation portal becomes devitalized and exposed for more than 3 months without any signs of healing in absence of recurrence. The rough surface of exposed bone sometimes causes further abrasion of adjacent soft tissue leading to discomfort, pain and in untreated cases leading to cellulitis. There may be also chances of food impaction, fetor oris and leading to functional limitations of mouth.

The diagnosis or ORN first needs recurrence to be ruled out. So proper clinical examination and panoramic and tomographic imaging may be performed. Imaging will confirm osteolysis consistent with bone loss and confirmatory for diagnosis of ORN. Tumor recurrence commonly presents as osteolytic lesions with associated soft-tissue mass. MRI can sometimes detect ORN at an earlier stage than CT by assessing soft tissue changes adjacent to the mandible. Dynamic contrast-enhanced MRI demonstrates quantitative differences in vascular leakiness in areas of bone with advanced ORN compared with normal bone [21]. PET can sometimes show false positive because of ORN induced inflammation.

There is no consensus for standard imaging based screening for ORN however high risk of ORN (based upon mandibular radiation dose) could be screened annually with radiographs and/or cone beam computed tomography imaging [22]. There is no need of biopsy unless recurrence is suspected. If biopsy is required, a portion of the area biopsied should also be submitted for microbial analysis to identify any potential source of secondary infections.

11.5 Management of Complications

A good communication and team work is required between oncologic and dental care for the optimal management of ORN. Prevention is always better than cure also holds true in clinical situation of ORN. Review of literature shows no difference in rates of ORN for extractions done before or after Radiation therapy [19, 20] however preferably all loose, caries teeth should be removed before the start of Radiation therapy. Radiation therapy should be started preferably 2 weeks later to dental extractions to allow for proper healing. Patient should always be explained about ORN and its sequelae and to be involved thoroughly in decision making for which teeth should be removed or salvaged. Loose, unwanted, caries tooth should be always knocked down during the major oral surgery only so as to allow adequate healing time before the post operative radiotherapy starts 4–6 weeks later to surgery.

Oral hygiene should always be emphasized and measures for it should be meticulously explained to patients with clear understanding that a good oral hygiene will enhance local control rates by making the patient compliant for radiation along with reduction in complications as well. Along with Benzydamine gargles, patient should also be educated to rinse with basic salt and soda gargles for better oral care. Dental extractions if needed should be avoided for at least 1 year after radiation therapy completion. Better conformal plans IMRT vs. 3DCRT also decreases the risk of ORN [15]. Usually in RT planning *D*max of 50 Gy is kept as constraint for mandible but off-late it has been realized that maximum dose to the mandible has not shown to correlate well with the risk of ORN. S Aarup-Kristensen et al. [23] showed that D_{mean} seems a more appropriate parameter to be considered in planning and dose to the mandible should be kept as low as possible so as to reduce the risk of ORN. In his study D_{mean} was significantly higher in cases as compared to controls indicating that higher radiation dose levels to mandibular volumes increased the risk of ORN.

Mohamed ASR et al. [24] from MD Anderson Head and Neck Cancer Symptom Working Group showed that volume of the mandibular irradiation was also a better parameter for predicting the risk of ORN. Even larger volumes though of lower dose radiation contribute to ORN more significantly than a maximum point dose which was consistent with pathogenesis of ORN-a larger volume of microvascular damage is more likely to lead to hypocellularity, fibrosis, and tissue hypoxia than a higher focal point dose. Dose volume histogram (V35 to V73) were significantly higher in ORN patients. There was significant differences in mean mandibular dose between who did and did not develop ORN (48.1 Gy vs. 43.6 Gy, $P < .0001$) with no difference in maximum dose (74 Gy vs. 73.2 Gy). Zhang et al. [25] showed more better sparing of mandible with proton therapy (significantly lower mandibular doses as compared with IMRT mean dose 41.2 Gy vs. 25.6 Gy with IMPT, ORN rates of 2% compared with 7.7%). There was no difference in maximum dose (71.3 Gy for IMPT vs. 71.7 Gy for IMRT). In cases where reirradiation is indicated the cumulative dose to the mandible should be considered as the chances of ORN have been seen upto 20% in cases of irradiation.

If ORN is diagnosed then treatment should start with conservative measures like analgesics, saline irrigation and antibiotics according to the culture reports. Pentoxifylline helps in healing by increasing collagenase activity, reduces fibroblast proliferation, increases oxygen saturation and lowers blood viscosity. It also causes vasodilation, decreased platelet aggregation, inhibition of inflammation, and increased erythrocyte membrane flexibility with a hypothesized overall effect of improving blood flow in tissue. It also has anti-tumor necrosis factor properties that may contribute to decreased fibrosis. The dose of pentoxifylline is 800 mg daily along with vitamin E 500 IU BID for at least 6 months. Vitamin E has antioxidant properties that can limit free radical damage. Both vitamin E and pentoxifylline acts synergistically as potent antifibrotic agents [26]. It can also be combined with clodronate which acts by inhibiting macrophages and increasing bone formation. It is commonly dosed at 1600 mg daily Monday through Friday to limit effects on calcium levels [27].

A systematic review [28] of the literature and meta-analysis in 2019 (7 retrospective and prospective studies with 211 patients) using pentoxifylline-tocopherol with or without clodronate showed full recovery from ORN or significant improvement precluding the need for additional intervention. (60% met the defined response criteria ~30% remained stable). Common side effect—gastrointestinal disturbance including nausea (managed with antiemetics). Dissard et al [29] recently published his experience of 27 patients treated in a similar manner with cure rate of 76.5% at an average of 9.6 months, 55% decrease in exposed bone area after 6 months, 92% decrease at 24 months. One of our patient who developed ORN at 6 months was given option of pentoxifylline 800 mg along daily with good healing of ORN at 3 months (Fig. 11.1 is clinical picture at diagnosis of ORN and Fig. 11.2 is clinical picture after 3 months of pentoxifylline). Role of biphosphonates is not very clear but it claims to reduce osteoclastic activity and thus is used in treatment of ORN [30, 31].

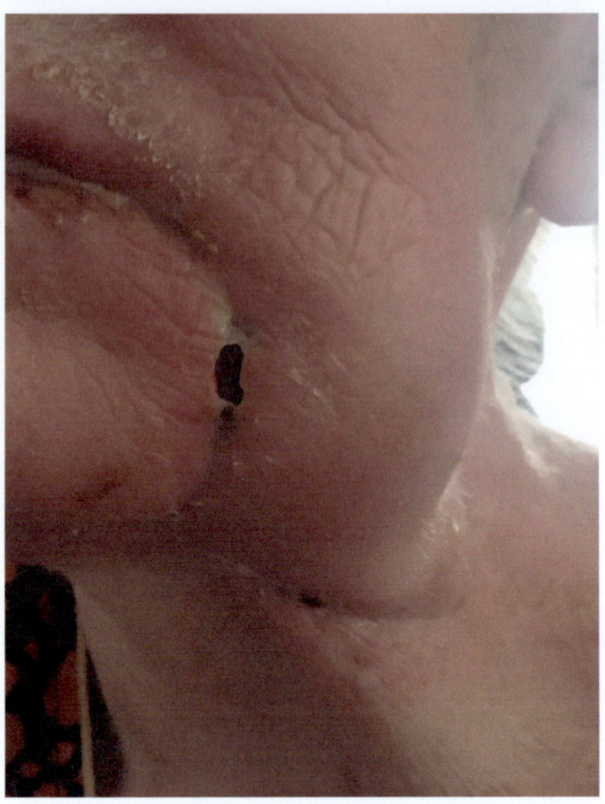

Fig. 11.1 Clinical picture at diagnosis of ORN

Ultrasound therapy tried in 1990s combined with metronidazole and local débridement induces neovascularity and cellularity in the irradiated volume has never gained much popularity [32]. Patients failing on conservative therapy can be taken for hyperbaric oxygen therapy (HBO). HBO historically has been used to reverse microvascular damage and associated impaired oxygenation. Despite its widespread use there has been significant debate about the efficacy [33]. Systematic review by Annane et al. from 2004 did not show a benefit to HBO [34]. Cochrane review [35] in 2016 identified 3 articles assessing the achievement of mucosal coverage in patients with ORN and found a modest improvement in this endpoint with the use of HBO compared with controls (having risk of bias).

A 2017 multidisciplinary guideline from the Dana-Farber Cancer Institute and Brigham and Women's Hospital [36] did not support HBO for the prevention or management of ORN except in select cases refractory to other treatments. Even DAHANCA 21 & NWHHT2009-1 [37] showed that HBO did not significantly improve the healing outcome of ORN after surgical removal of necrotic bone as compared to standard care (70% vs. 51%). This effect is not statistically significant due to the fact that the study was underpowered. Patients failing with conservative treatment can be given option of surgical interventions depending on the degree of damage present, ORN location, and individual patient characteristics. The common

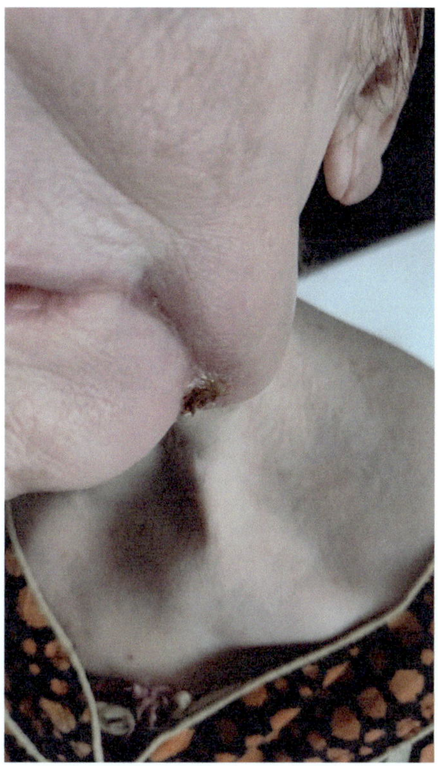

Fig. 11.2 Clinical picture after 3 months of pentoxiphylline

approaches are sequestrectomy of isolated islands of necrotic bone with either soft tissue or bone reconstruction. Major goals of surgery include relief of discomfort, infection management, restoration of bone continuity, repair of functional and cosmetic defects, and improvement of quality of life [38].

More extensive surgeries like marginal or segmental mandibulectomy are advocated in cases of deep involvement of bone or presence of pathologic fracture with the aim to remove bone and soft tissue with compromised perfusion and to enhance or maintain viable bleeding tissue for the highest chance of healing. The surgical approach is determined by the type of defect. Bone defects owing to resection of large portions of the mandible are addressed with bone grafts but associated with a higher complication rate than soft tissue grafts. Complex wounds are better addressed by soft tissue reconstruction with similar functional and esthetic outcomes compared with bone grafting [38].

11.6 TIPS and Tricks to Prevent Complications

ORN is every Radiation Oncologists' worst nightmare and the best way to manage is to start right from the prevention level. Dental evaluation, prohylactic dental extraction and pre RT, during RT and post RT good dental hygiene are the key steps to start with. Better conformal radiation plans aiming to reduce not only the D_{max} but also D_{mean} should be thrived for. Radiation plans should be planned with as much as sparing of volume of mandible possible. NCCN even recommends dental examinations at least every 6 months after radiation therapy for ORN prevention. The treatment should start with conservative management failing which to HBO and surgical intervention as the last method.

11.7 Conclusion

Head and neck cancer patients will always be a challenge for oncologists both surgical and radiation at majority of the times. Multidisciplinary management with proper dental evaluation right from start is the first step to prevent ORN. Better conformal radiotherapy plans and proper dental hygiene throughout the radiation treatment will help further to decrease chances of ORN. Dental extractions when unavoidable should be done with thorough consultation with Radiation Oncologists and enough time constraints to pre and post RT should be respected. Once having diagnosed the most unwanted complication start treatment with conservative measures followed by HBO or surgical intervention in multidisciplinary setting.

Ten Key Points

1. Prevention is better than cure. Follow all steps at the preventive level like proper dental evaluation pre surgery and pre RT time.
2. Dental extractions if required should be done along with the major surgery planned only so as to give adequate time for healing.
3. Pre radiation extraction of non restorable (loose, caries, sharp) tooth with attempted primary closure at the time of extraction.
4. Dental extractions if done before RT then minimum 2 weeks to wait before starting the radiation treatment.
5. Better conformal radiation plans with importance to D_{max}, D_{mean} and volume of mandible in radiation portal should be ascertained properly. Keep the mean dose as low as possible and keep as low volume of mandible in the radiotherapy portal.
6. Dental hygiene should be thoroughly managed during radiation therapy including the most simple salt and soda gargles along with benzydamine gargles.
7. Dental extractions post radiation should be done with minimum difference of 1 year post radiation treatment.
8. NCCN also recommends dental examinations at least every 6 months after radiation therapy for ORN prevention.
9. Diagnosis of ORN is more clinical along with simpler imaging tools and avoiding PET unless to rule out recurrence.
10. Start the treatment with conservative measures failing which to HBO and surgical intervention.

References

1. Rogers SN, D'Souza JJ, Lowe D, et al. Longitudinal evaluation of health-related quality of life after osteoradionecrosis of the mandible. Br J Oral Maxillofac Surg. 2015;53:854–7.
2. Pereira IF, Firmino RT, Meira HC, et al. Osteoradionecrosis prevalence and associated factors: a ten years retrospective study. Med Oral. 2018;23:e633–8.
3. Kojima Y, Yanamoto S, Umeda M, et al. Relationship between dental status and development of osteoradionecrosis of the jaw: a multicenter retrospective study. Oral Surg Oral Med Oral Pathol Oral Radiol. 2017;124:139–45.
4. Wang TH, Liu CJ, Chao TF, et al. Risk factors for and the role of dental extractions in osteoradionecrosis of the jaws: a national based cohort study. Head Neck. 2017;39:1313–21.
5. Renda L, Tsai TY, Huang JJ, et al. A nomogram to predict osteoradionecrosis in oral cancer after marginal mandibulectomy and radiotherapy. Laryngoscope. 2019;130(1):101–7.
6. Raguse JD, Hossamo J, Tinhofer I, et al. Patient and treatment related risk factors for osteoradionecrosis of the jaw in patients with head and neck cancer. Oral Surg Oral Med Oral Pathol Oral Radiol. 2016;121:215–21.
7. Owosho AA, Tsai CJ, Lee RS, et al. The prevalence and risk factors associated with osteoradionecrosis of the jaw in oral and oropharyngeal cancer patients treated with intensity-modulated radiation therapy (IMRT): The Memorial Sloan Kettering Cancer Center experience. Oral Oncol. 2017;64:44–51.
8. Ben-David MA, Diamante M, Radawski JD, et al. Lack of osteoradionecrosis of the mandible after intensity-modulated radiotherapy for head and neck cancer: likely contributions of both dental care and improved dose distributions. Int J Radiat Oncol Biol Phys. 2007;68:396–402.
9. Caparrotti F, Huang SH, Lu L, et al. Osteoradionecrosis of the mandible in patients with oropharyngeal carcinoma treated with intensity-modulated radiotherapy. Cancer. 2017;123:3691–700.
10. Sathasivam HP, Davies GR, Boyd NM. Predictive factors for osteoradionecrosis of the jaws: a retrospective study. Head Neck. 2018;40:46–54.
11. Xu J. Early-stage pathogenic sequence of jaw osteoradionecrosis in vivo. J Dent Res. 2012;91:702–8.
12. Dekker H. The irradiated human mandible: a quantitative study on bone vascularity. Oral Oncol. 2018;87:126–30.
13. Shuster A. Comparison of the histopathological characteristics of osteomyelitis, medication-related osteonecrosis of the jaw, and osteoradionecrosis. J Oral Maxillofac Surg. 2019;48:17–22.
14. Marx RE. Osteoradionecrosis: a new concept of its pathophysiology. J Oral Maxillofac Surg. 1983;41:283–8.
15. Moon DH. Incidence of, and risk factors for, mandibular osteoradionecrosis in patients with oral cavity and oropharynx cancers. Oral Oncol. 2017;72:98–103.
16. Owosho AA. The prevalence and risk factors associated with osteoradionecrosis of the jaw in oral and oropharyngeal cancer patients treated with intensity-modulated radiation therapy (IMRT): The Memorial Sloan Kettering Cancer Center experience. Oral Oncol. 2017;64:44–51.
17. De Felice F. Osteoradionecrosis following treatment for head and neck cancer and the effect of radiotherapy dosimetry: the Guy's and St Thomas' Head and Neck Cancer Unit experience. Oral Surg Oral Med Oral Pathol Oral Radiol. 2016;122:28–34.
18. Studer G. Risk profile for osteoradionecrosis of the mandible in the IMRT era. Strahlenther Onkol. 2016;192:32–9.
19. Sulaiman F, Huryn JM, Zlotolow IM. Dental extractions in the irradiated head and neck patient: a retrospective analysis of memorial Sloan-Kettering cancer center protocols, criteria and end results. J Oral Maxillofac Surg. 2003;61:1123–31.
20. Reuther T, Schuster T, Mende U, Kubler A. Osteoradionecrosis of the jaws as a side effect of radiotherapy of head and neck tumor patients: a report of a thirty year retrospective review. Int J Oral Maxillofac Surg. 2003;32:289–95.

21. Mohamed ASR. Quantitative dynamic contrast enhanced MRI identifies radiation-induced vascular damage in patients with advanced osteoradionecrosis: results of a prospective study. Int J Radiat Oncol Biol Phys. 2020;108:1319–28.
22. Owosho AA. Radiographic osteoradionecrosis of the jaw with intact mucosa: proposal of clinical guidelines for early identification of this condition. Oral Oncol. 2015;51:e93–6.
23. Aarup- KS. Osteoradionecrosis of the mandible after radiotherapy for head and neck cancer: risk factors and dose-volume correlations. Acta Oncol. 2019;58:1373–7.
24. Mohamed ASR. Dose-volume correlates of mandibular osteoradionecrosis in Oropharynx cancer patients receiving intensity-modulated radiotherapy: results from a case-matched comparison. Radiother Oncol. 2017;124:232–9.
25. Zhang W. Intensity-modulated proton therapy and osteoradionecrosis in oropharyngeal cancer. Radiother Oncol. 2017;123:401–5.
26. Patel V. Use of pentoxifylline and tocopherol in the management of osteoradionecrosis. Br J Oral Maxillofac Surg. 2016;54:342–5.
27. Delanian S, Chatel C, Porcher R. Complete restoration of refractory mandibular osteoradionecrosis by prolonged treatment with a pentoxifylline-tocopherol-clodronate combination (PENTOCLO): a phase II trial. Int J Radiat Oncol Biol Phys. 2011;80:832–9.
28. Kolokythas A. Management of osteoradionecrosis of the jaws with pentoxifylline-tocopherol: a systematic review of the literature and meta-analysis. Intern J Oral Maxillofac Surg. 2019;48:173–80.
29. Dissard A. Efficacy of pentoxifylline tocopherol- clodronate in mandibular osteoradionecrosis. Laryngoscope. 2020;130:E559–66.
30. Ruggiero S. American Association of Oral and Maxillofacial Surgeons position paper on medication-related osteonecrosis of the jaw–2014 update. J Oral Maxillofac Surg. 2014;72:1938–56.
31. Wan JT. Mitigating osteonecrosis of the jaw (ONJ) through preventive dental care and understanding of risk factors. Bone Res. 2020;8:14.
32. Harris M. Ultrasound therapy for osteoradionecrosis. Br J Maxillofac Surg. 1992;30:313–8.
33. Marx RE. Prevention of osteoradionecrosis: a randomized prospective clinical trial of hyperbaric oxygen versus penicillin. J Am Dent Assoc. 1985;111:49–54.
34. Annane D. Hyperbaric oxygen therapy for radionecrosis of the jaw: a randomized, placebo-controlled, double blind trial from the ORN96 study group. J Clin Oncol. 2004;22:4893–900.
35. Bennett MH. Hyperbaric oxygen therapy for late radiation tissue injury Cochrane Gynaecological, Neuro-oncology and Orphan Cancer Group, ed. Cochrane Database Syst Rev. 2016;4:CD005005.
36. Sultan A. The use of hyperbaric oxygen for the prevention and management of osteoradionecrosis of the jaw: A Dana-Farber/Brigham and Women's Cancer Center multidisciplinary guideline. Oncologia. 2017;22:343–50.
37. Forner L. Hyperbaric oxygen treatment of mandibular osteoradionecrosis: Combined data from the two randomized clinical trials DAHANCA-21 and NWHHT2009-1. Radiother Oncol. 2022;166:137–44.
38. Baumann DP. Free flap reconstruction of osteoradionecrosis of the mandible: A 10-year review and defect classification. Head Neck. 2011;33:800–7.

Managing Chronic Non-healing Ulcers After Definitive Radiation Therapy—Role of Hyperbaric Oxygen Therapy

12

Tarun Kumar Sahni and Manuj Goel

12.1 Introduction

Cancer treatment has improved significantly over the past decade and there is an ongoing focus on not only finding more and better ways to treat cancers but also to improve quality of life of the cancer survivor.

Surgery, radiation therapy and cytotoxic chemotherapy are the principal methods employed in the treatment of cancer. One-half of the estimated 1.2 million new cases of invasive cancer will receive radiation therapy as a part of their cancer treatment and despite best efforts, 5% of patients will develop severe reactions to radiation therapy [1].

The goal of radiation therapy is to eradicate tumour's with minimal, if any, adverse effects. However despite preventive measures permanent damage may occur. This leads often, to painful and disabling conditions. Conventional treatment of these lesions often has frustrating results.

Radiation therapy differs from the other two modes of treatment in that its most serious associated morbidity tends to occur months or years after treatment when management is often difficult and unsatisfactory.

Because a dominant feature of post-radiation change is the obliteration of small blood vessels leading to hypoxia, hyperbaric oxygen has been employed in the care of these patients. In the past 40 years there have been many publications reporting benefit in studies, which have included some thousands of patients [2].

T. K. Sahni (✉) · M. Goel
Department of Hyperbaric Medicine, Indraprastha Apollo Hospital, New Delhi, India
e-mail: tarun.sahni@adventhcg.com; drmanuj_g@apollohospitalsdelhi.com

K. Sood Sharma et al. (eds.), *Complications of Cancer Therapy: Best Practices in Prevention and Management*, https://doi.org/10.1007/978-981-99-0984-1_12

Hyperbaric Oxygenation (HBO2) has been proposed as a part of the overall treatment since the mid 1960s and several studies have reported beneficial effects. Hyperbaric oxygen helps reduce morbidity, disfiguring sequelae and further need for corrective surgery. It is also being evaluated for its role in enhancing radiosensitivity in selected head and neck tumors.

This article reviews the role of Hyperbaric oxygen in the management of wounds in patients who have received radiation for any form of cancers and are as a result the sequalae of side effects due to radiation [2].

12.2 Burden of Disease

12.2.1 Global Cancer Burden

Overall, cancer rates are projected to increase from approximately 9 million in 2017 to approximately 26 million new cancer cases by 2030 [3]. About 30% to 50% of all cancer patients receive irradiation either alone or with chemotherapy and surgery [4].

Therefore, around 7 million patients receive radiotherapy worldwide every year. Improved cure rates of all malignancies have resulted in more providers being confronted with a large number of patients with a wide range of chronic morbidities in long-term survivors. Hence all providers must be aware of the common adverse effects of radiation therapy.

12.2.2 Incidence of Radiation Induced Lesions in Normal Tissues

A large number of cancer patients receive radiation as part of their treatment. The incidence figures of radio-induced chronic lesions vary widely according to definition and site. Despite best efforts, 5% of patients develop severe reactions to radiation therapy often leading to painful and disabling conditions. Of these, about 1% may have serious problems, requiring major surgery and prolonged hospital care. Personal and social problems may be very distressing and commonly those affected are unable to pursue gainful employment [4].

12.3 The Nature of Radiation Injury

The risk factors for development of late radiation morbidity are similar over all sites and include the total radiation dose, the overall time, the biological effective dose which takes into account fraction size and the overall time, the volume irradiated, the use of a combination of external beam with an implantation or intracavitary procedure, a high dose rate with brachytherapy, tumours adjacent to or involving bone, the presence of infection, the use of surgery and the occurrence of trauma. Patients, who have received 2000 to 5000 rads or more, may have difficulties with any subsequent surgical healing. "Conformal" radiotherapy has encouraged the attainment of higher tumour doses and inevitably some normal tissues will be included.

The concomitant administration of cytotoxic and increasing use of major surgery for restoration of function or for salvage of advanced recurrent disease is also associated with a high risk of morbidity when a heavily irradiated area is operated upon [1].

Radiation injuries should be further sub classified as acute, subacute, or delayed complications [5].

Acute injuries are due to direct and essentially immediate cellular toxicity to normal tissues and are usually self-limited within a few weeks and are treated symptomatically. However, they can be very debilitating during their duration.

Subacute injuries are typically identifiable in only a few organ systems such as in the lung with a clinical syndrome mimicking bronchitis (radiation pneumonitis), in the spinal cord as the result of temporary demyelinization that causes the so-called Lhermitte's syndrome These, too, are generally self-limited but occasionally evolve to become delayed injuries. Some subacute injuries may persist for several months. No specific treatment is especially effective, although steroids are commonly employed.

Delayed radiation complications are typically seen after a latent period of 6 months or more and may occasionally develop many years after the radiation exposure. Sometimes acute injuries are so severe that they never resolve and evolve to become chronic injuries indistinguishable from other delayed radiation injuries. These are termed "consequential effects" and are not characterized by a symptom free latent period. Often, delayed injuries are precipitated by an additional tissue insult such as surgery within the radiation field [6].

A role for hyperbaric oxygen in acute and subacute radiation injuries has not been well studied or established, however is has a role in delayed radiation injuries [7].

12.3.1 The Aetiology of Delayed Radiation Injury

The exact causes and biochemical processes leading to delayed radiation injury are complex. In virtually all organ systems that demonstrate radiation damage, we observe vascular changes characterized by obliterative endarteritis.

Radiation researchers now appreciate that the process of radiation injury begins at the time of radiation treatment and involves the elaboration and release of many bioactive substances including, very prominently, fibrogenetic cytokines [8].

A major mechanism whereby therapeutic radiation inflicts damage on normal tissues has been termed the fibroatrophic effect. This model emphasizes the consequences of the observed depletion of parenchymal and stem cells and deemphasizes the impact of vascular damage. It also highlights the exuberant fibrosis usually found in severely damaged irradiated tissues. In this model, vascular damage and stenosis continue to be recognized as a consistent finding in tissues exhibiting radiation damage including frank necrosis; however, endarteritis as a causative factor for delayed radiation injuries is de-emphasized.

The negative impact of ionising radiation on stem cells is documented as another mechanism leading to the delayed radiation tissue damage. Research supports that Hyperbaric Oxygen can help increase the number of stem cells at these radiation injury sites.

Presently, we are not able to make practical clinical application of these observed associations. No single marker is likely to provide us with a reliable estimate of future radiation damage [9]. Similarly, no practical strategies have as yet been developed to prevent or reduce the production of these cytokines or reduce their impact in a prophylactic fashion.

12.4 Phases of Normal Wound Healing

Before discussing how HBO2 may improve wound healing, it is important to review the phases of normal wound healing. These phases are hemostasis, inflammation, proliferation, and maturation [10]. Immediately after injury, platelets attach to the injured endothelium, and the subsequent coagulation cascade triggers the formation of a provisional wound matrix to achieve hemostasis. This process also activates the inflammatory response, which includes leukocyte, neutrophil, and macrophage migration and activation. The inflammatory phase ends a few days after the initial injury, with apoptosis of the aforementioned inflammatory response cells [11, 12].

The proliferative phase begins as the inflammatory phase subsides. During the proliferative phase, neovascularization occurs via vasculogenesis, the recruitment of endothelial progenitor cells from the bone marrow that differentiate into capillary forming endothelial cells, and via angiogenesis, the formation of new blood vessels from existing endothelial cells in the wound capillary network [13]. Robust neovascularization is vital to the formation of granulation tissue because it supplies the migrating and proliferating dermal and epidermal cells in the wound bed with oxygen and nutrients. Key proliferating cells are fibroblasts, which create a new matrix of connective tissue to close wound gaps and restore mechanical strength to the wound (Fig. 12.1) [10].

In the final phase, wound contraction and matrix remodelling occur, resulting in scar tissue with 80% the tensile strength of unwounded skin.

Chronic wounds are characterized by a prolonged inflammatory phase, with an inability to progress to the proliferative phase or form newly vascularized granulation tissue.

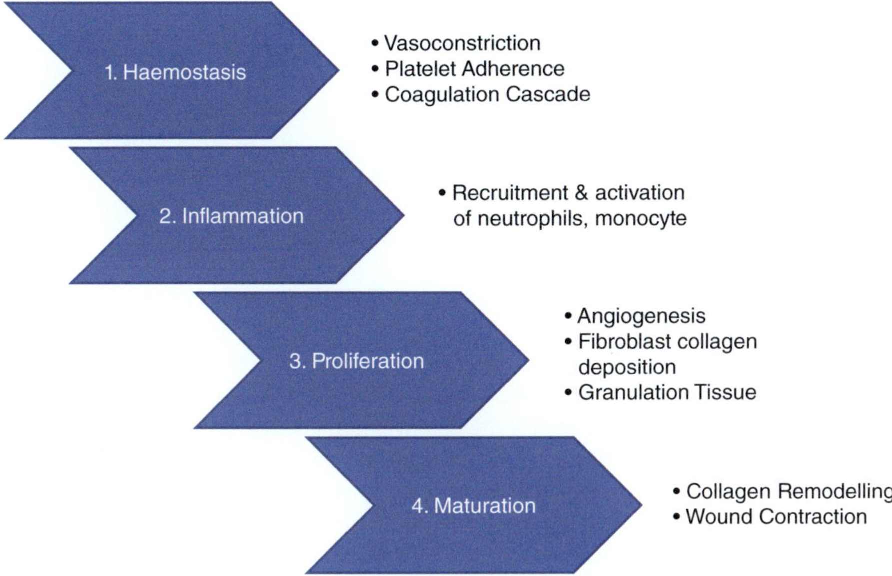

Fig. 12.1 The four phases of normal wound healing

12.5 Measurement of Wound Hypoxia

Transcutaneous oxygen tension (PtcO2) measurements provide a direct, quantitative assessment of oxygen availability to the periwound skin and an indirect measurement of periwound microcirculatory blood flow. Using PtcO2 measurement in the assessment of Peripheral Arterial Obstructive Disease has been well described by Scheffler [14] and its application to wound healing by Sheffield [15].

This technology allows objective determination of the presence and degree of local periwound hypoxia and serves as a screening tool to identify patients at risk for failure of primary wound or amputation flap healing. Fife et al. review in detail the value of PtcO2 in predicting response to HBO2 [16].

Although several tests intended to identify significant wound hypoxia and/or ischemia have been used, including ankle-brachial index (ABI), skin perfusion pressure (SPP), and laser Doppler flowmetry, PtcO2 is generally accepted as most useful for predicting wound healing failure without intervention, failure to heal an amputation incision, and failure to respond to HBO2. PtcO2 can be used to evaluate the success of revascularization. When comparing wound healing rates to ABI, toe blood pressure, and PtcO2, Löndahl et al. demonstrated PtcO2 to be a sensitive predictor of ulcer healing after HBO2 treatment. They noted that lower baseline PtcO2 levels correlated with lower rates of healing [17].

There is some variability in PtcO2 values obtained based upon the type of electrode and electrode temperature used. In a broad range, values below 25–40 mm Hg have been associated with poor healing of wound and amputation flaps; the lower the value, the greater the predicted degree of healing impairment.

Laboratory evidence linking hypoxia to wound healing failure is not in dispute. Clinical studies identifying the risks of wound or amputation flap healing failure define periwound hypoxia as the primary determinant of wound closure failure. Pecoraro reported that when periwound PtcO2 values were below 20 mm Hg, they were associated with a 39-fold increased risk of primary healing failure [18]. In clinical practice hyperbaric medicine physicians routinely measure PtcO2 and use the information obtained in order to make patient selection and treatment decisions.

12.6 Accelerating Impaired Wound Healing with HBO2

There are numerous primary pathologies that lead to non-healing or problem wounds including venous or arterial insufficiency, diabetes, and pressure. Regardless of the aetiology, a common underlying pathway that often exists in non-healing wounds is the interplay between tissue hypoperfusion, hypoxia, and infection.

A large body of evidence exists demonstrating that intermittent oxygenation of hypoperfused wound beds achieved by HBO2 treatment mitigates many of these impediments and sets into motion a cascade of cellular and biochemical events that lead to wound healing [19].

Hyperbaric oxygenation is achieved when a patient breathes 100% oxygen at an elevated atmospheric pressure in a special equipment called the Hyperbaric Chamber. There are two types of Hyperbaric Chambers: Monoplace chambers in which one patient is treated at a time and Multiplace chambers where multiple patients are treated at the same time (Fig. 12.2) [10].

Physiologically, this produces a directly proportional increase in the amount of oxygen dissolved in plasma that is readily available for cellular metabolism. Increase in pressure results in an increase in oxygen dissolved in plasma. This additional dissolved oxygen is responsible for the beneficial effects of Hyperbaric Oxygen Availability of substrate for oxygen-dependent enzymatic reactions that are critical to repair and resistance to infection is even more important than normalizing metabolic rate. Furthermore, oxidants appear to be among the most important signals that control the healing process. This may be another benefit of HBO2 in hypoxic

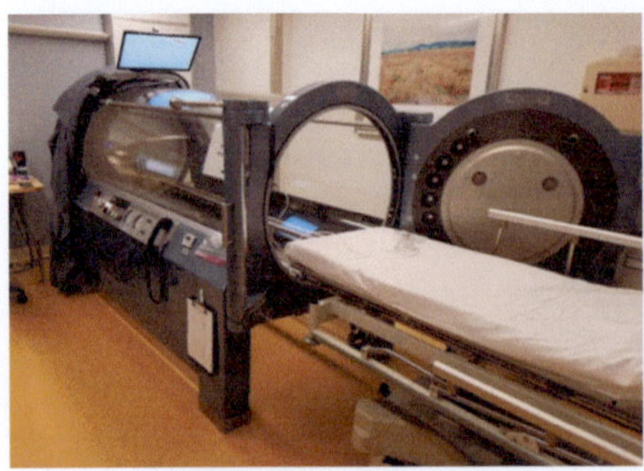

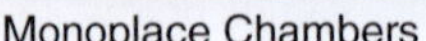

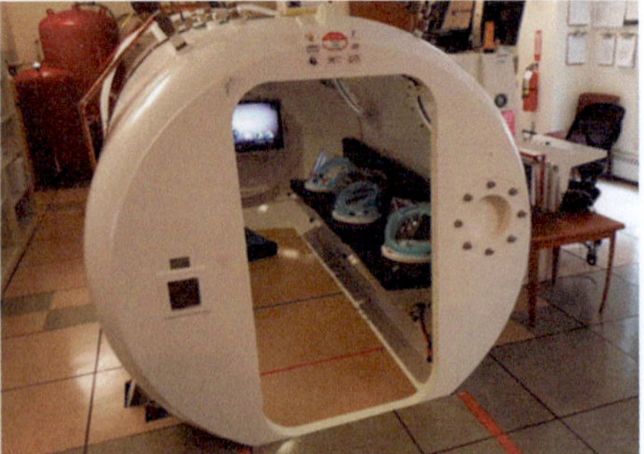

Fig. 12.2 Types of hyperbaric treatment chambers

wounds. Arterial PO2 elevations to 1500 mm Hg or greater are achieved at 2–2.5 ATA (202.65–253.32 k Pa) (Fig. 12.3) [10].

Treatment with HBO2 consists of three components. Firstly the pressure at which treated. This is measured in ATA which is the average atmospheric pressure exerted at sea level, or 14.7 psi. Most treatment for delayed wound healing due to radiation is treated at 2.4 or 2.8 ATA. Secondly the duration of each session. This is usually 60–90 min of Oxygen breathing time. Thirdly the number of sessions. 30–40 sessions are usually required for each patient in these conditions.

Hyperbaric Oxygen is an accepted treatment modality for the 14 Indications which is evidence based. These indications are recognised by the FDA and other regulatory bodies. Insurance Companies will reimburse the costs of treatment with Hyperbaric Oxygen for these conditions [19].

During tissue repair and wound healing, oxygen demand and utilization rates are increased, and chronic hypoxia in a wound is associated with reduced or absent wound healing [20]. Conversely increased oxygen supply to hypoxic tissues has multiple beneficial effects on wound healing [13]. Because oxygen cannot be stored in tissue, daily HBO2 supports an adequate oxygen supply to the site of injury to promote wound healing progression from the inflammatory phase to the proliferative phase.

Increased oxygen concentrations lead to an increased production of reactive oxygen species (ROS) and reactive nitrogen species (RNS), which play important roles in signalling pathways for promoting neovascularization, matrix formation, and decreasing inflammation (Fig. 12.4) [21].

Hypoxia is a stimulus for angiogenesis. New blood vessel formation, however, is dependent on normal levels of oxygenation. Hyperbaric oxygen therapy creates a gradient between tissues of low oxygenation in the center to higher concentrations at the periphery, thus creating a driving force conducive to neovascularization.

Improved neovascularization occurs through both local and distant processes. Locally, reactive oxygen species and reactive nitrogen species signal an increased production of wound growth factors, such as vascular endothelial growth factor (the most specific factor for neovascularization), transforming growth factor, and angiopoietin 2. Endothelial cells exposed to hyperbaric oxygen exhibit enhanced capillary tube formation and enhanced oxidative stress resistance. Although hypoxia stimulates neovascularization, chronic hypoxia actually inhibits new vessel formation. For this reason, hyperoxia induced by HBO2 promotes the neovascularization and healing of chronic wounds. In addition, it is important to distinguish between oxidative stress and oxygen toxicity.

Excessive reactive oxygen species are associated with harmful effects; however, studies have shown that the body's antioxidant defences protect against the limited number of reactive oxygen species generated by HBO2 treatment sessions. Hyperbaric oxygen therapy improves neovascularization by acting more distantly from the wound site. Increased oxygen leads to increased production of nitric oxide in the bone marrow, and multiple studies have shown that this stimulates increased vasculogenic stem/progenitor cell mobilization from the bone marrow in healthy human subjects, diabetic patients, and patients previously treated with radiation therapy, leading to more stem cells recruited to skin wounds and accelerated blood vessel formation.

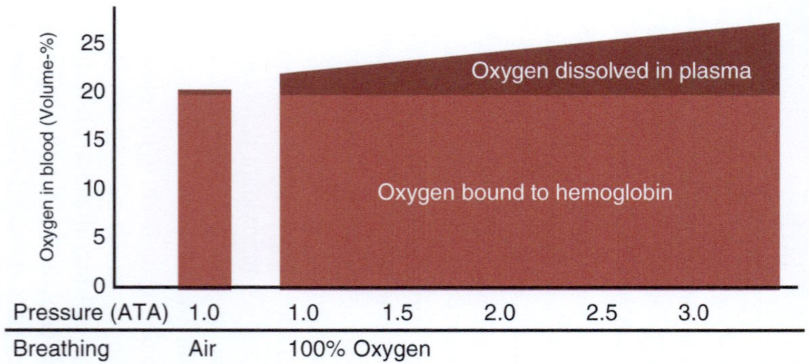

Value of Oxygen dissoloved in plama at different pressures			
ATA	MmHg	Breathing Air	100% Oxygen
1	760	0.32	**2.09**
1.5	1140	0.61	**3.26**
2	1520	0.81	**4.44**
2.5	1900	1.06	**5.62**
3	2280	1.31	**6.80**

1 ATA Is Atmosphere Absolute is the average atmospheric pressure exerted at sea level

Fig. 12.3 Mechanism of action of hyperbaric oxygen therapy

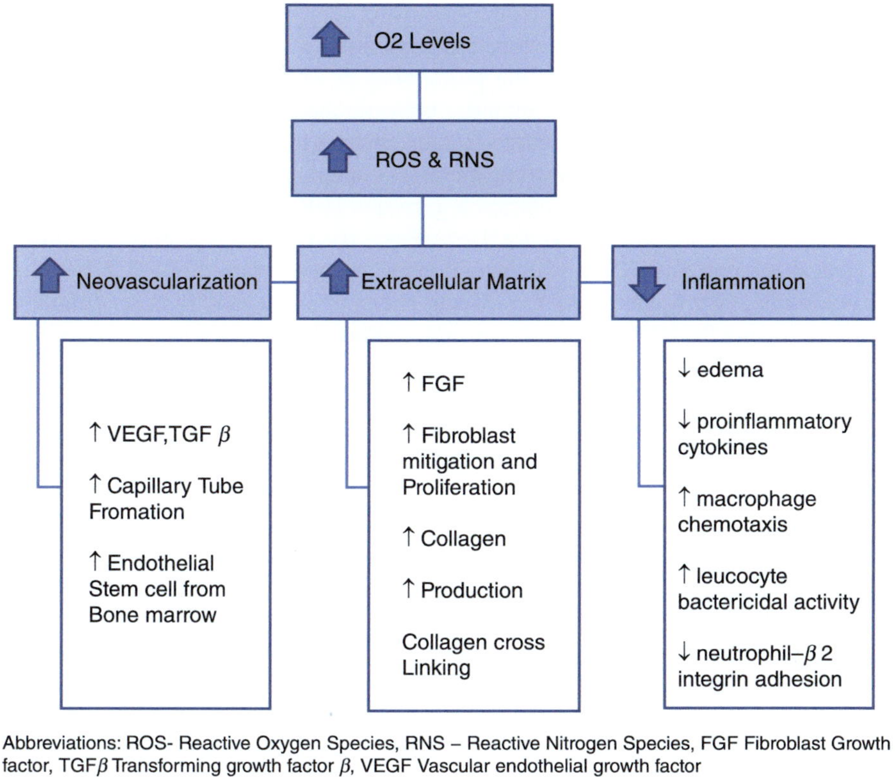

O2 Levels

ROS & RNS

Neovascularization

↑ VEGF,TGF β

↑ Capillary Tube Fromation

↑ Endothelial Stem cell from Bone marrow

Extracellular Matrix

↑ FGF

↑ Fibroblast mitigation and Proliferation

↑ Collagen

↑ Production

Collagen cross Linking

Inflammation

↓ edema

↓ proinflammatory cytokines

↑ macrophage chemotaxis

↑ leucocyte bactericidal activity

↓ neutrophil–β 2 integrin adhesion

Abbreviations: ROS- Reactive Oxygen Species, RNS – Reactive Nitrogen Species, FGF Fibroblast Growth factor, TGFβ Transforming growth factor β, VEGF Vascular endothelial growth factor

Fig. 12.4 Mechanism of action of hyperbaric oxygen in wound healing

Hyperoxia also improves the function of endothelial progenitor cells once they arrive at the wound site to differentiate into capillary-forming endothelial cells. Extracellular matrix formation is an oxygen-dependent process linked closely to neovascularization. Fibroblast growth factor production is also increased by HBO2, promoting fibroblast migration and proliferation [2, 12, 13]. Increased oxygen stimulates the proliferating fibroblasts to produce collagen at increased rates and also enhances collagen cross-linking to improve tissue tensile strengths [10].

Hyperoxia also promotes decreased inflammation by impacting three major inflammatory cell types: macrophages, leukocytes, and neutrophils and by inducing vasoconstriction to decrease local edema. Macrophages are impacted in two very different ways. First, HBO2 has been shown to reduce expression of pro-inflammatory cytokines by monocyte-macrophages in both animal and human studies. Second, HBO2 promotes macrophage chemotaxis to facilitate the clean-up of cellular debris at the wound site. Increased oxygen also enhances the bactericidal activity of leukocytes. Finally, HBO2 inhibits neutrophil 2 integrin adhesion in both animals and humans, and this mechanism has been shown to decrease tissue reperfusion injuries without reducing the neutrophils_ antibacterial function.

In summary, chronic wounds are characterized by hypoxia, impaired angiogenesis, and prolonged inflammation. Hyperbaric oxygen therapy is a successful adjunctive treatment for wound healing because it acts through diverse mechanisms to promote angiogenesis and decrease inflammation.

HBO2 undoubtedly escalates the production of reactive oxygen and nitrogen radicals (ROS and RNS), which underlie both the therapeutic and toxic effects of HBO2 on certain tissues. HBO2 paradoxically elevates the concentration of Hypoxia inducible factor (HIF)1 by diverting the HIF-1 degradation to pathways that are independent of the oxygen concentration. Elevated HIF-1 stimulates the production of different growth factors, boosting the healing process. HBO2 supports synthesis of Heat shock proteins (HSP), which are serving as chaperones of HIF-1. HBO2 has antimicrobial effect, increases the effectiveness of some antibiotics, stimulates fibroblasts growth, collagen synthesis and suppresses the activity of proteolytic enzymes like matrix metalloproteinases [22].

12.7 The Effects of Hyperbaric Oxygen on Irradiated Tissues

Because a consistent cause and manifestation of radiation injury is vascular obliteration and stromal fibrosis, the known impact of hyperbaric oxygen in stimulating angiogenesis is an obvious and important mechanism whereby hyperbaric oxygen is effective in radiation injury.

HBO2 induces neovascularization in hypoxic tissues. Marx has demonstrated the enhanced vascularity and cellularity in heavily irradiated tissues after hyperbaric oxygen therapy by comparing histologic specimens from patients pre- and post-hyperbaric oxygen [23]. Marx has also demonstrated the serial improvement in transcutaneous oxygen measurements of patients receiving hyperbaric oxygen as an indirect measure of increased vascular density [24]. Marx et al.(in an animal model) have shown increased vascularity in rabbit mandibles after exposure to hyperbaric oxygen.

Feldmeier and his colleagues, in a murine model of radiation damage to the small bowel, have shown that hyperbaric oxygen given 7 weeks after radiation can reduce the degree and mechanical effects of fibrosis by being applied prior to the manifestation of radiation injury [25].

The hyperbaric study group headed up by Dr. Goldstein who, while at the University of Pennsylvania, had published studies demonstrating the mobilization of stem cells mediated through nitric oxide with HBO2 [26]. These papers include a group of head and neck cancer patients who had received radiation treatments. A putative effect on increasing stem cells at the site of radiation injury is confirmed to some extent by Marx's [24] demonstration of increased cellular density in histologic preparations from patients who have received hyperbaric oxygen for mandibular osteoradionecrosis (ORN).

The impact of hyperbaric oxygen in terms of its beneficial effects is likely to involve all three of these mechanisms in irradiated tissues: HBO2 stimulates angiogenesis and secondarily improves tissue oxygenation; it reduces fibrosis; and it mobilizes and induces an increase of stem cells within irradiated tissues. Figure 12.5 is the treatment algorithm for Radiation necrosis with external wounds [27].

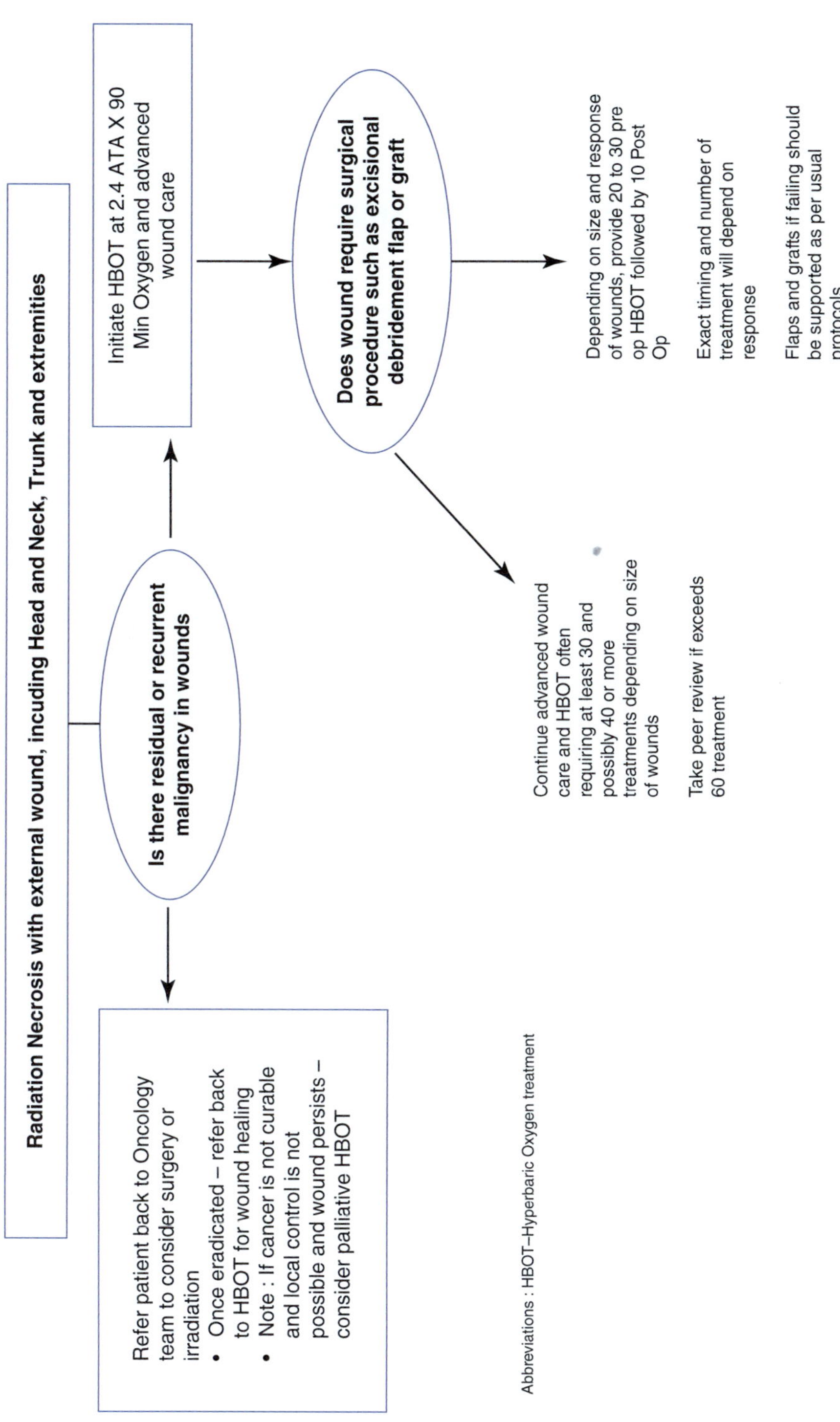

Fig. 12.5 Management of radiation induced wound with hyperbaric oxygen therapy

Hyperbaric oxygen has been applied as a therapy for delayed radiation injury for more than 30 years. Hyperbaric oxygen also has a frequent application in the prevention of mandibular ORN when dental extractions are required from heavily irradiated mandibles.

12.8 Potential Carcinogenesis with HBO2

A frequently expressed concern by those considering hyperbaric oxygen for a patient with radiation injury is the fear that hyperbaric oxygen will somehow accelerate malignant growth or cause a dormant malignancy to be reactivated.

In Marx's [24] very large group of patients treated with HBO2 for radiation injury of the mandible there was no increased likelihood of tumor recurrence or second tumor development. In 1994, Feldmeier and his colleagues reviewed the available literature related to this issue. An overwhelming majority of both clinical reports and animal studies reviewed in this paper showed no enhancement of cancer growth [28]. A small number of reports actually showed a decrease in growth or rates of metastases. Feldmeier updated this material for the Consensus Conference held in 2001, jointly sponsored by the European Society of Therapeutic Radiology and Oncology (ESTRO) and the European Committee for Hyperbaric Medicine (ECHM). In this update, Feldmeier emphasized the differences known in tumor and wound healing angiogenesis with similar but distinct processes operative in each case. He also showed that there are significant differences in the growth and inhibition factors, which modulate angiogenesis, in both circumstances [29].

He summarized the literature demonstrating that tumors that are hypoxic are less responsive to treatment, less subject to death by apoptosis, and more prone to aggressive growth and lethal metastases.

Most experienced practitioners of hyperbaric oxygen no longer fear that hyperbaric oxygen will promote malignant growth.

12.9 Risks and Contraindications

Hyperbaric oxygen therapy is a safe treatment modality with few serious adverse effects and contraindications (Fig. 12.6). Most adverse effects are minor and reversible. Patients may experience progressive myopia during treatment due to pressure-induced lens deformity, but this typically reverses within 6 weeks of treatment termination.

Hyperbaric oxygen therapy can also cause cataracts to mature more quickly but does not cause new cataract formation. Barotrauma to the ear and sinuses is another common adverse effect, particularly in older patient populations, but most cases are mild and reversible. Serious adverse effects of HBO2, resulting from oxygen toxicity, are seizures, congestive heart failure (CHF) exacerbation, pulmonary edema, and retinal changes, but these are rare. For example, reported incidences of grand

Minor Adverse Events
- Barotrauma to ears and sinuses
- Myopia
- Accelerated cataract maturation

Major Adverse Events
- Seizures
- Congestive heart failure (CHF) exacerbation
- Pulmonary edema
- Retinal changes

Relative Contraindications
- Febrile illness
- Seizure disorder
- Hyperthyroidism
- Congestive Heart Failure

Absolute Contraindication
- Pneumothorax

Fig. 12.6 Adverse events and contraindications of hyperbaric oxygen therapy

mal seizures following HBO2 range from 1 to 4 cases in 10,000 patient treatments. The most serious contraindication to HBO2 is an unrecognized and/or untreated pneumothorax, which would worsen under chamber pressure. Relative contraindications to HBO2 include febrile illness, which lowers the central nervous system seizure toxicity threshold, poorly controlled seizure disorder, and hyperthyroidism. Because oxygen is a vasoconstrictor, and HBO2 may increase cardiac afterload, CHF is also a relative contraindication for anyone with an ejection fraction of less than 30%.Other relative contradictions include patients with underlying pulmonary disease, such as chronic obstructive pulmonary disease, and severe claustrophobia [10].

12.10 Treatment Protocols

Treatment protocols vary depending on the severity of the problem and the type of hyperbaric chamber used. HBO2 treatments are delivered at 2–2.5 ATA (202.65–253.32 kPa) for 90 to 120 min of oxygen breathing once or twice daily. Patients with serious infections may require hospitalization for intravenous antibiotics, aggressive surgical intervention, and better diabetes control. For wound care, HBO treatment regimens consist of 20 to 40 treatments, and up to 60 treatments may be required .

HBO2 in some cases can be rendered twice daily until the condition stabilizes. Once stabilized, most of these patients are treated on a once daily basis as outpatients. HBO2 is an adjunctive therapy that depends on meticulous management of other comorbidities to the affected extremity. Infection control, optimized arterial blood flow, surgical debridement, offloading, and appropriate use of bioengineered tissue or surgical closure are mainstays of limb salvage therapy.

12.11 Cost Impact

Soft tissue and bony radiation necrosis are fortunately uncommon sequelae of therapeutic irradiation. By either avoiding surgery or supporting surgical healing, HBO2 therapy can significantly reduce the dollar and human costs of radiation complications. Marx accomplished a dollar cost estimate of the treatment of mandibular osteoradionecrosis [30]. In 1992 U.S. dollars, the cost of management is reduced from about $140,000 when HBO2 is not utilized to about $42,000 when HBO2 and surgery are combined in optimal fashion. Similar cost advantages are anticipated in the treatment of radiation injuries of other tissues.

12.12 Tips and Tricks to Prevent Complications

12.12.1 Predictors of Susceptibility to Radiation Injury

It is well known that there is a wide range of tolerance to radiation by different patients and that some patients are much more sensitive to radiation injury. If reliable predictors of delayed radiation injury were available during or before treatment, adjustments to the radiation-dosing scheme could be made for the radiosensitive patient. Some patients might be advised to seek alternative therapies instead of radiation. However as of now there are no well-defined parameters to predict.

In such patient prophylactic interventions such as hyperbaric oxygen or other yet-to-be-developed pharmacologic interventions could possibly be applied during the latent period but before the manifestation of the chronic injury. The hope and expectation would be that by identifying a group at risk and intervening in this group before manifestation of the injury, delayed radiation injury could be prevented or at least reduced in its severity.

Obviously, this postulate will have to be subjected to clinical trials, and the most important consideration is to do nothing that jeopardizes tumour control.

12.12.2 Hyperbaric Oxygen as Prophylaxis for Radiation Injury

A growing body of literature supports the use of HBO2 in the prevention of radiation injury, usually in the setting of surgery within an irradiated field where the likelihood of complications is very high.

The first published clinical report investigating prophylactic HBO2 is that by Marx where hyperbaric oxygen has been shown to decrease the incidence of mandibular osteoradionecrosis from 29.9% to 5.4% when a course of 20 daily HBO2 treatments was delivered prior to dental extractions from heavily irradiated mandibles. In this protocol, an additional 10 treatments are delivered after extractions to support tissue metabolic demands after surgical wounding. Marx has also reported the benefit of hyperbaric oxygen in the enhancement of osseointegration of dental implants in irradiated bone.

Feldmeier et al. have reported the utility of hyperbaric oxygen in preventing serious wound complications in patients with recurrent head and neck cancer who had salvage procedures including radical resection within irradiated fields. In that report, 87.5% of patients had prompt wound healing without complication whereas previous publications report up to a 60% incidence of serious complications in this setting without prophylactic HBO2 [31]. Pomeroy and his associates have reported their results in applying preoperative hyperbaric oxygen as an adjunct to surgery for soft tissue injuries of the pelvis. All five patients in this report had an uneventful postoperative course, although two of five required a second surgical procedure to resolve the radiation injury [32].

A promising area for clinical application will be the further definition of prophylactic hyperbaric oxygen in the prevention of radiation injury. The development of reliable biochemical predictors of radiation injury would permit the identification of the population at risk for development of radiation injury. At the present time, a reasonable approach is to provide adjunctive HBO2 when surgery is planned to occur in a heavily irradiated bed. The medical literature is consistent in demonstrating a high rate of serious complications and even death when radical surgical procedures are required in irradiated tissues without prophylactic HBO2 [33].

Third-party insurance carriers must be convinced that such prophylactic intervention is not only valuable for humanistic reasons but also for financial reasons. Hyperbaric oxygen in a preventative setting is likely to be more cost effective than a prolonged course of rehabilitation and reconstructive surgeries in a corrective fashion.

In summary, the use of hyperbaric oxygen prior to surgery in an irradiated field may prevent or decrease the incidence of catastrophic events such as wound breakdown with bony or hardware exposure, vascular rupture, infection, fistula formation, and/or flap loss and prevent further surgical intervention in an already compromised patient.

12.13 Conclusions

Hyperbaric oxygen therapy has been in medical use for half a century. Its mechanisms of action in the healing of chronic wounds include promoting neovascularization and decreasing inflammation. Clinical studies have demonstrated its efficacy in treating various conditions, and it is currently used for 14 different indications.

Radiation induces endarteritis obliterans and fibrosis and leads to delayed healing of wounds. These respond well to the use of Hyperbaric Oxygen therapy.

There is also a role of Hyperbaric Oxygen as a prophylactic in patients undergoing Surgery in previously irradiated tissue especially if the patient is immune compromised due to other comorbidities such as advanced age, diabetes etc..

12.14 Case Reports

12.14.1 Case Report 1

54 year lady with no known comorbidity referred for hyperbaric oxygen for a non healing ulcer in the Right Axilla of 2 years duration post radiation treatment. HBO2 was combined with standard treatment of debridement's, dressings and antibiotics (Fig. 12.7).

12.14.2 Case Report 2

58 year old male with history of Ca Prostate and spine metastasis treated with Radiation and developed non healing radiation ulcer and referred for HBO2 (Fig. 12.8).

Ten Key Points

1. The goal of radiation therapy is to eradicate residual tumour tissue with minimal, if any, adverse effects. However despite all preventive measures damage may occur. This leads often, to painful and disabling conditions. Conventional treatment of these lesions often has frustrating results.

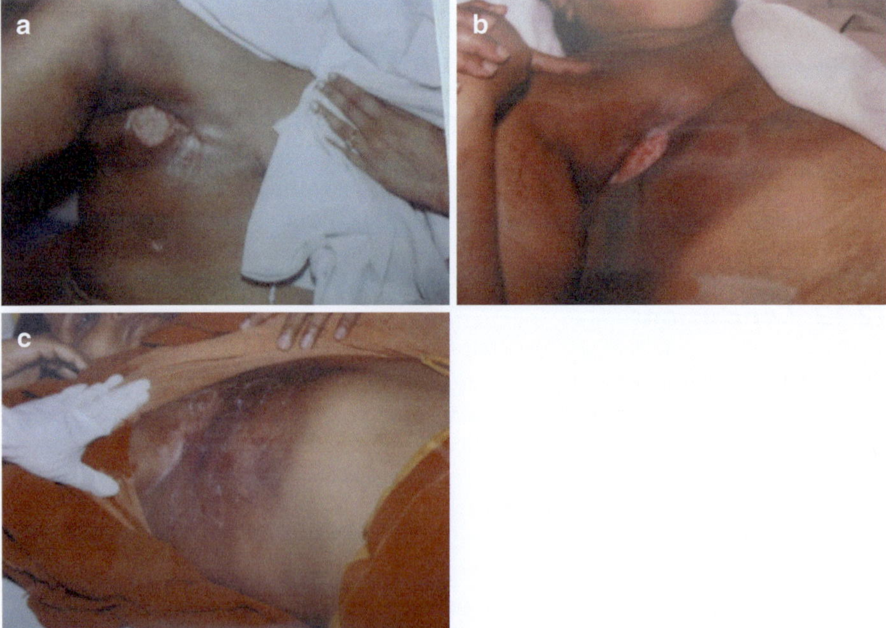

Fig. 12.7 (**a**) Day 0 of HBO2 showing pale wound base. (**b**) Day 10 of HBOT showing health granulation tissue. (**c**) Day 25 of HBO2 showing complete healing

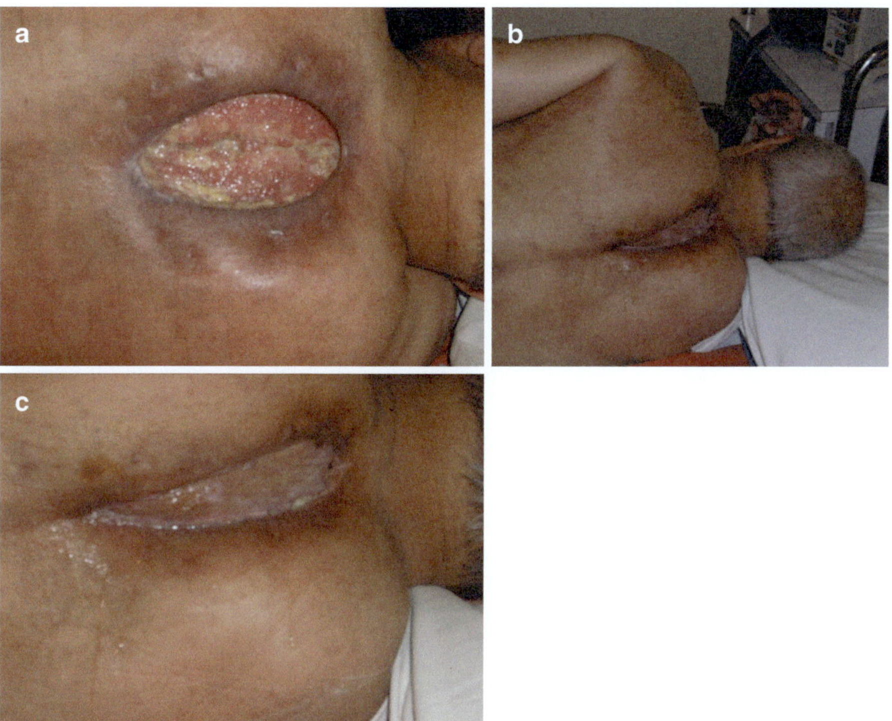

Fig. 12.8 (**a**) Day 10 of HBOT showing gaping non healing wound with healthy granulation. (**b**) Day 15 of HBOT showing graft in place over the wound. (**c**) Day 30 of HBOT showing complete healing of the graft

2. The delayed effects of radiation can cause significant morbidity which may occur months or years after treatment. Management is often difficult and unsatisfactory. Surgical wounds heal poorly in previously irradiated tissues. This is compounded if the patient has other comorbidities.
3. Because a dominant feature of post-radiation change is the obliteration of small blood vessels leading to hypoxia, and fibrosis, hyperbaric oxygen has been employed in the care of these patients. Hyperbaric oxygen helps reduce morbidity, disfiguring sequelae and further need for corrective surgery.
4. The impact of hyperbaric oxygen in terms of its beneficial effects is likely to involve all three of these mechanisms in irradiated tissues: HBO2 stimulates angiogenesis and secondarily improves tissue oxygenation; it reduces fibrosis; and it mobilizes and induces an increase of stem cells within irradiated tissues.
5. Hyperbaric oxygen therapy is a treatment in which patients breathe 100% oxygen while inside a pressurized hyperbaric chamber.
6. For wound care, HBO treatment regimens consist of 1.5 to 2 h per treatment for 20 to 40 treatments, and up to 60 treatments if needed.
7. The Undersea and Hyperbaric Medical Society maintains an evidence-based list of indications for HBO2; there are currently 14 indications. These 14 indi-

cations include arterial insufficiency wounds (i.e., ischemic diabetic ulcers), delayed radiation injury (i.e., to the soft tissue, osteoradionecrosis, cystitis, Proctitis), and chronic refractory osteomyelitis.

8. Common and reversible adverse effects of HBO2 include barotrauma to the ear and myopia. Serious adverse events are rare but include seizures, CHF exacerbation, pulmonary edema, and retinal changes. Untreated pneumothorax is an absolute contraindication to HBO2.
9. Evidence demonstrated that Hyperbaric Oxygen does not accelerate malignant growth or cause a dormant malignancy to be reactivated.
10. Hyperbaric Oxygen is a cost effective treatment for reducing mortality and morbidity in patients with radiation induced wounds in any area of the body and should be used as an adjunct to standard line of treatment with antibiotics and surgical debridement's.

References

1. Thun MJ, DeLancey JO, Center MM, Jemal A, Ward EM. The global burden of cancer: priorities for prevention. Carcinogenesis. 2010;31(1):100–10.
2. Sahni T, Jain M, Hukku S, Jadhav GK. Role of hyperbaric oxygen in oncology and radiation induced tissue damage. Apollo Med. 2004;1:P186–9.
3. Hayes NS, Hohman K, Vinson C, Pratt-Chapman M. Comprehensive cancer control in the U.S.: summarizing twenty years of progress and looking ahead. Cancer Causes Control. 2018;29(12):1305–9.
4. Barton MB, Jacob S, Shafiq J, Wong K, Thompson SR, Hanna TP, Delaney GP. Estimating the demand for radiotherapy from the evidence: a review of changes from 2003 to 2012. Radiother Oncol. 2014;112(1):140–4.
5. Rubin P, Casarrett GW. Clinical radiation pathology, vol. I. Philadelphia: WB Saunders; 1968. p. 58–61.
6. Dorr W, Hendry H. Consequential late effects in normal tissues. Radiother Oncol. 2001;61:223–31.
7. Carl UM, Hartmann KA. Hyperbaric oxygen treatment for symptomatic breast edema after radiation therapy. Undersea Hyperb Med. 1998;25:233–4.
8. Fleckenstein K, Gauter-Fleckenstein B, Jackson IL, Rabbani Z, Anscher M, Vujaskovic Z. Using biological markers to predict risk of radiation injury. Semin Radiat Oncol. 2007;17:89–98.
9. Trott KR. Chronic damage after radiation therapy: challenge to radiation biology. Int J Radiat Oncol Biol Phys. 1984;10:907–13.
10. Greti L, Rocky F, Frank LR, Chiu ES. Hyperbaric oxygen therapy: exploring the clinical evidence. Adv Skin Wound Care. 2017;30(4):181–90.
11. Demidova-Rice TN, Hamblin MR, Herman IM. Acute and impaired wound healing: pathophysiology and current methods for drug delivery, part 1: normal and chronic wounds: biology, causes, and approaches to care. Adv Skin Wound Care. 2012;25:304–14.
12. Reinke JM, Sorg H. Wound repair and regeneration. Eur Surg Res. 2012;49:35–43.
13. Stavrou D. Neovascularization in wound healing. J Wound Care. 2008;17:298–300.
14. Scheffler A, Rieger H. Clinical information content of transcutaneous oxymetry (PtcO2) in peripheral arterial occlusive disease (a review of the methodological and clinical literature with a special reference to critical limb ischemia). Vasa. 1992;21:111–26.
15. Sheffield PJ. Measuring tissue oxygen tension: a review. Undersea Hyperb Med. 1998;25:179–88.

16. Fife CE, Smart DR, Sheffield PJ, Hopf HW, Hawkins G, Clarke D. Transcutaneous oximetry in practice: consensus statements from an expert panel based on evidence. Undersea Hyperb Med. 2009;36(1):43–53.
17. Löndahl M, Katzman P, Hammarlund C, Nilsson A, Landin-Olsson M. Relationship between ulcer healing after hyperbaric oxygen therapy and transcutaneous oximetry, toe blood pressure and ankle-brachial index in patients with diabetes and chronic foot ulcers. Diabetologia. 2011;54(1):65–8.
18. Pecoraro RE, Ahroni JH, Boyko EJ, Stensel VL. Chronology and determinants of tissue repair in diabetic lower—extremity ulcers. Diabetes. 1991;40:1305–13.
19. Worth ER, Tettelbach WH, Harriet W. Arterial insufficiencies: enhancement of healing in selected problem wounds. In: Hyperbaric oxygen therapy indications. 13th ed. Undersea and Hyperbaric Medical Society; 2014. p. 52–8.
20. Howard MA, Asmis R, Evans KK, Mustoe TA. Oxygen and wound care: a review of current therapeutic modalities and future direction. Wound Repair Regen. 2013;21:503–11.
21. Thom SR. Hyperbaric oxygen: its mechanisms and efficacy. Plast Reconstr Surg. 2011;127(Suppl 1):131S–41S.
22. Ruzicka J, Dejmek J, Bolek L, Benes J, Kuncova J. Hyperbaric oxygen influences chronic wound healing—a cellular level review. Physiol Res. 2021;70(Suppl. 3):S261–73.
23. Marx RE, Ehler WJ, Tayapongsak P, Pierce LW. Relationship of oxygen dose to angiogenesis induction in irradiated tissue. Am J Surg. 1990;160:519–24.
24. Marx RE. Radiation injury to tissue. In: Kindwall EP, editor. Hyperbaric medicine practice. 2nd ed. Flagstaff: Best Publishing Co.; 1999. p. 665–723.
25. Feldmeier JJ, Jelen I, Davolt DA, Valente PT, Meltz ML, Alecu R. Hyperbaric oxygen as a prophylaxis for radiation induced delayed enteropathy. Radiother Oncol. 1995;35:138–44.
26. Goldstein LJ, Gallagher KA, Bauer SM, et al. Endothelial progenitor cell release into circulation is triggered by hyperoxia-induced increases in bone marrow nitric oxide. Stem Cells. 2006;24:2309–18.
27. Feldmeir JJ, Gesell LBG. Delayed radiation injuries Chapter 8. In: Hyperbaric oxygen therapy indications. 14th ed. Undersea and Hyperbaric Medicine Society; 2019. p. 163–93.
28. Feldmeier JJ, Heimbach RD, Davolt DA, Brakora MJ, Sheffield PJ, Porter AT. Does hyperbaric oxygen have a cancer causing or promoting effect? A review of the pertinent literature. Undersea Hyperb Med. 1994;21:467–75.
29. Feldmeier JJ. Hyperbaric oxygen: does it have a cancer causing or growth enhancing effect. In: Proceedings of the consensus conference sponsored by the European society for therapeutic radiology and oncology and the European Committee for hyperbaric medicine. Portugal; 2001. p. 129–146.
30. Vudiniabola S, Pirone C, Williamson J, Goss AN. Hyperbaric oxygen in the prevention of osteoradionecrosis of the jaws. Aust Dent J. 1999;44(4):243–7.
31. Feldmeier JJ, Newman R, Davolt DA, Heimbach RD, Newman NK, Hernandez LC. Prophylactic hyperbaric oxygen for patients undergoing salvage for recurrent head and neck cancers following full course irradiation (abstract). Undersea Hyper Med. 1998;25(Suppl):10.
32. Pomeroy BD, Keim LW, Taylor RJ. Preoperative hyperbaric oxygen therapy for radiation induced injuries. J Urol. 1998;159:1630–2.
33. Neovius EB, Lind MG, Lind FG. Hyperbaric oxygen for wound complications after surgery in the irradiated head and neck: a review of the literature and a report of 15 consecutive cases. Head Neck. 1997;19:315–22.

Prevention and Management of Aspiration Pneumonitis in Patients Undergoing Radiotherapy for Head and Neck Malignancies

13

Kundan Singh Chufal, Irfan Ahmad, Muhammed Ismail Sharief, and Rahul Lal Choudhary

13.1 Introduction

Aspiration pneumonia (AsP) is a common complication among cancer patients, causing significant morbidity [1, 2]. The reported incidence rates vary based on the underlying tumor location and treatment modality [3–5]. In head and neck cancer patients treated with concurrent chemoradiation, incidence rates for AsP range widely and are frequently under-reported [3–8]. Higher rates tend to be associated with tumors originating from the hypopharynx or nasopharynx compared to other head and neck (HNC) sites [2, 7]. Precise figures remain difficult to ascertain given the challenges in diagnosing subclinical or "silent" aspiration events [9].

In general, pneumonia is an inflammation of the alveoli and the surrounding tissue, usually caused by bacteria and classified based on the setting in which it is acquired or the presumed etiology (Fig. 13.1) [1, 10, 11]. Aspiration Pneumonitis (Mendelson's syndrome; originally described in 1946 as a frequent occurrence during obstetric anesthesia) occurs when sterile gastric contents are inhaled, leading to acute lung injury [12]. In contrast, AsP involves inhaling colonized oropharyngeal material, causing an acute bacterial inflammatory response [13]. This condition is

K. S. Chufal (✉) · I. Ahmad
Department of Radiation Oncology, Rajiv Gandhi Cancer Institute & Research Centre, New Delhi, India

M. I. Sharief
Department of Radiation Oncology, American Oncology Institute, Jalandhar, Punjab, India

R. L. Choudhary
Department of Radiation Oncology, Malnad Hospital & Institute of Oncology, Shimoga, Karnataka, India

K. Sood Sharma et al. (eds.), *Complications of Cancer Therapy: Best Practices in Prevention and Management*, https://doi.org/10.1007/978-981-99-0984-1_13

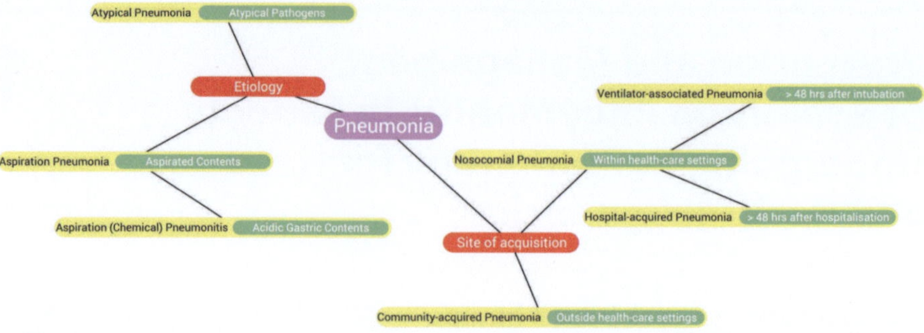

Fig. 13.1 Classification of Pneumonia based on etiology and site of acquisition

more common in elderly individuals with swallowing difficulties or gastric dysmotility. While Aspiration Pneumonitis initially presents with sterile bacteriologic findings, AsP is associated with various bacteria, including gram-positive cocci and gram-negative rods [1, 10, 14].

As their names suggest, the common precursor of both aspiration pneumonitis and pneumonia is the occurrence of aspiration, which is in itself a multifactorial, anatomically defined event, often preceded by a phase of swallowing dysfunction [15–17].

13.1.1 Swallowing Dysfunction: The Link Between HNC, Its Treatment and AsP

Swallowing dysfunction is common among patients with HNC at diagnosis [18, 19]. Decreased base of the tongue and posterior pharyngeal contraction due to involvement by the disease impairs the food bolus transport through the pharynx, and chemoradiotherapy may lead to further deterioration in swallowing function [20]. The function of swallowing muscles before radiation and the radiation dose they receive has been established as the causal link between radiotherapy and AsP [21]. The radiotherapy dose received by DARS has also been shown to be associated with a higher risk of malnutrition and tube-feeding dependence, resulting in inferior health-related quality of life (HRQoL) [22, 23].

13.1.2 AsP in HNC Patients: Problem Statement

Since HNC constitutes a significant proportion of the cancer burden in lower- and middle-income countries and most patients present to oncology clinics in a locally advanced stage, concurrent chemoradiotherapy is often the treatment modality used to treat them [24–26]. The inherent swallowing dysfunction associated with HNC, combined with chemoradiotherapy, increases the risk of AsP [3, 18, 19, 27].

Specifically, AsP after radiation is likely caused by a combination of contributing factors, including acute and chronic radiation-induced mucosal changes, muscle fibrosis, and xerostomia, making swallowing difficult and dysfunctional.

The incidence of AsP reported in the literature ranges from 5% to 47%, with a mortality rate of up to 32% [5, 28–31]. In a post-hoc analysis of a phase 3 trial in HNC, out of 536 patients, 28.3% developed AsP, and the median time to its development after initiating chemoradiation was 39 days [32]. In a SEER database analysis of 3513 HNC patients, 22.8% developed AsP with a median time of 5 months from treatment initiation [29].

As a late effect, the risk of AsP associated with dysphagia remains a concern, as highlighted by the findings of a longitudinal cohort study [33]. After 6 years of follow-up, up to 71% of long-term survivors had persistent swallowing difficulties, 28% had a history of chest infection requiring antibiotics in the preceding 2 years, and 22% had silent aspiration.

13.1.3 Classification of AsP After Radiotherapy

AsP after radiation can be further classified as an acute and chronic condition. AsP diagnosed during or within 6 weeks of treatment is acute, and if developing 6 weeks or more after treatment completion is labeled as chronic. Acute AsP leads to gaps in chemoradiotherapy, resulting in poorer oncological outcomes [34]. It is the consequence of treating patients who already have an advanced degree of swallowing dysfunction prior to treatment [28].

Chronic AsP is a late effect seen after radiotherapy, a direct consequence of chronic edema and increased fibroblast proliferation leading to the overproduction of collagen, causing scarring and fibrosis [35, 36]. Tissues lose their elasticity, and the swallowing musculature becomes atrophic and loses strength, leading to altered oropharyngeal anatomical relationships and restricting the complex interplay of movements for adequate swallowing [37, 38]. This is further complicated by sensory impairment (which blunts the cough response) and infrequently lower cranial nerve palsies (CN IX, X, and XII) (due to compression or direct nerve damage) [39, 40].

13.1.4 Importance from the Radiation Oncologist's Perspective

From the perspective of a radiation oncologist, AsP represents a particularly concerning complication of chemoradiation therapy for head and neck cancers. Aspiration events often necessitate treatment delays or interruptions which can compromise tumor control and cure rates [34]. AsP contributes to increased length of hospital stays, escalations in care, use of intravenous antibiotics, and overall financial toxicity. Therefore, understanding predisposing risk factors and implementing preventive measures are paramount for the radiation oncologist treating head and neck malignancies.

13.2 Pathophysiology of Aspiration Pneumonia and Pneumonitis

13.2.1 Mechanism of Swallowing

Swallowing is a coordinated process that swiftly moves food into the digestive tract, involving voluntary and reflexive actions [41–43]. Initially, during the voluntary oral preparatory phase, the tongue, primarily through the action of intrinsic muscles and the powerful genioglossus muscles, shapes the food into a bolus [44]. As this bolus is moved towards the back of the mouth, it triggers pressure receptors at the base of the tongue and pharyngeal arches, initiating the involuntary pharyngeal phase of swallowing [45, 46]. The key movement of the reflexive phase is the hyolaryngeal elevation (HLE), which is an upward and forward motion of the hyoid bone and larynx, leading to the closure of the laryngeal entrance and allowing the bolus to move into the esophagus [47–49].

Swallowing muscles are grouped into Functional Swallowing Units (FSUs) based on function and location [27, 50]. Four primary FSUs drive HLE:

1. Floor of Mouth (FOM) (Geniohyoid, Anterior Digastric & Mylohyoid muscles)
2. Posterior Digastric/Stylohoid muscles (PDS)
3. Longitudinal Pharyngeal Muscles (LPM) (Palatopharyngeus, Salpingopharyngeus, Stylopharyngeus muscles)
4. Thyrohyoid muscle (THM)

The FOM and PDS create the anterior sling, and the LPM forms the posterior sling (assisted by the THM). The anterior sling facilitates the upward and forward movement of the hyoid and larynx, while the posterior sling and THM elevate the larynx towards the hyoid [51]. Since many of these muscles get unintentionally affected during Head and Neck Cancer (HNC) treatment, it disrupts the pharyngeal swallowing phase, increasing the risk of aspiration [21].

13.2.2 Mechanism of Aspiration

The pathophysiologic mechanism of AsP first involves the entry of foreign materials [1, 10]. The lack of adequate shunting of the food bolus around the larynx, pharyngeal stasis, poor hypopharyngeal transit, and loss of supraglottic and glottic sensation all play a role in permitting aspiration, with the final two factors ultimately permitting food entry into the lower respiratory tract [52, 53]. If impaired, the final critical pathway, which is the reflexive closure of the true and false vocal cords, ultimately allows foreign materials to descend past the cords into the trachea and main bronchi, setting in motion the inflammatory reaction and subsequent lung parenchymal damage [1].

13.2.3 Commonly Aspirated Materials

Typical materials aspirated into the lung include saliva, gastric acid, foods and fluids, and oral bacteria inhabiting the oropharynx and gingiva [1, 10, 14]. Gastric contents are particularly damaging when aspirated due to its highly acidic pH, which can cause caustic burns to the bronchial mucosa [10]. Additional sources of aspirated material in cancer patients are secretions and/or blood from ulcerated tumors.

13.2.4 Pulmonary Reactions to Aspiration

Pre-clinical studies have played a pivotal role in exploring the pathophysiology of aspiration pneumonitis [54, 55]. These studies used the intratracheal installation of acid, demonstrating that contents with a pH of 2.5 or lower and a substantial volume (usually 1–4 mL/kg) cause chemical pneumonitis. Translated to adult humans, this amounts to at least 70 mL of gastric acid. Smaller volumes may lead to milder or undetected forms of pneumonitis, and in that clinical context, patients with gastroesophageal reflux disease (GERD) have been observed to experience recurrent bouts of pneumonitis, potentially progressing to pulmonary fibrosis [56, 57].

Once aspirated, foreign particulates initiate an inflammatory response in the lung parenchyma, leading to edema, hemorrhage, and necrosis of the bronchial mucosa [54]. Bacterial proliferation frequently follows (up to 25%), causing infectious pneumonia superimposed on the chemical injury [58, 59]. Neutrophil recruitment and activation release proteases and reactive oxygen species, exacerbating tissue damage [60]. Outcomes range from acute exudative pneumonitis to abscess formation or chronic pulmonary fibrosis. Similar findings have been confirmed in human autopsy cases of fatal aspiration pneumonitis, with the presumed mechanism attributed to the release of proinflammatory cytokines, such as TNF-alpha and IL-8 [61].

13.3 Risk Factors for AsP

Risk factors for AsP can be classified under three broad headings (Fig. 13.2).

13.3.1 General Risk Factors

Several factors universally predispose patients to an increased risk of AsP. These include advanced age, sedative use, poor dental health, smoking, alcoholism, and loss of consciousness [62–64]. Critically ill patients are particularly susceptible [65].

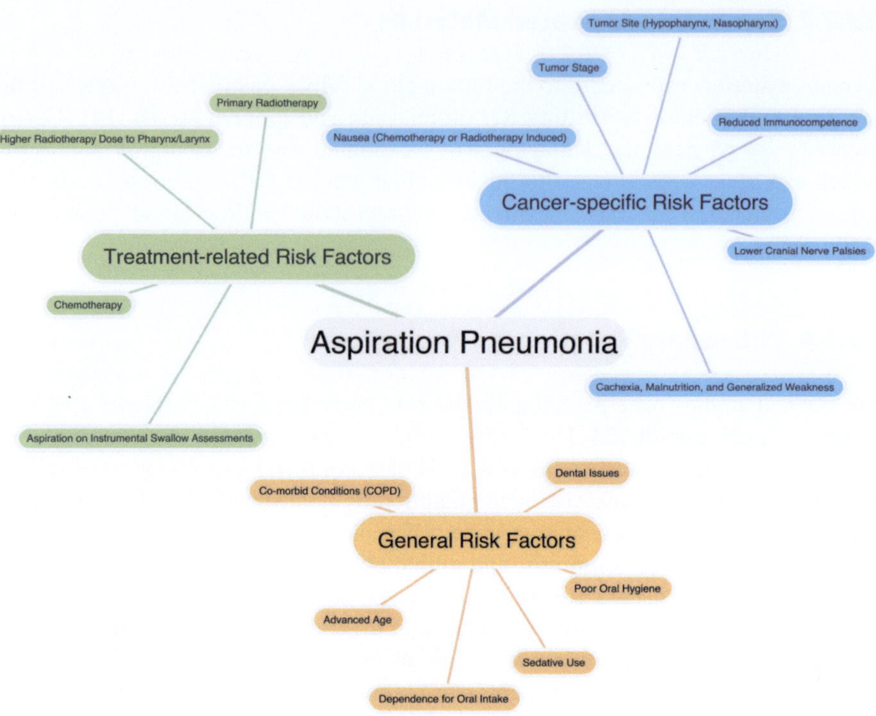

Fig. 13.2 Risk factors for AsP

13.3.2 Cancer-Specific Factors

Head and neck cancer patients possess additional risk factors imparted by direct tumor effects on regional anatomy. Bulky lesions obstructing vital swallowing structures like the larynx, pharynx, tongue base, and esophagus lead to dysphagia and impaired airway protection [3, 27]. Perineural invasion can cause cranial neuropathies affecting the cranial nerves IX, X, and XII, further compromising the swallowing mechanism [39]. Cachexia, malnutrition, and generalized weakness increase fatigue and incoordination during feeding [66]. Nausea from chemotherapy or radiotherapy may also contribute. Immune suppression secondary to alcohol intake (a frequently associated risk factor for HNC) and chemoradiotherapy render these patients more susceptible to infections when aspiration occurs [67].

13.3.3 Treatment-Related Factors

Cancer treatment modalities exacerbate dysfunction of the intricate muscles involved in swallowing, airway protection, and precise upper aerodigestive tract coordination [19, 21]. Details are provided elsewhere in this book. Specifically, dose-escalated radiotherapy leads to fibrosis, edema, neuropathy, and xerostomia, predisposing patients to AsP [22].

13.4 Clinical Presentation and Diagnosis

In AsP, the initial symptoms and findings can differ widely. This variation depends on the timing of the patient's examination relative to the infection's course, the type of bacteria involved, and the host's condition [1, 10, 11, 14]. Most patients exhibit standard symptoms of pneumonia, including cough, fever, purulent sputum, and shortness of breath [13]. Unlike most cases of community-acquired pneumonia, AsP involving anaerobes often develops more gradually [65]. Fever is common, but rigors and chills are typically absent. Hospital-acquired AsP frequently involves bacteria such as *S. aureus* or gram-negative bacilli, often found in hospitalized patients' oral cavities [63].

Distinct clinical features of bacterial AsP include:

1. Gradual symptom onset and lack of rigors.
2. Foul-smelling sputum, indicative of anaerobic infection, though not excluding aerobic pathogens.
3. Diffuse crackles or wheezes on lung auscultation.

The diagnostic evaluation of bacterial AsP focuses on patients showing new or worsening respiratory difficulties after an aspiration event or those at risk of aspiration. Considerations include:

1. History: Coughing during eating or drinking can suggest aspiration, although it may also be silent.
2. Microbiologic studies: Depending on the illness's severity, similar to community-acquired pneumonia, studies are obtained, including blood cultures, sputum Gram stain, and culture for hospitalized patients.
3. For most non-critically ill hospitalized patients, sputum studies are usually sufficient, with bronchoscopy for those needing mechanical ventilation.
4. Thoracentesis may be needed if parapneumonic pleural fluid is detected on clinical examination or imaging.
5. Procalcitonin: Not a reliable marker for determining bacterial lung infection post-aspiration [68].

The only differentiating clinical feature of aspiration pneumonitis versus bacterial AsP is the sudden onset of symptoms.

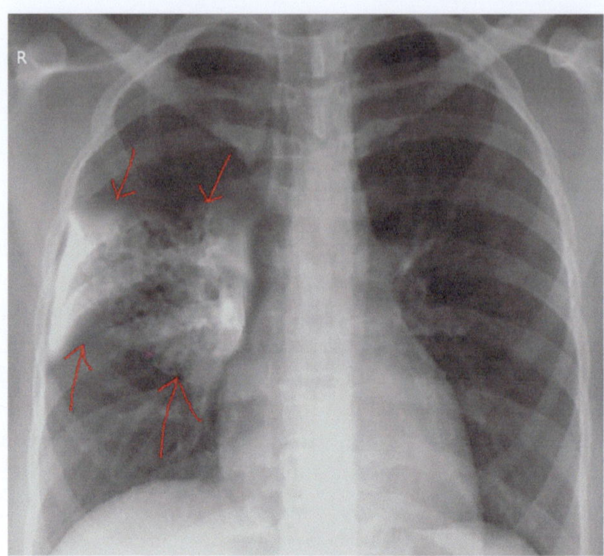

Fig. 13.3 Aspiration Pneumonia (Image courtesy O.Chaigasame. Obtained by a CC BY-NC-ND 4.0 license from Sanivarapu RR, Gibson J. Aspiration Pneumonia. (Updated 2023 May 8). In: StatPearls [Internet]. Treasure Island, FL: StatPearls Publishing; 2023 Jan. Available from: https://www.ncbi.nlm.nih.gov/books/NBK470459/) (Image unaltered)

13.4.1 Imaging Findings

Chest radiography (CXR) represents the most routine initial imaging modality to discern features consistent with AsP from alternative diagnoses. Findings classically include basilar-predominant patchy or confluent airspace opacities due to the gravity-dependent distribution deeper within lung segments (Fig. 13.3) [69]. Air bronchograms are often present within areas of consolidation. Pleural effusions frequently occur as a secondary inflammatory phenomenon. A CXR may be negative early on, but chest computed tomography (CT) scans can identify or exclude pneumonia, and they play a vital role in evaluating abscesses and pleural disease, including empyema [70]. As such, CT is more sensitive and provides superior pulmonary parenchymal and airway detail. It also better depicts fat stranding in the bronchi and multifocal ground-glass or tree-in-bud opacities suggestive of aspiration [71].

13.4.2 Role of the Radiation Oncologist

The radiation oncologist plays a vital role in promptly recognizing and having a high clinical suspicion for AsP in cancer patients undergoing concurrent chemoradiation therapy based on the acute development of suggestive symptoms, focused physical exam maneuvers tailored toward swallowing and respiration, and familiarity with characteristic imaging findings described above. The complex multisystem sequelae of chemoradiation, asthma, COPD, pulmonary embolism, radiation pneumonitis, and cardiogenic pulmonary edema are important in the differential diagnosis. Early engagement of medical oncology, pulmonary medicine, and critical care services is crucial.

13.5 Prevention Strategies: Modern RT Planning

Swallowing dysfunction is the causal link between HNC, its treatment, and AsP [19, 21, 22]. Covered in more detail elsewhere, a summary is vital to provide context on arguably the single most important preventable factor for AsP.

Delineation Guidelines for the organs at risk (OARs) involved in swallowing have been developed and can be contoured during RT planning [72–74]. The guidelines cover the larynx, pharyngeal constrictor muscles, cricopharyngeus muscles, esophageal inlet muscles, and the base of the tongue. Once delineated Dysphagia-Sparing Radiotherapy Techniques using Intensity-modulated radiotherapy (IMRT) allow for highly conformal dose distributions with rapid dose fall-off, thereby selectively reducing doses to the swallowing OARs [17, 75–77]. Reducing mean doses to these structures appears more consistent than using dose-volume constraints based on existing data [78]. Adaptive replanning during treatment may further enhance OAR sparing.

The collective evidence from prospective trials demonstrates the potential benefits of Dysphagia-Sparing IMRT in improving swallowing function and possibly lowering AsP risk in head and neck cancer patients. Additional studies are needed to confirm the magnitude of this potential impact.

13.5.1 Phase 2 Trials

Two separate single-arm phase 2 trials were conducted without randomization or control groups. Feng et al. enrolled 73 patients with stage III-IV oropharyngeal cancer, treating them with definitive chemoradiotherapy [79]. In contrast, Schwartz et al. enrolled 31 patients with the same cancer stage, treating them with definitive chemoradiotherapy but using a split-field Intensity Modulated Radiation Therapy (IMRT) technique [80]. Both trials focused on sparing specific structures. Feng et al. aimed to spare the medial retropharyngeal lymph nodes, with dose constraints set at less than 50 Gy mean dose for partial volumes of PCM and SGL in the targeted region. Schwartz et al. spared the oral cavity and superior PCM using a split-field IMRT technique, with dose constraints of 30–40 Gy to the oral cavity and less than 50 Gy to the superior PCM.

Additionally, a larynx block was employed to spare the larynx. The outcomes were promising. Feng et al. achieved mean doses of 48 Gy to spare PCM and 42 Gy to spare SGL. Swallowing outcomes only slightly deteriorated compared to baseline, and no local recurrences were observed. On the other hand, Schwartz et al. reported a significantly lower 4% aspiration rate compared to historical rates exceeding 40%, with the locoregional control rate being 100% at 2 years. Both studies concluded that sparing PCM and SGL through IMRT is feasible and safe without any increased risk of recurrence. Swallowing outcomes improved compared to historical data, suggesting the possibility of reducing dysphagia.

Strengths:

1. Demonstrated feasibility of dysphagia-sparing IMRT techniques
2. Showed promising results in terms of reduced aspiration rates and improved swallowing outcomes
3. Provided initial prospective evidence that sparing swallowing structures with IMRT is safe and does not increase recurrence risk

Weaknesses:

1. Small sample sizes
2. Lack of control or comparison group
3. Limited follow-up time
4. Single institution experiences
5. Potential bias without blinded assessments

13.5.2 The DARS Phase 3 Randomized Trial

The DARS trial furthered the phase 2 studies and randomized 112 patients diagnosed with oropharyngeal or hypopharyngeal cancer into two arms: standard IMRT (control) and dysphagia-optimized IMRT (DO-IMRT) [81]. The primary endpoint was the MD Anderson Dysphagia Inventory (MDADI) score at 12 months, with patients and speech therapists masked to treatment allocation. In this phase 3 trial, the superior/middle and inferior PCM were delineated as organs at risk. Specifically, for the DO-IMRT arm, mean dose constraints of less than 50 Gy were applied to PCM outside the high-dose Clinical Target Volume (CTV). IMRT optimization was performed to meet these constraints. The DARS trial achieved a significant reduction in mean PCM doses with DO-IMRT. Patients receiving DO-IMRT reported significantly higher MDADI scores at 12 months than those on standard IMRT. Additional patient-reported and clinician-reported secondary endpoints also favored DO-IMRT. Improving mean PCM dose with DO-IMRT led to better swallowing outcomes, and DO-IMRT emerged as a new standard of care for pharyngeal cancer patients receiving IMRT.

Although the DARS trial did not specifically report on AsP outcomes, inferences can be made. DO-IMRT's reduction of dysphagia is expected to decrease the risk of aspiration events, and the significant improvements in swallowing outcomes suggest likely reductions in aspiration frequency and related complications. However, the trial was not designed to compare AsP rates directly, and further studies with objective assessments like videofluoroscopy are required.

Strengths:

1. Randomized, controlled trial design
2. Adequate sample size to detect differences in the primary outcome
3. Multicenter trial—increasing generalizability
4. Blinded speech therapist assessments
5. Multiple swallowing outcome measures
6. Mature follow-up time of 3+ years

Weaknesses:

1. Lack of pre-treatment swallowing assessments
2. The primary outcome is patient-reported rather than objective measures
3. Limited to primarily oropharyngeal cancer patients
4. Prophylactic swallowing exercises not standardized across centers

13.6 Prevention Strategies: General Measures

13.6.1 Surveillance Protocols

During routine follow-up visits after chemoradiation, radiation oncologists should maintain vigilance and a low threshold to screen for subtle symptoms or signs potentially attributable to evolving dysphagia and aspiration risk. A few risk factors are associated with a decreased time to aspiration pneumonia, which are: male sex; hypopharynx and nasopharynx primary sites; radiotherapy ± chemotherapy vs. surgery alone; surgery followed by chemoradiotherapy vs. surgery alone, and reirradiation [29]. Contrary to expectations, placement of gastrostomy or jejunostomy feeding tubes does not reduce the risk of AsP [82]. Prophylactic metoclopramide and domperidone have shown benefit in preventing AsP in patients with neurological deficits, but their utility in HNC patients is currently unknown [83, 84].

Evaluation starts with a thorough history of any new cough, change in voice or breathing, choking episodes, or swallowing difficulties. Formal swallowing assessments can be obtained for concerning symptoms [85]. Flexible laryngoscopy provides a valuable direct examination of laryngeal anatomy and function. Pulmonary imaging with a chest x-ray or CT should be obtained for any respiratory concerns to evaluate for new infiltrates. Late side effects such as esophageal strictures, pharyngeal fibrosis and scarring, laryngeal immobility, and generalized dysphagia or frank aspiration can manifest months to years after radiation as delayed effects [36]. Therefore, maintaining vigilance and repeat assessments for these late toxicities facilitates earlier interventions to optimize long-term swallowing outcomes and prevent aspiration.

13.6.2 Swallowing Assessments

Performing baseline videofluoroscopic or functional endoscopic evaluations of swallowing for dysphagia and airway protection deficits allows stratification of aspiration risk severity [85, 86]. Patients identified as high-risk can then undergo more intensive surveillance and management during therapy [87]. Additionally, serial monitoring assessments for signs of evolving swallowing impairment enables earlier detection and interventions before severe aspiration or pneumonia develops.

13.6.3 Nutritional Considerations

Optimization of nutrition prior to and during cancer treatment helps compensate for the catabolic state induced by malignancy and treatment, which directly contribute to debility and aspiration events [66]. Thickened liquids and pureed or minced foods (and alternating liquid/solid bolus swallows) are better tolerated by those with identified chewing and swallowing difficulties [88]. Coordinated care with a dietician and physiotherapist trained in addressing swallowing dysfunction may minimize the risk of aspiration [86].

13.6.4 Postural and Behavioural Modifications

Educating patients and their care providers on proper positioning, swallowing precautions, and pragmatic dietary adjustments provides a simple yet effective approach to reducing aspiration risk. Sitting upright with the chin tucked brings the oral cavity and pharynx into optimal alignment for gravity to assist swallowing and prevent the misdirection of food [89–92]. Taking small boluses and deliberate swallows instead of continuous eating gives the pharynx time to clear completely before the next bite. These pragmatic steps can significantly reduce aspiration if implemented consistently.

13.6.5 Patient's Perspective

Themes that have emerged from interviews with patients who underwent rehabilitation after HNC treatment were: patients valued having a supportive network of family, friends, peers, and healthcare staff during their recovery; they appreciated the expertise, empathy, communication skills, and holistic approach of the rehabilitation staff which provided reassurance; patients relied heavily on their own motivation and resilience in addition to support from others; receiving education tailored to their individual needs at each stage was important; and despite completing treatment, patients continue to experience distress about their diagnosis [93].

Oncologists treating HNC should ensure patients have access to peer support groups and psychological services to help address the significant emotional impacts of a cancer diagnosis and treatment [94]. Providing education tailored to each patient's needs at all stages of treatment and recovery is also critical to prepare patients for potential side effects and empower them to take an active role in their rehabilitation [95, 96]. All care team members should strive to provide compassionate, empathetic care focused on the whole patient, not just the disease. This includes strong communication skills, recognizing patients' resilience, and coordinating holistic care that goes beyond treating physiological symptoms [97].

13.7 Treatment Approaches

After a witnessed aspiration event, initial management involves patient positioning and airway suctioning to clear fluids and particulates. However, this does not reverse the chemical injury that occurs with acid aspiration. Moreover, most aspiration events do not occur in hospitals, and the patient (as well as their care providers) often cannot identify the event. Given that the patient then presents to the hospital after a significant delay, if AsP is clinically suspected, hospitalization for close monitoring should be considered, given the potential for rapid deterioration. Supportive measures, including supplemental oxygenation, intravascular fluid management, sputum clearance techniques like chest physiotherapy, and close trending of laboratory parameters, are critical adjuncts to antibiotic therapy (which may be instituted empirically, but consultation with a respiratory physician and infectious disease physician is strongly suggested; Fig. 13.4) [98]. The prognosis relates strongly to the number of comorbid conditions and severity of illness at presentation.

Aspiration pneumonitis due to gastric acid aspiration is managed supportively with oxygenation support and mechanical ventilation as needed. Corticosteroids are generally not routinely used as studies have not shown clear benefit [99]. Unless a secondary infection is imminent (based on a deteriorating clinical condition), prophylactic antibiotics are usually not recommended.

13.7.1 Multidisciplinary Approach

Close coordination between radiation, medical and surgical oncology services, chest physicians, infectious disease physicians, gastroenterology, speech pathology, nursing, and dedicated nutritional support forms a comprehensive multidisciplinary team needed to optimize outcomes and quality of life in this complex cohort. Patients developing recurrent AsP may require a tracheostomy as a significant proportion have absent cough reflexes [100].

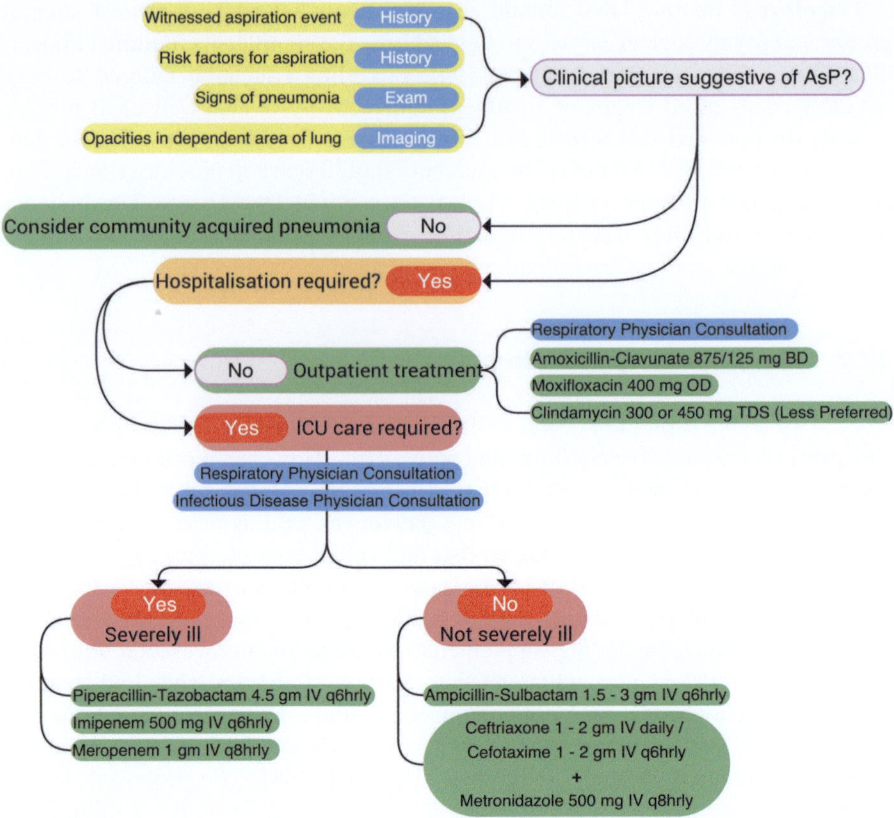

Fig. 13.4 Suggested risk assessment and management algorithm for bacterial AsP. Consideration should be given to local antibiotic resistance patterns; therefore, consultation with a respiratory and infectious disease physician is strongly recommended. An infectious disease physician should perform an additional risk assessment for *Pseudomonas* and MRSA

13.8 Complications

13.8.1 End-of-Life Considerations

In patients with end-stage cancer and poor functional status, AsP may represent a terminal complication warranting primarily comfort-directed care. The decision to pursue mainly palliative measures or continue more aggressive management requires careful discussion of prognosis and aligned care goals with patients and care providers. This includes judicious use of narcotics, benzodiazepines, and anxiolytics for dyspnea and anxiety. Hospice referral for end-of-life support is reasonable for appropriate patients.

13.9 Follow-Up and Surveillance

13.9.1 Monitoring for Recurrent Aspiration Pneumonia

Surveillance for recurrent or persistent AsP is similar to the initial diagnosis and requires continued meticulous symptom assessment at follow-up appointments. Repeat chest imaging can confirm resolution or identify radiographic signs concerning chronic aspiration injury. Sputum or bronchoscopy cultures also assist in differentiating persistent pneumonia from new events. Close collaboration with a respiratory physician is encouraged.

13.10 Future Directions and Research

13.10.1 Advances in Radiation Techniques

While conventional 2D radiation has essentially been replaced by 3D conformal and intensity-modulated approaches, continued research into emerging technologies such as proton beam therapy may further improve the sparing of critical swallowing anatomy and minimize dysphagia/aspiration risk [101]. However, clinical data remain limited, and large collaborative datasets and well-designed prospective trials are needed to validate any benefits in aspiration outcomes with proton therapy compared to modern photon techniques.

13.10.2 Future Research Directions

Other priority areas for ongoing research include studying the effectiveness of prophylactic swallowing therapy programs before cancer treatment and identifying patient and tumor factors associated with the highest post-treatment aspiration risk to target more intensive interventions. Cost-effectiveness studies analyzing prevention strategies are also lacking.

13.11 Conclusion

Aspiration pneumonia remains one of the most severe treatment-associated complications facing head and neck cancer patients undergoing chemoradiation therapy. Radiation oncologists are uniquely positioned to play vital multifaceted roles in mitigating aspiration risk through meticulous treatment planning focused on reducing the dose to dysphagia-related anatomy, maintaining vigilant surveillance for subtle symptoms during follow-up, providing prompt, coordinated care once diagnosed, and educating at-risk patients on preventive strategies.

Key Messages

1. Aspiration pneumonia is a common but under-reported complication of chemoradiotherapy for head and neck cancers
2. Dysphagia leading to aspiration events is the primary precursor
3. Radiation dose to swallowing anatomy links therapy to aspiration risk
4. Reducing the dose to swallowing structures via Intensity-modulated radiotherapy may lower the risk of AsP, though direct evidence is lacking
5. Additional prevention strategies include swallowing therapy, postural and dietary changes
6. Diagnosis requires high clinical suspicion and characteristic imaging findings
7. Supportive care and antibiotics are the mainstays of treatment. Guidance from pulmonologists, critical care specialists, and infectious disease physicians should be sought.
8. Radiation oncologists play vital roles from radiotherapy planning to surveillance, diagnosis, management, and care coordination.
9. Future research priorities include emerging radiation techniques like proton beam treatment.

References

1. Mandell LA, Niederman MS. Aspiration pneumonia. N Engl J Med. 2019;380:651–63. https://doi.org/10.1056/NEJMra1714562.
2. Reddy PD, Yan F, Nguyen SA, et al. Factors influencing the development of pneumonia in patients with head and neck cancer: a meta-analysis. Otolaryngol Neck Surg. 2021;164:234–43. https://doi.org/10.1177/0194599820938011.
3. Nguyen NP, Frank C, Moltz CC, et al. Aspiration rate following chemoradiation for head and neck cancer: an underreported occurrence. Radiother Oncol. 2006;80:302–6. https://doi.org/10.1016/j.radonc.2006.07.031.
4. Mortensen HR, Jensen K, Grau C. Aspiration pneumonia in patients treated with radiotherapy for head and neck cancer. Acta Oncol. 2013;52:270–6. https://doi.org/10.3109/0284186X.2012.742205.
5. Hunter KU, Lee OE, Lyden TH, et al. Aspiration pneumonia after chemo-intensity-modulated radiation therapy of oropharyngeal carcinoma and its clinical and dysphagia-related predictors: aspiration pneumonia after chemo-intensity-modulated radiation therapy. Head Neck. 2014;36:120–5. https://doi.org/10.1002/hed.23275.
6. Szczesniak MM, Maclean J, Zhang T, et al. Persistent dysphagia after head and neck radiotherapy: a common and under-reported complication with significant effect on non-cancer-related mortality. Clin Oncol. 2014;26:697–703. https://doi.org/10.1016/j.clon.2014.08.009.
7. Xiong J, Krishnaswamy G, Raynor S, et al. Risk of swallowing-related chest infections in patients with nasopharyngeal carcinoma treated with definitive intensity-modulated radiotherapy: risk of swallowing-related chest infections in NPC. Head Neck. 2016;38:E1660–5. https://doi.org/10.1002/hed.24296.
8. Motz K, Herbert RJ, Fakhry C, et al. Short- and long-term outcomes of oropharyngeal cancer care in the elderly: functional outcomes of oropharyngeal cancer care in the elderly. Laryngoscope. 2018;128:2084–93. https://doi.org/10.1002/lary.27153.

9. Smith HC. Cough and aspiration of food and liquids due to oral pharyngeal dysphagia. Lung. 2008;186:35–40. https://doi.org/10.1007/s00408-007-9064-4.
10. Marik PE. Aspiration pneumonitis and aspiration pneumonia. N Engl J Med. 2001;344:665–71. https://doi.org/10.1056/NEJM200103013440908.
11. Bartlett JG. Aspiration pneumonia. In: Netter's infectious diseases. Elsevier; 2012. p. 153–6. https://doi.org/10.1016/B978-1-4377-0126-5.00029-X.
12. Mendelson CL. The aspiration of stomach contents into the lungs during obstetric anesthesia. Am J Obstet Gynecol. 1946;52:191–205. https://doi.org/10.1016/S0002-9378(16)39829-5.
13. Yoshimatsu Y, Melgaard D, Westergren A, et al. The diagnosis of aspiration pneumonia in older persons: a systematic review. Eur Geriatr Med. 2022;13:1071–80. https://doi.org/10.1007/s41999-022-00689-3.
14. DePaso WJ. Aspiration pneumonia. Clin Chest Med. 1991;12:269–84. https://doi.org/10.1016/S0272-5231(21)00743-7.
15. Ursino S, D'Angelo E, Mazzola R, et al. A comparison of swallowing dysfunction after three-dimensional conformal and intensity-modulated radiotherapy: a systematic review by the Italian Head and Neck Radiotherapy Study Group. Strahlenther Onkol. 2017;193:877–89. https://doi.org/10.1007/s00066-017-1160-7.
16. Caglar HB, Tishler RB, Othus M, et al. Dose to larynx predicts for swallowing complications after intensity-modulated radiotherapy. Int J Radiat Oncol. 2008;72:1110–8. https://doi.org/10.1016/j.ijrobp.2008.02.048.
17. Feng FY, Kim HM, Lyden TH, et al. Intensity-modulated radiotherapy of head and neck cancer aiming to reduce dysphagia: early dose–effect relationships for the swallowing structures. Int J Radiat Oncol. 2007;68:1289–98. https://doi.org/10.1016/j.ijrobp.2007.02.049.
18. Robbins KT. Barriers to winning the battle with head-and-neck cancer. Int J Radiat Oncol. 2002;53:4–5. https://doi.org/10.1016/S0360-3016(02)02713-X.
19. Eisbruch A, Lyden T, Bradford CR, et al. Objective assessment of swallowing dysfunction and aspiration after radiation concurrent with chemotherapy for head-and-neck cancer. Int J Radiat Oncol. 2002;53:23–8. https://doi.org/10.1016/S0360-3016(02)02712-8.
20. Mittal BB, Pauloski BR, Haraf DJ, et al. Swallowing dysfunction—preventative and rehabilitation strategies in patients with head-and-neck cancers treated with surgery, radiotherapy, and chemotherapy: a critical review. Int J Radiat Oncol. 2003;57:1219–30. https://doi.org/10.1016/S0360-3016(03)01454-8.
21. Starmer HM, Quon H, Kumar R, et al. The effect of radiation dose on swallowing: evaluation of aspiration and kinematics. Dysphagia. 2015;30:430–7. https://doi.org/10.1007/s00455-015-9618-1.
22. Dornfeld K, Simmons JR, Karnell L, et al. Radiation doses to structures within and adjacent to the larynx are correlated with long-term diet- and speech-related quality of life. Int J Radiat Oncol. 2007;68:750–7. https://doi.org/10.1016/j.ijrobp.2007.01.047.
23. Vainshtein JM, Moon DH, Feng FY, et al. Long-term quality of life after swallowing and salivary-sparing chemo–intensity modulated radiation therapy in survivors of human papillomavirus–related oropharyngeal cancer. Int J Radiat Oncol. 2015;91:925–33. https://doi.org/10.1016/j.ijrobp.2014.12.045.
24. Sung H, Ferlay J, Siegel RL, et al. Global Cancer Statistics 2020: GLOBOCAN estimates of incidence and mortality worldwide for 36 cancers in 185 countries. CA Cancer J Clin. 2021;71:209–49.
25. Patterson RH, Fischman VG, Wasserman I, et al. Global burden of head and neck cancer: economic consequences, health, and the role of surgery. Otolaryngol Neck Surg. 2020;162:296–303. https://doi.org/10.1177/0194599819897265.
26. Chaturvedi P, Singhavi H, Malik A, et al. Outcome of head and neck squamous cell cancers in low-resource settings. Otolaryngol Clin N Am. 2018;51:619–29. https://doi.org/10.1016/j.otc.2018.01.008.
27. Pearson WGJ, Davidoff AA, Smith ZM, et al. Impaired swallowing mechanics of post-radiation therapy head and neck cancer patients: a retrospective videofluoroscopic study. World J Radiol. 2016;8:192. https://doi.org/10.4329/wjr.v8.i2.192.

28. Madan R, Kairo AK, Sharma A, et al. Aspiration pneumonia-related deaths in head and neck cancer patients: a retrospective analysis of risk factors from a tertiary care center in North India. J Laryngol Otol. 2015;129:710–4. https://doi.org/10.1017/S0022215115001450.
29. Xu B, Boero IJ, Hwang L, et al. Aspiration pneumonia after concurrent chemoradiotherapy for head and neck cancer: aspiration pneumonia after radiation. Cancer. 2015;121:1303–11. https://doi.org/10.1002/cncr.29207.
30. Kawai S, Yokota T, Onozawa Y, et al. Risk factors for aspiration pneumonia after definitive chemoradiotherapy or bio-radiotherapy for locally advanced head and neck cancer: a monocentric case-control study. BMC Cancer. 2017;17:59. https://doi.org/10.1186/s12885-017-3052-8.
31. Wang J-J, Jiang R-S, Yen T-T, et al. Risk factors for recurrent pneumonia in post-irradiated patients with nasopharyngeal carcinoma. J Chin Med Assoc. 2017;80:558–62. https://doi.org/10.1016/j.jcma.2017.01.006.
32. Patil V, Noronha V, Shrirangwar S, et al. Aspiration pneumonia in head and neck cancer patients undergoing concurrent chemoradiation from India: findings from a post hoc analysis of a phase 3 study. Cancer Med. 2021;10:6725–35. https://doi.org/10.1002/cam4.4210.
33. Patterson JM, McColl E, Carding PN, et al. Swallowing beyond six years post (chemo)radiotherapy for head and neck cancer: a cohort study. Oral Oncol. 2018;83:53–8. https://doi.org/10.1016/j.oraloncology.2018.06.003.
34. Shirasu H, Yokota T, Hamauchi S, et al. Risk factors for aspiration pneumonia during concurrent chemoradiotherapy or bio-radiotherapy for head and neck cancer. BMC Cancer. 2020;20:182. https://doi.org/10.1186/s12885-020-6682-1.
35. Nguyen NP, Moltz CC, Frank C, et al. Long-term aspiration following treatment for head and neck cancer. Oncology. 2008;74:25–30. https://doi.org/10.1159/000138976.
36. Dong Y, Ridge JA, Li T, et al. Long-term toxicities in 10-year survivors of radiation treatment for head and neck cancer. Oral Oncol. 2017;71:122–8. https://doi.org/10.1016/j.oraloncology.2017.05.009.
37. Meheissen MAM, Mohamed ASR, Kamal M, et al. A prospective longitudinal assessment of MRI signal intensity kinetics of non-target muscles in patients with advanced stage oropharyngeal cancer in relationship to radiotherapy dose and post-treatment radiation-associated dysphagia: preliminary findings from a randomized trial. Radiother Oncol. 2019;130:46–55. https://doi.org/10.1016/j.radonc.2018.08.010.
38. Pigorsch SU, May C, Kessel KA, et al. MRI- and CT-determined changes of dysphagia/aspiration-related structures (DARS) during and after radiotherapy. PLoS One. 2020;15:e0237501. https://doi.org/10.1371/journal.pone.0237501.
39. Hutcheson KA, Yuk M, Hubbard R, et al. Delayed lower cranial neuropathy after oropharyngeal intensity-modulated radiotherapy: a cohort analysis and literature review. Head Neck. 2017;39:1516–23. https://doi.org/10.1002/hed.24789.
40. Hutcheson KA, Barrow MP, Warneke CL, et al. Cough strength and expiratory force in aspirating and non aspirating post-radiation head and neck cancer survivors: expiratory function and aspiration in HNC. Laryngoscope. 2018;128:1615–21. https://doi.org/10.1002/lary.26986.
41. Dua K, Ren J, Bardan E, et al. Coordination of deglutitive glottal function and pharyngeal bolus transit during normal eating. Gastroenterology. 1997;112:73–83. https://doi.org/10.1016/S0016-5085(97)70221-X.
42. Pouderoux P, Logemann JA, Kahrilas PJ. Pharyngeal swallowing elicited by fluid infusion: role of volition and vallecular containment. Am J Physiol-Gastrointest Liver Physiol. 1996;270:G347–54. https://doi.org/10.1152/ajpgi.1996.270.2.G347.
43. Martin RE, Sessle BJ. The role of the cerebral cortex in swallowing. Dysphagia. 1993;8:195–202. https://doi.org/10.1007/BF01354538.
44. Kahrilas PJ, Lin S, Logemann JA, et al. Deglutitive tongue action: volume accommodation and bolus propulsion. Gastroenterology. 1993;104:152–62. https://doi.org/10.1016/0016-5085(93)90847-6.

45. Kahrilas PJ, Logemann JA, Lin S, et al. Pharyngeal clearance during swallowing: a combined manometric and videofluoroscopic study. Gastroenterology. 1992;103:128–36. https://doi.org/10.1016/0016-5085(92)91105-D.
46. Kahrilas P, Lin S, Chen J, et al. Oropharyngeal accommodation to swallow volume. Gastroenterology. 1996;111:297–306. https://doi.org/10.1053/gast.1996.v111.pm8690194.
47. Shaker R, Dodds WJ, Dantas RO, et al. Coordination of deglutitive glottic closure with oropharyngeal swallowing. Gastroenterology. 1990;98:1478–84. https://doi.org/10.1016/0016-5085(90)91078-K.
48. Logemann JA, Kahrilas PJ, Cheng J, et al. Closure mechanisms of laryngeal vestibule during swallow. Am J Physiol-Gastrointest Liver Physiol. 1992;262:G338–44. https://doi.org/10.1152/ajpgi.1992.262.2.G338.
49. Cook IJ, Dodds WJ, Dantas RO, et al. Opening mechanisms of the human upper esophageal sphincter. Am J Physiol-Gastrointest Liver Physiol. 1989;257:G748–59. https://doi.org/10.1152/ajpgi.1989.257.5.G748.
50. Gawryszuk A, Bijl HP, Holwerda M, et al. Functional swallowing units (FSUs) as organs-at-risk for radiotherapy. Part 1: Physiology and anatomy. Radiother Oncol. 2019;130:62–7. https://doi.org/10.1016/j.radonc.2018.10.028.
51. Pearson WG, Hindson DF, Langmore SE, et al. Evaluating swallowing muscles essential for hyolaryngeal elevation by using muscle functional magnetic resonance imaging. Int J Radiat Oncol. 2013;85:735–40. https://doi.org/10.1016/j.ijrobp.2012.07.2370.
52. Cook IJ, Kahrilas PJ. AGA technical review on management of oropharyngeal dysphagia. Gastroenterology. 1999;116:455–78. https://doi.org/10.1016/S0016-5085(99)70144-7.
53. Fullerton A, Mou Y, Silver N, et al. Reflex vs. volitional cough differences amongst head and neck cancer survivors characterized by time since treatment and aspiration status. Respir Physiol Neurobiol. 2021;293:103702. https://doi.org/10.1016/j.resp.2021.103702.
54. Fisk RL, Symes JF, Aldridge LL, et al. The pathophysiology and experimental therapy of acid pneumonitis in ex vivo lungs. Chest. 1970;57:364–70. https://doi.org/10.1378/chest.57.4.364.
55. Fisk RL, Symes JF, Brown DR, et al. Aspiration pneumonitis: studies in the isolated perfused lung. Surg Forum. 1968;19:252–3.
56. Mays EE, Dubois JJ, Hamilton GB. Pulmonary fibrosis associated with tracheobronchial aspiration. Chest. 1976;69:512–5. https://doi.org/10.1378/chest.69.4.512.
57. Khoma O, Park J, Lee FM, et al. Different clinical symptom patterns in patients with reflux micro-aspiration. ERJ Open Res. 2022;8:00508–2021. https://doi.org/10.1183/23120541.00508-2021.
58. Cameron JL. Aspiration pneumonia: clinical outcome following documented aspiration. Arch Surg. 1973;106:49. https://doi.org/10.1001/archsurg.1973.01350130051011.
59. Dines DE, Titus JL, Sessler AD. Aspiration pneumonitis. Mayo Clin Proc. 1970;45:347–60.
60. Alexander IGS. The Ultrastructure Of The Pulmonary Alveolar Vessels In Mendelson's (acid pulmonary aspiration) syndrome. Br J Anaesth. 1968;40:408–14. https://doi.org/10.1093/bja/40.6.408.
61. Goldman G, Welbourn R, Kobzik L, et al. Tumor necrosis factor-α mediates acid aspiration-induced systemic organ injury. Ann Surg. 1990;212:513–20. https://doi.org/10.1097/00000658-199010000-00013.
62. Terpenning MS, Taylor GW, Lopatin DE, et al. Aspiration pneumonia: dental and oral risk factors in an older veteran population. J Am Geriatr Soc. 2001;49:557–63. https://doi.org/10.1046/j.1532-5415.2001.49113.x.
63. DiBardino DM, Wunderink RG. Aspiration pneumonia: a review of modern trends. J Crit Care. 2015;30:40–8. https://doi.org/10.1016/j.jcrc.2014.07.011.
64. Makhnevich A. Aspiration pneumonia in older adults. J Hosp Med. 2019;14:429. https://doi.org/10.12788/jhm.3154.
65. Marik PE, Careau P. The role of anaerobes in patients with ventilator-associated pneumonia and aspiration pneumonia. Chest. 1999;115:178–83. https://doi.org/10.1378/chest.115.1.178.
66. Matsuo H, Sakuma K. Dysphagia of cachexia and sarcopenia. In: Sarcopenia. Elsevier; 2021. p. 267–93. https://doi.org/10.1016/B978-0-12-822146-4.00013-2.

67. Happel KI. Alcohol, immunosuppression, and the lung. Proc Am Thorac Soc. 2005;2:428–32. https://doi.org/10.1513/pats.200507-065JS.
68. El-Solh AA, Vora H, Knight PR, et al. Diagnostic use of serum procalcitonin levels in pulmonary aspiration syndromes*. Crit Care Med. 2011;39:1251–6. https://doi.org/10.1097/CCM.0b013e31820a942c.
69. Franquet T, Giménez A, Rosón N, et al. Aspiration diseases: findings, pitfalls, and differential diagnosis. Radiographics. 2000;20:673–85. https://doi.org/10.1148/radiographics.20.3.g00ma01673.
70. Komiya K, Ishii H, Umeki K, et al. Computed tomography findings of aspiration pneumonia in 53 patients: CT findings of aspiration pneumonia. Geriatr Gerontol Int. 2013;13:580–5. https://doi.org/10.1111/j.1447-0594.2012.00940.x.
71. Ryu AJ, Navin PJ, Hu X, et al. Clinico-radiologic features of lung disease associated with aspiration identified on lung biopsy. Chest. 2019;156:1160–6. https://doi.org/10.1016/j.chest.2019.07.018.
72. Christianen MEMC, Langendijk JA, Westerlaan HE, et al. Delineation of organs at risk involved in swallowing for radiotherapy treatment planning. Radiother Oncol. 2011;101:394–402. https://doi.org/10.1016/j.radonc.2011.05.015.
73. Brouwer CL, Steenbakkers RJ, Bourhis J, Budach W, Grau C, Grégoire V, Van Herk M, Lee A, Maingon P, Nutting C, O'Sullivan B. CT-based delineation of organs at risk in the head and neck region: DAHANCA, EORTC, GORTEC, HKNPCSG, NCIC CTG, NCRI, NRG Oncology and TROG consensus guidelines. Radiother Oncol J Eur Soc Ther Radiol Oncol. 2015;117:83–90. https://doi.org/10.1016/j.radonc.2015.07.041.
74. Eisbruch A, Schwartz M, Rasch C, Vineberg K, Damen E, Van As CJ, Marsh R, Pameijer FA, Balm AJ. Dysphagia and aspiration after chemoradiotherapy for head-and-neck cancer: which anatomic structures are affected, and can they be spared by IMRT? Int J Radiat Oncol Biol Phys. 2004;60:1425–39. https://doi.org/10.1016/j.ijrobp.2004.05.050.
75. Van Der Laan HP, Christianen MEMC, Bijl HP, et al. The potential benefit of swallowing sparing intensity-modulated radiotherapy to reduce swallowing dysfunction: an in silico planning comparative study. Radiother Oncol. 2012;103:76–81. https://doi.org/10.1016/j.radonc.2011.11.001.
76. Van Der Laan HP, Gawryszuk A, Christianen MEMC, et al. Swallowing-sparing intensity-modulated radiotherapy for head and neck cancer patients: treatment planning optimization and clinical introduction. Radiother Oncol. 2013;107:282–7. https://doi.org/10.1016/j.radonc.2013.05.004.
77. Christianen MEMC, Van Der Schaaf A, Van Der Laan HP, et al. Swallowing sparing intensity-modulated radiotherapy (SW-IMRT) in head and neck cancer: clinical validation according to the model-based approach. Radiother Oncol. 2016;118:298–303. https://doi.org/10.1016/j.radonc.2015.11.009.
78. Batth SS, Caudell JJ, Chen AM. Practical considerations in reducing swallowing dysfunction following concurrent chemoradiotherapy with intensity-modulated radiotherapy for head and neck cancer. Head Neck. 2013;36:291–8. https://doi.org/10.1002/hed.23246.
79. Feng FY, Kim HM, Lyden TH, et al. Intensity-modulated chemoradiotherapy aiming to reduce dysphagia in patients with oropharyngeal cancer: clinical and functional results. J Clin Oncol. 2010;28:2732–8. https://doi.org/10.1200/JCO.2009.24.6199.
80. Schwartz DL, Hutcheson K, Barringer D, et al. Candidate dosimetric predictors of long-term swallowing dysfunction after oropharyngeal intensity-modulated radiotherapy. Int J Radiat Oncol. 2010;78:1356–65. https://doi.org/10.1016/j.ijrobp.2009.10.002.
81. Nutting C, Finneran L, Roe J, Sydenham MA, Beasley M, Bhide S, Boon C, Cook A, De Winton E, Emson M, Foran B, Frogley R, Petkar I, Pettit L, Rooney K, Roques T, Srinivasan D, Tyler J, Hall E. Dysphagia-optimized intensity-modulated radiotherapy versus standard intensity-modulated radiotherapy in patients with head and neck cancer (DARS): a phase

3, multicentre, randomized, controlled trial. Lancet Oncol. 2023;24:868–80. https://doi.org/10.1016/s1470-2045(23)00265-6.
82. Fox KA, Mularski RA, Sarfati MR, et al. Aspiration pneumonia following surgically placed feeding tubes. Am J Surg. 1995;170:564–7. https://doi.org/10.1016/S0002-9610(99)80016-6.
83. Warusevitane A, Karunatilake D, Sim J, et al. Safety and effect of metoclopramide to prevent pneumonia in patients with stroke fed via nasogastric tubes trial. Stroke. 2015;46:454–60. https://doi.org/10.1161/STROKEAHA.114.006639.
84. Allami A, Kianimajd S, Mavandadi S, et al. Evaluation of domperidone efficacy to prevent aspiration pneumonia in patients with acute ischemic stroke: a randomized clinical trial. Acta Neurol Belg. 2022;122:1337–42. https://doi.org/10.1007/s13760-022-01925-0.
85. Logemann JA. The evaluation and treatment of swallowing disorders. Curr Opin Otolaryngol Head Neck Surg. 1998;6:395–400. https://doi.org/10.1097/00020840-199812000-00008.
86. Logemann JA, Pauloski BR, Rademaker AW, Lazarus CL, Gaziano J, Stachowiak L, Newman L, MacCracken E, Santa D, Mittal B. Swallowing disorders in the first year after radiation and chemoradiation. Head Neck. 2008;30:148–58. https://doi.org/10.1002/hed.20672.
87. Nguyen NP, Moltz CC, Frank C, et al. Impact of swallowing therapy on aspiration rate following treatment for locally advanced head and neck cancer. Oral Oncol. 2007;43:352–7. https://doi.org/10.1016/j.oraloncology.2006.04.002.
88. Newman R, Vilardell N, Clavé P, et al. Effect of bolus viscosity on the safety and efficacy of swallowing and the kinematics of the swallow response in patients with oropharyngeal dysphagia: white paper by the European Society for Swallowing Disorders (ESSD). Dysphagia. 2016;31:232–49. https://doi.org/10.1007/s00455-016-9696-8.
89. Shanahan TK, Logemann JA, Rademaker AW, et al. Chin-down posture effect on aspiration in dysphagic patients. Arch Phys Med Rehabil. 1993;74:736–9. https://doi.org/10.1016/0003-9993(93)90035-9.
90. Rasley A, Logemann JA, Kahrilas PJ, et al. Prevention of barium aspiration during videofluoroscopic swallowing studies: value of change in posture. AJR Am J Roentgenol. 1993;160:1005–9. https://doi.org/10.2214/ajr.160.5.8470567.
91. Welch MV, Logemann JA, Rademaker AW, et al. Changes in pharyngeal dimensions effected by chin tuck. Arch Phys Med Rehabil. 1993;74:178–81.
92. Logemann JA, Rademaker AW, Pauloski BR, et al. Effects of postural change on aspiration in head and neck surgical patients. Otolaryngol Head Neck Surg Off J Am Acad Otolaryngol-Head Neck Surg. 1994;110:222–7. https://doi.org/10.1177/019459989411000212.
93. Checkin M, Bain J, Bath L, et al. Patients' perspectives on what makes a better care experience while undergoing treatment for oropharyngeal dysphagia secondary to head and neck cancer. Dysphagia. 2020;35:702–16. https://doi.org/10.1007/s00455-019-10077-y.
94. Bonomo P, Paderno A, Mattavelli D, et al. Quality assessment in supportive care in head and neck cancer. Front Oncol. 2019;9:926. https://doi.org/10.3389/fonc.2019.00926.
95. Kaasa S, Loge JH, Aapro M, et al. Integration of oncology and palliative care: a Lancet Oncology Commission. Lancet Oncol. 2018;19:e588–653. https://doi.org/10.1016/S1470-2045(18)30415-7.
96. Goyal N, Day A, Epstein J, et al. Head and neck cancer survivorship consensus statement from the American Head and Neck Society. Laryngoscope Investig Otolaryngol. 2022;7:70–92. https://doi.org/10.1002/lio2.702.
97. Söllner W, DeVries A, Steixner E, et al. How successful are oncologists in identifying patient distress, perceived social support, and the need for psychosocial counseling? Br J Cancer. 2001;84:179–85. https://doi.org/10.1054/bjoc.2000.1545.
98. Klompas M. Aspiration pneumonia in adults. In: UpToDate. Waltham, MA; 2023. https://www.uptodate.com/contents/aspiration-pneumonia-in-adults?search=aspiration%20pneumonia%20treatment%20adult&source=search_result&selectedTitle=1~150&usage_type=default&display_rank=1#H8 (accessed 23 Aug 2023).

99. Wolfe JE, Bone RC, Ruth WE. Effects of corticosteroids in the treatment of patients with gastric aspiration. Am J Med. 1977;63:719–22. https://doi.org/10.1016/0002-9343(77)90157-7.
100. Nguyen NP, Moltz CC, Frank C, et al. Effectiveness of the cough reflex in patients with aspiration following radiation for head and neck cancer. Lung. 2007;185:243–8. https://doi.org/10.1007/s00408-007-9016-z.
101. Van Der Laan HP, Van De Water TA, Van Herpt HE, et al. The potential of intensity-modulated proton radiotherapy to reduce swallowing dysfunction in the treatment of head and neck cancer: a planning comparative study. Acta Oncol. 2013;52:561–9. https://doi.org/10.3109/0284186X.2012.692885.

Oral Mucositis Management in Patients Receiving Radiation Therapy or Dose Intense Chemotherapy

14

Gagan Saini and Rashmi Shukla

14.1 Introduction

The mucosal lining of the oral mucosa has a rapid rate of cell turnover and is therefore afflicted by cytotoxic cancer treatments in up to 90 percent of cancer patients [1]. Systemic cytotoxic agents can cause mucositis from mouth to anus whereas it is confined to the geographic radiation area when caused by radiation therapy [2]. Oral mucosa is also at a high risk due to its microbiota and regular trauma during normal use.

Even an uncomplicated mucositis can result in intense discomfort and can adversely affect the quality of life.

Pain is common in patients with Head and Neck Cancers (HNC) and can be seen in up to 50% of patients before cancer treatments, 81% during treatments, 70% at the completion of treatment and 36% at 6 months after completion of treatment [3]. Dysguesia can happen in up to 56% patients with chemotherapy (CT), 66% with Radiotherapy (RT) and in up to three quarters of patients receiving combined radiation and chemotherapy [4]. Superadded or primary fungal infections can be seen in 7.5% patients before cancer treatments and in up to one-third patients during and post treatments [5]. On the other hand viral infections are almost non-existent in RT patients but can be seen in up to half the patients on CT for haematological malignancies [6]. The most common dental disease seen in patients on cancer treatments is caries and can be seen in up to one-fourth of the patients [7]. Xerostomia is a complex symptom and is not just the result of hypofunction of salivary glands but also due to loss of minor salivary glands of the mucosa afflicted by the disease and its treatment. Overall incidence of the same is up to 93% which decreases over

G. Saini (✉) · R. Shukla
Department of Radiation Oncology, Max Institute of Cancer Care, Max Hospital, Vaishali and Patparganj, India

K. Sood Sharma et al. (eds.), *Complications of Cancer Therapy: Best Practices in Prevention and Management*, https://doi.org/10.1007/978-981-99-0984-1_14

months post RT and stabilises after 1 year. It is much higher with conventional techniques and technology of RT and decreases significantly with use of Intensity Modulated Radiation Therapy (IMRT). However, the prevalence continues to be in about two-third patients with IMRT even after a year [8].

14.2 Pain and Mucositis

Painful mucositis is perhaps the most common effect of cancer therapies. The same has been objectively graded by Visual Analogue Scale (VAS), Verbal Rating Scale (VRS) and Numerical Rating Scale (NRS) [9, 10]. These are used widely by medical professionals practicing in fields not dealing with cancer treatments. For an oncologist, the assessment of oral mucositis related pain is not just a function of pain levels but also that of functional status and therefore WHO, RTOG, and CTCAE scores are considered better for a comprehensive assessment [11–13] (Table 14.1). A reasonable concordance is also observed in these scales especially in the moderate grades [14].

The patients must always be evaluated by multi-disciplinary teams including dentistry to explain to them of the possibility of pain and dysfunction and their access to the treatments. The pain is not preventable in most cases but a clear understanding changes their outlook positively and improves the compliance and outcomes [9]. The approach towards pain must be expectant and not reactionary. Regular reviews of patients on cancer treatments must be instituted to educate the patients about pain and make clinical observations of the oral mucosa (Table 14.1). We recommend at least once a week evaluation of patients on RT. Before start CT that may cause mucositis, an oral examination to assist in risk assessment at baseline must be performed to aid future clinical decision in terms of worsening of grade and interventions.

Table 14.1 Oral mucositis scales (including the comparison between NCI-CTCAE v2 and v4)

	Grade 0	Grade I	Grade II	Grade III	Grade IV	Grade V
WHO	No findings	Erythema and soreness; no ulcers	Oral erythema, ulcers, solid diet tolerated	Oral ulcers, liquid diet only	Not able to tolerate a solid or liquid diet	NA
RTOG	No findings	Painless ulcers, erythema or mild soreness	Painful erythema, edema or ulcers, but can eat	Painful erythema, edema or ulcers and cannot eat	Requires parenteral or enteral support	NA
NCI-CTCAE v4	No findings	Asymptomatic or mild symptoms; intervention not indicated	Moderate pain or ulcer that does not interfere with oral intake; modified diet indicated	Severe pain; interfering with oral intake	Life-threatening consequences, urgent intervention indicated	Death related to toxicity
NCI-CTCAE v2	None	Erythema of the mucosa	Patchy pseudomembranous reaction (patches generally ≤ 1.5 cm in diameter and noncontiguous)	Confluent pseudomembranous reaction (contiguous patches generally >1.5 cm in diameter)	Necrosis or deep ulceration; may include bleeding not induced by minor trauma or abrasion	NA

Abbreviations: *WHO* World Health Organization, *RTOG* Radiation Therapy Oncology Group, *NCI* National Cancer Institute, *CTCAE* common terminology criteria for adverse evens

14.3 Preventive Measures

Using a soft toothbrush for brushing twice a day, flossing and rinsing with bland solutions.

Rinse mouth with salt plus sodium bicarbonate solution 4 to 6 times a day [15].

Dental assessment for prophylactic care and treatment of caries with extraction of compromised teeth [16].

e prophylactic.

Sucking ice chips where patients should hold ice chips in their mouth for half an hour before 5FU infusion [15].

Also important for preventing radiation-induced mucositis is to limit the mucosal exposure to RT by using good techniques and technology like IMRT [8].

Prophylactic dietary modifications to avoid acidic and sharp foods Benzydamine mouthwashes are useful for patients with head and neck cancer [17].

Prophylactic placement of a percutaneous endoscopic gastrostomy tube in patients at high risk can be helpful [15].

14.4 Treatment of Established Radiation Induced Mucositis

Bland rinses with salt and sodium bicarbonate to be used up to four times a day (One litre of water with one teaspoon of salt with one teaspoon of sodium bicarbonate). Topical anaesthetics, such as 2% viscous lignocaine (or Lidocaine) swish and spit.

The interventions needed in the early grade of mucositis is to modify their diet. At the minimum, patients need to give up on spices and chillies. A grade 3 mucositis generally means that the patient is put on a liquid diet [18].

Grade 3 mucositis also means that the pain killers need to be escalated as per the WHO ladder [5, 9]. It is imperative that a more frequent review of patients be done when they develop grade 3 mucositis to assess their oral intake and institute a feeding procedure like a feeding tube or a PEG tube when deemed fit.

Institution of gabapentin in radiation induced mucositis especially in T3/T4 infiltrating tumours receiving curative radiation therapy may decrease the need for opiates.

14.5 Treatment of Chemotherapy Induced Mucositis

This typically occurs within 5 to 14 days of receiving chemotherapy [5]. The dose dense regimens or the regimens containing fluorouracil, methotrexate, or etoposide put the patient at a higher risk of mucositis [19].

Most of what has been discussed above is applicable for CT induced mucositis as well. However since these afflictions are often not limited to just the oral mucosa [2] and are often associated with low blood counts the need to institute other supportive treatments like systemic antibiotics and colony stimulating factors is considered and is beyond the scope of this discussion.

In our opinion the magic mouthwashes (which contain mixture of topical anaesthetics, antihistamines, steroids and/or antibiotics) are not recommended because they do not contain standardised ingredients with respect to the ratios and pharmacokinetics (for e.g. a crushed tablet applied on mucosa will likely not have enough bioavailability of an ingredient). These are therefore not more beneficial than bland rinses with salt and sodium bicarbonate. Along with they carry an additional risk of systemic toxicity [15, 20].

Chlorhexidine as a mouthwash is recommended only when oral hygiene is not possible since the studies have not shown a consistent benefit compared with a placebo [21]. Sucralfate [5], calcium phosphate rinses [22, 23], Mucoadhesive hydrogel rinses or any other mucosa-coating agents [24] are also not recommended for chemotherapy-induced mucositis or radiation therapy induced mucositis.

14.6 Dysgeusia

Dysgeusia with RT is associated with damage to taste buds, xerostomia. CT causes an unpleasant taste due to diffusion of the drug into the oral cavity and that is why the same happens after a time interval following administration of CT and is also reversible over the course of months. Treatment of oral tongue by fractionated radiation dose higher than 30 Gy decreases the acuity of sweet, sour, bitter, and salt tastes [25]. Radiation induced mucositis leading to the damage to the microvilli the taste cells has been proposed as the principal mechanism [26]. While there is a possibility of the acuity of taste to recover after a few months the same remains low in head and neck patients who are mostly chronic tobacco chewers and are nutritionally compromised [27, 28]. Tobacco users have been known to have a compromised gustatory function which may contribute to delayed recovery [29]. Studies have shown that Zinc supplementation (zinc sulphate 220 mg 2 times a day) has been useful in some patients [25, 30]. The benefit of saving tongue from a low dose of 30Gy remains the primary modality to avoid radiation induced dysgeusia.

14.7 Superadded or Primary Candidiasis

Candidiasis is the most common fungal infection in these patients. Pseudomembranous and erythematous candidiasis are the two most common patterns of affliction reported. While the former is easily diagnosed with clinical examination the latter may need lab tests for diagnosis.

The common clinical symptoms are pain with taste changes.

Although topical agents with clotrimazole may be helpful, systemic treatment with fluconazole remains the best treatment with a low prevalence of 1.9% of infection in the treated population [31, 32].

References

1. Brown TJ, Gupta A. Management of cancer therapy–associated oral mucositis. JCO Oncol Pract. 2020;16(3):103–9.
2. Al-Dasooqi N, Sonis ST, Bowen JM, et al. Emerging evidence on the pathobiology of mucositis. Support Care Cancer. 2013;21:3233–41.
3. Epstein JB, Hong C, Logan RM, et al. A systematic review of orofacial pain in patients receiving cancer therapy. Support Care Cancer. 2010;18(8):1023–31.
4. Hovan AJ, Williams PM, Stevenson-Moore P, et al. A systematic review of dysgeusia induced by cancer therapies. Support Care Cancer. 2010;18(8):1081–7.
5. Lalla RV, Latortue MC, Hong CH, et al. A systematic review of oral fungal infections in patients receiving cancer therapy. Support Care Cancer. 2010;18(8):985–92.
6. Elad S, Zadik Y, Hewson I, et al. A systematic review of viral infections associated with oral involvement in cancer patients: a spotlight on Herpesviridea. Support Care Cancer. 2010;18(8):993–1006.
7. Hong CH, Napeñas JJ, Hodgson BD, et al. A systematic review of dental disease in patients undergoing cancer therapy. Support Care Cancer. 2010;18(8):1007–21.
8. Jensen SB, Pedersen AM, Vissink A, et al. A systematic review of salivary gland hypofunction and xerostomia induced by cancer therapies: prevalence, severity and impact on quality of life. Support Care Cancer. 2010;18(8):1039–60.
9. Ripamonti CI, Santini D, Maranzano E, Berti M, Roila F, ESMO Guidelines Working Group. Management of cancer pain: ESMO Clinical Practice Guidelines. Ann Oncol. 2012;23(Suppl 7):139–54. https://doi.org/10.1093/annonc/mds233.
10. Sonis ST. A comparison and assessment of scoring scales for mucositis. Oral mucositis. Tarporley: Springer Healthcare Ltd.; 2012. p. 39–46.
11. World Health Organization. WHO handbook for reporting results of cancer treatment. Geneva: World Health Organization; 1979.
12. NCI Common Terminology Criteria for Adverse Events (CTCAE) version 4. Retrieved from: https://evs.nci.nih.gov/ftp1/CTCAE/CTCAE_4.03/.
13. Trotti A, Byhardt R, Stetz J, Gwede C, Corn B, Fu K, Gunderson L, McCormick B, Morris M, Rich T, Shipley W, Curran W. Common toxicity criteria: version 2.0. an improved reference for grading the acute effects of cancer treatment: impact on radiotherapy. Int J Radiat Oncol Biol Phys. 2000;47:13–47.
14. Villa A, Vollemans M, De Moraes A, et al. Concordance of the WHO, RTOG, and CTCAE v4.0 grading scales for the evaluation of oral mucositis associated with chemoradiation therapy for the treatment of oral and oropharyngeal cancers. Support Care Cancer. 2021;29:6061–8.
15. Bensinger W, Schubert M, Ang KK, et al. NCCN Task Force Report. Prevention and management of mucositis in cancer care. J Natl Compr Canc Netw. 2008;6:S1–S21, quiz S22-S24
16. Hong CHL, Gueiros LA, Fulton JS, et al. Systematic review of basic oral care for the management of oral mucositis in cancer patients and clinical practice guidelines. Support Care Cancer. 2019;27:3949–67.
17. Lalla RV, Bowen J, Barasch A, et al. MASCC/ISOO clinical practice guidelines for the management of mucositis secondary to cancer therapy. Cancer. 2014;120:1453–61.
18. Mallick S, Benson R, Rath GK. Radiation induced oral mucositis: a review of current literature on prevention and management. Eur Arch Otorhinolaryngol. 2016;273:2285–93.
19. Jones JA, Avritscher EB, Cooksley CD, et al. Epidemiology of treatment-associated mucosal injury after treatment with newer regimens for lymphoma, breast, lung, or colorectal cancer. Support Care Cancer. 2006;14:505–15.
20. Uberoi AS, Brown TJ, Gupta A. Magic mouthwash for oral mucositis: a teachable moment. JAMA Intern Med. 2019;179:104–5.
21. Dodd MJ, Dibble SL, Miaskowski C, et al. Randomized clinical trial of the effectiveness of 3 commonly used mouthwashes to treat chemotherapy-induced mucositis. Oral Surg Oral Med Oral Pathol Oral Radiol Endod. 2000;90:39–47.

22. Murdock JL, Reeves DJ. Chemotherapy-induced oral mucositis management: A retrospective analysis of MuGard, Caphosol, and standard supportive care measures. J Oncol Pharm Pract. 2020;26(3):521–8. https://doi.org/10.1177/1078155219850298.
23. Lambrecht M, Mercier C, Geussens Y, et al. The effect of a supersaturated calcium phosphate mouth rinse on the development of oral mucositis in head and neck cancer patients treated with chemo radiation: a single-center, randomized, prospective study of a calcium phosphate mouth rinse 1 standard of care versus standard of care. Support Care Cancer. 2013;21:2663–70.
24. Allison RR, Ambrad AA, Arshoun Y, et al. Multi-institutional, randomized, double-blind, placebo-controlled trial to assess the efficacy of a mucoadhesive hydrogel (MuGard) in mitigating oral mucositis symptoms in patients being treated with chemoradiation therapy for cancers of the head and neck. Cancer. 2014;120:1433–40.
25. Deshpande TS, Blanchard P, Wang L, Foote RL, Zhang X, Frank SJ. Radiation-related alterations of taste function in patients with head and neck cancer: a systematic review. Curr Treat Options in Oncol. 2018;19(12):72. https://doi.org/10.1007/s11864-018-0580-7.
26. Irune E, Dwivedi RC, Nutting CM, Harrington KJ. Treatment-related dysgeusia in head and neck cancer patients. Cancer Treat Rev. 2014;40(9):1106–17. https://doi.org/10.1016/j.ctrv.2014.06.011. Epub 2014 Jul 5
27. Deems DA, Yen DM, Kreshak A, Doty RL. Spontaneous resolution of dysgeusia. Arch Otolaryngol Head Neck Surg. 1996;122(9):961–3. https://doi.org/10.1001/archotol.1996.01890210037009.
28. Munshi A, Pandey MB, Durga T, Pandey KC, Bahadur S, Mohanti BK. Weight loss during radiotherapy for head and neck malignancies: what factors impact it? Nutr Cancer. 2003;47(2):136–40. https://doi.org/10.1207/s15327914nc4702_5.
29. Kale YS, Vibhute N, Belgaumi U, Kadashetti V, Bommanavar S, Kamate W. Effect of using tobacco on taste perception. J Family Med Prim Care. 2019;8(8):2699–702. https://doi.org/10.4103/jfmpc.jfmpc_457_19.
30. Ripamonti C, Zecca E, Brunelli C, et al. A randomized, controlled clinical trial to evaluate the effects of zinc sulfate on cancer patients with taste alterations caused by head and neck irradiation. Cancer. 1998;82(10):1938–45.
31. Nicolatou-Galitis O, Velegraki A, Sotiropoulou-Lontou A, et al. Effect of fluconazole antifungal prophylaxison oral mucositis in head and neck cancer patients receiving radiotherapy. Support Care Cancer. 2006;14(1):44–51.
32. Lalla RV, Latortue MC, Hong CH, Ariyawardana A, D'Amato-Palumbo S, Fischer DJ, Martof A, Nicolatou-Galitis O, Patton LL, Elting LS, Spijkervet FK, Brennan MT, Fungal Infections Section, Oral Care Study Group, Multinational Association of Supportive Care in Cancer (MASCC)/International Society of Oral Oncology (ISOO). A systematic review of oral fungal infections in patients receiving cancer therapy. Support Care Cancer. 2010;18(8):985–92. https://doi.org/10.1007/s00520-010-0892-z.

15 Prevention and Management of Cutaneous Toxicity Encountered in Patients Undergoing Radiation Therapy

Manisha Himthani, Kanika Sood Sharma, and Nikhil Himthani

15.1 Introduction

Radiotherapy (RT) is the one of the primary treatment modality for many cancers of various subsites. But along with its tumoricidal effect, it has various side effects on normal tissues as well. Radiation-induced skin reactions (RISR) or Radiation induced dermatitis (RID) is one of the well-established adverse effects of radiation. Radiation dermatitis is often misinterpreted as radiation burn, but unlike burn, which occurs immediately after the infliction of trauma, pathophysiology behind radiation dermatitis is imbalance between damage and restoration of basal layer of skin and can occur months to years later after receiving radiation therapy. Hence, RISR's are classified as acute or chronic. Acute reactions are predominantly in the form of erythema and desquamation and late effects manifest as fibrosis, telangiectasia, skin atrophy, radiation-induced keratosis and even skin cancers [1, 2] (Figs. 15.1, 15.2, 15.3, and 15.4). The overall incidence of acute erythematous reactions is to the tune of 80–90%, whereas moist desquamation is encountered in 10–15% of the patients at radical doses of radiation [3]. The factors that play a role in manifestation of RISR's are patient related factors [4] and treatment related factors. Patient parameters are age, body mass index (BMI), smoking status, comorbid conditions like diabetes, fanconi anemia, ataxia telangiectasia, nutritional status

M. Himthani (✉)
Dharamshila Narayana Superspeciality Hospital, New Delhi, India
e-mail: manisha.himthani.dr@narayanahealth.org

K. Sood Sharma
Department of Radiation Oncology, Dharamshila Narayana Superspeciality Hospital, New Delhi, India

N. Himthani
Batra Hospital, Delhi, India

K. Sood Sharma et al. (eds.), *Complications of Cancer Therapy: Best Practices in Prevention and Management*, https://doi.org/10.1007/978-981-99-0984-1_15

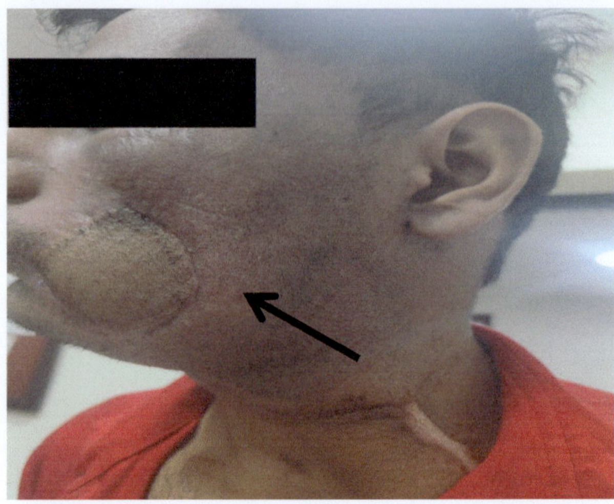

Fig. 15.1 Post 2 weeks radiation, skin presenting with erythematous changes depicting Grade 1 skin reactions

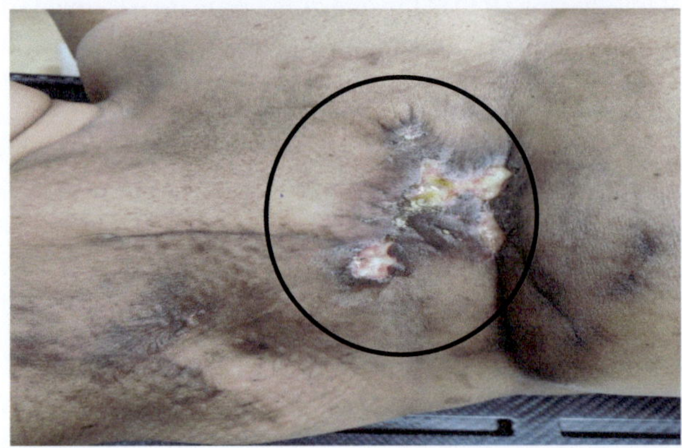

Fig. 15.2 Moist desquamation in a patient undergoing hypo fractionated adjuvant radiation therapy for carcinoma breast

before and during treatment, presence of a pre-existing skin or connective tissue disorders disease and genetic susceptibility. Treatment factors depends on total dose, higher dose per fraction, use of bolus, kilo voltage radiation, treatment techniques deployed, location of the primary [5], use of concurrent chemotherapy [6, 7] size of radiation portal, dose hotspots or overlapping fields.

When acute in nature, not only they cause pain and discomfort to the patient but also hamper the treatment continuity that leads to unplanned gaps. It is therefore, crucial to review patients on regular intervals and take necessary measures to alleviate the adverse effects of acute radiation induced skin toxicity. While chronic RISR's have to be diagnosed clinically with elaborate history of previous irradiation, careful local examination and have to be treated accordingly.

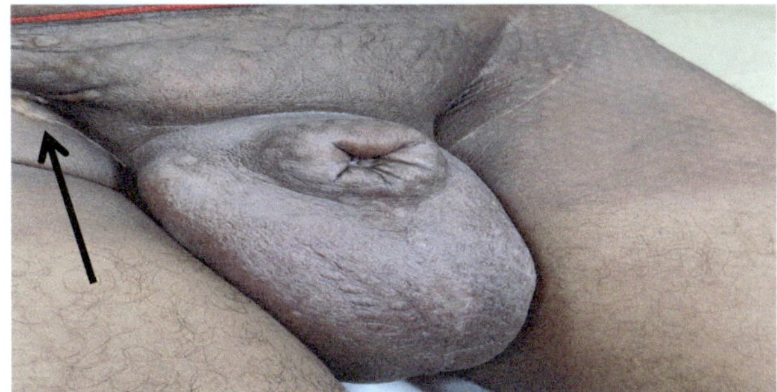

Fig. 15.3 Patchy dry desquamation in patient treated with post op radiotherapy for a case of carcinoma penis. The reactions are more pronounced near groin folds due to unavoidable constant friction

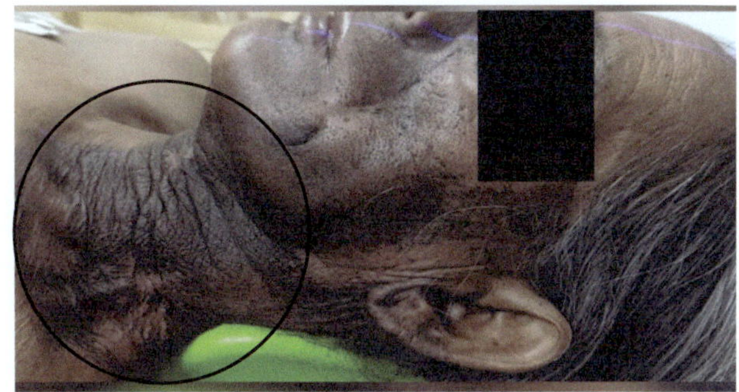

Fig. 15.4 Pigmentation and Grade 2 skin reactions predominantly in neck region due irregular tissue distribution in that region

15.2 Types of Complications

Acute RISR's are encountered up to 90 days (3 months) of radiation treatment whereas CISR's occur post 90 days of radiation therapy (Fig. 15.5) Overall Incidence of complications is summarised below [8, 9] (Table 15.1).

At doses above 60 Gy, risk for ulceration and necrosis increases [10].

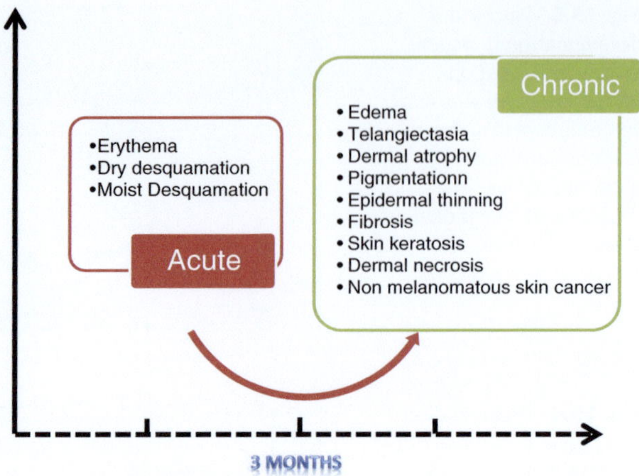

Fig. 15.5 Acute and chronic radiation induced side effects

Table 15.1 Overall incidence of complications [8, 9]

Grade	Complication	Incidence rate	Threshold dose (Gy)
Grade 1	Erythema	60%	20 Gy
Grade 2	Dry desquamation	32%	45 Gy
Grade 3	Moist desquamation	8%	50–60 Gy

15.3 Risk Factors

The overall incidence of grade 1–2 acute erythematous reactions is 80–90%, while moist desquamation is seen in 10–15% of the patients undergoing radiation at radical doses [11] and the variation is attributed to multiple patient and treatment related factors (Tables 15.2 and 15.3).

Table 15.2 Patient related factors for increased risk of RID's

Patient related factors	Remarks
Age	• Cell aging
	• Epidermis thickening
	• Loss of collagen in senile population
	• Poor capillary networking
	• Poor healing due to other comorbidities
Addiction status	• Smoking leads to reduced oxygenation and increased carboxy-hemoglobin causing delayed recovery of cells
	• Alcohol causes depletion of anti-oxidants, vitamins and minerals that promote healing
Genetic susceptibility	• Blooms syndrome
	• Ataxia telangiectasia
	• Xeroderma pigmentosa: faulty DNA repair mechanism conditions impair normal tissue healing from radiation damage
Co-morbidities	• Diabetes
	• Vascular disorders
	• Autoimmune conditions may cause delayed wound healing and lead to super imposed infections
Skin and connective tissue disorders	• Psoriasis
	• Eczema
	• Acne
	Aforementioned conditions of skin: Reason for increased probability of acute skin reactions
	• Systemic lupus erythematosus
	• Rheumatoid arthritis
	• Scleroderma
	Aforementioned connective tissue disorders: Reason for increased risk of chronic skin reactions
Nutrition status	• Poor nutrition status leads to loosening of thermoplastic masks causing increased risk of skin reactions
	• Poor nutrition status depletes body stores required for healing of normal tissues from radiation damage

Table 15.3 Treatment related factors for increased risk of RID

Treatment related factors	Remarks
Radiation dose	• Doses upto 60 Gy increases the risk of Grade 1–3 skin reactions
	• Doses more than 60 Gy increases the risk of Grade 4 reactions
Radiation type	• Photons deposit energy at Dmax depth
	• Electrons deposit energy at skin surface
	• Protons exhibit Bragg peak phenomenon causing maximum dose deposition at a certain depth
Energy of incident beam	• Higher photon energy has skin sparing effect
	• Higher electron energy causes increased dose at skin surface
Radiation fractionation	• Hyperfractionation causes increased risk of Acute Radiation reactions
	• Hypofractionation poses risk for chronic toxicities
Location of radiation field	• Skin folds
	• Hairy skin
	• Loose skin
	• Sweaty areas have higher risk of friction and more proportion of skin and henceforth increased risk of toxicities
Treatment technique	• Conventional 2D portals increase volume of skin irradiated
	• Conformal techniques increase dose homogeneity and decreases hotspots and hence decreased skin reactions
Volume of irradiated field	• Larger treatment fields predisposes larger area to skin reactions
Use of beam modifying devices	• Tissue equivalent bolus increases surface dose
Use of concurrent chemotherapy/targeted therapy	• Doxorubicin
	• 5-fluorouracil
	• Bleomycin
	• Cisplatin
	• Cetuximab
	Such agents are notorious for causing radiation recall reactions and skin rashes

15.4 Diagnostic Work Up

The most commonly used systems to grade skin reactions by the oncologists are CTCAE and RTOG (Table 15.4).

Table 15.4 Grading systems for RISR's

Grade	0	1	2	3	4	5
CTCAE v 5.0	No change	Faint erythema or dry desquamation	Moderate to brisk erythema; patchy moist desquamation, mostly confined to skin folds and creases; moderate edema	Moist desquamation in areas other than skin folds and creases; bleeding induced by minor trauma or abrasion	Life-threatening consequences; skin necrosis or ulceration of full thickness dermis; spontaneous bleeding from involved site; skin graft indicated	Death
RTOG acute	No change	Faint erythema, dry desquamation, epilation, diminished sweating	Moderate, brisk erythema, exudative dermatitis in plaques and moderate edema	Exudative dermatitis, besides cutaneous folds and intense edema	Ulceration, hemorrhage, necrosis	
RTOG chronic	No change	Slight atrophy, pigmentation change, some hair loss	Patchy atrophy, Moderate telangiectasia, total hair loss	Marked atrophy, Gross telangiectasia	Ulceration	

15.5 Management of Complications

The management of RISR's is not backed up by robust data despite its high prevalence. It is of utmost importance to maintain skin hydration and prevent escalation of grade of dermatitis. Severe desquamation needs special attention in order to prevent secondary infections. Withholding radiation, although not preferred, is also one of the methods to allow time for tissue healing and repair. However, due to the radio-biological process of accelerated repopulation, treatment gaps should be best avoided. Although, multiple RCT's have given recommendations for different sub sites on prevention or management of RID's. deriving data from them has helped classifying the management that includes:

- Regular Washing
- Medical Therapy
  - Pharmaceutical agents
    - Topical
    - Systemic
  - Non Pharmaceutical agents
- Interventional therapy

  - Laser therapy
  - Hyper Baric Oxygen Therapy(HBOT) therapy
  - Surgical intervention
- Research options

15.6 Regular Washing

Maintaining proper hygiene is the first step towards prevention of RISR's. Washing the radiation area with lukewarm water and using mild soaps is found to have lesser chances of pruritus [12].

15.7 Medical Therapy

15.7.1 Pharmaceutical Agents

15.7.1.1 Topical Agents

Silver Sulfadiazine

Due to its antibacterial properties, dressings coated with silver sulfadiazine are found to have protective effect on RISR's by attenuating the severity of reactions. Similar findings are seen with silver nylon dressings.

15.7.1.2 Topical Steroids

The pathophysiology behind radiation induced skin reactions is mediated via pro inflammatory cytokines.

Using topical steroids have their own good, bad and the ugly aspect to them. Attributing to their anti-inflammatory properties they act as a good modality to ameliorate the severity of skin reactions [13], but their skin thinning properties may be a downside later in the course of treatment. Also, they increase the chances of secondary infections which might add on to the healing time of the basal layer of skin.

Topical 0.1% mometasone furoate and 1% methylprednisone are the most commonly prescribed steroids in the form of ointments.

15.7.1.3 Doxepin

When used in cream formulation, it has proven beneficial effect in reducing dermatitis risk in patients undergoing radiation for breast cancer.

15.7.1.4 Silicone Based Agents

Film forming agents when applied locally delay the onset of skin reactions.

15.7.2 Emolient Creams

Ingredients like sucralfate, trolamine, azelastine, prostaglandin E1, essential fatty acids have been commonly used in various studies with equivocal results. Sucralfate is an anti-inflammatory, acts as a barrier and promotes angiogenesis. Despite these properties, it does not yield any substantial benefit with its application. Similarly, trolamine is supposed to act as a non-steroidal anti-inflammatory agent but its role too, is not well established.

15.8 Biological Agents

Certain agents with GM CSF and EGF promoting capabilities have some role in diminishing the severity of skin reactions by promoting macrophage maturation and proliferation of fibroblast, human epidermal stem cells respectively [14, 15].

15.9 Systemic Agents

15.9.1 Amifostine

Subcutaneous administration WR-2721, to a dose of 500 mg, diluted in 2.5 ml normal saline, 20 minutes before each fraction of radiation has significant results in reducing incidence of RISR's [16]. The preferred mode of administration is subcutaneous over intravenous as it is more time efficient.

15.9.2 Pentoxifylline

Along with vitamin E supplements, it has shown benefits in treating post radiation fibrosis of breast and cases of osteo-radionecrosis. It acts by increasing microcirculation and subsequently better oxygenation [17].

15.10 Non-Pharmaceutical Agents

15.10.1 Aloe Vera

Acts as a hydrating agent and has anti-infective properties. Diminishes radiation induced dryness and itching. Has been shown to reduce pigmentation from radiation in head and neck cancers. The role in preventive RID is still subjective.

15.10.2 Hyaluronic Acid and Amniotic Membrane

A double blind RCT supports the use of topical HA in reducing the severity of RID in head and neck, breast or pelvic malignancies. If used as conjugated high molecular weight and low molecular weight, its efficacy increases [18].

Cryopreserved human amniotic membrane adheres over moist desquamation area and acts as barrier against trauma. It impedes microbial invasion and promotes healing. Has limited use in infection scenarios.

15.11 Gentian Violet

Cost efficient, antiseptic dye with astringent properties has been widely used in moist desquamation when applied locally. However, it is cosmetically unappealing and has drawbacks like staining of clothes along with wound masking and few reports of potential carcinogenic effects.

15.12 Hydrocolloid Dressing

Best indicated post completion of radiation therapy. They are transparent so there is an added advantage of wound observation. Less beneficial in highly exudative wounds because of their poor absorbent properties.

Hydrocolloid occlusive dressing (Duoderm) and other dressings like silicine and polyurethane based Mepitel® film, StrataXRT®, a silicone-based film are effective in terms of healing, comfort and potential to prevent infections,

15.13 Oils

The advantages of olive oil and cream containing sandalwood and turmeric oil have also been explored. While the former has a role in decreasing the intensity of radiation induced reactions, the latter has a role in delaying the onset.

15.13.1 *Calendula officinalis*

It has a spectrum of anti inflammatory, anti bacterial, anti fungal properties. Use of this resulted in statistically significant decreased incidence of grade 2 radio dermatitis when compared to essential fatty acids in literature [19].

15.13.2 Interventional Therapy

15.13.2.1 Laser Therapy

Also known as photo biomodulation therapy or low level laser therapy revealed lower reports grade 3 radiation dermatitis when compared to a placebo group. It is a technique that deploys use of low power infrared rays to reduce radiation induced inflammation and pain to promote healing.

15.13.2.2 Hyperbaric Oxygen Therapy

As the name suggests, HBOT uses 100% oxygen at pressures much greater than the atmospheric level. It is used for chronic, non healing radiation dermatitis and radiation fibrosis. HBOT also reduces the chance of osteoradionecrosis following tooth extraction in an irradiated field. Its efficacy is backed up by multiple randomized trials that have found its use beneficial [20, 21].

15.13.2.3 Surgical Intervention

Often sought when underlying tissues are exposed due to ulceration. It usually involves excision of ulcer when they are large, else generous debridement with replacement of non irradiated vascularized tissue is done. Whenever feasible plastic reconstruction is done using skin grafts or flaps. It helps restoration of function, alleviates pain and prevents further chances of infection. Skin grafts usually perform inferior when compared to regional or free-flaps from non irradiated area.

15.13.3 Future Research

Epigallocatechin-3-gallate (EGCG), promotes healing of skin damage caused by UV light, has shown promising results in phase1/2 trials.

Topical keratin use for breast cancer also has a promising role as per the results published in 2020 updates.

15.14 Prevention of Complications

Certain factors that increase the risk of RISR should be kept in mind and carefully taken care of, to prevent skin reactions. The summary of certain do's and don'ts (Table 15.5) shall be explained to patient at the time of simulation.

Table 15.5 Preventive measures during the course of radiation

Categories	Do's	Don'ts
Clothes	• Encourage wearing loose cotton clothes to avoid excessive sweating	• Avoiding tight clothing • Avoid collared shirts/ t shirts to avoid friction induced peeling of skin
Nutritional status	• Proper nutrition intake with dietary supplements as advised by treating physician • Maintaining adequate hydration	• Avoiding oily/spicy food • Avoiding improperly cooked food/raw food
Skin care	• Keeping radiation treatment area dry before treatment • Maintaining hygiene by washing area with lukewarm water and avoiding secondary infections • Using soft cotton cloth to gently dab the area dry • Use gentle moisturizers/ oils to prevent dryness after the treatment • Use electric shaver to trim hair	• Avoid harsh soaps/ shampoos with high fragrance to clean the radiation area • Do not shave with razor blades • Do not rub/itch radiation site • Avoid direct sunlight • Avoiding strenuous activities or activities that cause excessive perspiration

15.15 Conclusion

Radiation dermatitis is one of the most common side effect encountered during the course of radiation. Its effects are more pronounced at radical doses and at low doses, the grades of dermatitis is often manageable on out patient basis. Multiple studies use different methods to prevent and treat RISR's but there are no fixed guidelines. Overall, in initial stages of acute reactions, maintaining proper hygiene, washing area with lukewarm water, using moisturizers and antibacterial ointments have shown beneficial outcomes. If the area is non infected, but is painful, addition of analgesics is usually preferred. For dry desqauamtion, use of antiseptic ointments with topical steroids is the most common practiced method. Once, moist desquamation sets in, steroids are generally avoided to prevent infection. Barrier dressings, oral antibiotics, gentian violet are generally used for later stages of RID. For, advanced stages like necrosis, surgical intervention or hyper baric oxygen plays a major role.

The primary objective should be to ameliorate patient's symptoms and to improve the patient's adherence to receive complete treatment. Use of topical agents is usually preferred as most cancer patients are already poly medicated. Preventive measures are also of utmost importance and should not be neglected as they delay the onset of RID's. Careful instructions before and during treatment and regular counseling during weekly follow ups are mandatory to assure compliance. Treatment related factors like using newer treatment techniques, using image guidance, practicing adaptive RT can cut down the incidence of RID's. Well-designed, randomized, multicentric clinical studies are warranted to derive a consensus and more streamlined management of RD.

Key Points

1. Maintain proper hygiene, hydration and nutritional status.
2. Wear loose fitting cotton clothes, avoid excessive temperatures and avoid rubbing area under treatment.
3. Regular follow ups in OPD's for accurate assessment of skin reactions and prompt intervention.
4. Using lukewarm water to wash radiation area after treatment and keeping it dry before radiation process.
5. Using higher end techniques to achieve skin sparing effect, utilizing image guidance for proper treatment setup and practicing planned adaptive RT.
6. Use of proper immobilization masks, using bolus with caution, using tissue compensators for inhomogeneous tissue sites.
7. Monitoring and managing comorbid conditions.
8. Avoiding altered fractionation in susceptible patients.
9. Proper monitoring when administering skin reaction precipitating concurrent chemotherapy agents.
10. Avoiding steroids creams in infective conditions.

References

1. Khanna NR, Kumar DP, Laskar SG, Laskar S. Radiation dermatitis: an overview. Indian J Burns. 2013;21(24):31.
2. Singh M, Alavi A, Wong R, Akita S. Radiodermatitis: a review of our current understanding. Am J Clin Dermatol. 2016;17:277–92.
3. Porock D, Kristjanson L. Skin reactions during radiotherapy for breast cancer: the use and impact of topical agents and dressings. Eur J Cancer Care (Engl). 1999;8:143–53.
4. Safwat A, Bentzen SM, Turesson I, Hendry JH. Deterministic rather than stochastic factors explain most of the variation in the expression of skin telangiectasias after radiotherapy. Int J Radiat Oncol Biol Phys. 2002;52:198–204.
5. Behroozian T, Milton L, Li N, Zhang L, Lou J, Karam I, et al. Predictive factors associated with radiation dermatitis in breast cancer. Cancer Treat Res Commun. 2021;28:100403.
6. Iacovelli NA, Torrente Y, Ciuffreda A, Guardamagna VA, Gentili M, Giacomelli L, et al. Topical treatment of radiation-induced dermatitis: current issues and potential solutions. Drugs Context. 2020;9:2020-4-7.
7. Sibaud V, Lebœuf NR, Roche H, Belum VR, Gladieff L, Deslandres M, et al. Dermatological adverse events with taxane chemotherapy. Eur J Dermatol. 2016;26:427–43.
8. Rzepecki AK, Cheng H, McLellan BN. Cutaneous toxicity as a predictive biomarker for clinical outcome in patients receiving anticancer therapy. J Am Acad Dermatol. 2018;79:545–55.
9. Burke G, Faithfull S, Probst H. Radiation induced skin reactions during and following radiotherapy: a systematic review of interventions. Radiography. 2022;28(1):232–9. https://doi.org/10.1016/j.radi.2021.09.006.
10. Talapatra K, Singh P, Jaiswal I, Rais S, Pandey S. Radiation dermatitis: a narrative review of the Indian perspective. Cancer Res Stat Treat. 2020;3:526–36.
11. Saini S, Pai V, Shukla P, Ranglani H. A study of clinical pattern of acute radiation dermatitis among patients attending dermatology outpatient department at tertiary center in Western India. Clin Dermatol Rev. 2018;2:8–12.

12. Roy I, Fortin A, Larochelle M. The impact of skin washing with water and soap during breast irradiation: a randomized study. Radiother Oncol. 2001;58(3):333–9. https://doi.org/10.1016/S0167-8140(00)00322-4.
13. Haruna F, Lipsett A, Marignol L. Topical management of acute radiation dermatitis in breast cancer patients: a systematic review and meta-analysis. Anticancer Res. 2017;37:5343–53.
14. Kang HC, Ahn SD, Choi DH, et al. The safety and efficacy of EGF-based cream for the prevention of radiotherapy-induced skin injury: results from a multicenter observational study. Rad Oncol J. 2014;32(3):156. https://doi.org/10.3857/roj.2014.32.3.156.
15. Kouvaris JR, Kouloulias VE, Plataniotis GA, et al. Topical granulocyte-macrophage colony-stimulating factor for radiation dermatitis of the vulva. Br J Dermatol. 2001;144:646–7. https://doi.org/10.1046/j.1365-2133.2001.04115.x.
16. Koukourakis MI, Kyrias G, Kakolyris S, Kouroussis C, Frangiadaki C, Giatromanolaki A, Retalis G, Georgoulias V. Subcutaneous administration of amifostine during fractionated radiotherapy: a randomized phase II study. J Clin Oncol. 2000;18(11):2226–33. https://doi.org/10.1200/JCO.2000.18.11.2226.
17. Pareek P, Sharma A, Thipparampalli JR, Nag P, Gupta N, Shekhar S, Kirubakaran R. Pentoxifylline and vitamin E alone or in combination for preventing and treating side effects of radiation therapy and concomitant chemoradiotherapy. Cochrane Database Syst Rev. 2016;2016(3):CD012117. https://doi.org/10.1002/14651858.CD012117.
18. Liguori V, Guillemin C, Pesce GF, et al. Double-blind, randomized clinical study comparing hyaluronic acid cream to placebo in patients treated with radiotherapy. Radiother Oncol. 1997;42(2):155–61. https://doi.org/10.1016/S0167-8140(96)01882-8.
19. Schneider F, Danski MT, Vayego SA. Usage of Calendula officinalis in the prevention and treatment of radiodermatitis: a randomized double-blind controlled clinical trial. Rev Esc Enferm USP. 2015;49(2):221–8. https://doi.org/10.1590/S0080-623420150000200006.
20. Craighead P, Shea-Budgell MA, Nation J, Esmail R, Evans AW, Parliament M, et al. Hyperbaric oxygen therapy for late radiation tissue injury in gynecologic malignancies. Curr Oncol. 2011;18:220–7.
21. Bennett MH, FeldmeierJ HNB, Smee R, Milross C. Hyperbaric oxygen therapy for late radiation tissue injury. Cochrane Database Syst Rev. 2016;4:CD005005.

Cutaneous Manifestation of Chemotherapeutic Agents

16

Chaturbhuj R. Agrawal, Kshitiz Domadia, and Silky Kothiwal

Abbreviations

5FU	5 Fluorouracil
ATP	Adenosine triphosphate
BEP	Bleomycin, etoposide, and platinum
CML	Chronic myeloid leukaemia
CLL	Chronic lymphocytic leukaemia
DMSO	Dimethyl sulfoxide
DPYD	dihydropyrimidine dehydrogenase
EGFR	Epidermal growth factor receptor
FDA	united states food and drug administration
GIST	Gastrointestinal stromal tumour
HFS	Hand foot syndrome
mAbs	Monoclonal antibodies
NSCLC	Non small cell lung cancer
PDGFR	Platelet derived growth factor receptor
PLD	Liposomal doxorubicin
RRD	Radiation recall reaction
SCLC	small cell lung cancer

C. R. Agrawal (✉)
Department of Medical Oncology, Bahrain Specialist Hospital and Clinics, Juffair, Kingdom of Bahrain

K. Domadia
Department of Medical Oncology, HCG Cancer Institute, Ahmedabad, India

S. Kothiwal
Department of Gynecology and Obstetrics, Bahrain Specialist Hospital and Clinics, Juffair, Kingdom of Bahrain

K. Sood Sharma et al. (eds.), *Complications of Cancer Therapy: Best Practices in Prevention and Management*, https://doi.org/10.1007/978-981-99-0984-1_16

TKI	Tyrosine kinase inhibitors
VEGFR	Vascular endothelial growth factor receptor
TYMS	Thymidylate synthetase

16.1 Introduction

Cancer patients are complex and when it comes to management of malignancy with systemic therapy, there is an unusual combination of general poor health, multidrug regimens, immunosuppressive status, and poor dietary intake with altered body milieu. Systemic cancer treatment causing cutaneous toxicities are common and seen in significant number of patients receiving cancer chemotherapy, targeted therapy, or immunotherapy. However, these adverse events may be dose-dependent or dose independent and often they require modification of drug doses, dose density and dose intensity.

There has been rapid development in cancer therapy in last decade with paradigm shift to targeted anti—cancer therapy rather than conventional chemotherapy. Considering the clinical deployment and speedy development of these agents, physicians, oncologists, and dermatologists are often not familiar with full spectrum of cutaneous toxicities of these agents and their management which often require multidisciplinary management. Further considering the lifesaving nature of emerging newer drugs, it seems unwise to discontinue the for minor alterations and wisely early recognition of clinical signs and symptoms of such toxicities with their management and continuation of these lifesaving drugs in most tolerable dose appears to be the need of hour.

This chapter will further classify and simplify various cutaneous manifestations seen with chemotherautic agents and their management.

16.2 Hyperpigmentation

One of the most common cutaneous side effects of Cancer therapy drugs including chemotherapy and targeted therapy is hyper pigmentation. The pathophysiology is assumed to be related to melanocyte destruction due to toxic effects of chemotherapy which can lead to increase melanin release and hence hyperpigmentation. This hyperpigmentation can manifest itself in skin, nails, teeth and even tongue.

Variety of hyperpigmentation have been described in association with different chemotherapeutic agents.

1. Irregular hyperpigmentation
   - 5 FU and cyclophosphamide usually causes irregular hyperpigmentation.

- 5 FU usually causes serpentine hyperpigmentation causing tree bark appearance at the infusion site through the course of vein through which drug is infused if given through peripheral IV line [1]. Cyclophosphamide usually causes generalized hyperpigmentation of face and extremities and nail pigmentation [2].

2. Supra-venous hyperpigmentation

   It is an unusual form of hyperpigmentation of superficial venous system after systemic chemotherapy. Although this term was first coined by Hrushesky to describe increased pigmentation of skin during 5 FU infusion and previously it has been reported more with CHOP based chemotherapy for lymphomas it can virtually happen with most of the chemotherapeutic drug in practice like antibiotics, proteasome inhibitors or alkylating agents [3].
3. Flagellate hyperpigmentation—It is an unusual rash that appear as "whip-like" linear streaks and occur usually with Bleomycin use. The rash has a characteristic and intermingled lacy appearance as if it has been whipped. Bleomycin hydrolase, the enzyme which cleaves ammonia group from Bleomycin (Fig. 16.1)

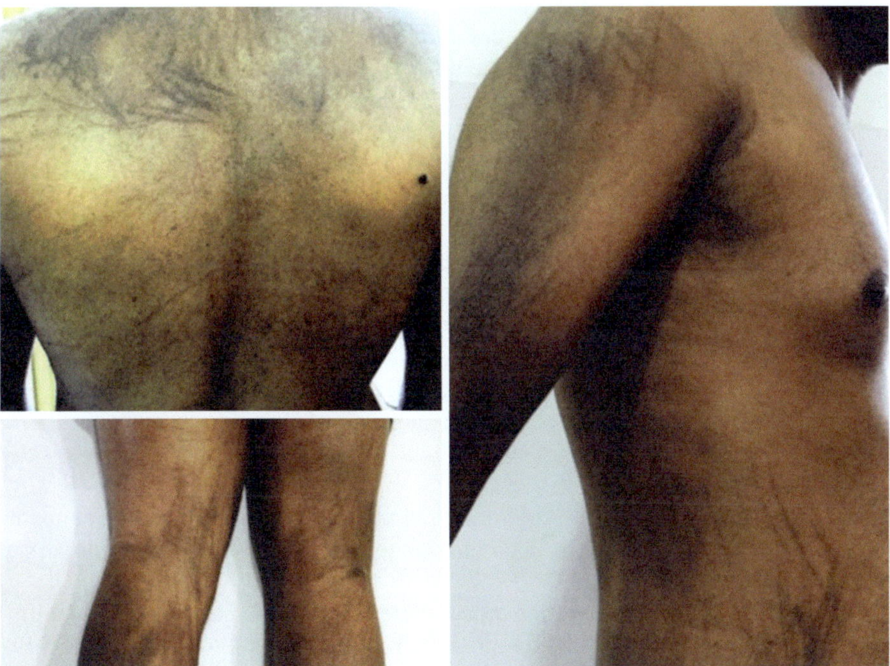

Fig. 16.1 Bleomycin associated flagellate rash over back, trunk and legs in a patient undergoing BEP chemotherapy for Germ cell tumour

and makes its inactive for most of the organs of body except skin and lung tissue causing toxicities in these two places. This rash has been described since 1996 but since then it is declining due to limited use of bleomycin in Germ cell tumours, Hodgkin's lymphoma and for pleurodesis. There is previously reported spectrum of skin disorders with bleomycin in form of skin peeling, hyperkeratosis, nail bed changes, Raynaud's phenomenon, and palmoplantar desquamation [4].

4. Nail hyperpigmentation—This will be covered in subsequent paragraph under "Nail disorders".
5. Others—Other forms of hyperpigmentation are drug specific and can occur with different characteristic pattern. E.g. Hydroxyurea may affect the face, neck, lower arms, palms and nails. Cisplatin can cause pressure induced hyperpigmentation in minority of patients. When methotrexate can rarely induce diffuse brown skin pigmentation, procarbazine can cause generalized melanosis [5].

16.3 Nail Disorders

Nail changes are one of the most common mucocutaneous adverse reactions of cancer chemotherapy and radiation therapy [6]. The changes in nail can vary from primary cosmetic change like discoloration to onycholysis and severe infection requiring systemic antibiotics. Non-specific nail disorders are commonly observed during systemic anti-cancer treatment. This includes transverse grooves on the nail plate (Beau's lines) and onychomadesis which are most common.

- Melanonychia refers to brownish or black pigmented bands which can be transverse, longitudinal, or diffuse and mostly appear 1–2 months after chemotherapy initiation. This occurs due to melanocyte activation in matrix epithelium [7]. The alternation dark and normal bands on nails are seen with docetaxel and anthracyclines like daunorubicin. However, these pigmentary changes are usually reversible, and they reverse few months after stoppage of chemotherapeutic agents.
- Paronychia refers to inflammation of nail fold and has seen characteristically with cetuximab [8].
- Leukonychia refers to white colouration of nail plate which can be true or apparent leukonychia. This can be apparent due to abnormalities of blood flow in the nail bed.
- Onycholysis refers to separation of nail plate from nail bed and it can be painful. This is commonly seen with administration of Taxanes, anthracyclines and 5 FU [9] (Fig. 16.2).

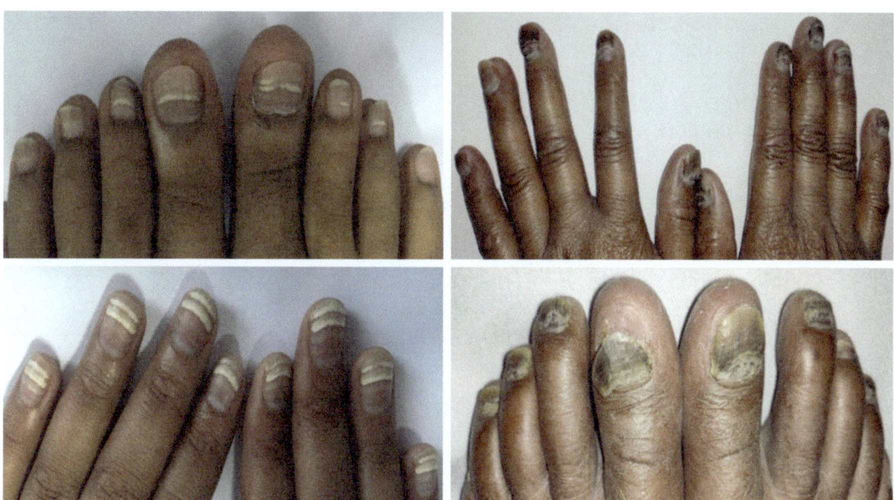

Fig. 16.2 Transverse grooves on nail plate and Onycholysis seen classically with Taxanes chemotherapy

16.4 Acral Erythema

Acral erythema also known by various terms like hand foot syndrome, toxic erythema of palms and soles, palmer planter erythrodysesthesia or Bergdorf reaction. It was first described with patients receiving high dose cytarabine for acute leukaemia and later, it has been described with many chemotherapeutic agents like Pegylated liposomal, doxorubicin. Capecitabine or Fluorouracil and with tyrosine kinase inhibitors like sorafenib, Sunitinib and regorafenib. It is most seen in clinical practice with fluoropyrimidines and capecitabine and it may be associated with genetic polymorphisms of dihydropyrimidine dehydrogenase (DPYD) and Thymidylate synthetase (TYMS) which are the enzymes involved in metabolism of capecitabine and other fluoropyrimidine. Although genetic tests are available to identify these enzyme deficiencies, It is not considered standard of care to test for these mutations or deficiencies prior to initiating fluoropyrimidine therapy. Moreover, it also varies with infusional versus bolus dose like in case of 5 FU it can be seen in up to 38% of patients receiving infusional 5 FU or oral capecitabine in fully recommended doses while only in less than 5% cases who receive bolus 5 FU infusion (Fig. 16.3).

Common chemo therapeutic agents causing HFS are summarized below in Table 16.1.

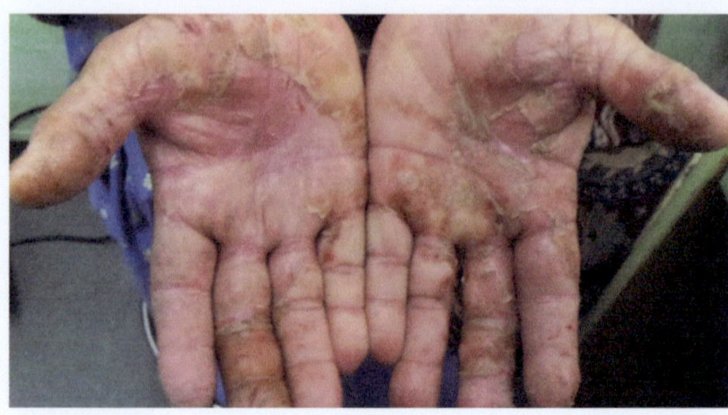

Fig. 16.3 Capecitabine induced HFS in a patient receiving palliative chemotherapy for metastatic colon cancer

Table 16.1 Common chemotherapeutic agents causing hand foot syndrome

Chemotherautic agents	Targeted agents
Cytarabine	Lapatinib
Capecitabine	Sorafenib
5 FU	Sunitinib
Idarubicin	Pazopanib
Liposomal doxorubicin (PLD)	Ixabepilone

Fingerprint loss is one of the very important consequences of Hand foot syndrome and patients on long term capecitabine or sorafenib or sunitinib therapy should be informed about this potential adverse effect. Although it can create short term troubles for patients in their legal matters, this complication is not permanent and there is complete recovery of fingerprints after resolution of hand Foot syndrome when these drugs are discontinued [10].

16.4.1 Prevention

16.4.1.1 Topical Urea Cream

For patients receiving Capecitabine,10% topical urea cream is recommended for prevention of hand foot syndrome. This cream is typically applied to both hand and feet three to four times per day and preferably after washing hands. The prophylactic benefit of topical urea treatment has not been demonstrated for other chemotherapeutic agents.

16.4.1.2 Pyridoxine

Use of oral pyridoxine has been tested widely for prevention of HFS however there are four phase III trials in which patient receiving capecitabine based chemotherapy or PLD were randomly assigned to either pyridoxine 150 or 200 mg daily or placebo and in these trials, it did not prevent this complication or even lessen its severity. Also, two separate meta-analysis also concluded the same. There is inadequate evidence to recommend use of pyridoxine for prevention of chemotherapy induced hand foot syndrome [11].

16.4.1.3 Celecoxib

In 2014, meta-analysis, oral celecoxib 200 to 400 mg twice daily for 12 to 18 weeks significantly decreased the risk of Grade II to III HFS. However, because of its potential cardiovascular side effects and upper gastrointestinal bleeding risk its use has been questioned.

16.4.2 Other Measures

1. Local application of cold therapy by applying ice packs to wrist and ankle may help by decreasing blood flow to hands and feet [12].
2. A trial of oral corticosteroids in reducing the frequency of hand foot syndrome has also been tested in two small series and found effective [13].

16.4.2.1 Treatment

The main treatment for hand foot syndrome is drug interruption or dose modification. Preliminary treatment involves topical corticosteroids to decrease inflammation, proper wound care for erosions and ulcerations to prevent supernumerary infections, topical keratolytic to prevent hyperkeratosis and analgesics for pain control.

16.5 Extravasation Injuries

Chemotherapy extravasation causing tissue injury is not new however now with use of more and more central access devices the incidence of extravasation injury is rapidly declining. Accidental extravasation of chemotherapy in surrounding tissues causes local tissue injury and necrosis. There are five brief categories of chemotherapy drugs as per their nature to cause extravasation injury (Table 16.2) out of which broad two categories are vesicants and irritants.

Table 16.2 Different nature of chemotherapeutic agents with respect to their extravasation hazard

Vesicants	Irritants	Exfoliants	Inflammitants	Neutrals
DNA binding Vesicants – Anthracyclines – Alkylating agents like nitrogen mustards Non-DNA binding Vesicants – Vinca alkaloids – Taxanes like Docetaxel and paclitaxel	Carboplatin Topotecan Etoposide Teniposide Cytarabine	Carboplatin Topotecan	Methotrexate Raltitrexed Bortezomib 5 Fluorouracil	Trastuzumab Gemcitabine Bevacizumab Bortezomib Bleomycin

1. Vesicants—Extravasation of a vesicant drug has potential to cause tissue necrosis (blistering, sloughing of tissues and various degrees of deep tissue damage) and more severe injury seen as compared to irritants chemotherapy. Vesicants are further classified as non-DNA binding and DNA binding. Non-DNA binding agents are metabolized and neutralized in tissues whereas DNA binding drugs they set up a continuous cycle of tissue damage that is mediated by cellular DNA causing more extensive injuries [14]. Anthracyclines are most notorious amongst these because of their widespread use and potential to cause severe tissue damage. Therefore, for infusion of these drugs, particularly in case of infusions rather than bolus, CVAD rather than peripheral IV line should be preferred [15].
2. Irritants—Irritants causes inflammation (warmth, erythema, tenderness) at administration site and along the veins, but they rarely cause direct tissue toxicity or necrosis. However, if large volumes of concentrated solution are extravasated, tissue necrosis can occur.

Risk factors from extravasation from CVAD device are –

1. Catheter migration from the vein into the tissue.
2. Presence of fibrin sheath or thrombus at catheter tip.
3. Deeply implanted port device increases risk that the length of access needle will not be sufficiently long to be correctly positioned.
4. Difficulty encountered during insertion of the device, such as probing or inability to advance the guidewire or catheter.
5. Long indwelling time (6 months or more).

Risk factors from extravasation from CVAD device are –

1. Obesity.
2. Sclerosed veins.
3. Excessive patient movement during chemo infusion.
4. Bolus infusion (for example, power injectors of radio contrast media).
5. Prolonged infusion duration.
6. Small and or fragile veins.
7. Sclerosed veins due to multiple prior chemotherapy sessions or numerous venepunctures.

16.5.1 Management of Extravasation

Once extravasation occur the most important step is to immediately stop the infusion and identify the extravasated agent and classify it as vesicant or irritant. The extravasation area should be marked and photographed, and the cannula needle should be removed. Analgesics may be given to manage the pain, and once initial measures are completed, it is very important to document the adverse drug reaction or medication error that has happened.

Application of local heat for 20 min, four times daily for 1–2 days for Vinca alkaloids while for other vesicant extravasation including anthracycline, the initial treatment is towards localizing and neutralizing the extra visited agents with cold compresses for 20 min four times daily for 1–2days, which limits the cellular uptake of these agents [16].

16.5.2 Pharmacological Treatment

16.5.2.1 DMSO

It is a common solvent which penetrates tissue and increases skin permeability and facilitate absorption of extravasated drug. It has free radical scavenging and antioxidant property when applied locally and causes speedy removal of extravasated drug. The efficacy of DMSO for treatment of chemotherapy extravasation was first described in several case reports and small studies. Oliver and Schwartz reported three cases of extravasation which were successfully resolved with DMSO, and the extravasation guidelines recommend use of DMSO 50–99% for use at discretion of the clinicians [17].

16.5.2.2 Hyaluronidase

Hyaluronidase can breakdown the extracellular matrix that underlies epithelial cells. It has been used for treatment of Vinca alkaloids and Taxanes extravasation, and the dose of hyaluronidase varies from 150 to 1500 units diluted in 1 ml of normal saline subcutaneously or intradermally within one hour of extravasation. There is rapid resolution of pain when patients are treated with hyaluronidase and several reports indicates its effectiveness in vinca alkaloids and Taxanes extravasation. The EONS extravasation guidelines recommend hyaluronidase may be considered as an potential option for these cases at discretion of physicians [16].

16.5.2.3 Sodium Thiosulfate

It prevents alkylation and tissue destruction by providing a substrate for alkylation in subcutaneous tissue. The recommended dose is 2 ML of 0.17 M (a solution of 4 ml 10% sodium thiosulphate and 6 mL sterile water for injection). However, due to lack of sufficient evidence, the EONS extravasation guidelines do not recommend this as an antidote [18].

16.5.2.4 Dexrazoxane

It has dual mechanism of action—(1) It stabilizes topoisomerase II and makes it inaccessible to anthracycline chemotherapy. It blocks the enzyme so that there is no longer affect by anthracycline and prevent damage to healthy cells. (2) It acts as an iron chelator and prevents formation of iron anthracycline complexes. The most common adverse events of dexrazoxane includes decreased white blood cell counts, decreased haemoglobin, thrombocytopenia, Increased liver enzymes and nausea.

16.6 Immune Mediated Infusion Reactions

All chemotherapeutic agents when administered systematically can induce infusion reaction but some are immune mediated infusion reaction. Briefly there are three types of immune mediated hypersensitivity reactions that can cause cutaneous manifestation during chemotherapy administration (Table 16.3).

1. Classic type 1 immunoglobulin E (Ig E) mediated allergic reactions—Most infusion reactions with Platinum drugs (cisplatin, carboplatin and oxaliplatin) are classical type 1 immunoglobulin E mediated allergic reactions which develop within 1 h of drug administration in form of urticaria, pruritus interior, angioedema, and other anaphylactic symptoms. However, they may offer up to 24 h following exposure but usually resolve spontaneously.
2. Type III reactions—These results from formation and tissue deposition of antigen-antibody complexes. Cutaneous vasculitis seen with methotrexate and serum sickness following infusion of rituximab are classical type 3 reactions.
3. Type IV Reactions—These are mediated by activated T cells. Classic example of Type IV allergic reaction is contact dermatitis to topical mechlorethamine (nitrogen mustard).

Table 16.3 Classification of allergic cutaneous reactions to chemotherapeutic agents

Type	Description	Mechanism	Clinical features
I	Anaphylactic, immediate type hypersensitivity	Antigen exposure causes release of vasoactive substances like histamine, prostaglandins, and leukotrienes from mast cells. This response is usually IgE mediated	Anaphylaxis Angioedema Bronchospasm Urticaria
II	Antibody dependent cytotoxicity	An antigen or hapten that is intimately associated with a cell bind to antibody and causes tissue injury	Hemolytic anemia Interstitial nephritis
III	Immune complex disease	Deposition of antigen-antibody complex causes tissue damage	Serum sickness
IV	Cell mediated/ delayed hypersensitivity	Antigen exposure sensitizes T cells which then mediates tissue injury	Contact dermatitis

16.7 Unique Drug Specific Reactions

Fludarabine has been reported to cause paraneoplastic pemphigus (PNP) which is characterized by painful mucosal ulcerations and polymorphous skin lesions that progress to blistering eruptions on trunk and extremities. The treatment involves treating the underlying malignancy itself and there is no standard therapy for PNP. Some patients may get benefited with immunosuppression and rituximab-based therapy [19].

Hydroxyurea can cause lichen planus like eruption in up to 35% of patients. Secondary non melanoma skin cancers may occur in patients taking hydroxyurea therapy and systemic retinoids have been used for treating such skin cancers [20].

Taxanes are usually associated with fluid retention syndrome which is more commonly seen with Docetaxel as compared to paclitaxel. Appropriate prophylaxis with 3–5 days of Glucocorticoids premedication can ameliorate this fluid retention [21]. Gemcitabine too can cause pedal oedema in up to 9% of patients [22].

Anthracyclines can induce pruritic erythematous macules, papules, and plaques, with or without vesicles which can appear 3–4 weeks after completion of chemotherapy. These eruptions usually resolve within weeks to months [23]. Estramustine can cause oestrogen related adverse events like gynecomastia [24].

EGFR inhibitors have been associated with altered hair growth & trichomegaly (Fig. 16.4). Although it has no correlation to response or rarely it required dose modification but its knowledge is important in relieving patient anxiety [25].

VEGF TKI (E.g., Sunitinib) can cause multiple dermatological side effects like hand foot syndrome, acral erythema, subungual splinter haemorrhages and generalized rashes but typical pattern of hair discolouration may occur which has succession of depigmented and normally pigmented bands of hair, and it may correlate with on and off periods of treatment [26].

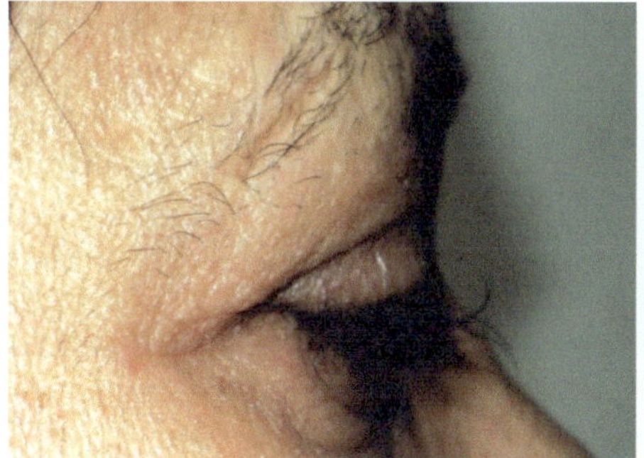
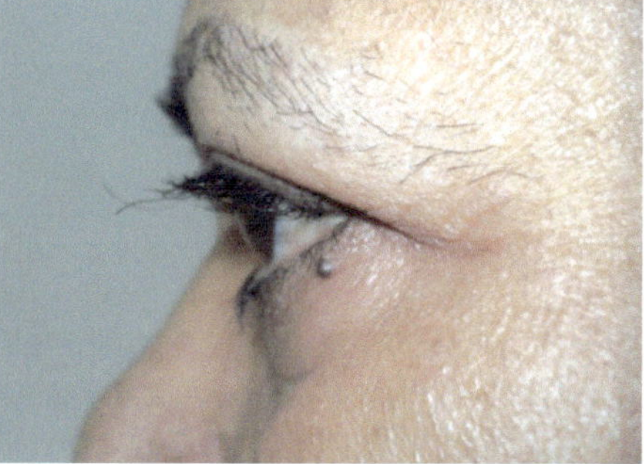

Fig. 16.4 Gefitinib induced eyelashes trichomegaly in a patient receiving palliative Gefitinib for EGFR positive metastatic NSCLC

Antiapoptotic agents particularly proteosome inhibitors like Bortezomib used in myeloma can cause cutaneous reaction in up to 10–24% of patients and varies in clinical presentation from erythematous nodules and plaques to morbilliform rash with ulcers. Rarely occurrence of acute febrile neutrophilic dermatosis (Sweet syndrome) has also been described with Bortezomib [27].

16.7.1 Tyrosine Kinase Inhibitors and Anti EGFR Monoclonal Antibodies

The mechanism through which EGFR inhibitors act is blocking of transduction pathway needed for cell proliferation, migration, and angiogenesis of tumour cells. Several generations of oral tyrosine kinase inhibitors are available now with wide variety of indications which are beyond the scope of this discussion, but they can cause severe cutaneous reactions in form of papulopustular rash, paronychia, hair changes, itchiness, and dryness. Monoclonal antibodies (Cetuximab, Panitumumab) on the other hand are given intravenously and can cause similar pattern of dermatological toxicity.

1. Papulopustular rash—The frequency differs between different EGFR TKI, and it is approximately 49% to 67% with erlotinib, 24 to 62% with Gefitinib and 75 to 91% with patients taking cetuximab [28]. Although initially thought to be a marker of response, multiple studies subsequently failed to establish any direct correlation between therapeutic efficacy of these drugs and occurrence of rashes. Treatment usually involved topical antibiotics like topical Clindamycin or erythromycin and oral Minocycline and Doxycycline for advanced cases along with topical steroids. Systemic isotretinoin can be useful in some cases that are not responding to antibiotic therapy [29].
2. Paronychia—Next most frequent reaction occurs in nails and digits and first digit being most affected. These occur in approximately 10–15% of patients and appear after 1–2 months of beginning treatment. Superinfection prevention with antibacterial soaks are important and warm compresses, silver nitrate, topical corticosteroids and systemic tetracyclines can also be used to reduce periungual inflammation [30].
3. Pruritus—Pruritus can have dramatic impact on patients HQOL although it rarely requires dose modifications or discontinuation of drug. It occurs in approx. 50% of EGFR TKI treated patients and often accompanies with Papulopustular rashes describe above. Underlying mechanism for pruritus has not been elucidated till date but histamine release has been suggested as one of the potential mechanisms. Topical anti-histaminic, topical steroids and gentle skin care with moisturizers has been suggested treatment [31].
4. Other reactions—Anaphylaxis can occur in 1–3% of patient taking cetuximab or panitumumab, but these are rare. Other reactions include increased propensity of oral aphthous ulcers, vasculitis, enhancement of radiation dermatitis, and transient acantholytic dermatosis [32].

16.8 Angiogenesis Inhibitors

Multi kinase inhibitors like sorafenib and sunitinib are specific angiogenesis inhibitors Via VEGFR, PDGFR and other kinases. Dermatological manifestations are very common with these inhibitors and are found in approximately 81% of patients taking sunitinib and 74% patients taking sorafenib. Most frequent amongst them are hand foot reactions and stomatitis. However. Other reactions in form of oral mucosal complications, alopecia, hair depigmentation, Facial erythema. Fingernail subungual splinter haemorrhages are also not uncommon [33]. Management of these rashes depends entirely on the severity and usually they resolve with use of topical corticosteroid cream without any interruption of treatment. Topically urea cream in combination with oral pyridoxal has been used for severe hand foot syndrome. Systemic corticosteroids, like Prednisone, are rarely required and reserved for severe life-threatening reactions like toxic epidermal necrolysis [34].

16.9 Radiation Recall Dermatitis

The inflammatory skin reaction that develops in an area of previously irradiated skin after administration of certain Chemotherapeutic agents is known as radiation recall dermatitis. The interval between the administration of. Chemotherapeutic, agent and appearance of RRD may vary [35]. However, the frequency of these reactions is unclear. The commonly associated agents with RRD are antimetabolites like gemcitabine and anthracyclines like daunorubicin. The usual manifestation is erythema which can be painful. However, vesiculation, desquamation and ulceration can also happen. It typically occurs with first dose of chemotherapy agent or combination and drug dose appears to be the most important factor in its occurrence [36].

It also requires minimum threshold radiation dose. In previously reported cases, the radiation recall reaction with bleomycin or docetaxel has occurred only in those skin site that has received highest radiation dose. Dose reductions and use of corticosteroids have been used as adjunctive measures to prevent recurrence of RRD [37].

16.10 Conclusions

1. Systemic & local conventional chemotherapy drugs and even targeted agents can cause several changes in skin, mucus membrane, hairs, or nails. Some of these are immune mediated non dose dependent while some of them are dose dependent and to identify and categorize this is very important so as not to reduce the dose unnecessarily compromising efficacy of that agent particularly in curative setting.
2. Pigmentary changes may involve skin, nails and mucus membrane and hyperpigmentation may be localized or diffuse or with distinctive patterns like Serpentine or flagellate depending upon the chemotherapeutic agent. However,

most of the time, hyperpigmentation has only cosmetic implication and may not require active management.

3. Nail changes such as hyperpigmentation or onycholysis may be induced by many medications including alkylating agents, Taxanes, Antimetabolites, anthracyclines, and antibiotics. Reassurance to patient and supportive care with dressing and prevention of secondary bacterial infection is important form of management for these nail changes.
4. HFS is important and common complications seen with commonly used drugs like Capecitabine, PLD, Fluorouracil and TKIs like Sunitinib & Sorafenib. In these patients, given the low risk of toxic effects, preventive application of topical 10% urea cream for prevention appears to be a wise decision. Reassurance to the patient that this side effect is dose related & it usually resolves within 2–4 weeks after discontinuation is very important and dose titration to be done wisely so as not to compromise therapeutic efficacy too.
5. Chemotherapy extravasation, although uncommonly seen in present era with more use of central venous access devices, is important and early detection of this condition can prevent further tissue damage. Identification and classification of the agent as Vesicant or Irritant will help in further management of this complication as per recommended guidelines.
6. Radiation recall dermatitis (RRD) is important dermatological toxicity related to both radiation therapy and concurrently administered chemotherapy. A knowledge of this side effect is important in selecting the subsequent chemotherapeutic agent particularly in those patients who are prone and have received higher doses of radiation.
7. Few anti neoplastic agents can cause severe cutaneous reactions like steven Johnson syndrome (SJS) or toxic epidermal necrolysis (TEN) which could be life threatening due to widespread epidermal detachment due to massive keratinocyte apoptosis. Those who develop this complication and recovered should never be re-exposed to the causative agent because of life threatening nature of this complication.

References

1. Agrawal CR. Unusual serpentine hyperpigmentation induced by 5-fluorouracil. Pigment Int. 2017;4(2):124.
2. Youssef M, Mokni S, Belhadjali H, Aouem K, Moussa A, Laatiri A, Zili J. Cyclophosphamide-induced generalised reticulated skin pigmentation: a rare presentation. Int J Clin Pharm. 2013;35(3):309–12.
3. Hrushesky WJ. Unusual pigmentary changes associated with 5-fluorouracil therapy. Cutis. 1980;26(2):181–2.
4. Agrawal C, Talwar V, Saini R, Babu P. Flagellate rash: An unusual complication of bleomycin therapy – a case report with brief review of literature. Indian J Med Paediatr Oncol. 2017;38:548–51.
5. Hendrix JD Jr, Greer KE. Cutaneous hyperpigmentation caused by systemic drugs. Int J Dermatol. 1992;31(7):458–66.

6. Naveed S, Thappa DM, Dubashi B, Pandjatcharam J, Munisamy M, Singh N. Mucocutaneous adverse reactions of cancer chemotherapy and chemoradiation. Indian J Dermatol. 2019;64(2):122.
7. Piraccini BM, Iorizzo M, Starace M, Tosti A. Drug-induced nail diseases. Dermatol Clin. 2006;24(3):387–91.
8. Monti M. Cutaneous toxicity induced by cetuximab. Am Soc Clin Oncol. 2003;21:4651–3.
9. Marrs J, Newton S. Chemotherapy-induced nail changes: an unsightly nuisance. Clin J Oncol Nurs. 2004;8(5):527–8.
10. Van Doorn L, Veelenturf S, Binkhorst L, Bins S, Mathijssen R. Capecitabine and the risk of fingerprint loss. JAMA Oncol. 2017;3(1):122–3.
11. Chen M, Zhang L, Wang Q, Shen J. Pyridoxine for prevention of hand-foot syndrome caused by chemotherapy: a systematic review. PLoS One. 2013;8(8):e72245.
12. Mangili G, Petrone M, Gentile C, De Marzi P, Viganò R, Rabaiotti E. Prevention strategies in palmar–plantar erythrodysesthesia onset: the role of regional cooling. Gynecol Oncol. 2008;108(2):332–5.
13. Drake RD, Lin WM, King M, Farrar D, Miller DS, Coleman RL. Oral dexamethasone attenuates Doxil®-induced palmar-plantar erythrodysesthesias in patients with recurrent gynecologic malignancies. Gynecol Oncol. 2004;94(2):320–4.
14. Hannon MG, Lee SK. Extravasation injuries. J Hand Surg Am. 2011;36:2060.
15. Kreidieh FY, Moukadem HA, El Saghir NS. Overview, prevention and management of chemotherapy extravasation. World J Clin Oncol. 2016;7:87.
16. Wengström Y, Margulies A. European oncology nursing society extravasation guidelines. Eur J Oncol Nurs. 2008;12(4):357–61.
17. Lebredo L, Barrie R, Woltering EA. DMSO protects against adriamycin-induced tissue necrosis. J Surg Res. 1992;53(1):62–5.
18. Gorski LA. Central venous access device occlusions: part 2: nonthrombotic causes and treatment. Home Healthcare Now. 2003;21(3):168–71.
19. Schadlow MB, Anhalt GJ, Sinha AA. Using rituximab (anti-CD20 antibody) in a patient with paraneoplastic pemphigus. J Drug Dermatol. 2003;2(5):564–7.
20. Sanchez-Palacios C, Guitart J. Hydroxyurea-associated squamous dysplasia. J Am Acad Dermatol. 2004;51(2):293–300.
21. Goh ML, Lim HL, Ng AWK, Chan CC, Kong HL, Lee SC, Joseph Wee ET, Chua JEL, Wong BC. Phase II trial of docetaxel in Asian patients with inoperable stage III non-small cell lung cancer. Acta Oncol. 2000;39(2):225–9.
22. Halme M, Jekunen A, Tamminen K, Mattson K. Phase II study of weekly gemcitabine in advanced non-small cell lung cancer. Respir Med. 1997;91(7):423–6.
23. Skelton H, Linstrum J, Smith K. Host-vs.-altered-host eruptions in patients on liposomal doxorubicin. J Cutan Pathol. 2002;29(3):148–53.
24. Sinibaldi VJ, Carducci MA, Moore-Cooper S, Laufer M, Zahurak M, Eisenberger MA. Phase II evaluation of docetaxel plus one-day oral estramustine phosphate in the treatment of patients with androgen independent prostate carcinoma. Cancer. 2002;94(5):1457–65.
25. Agrawal CR, Goyal P, Doval DC, Dutta K, Domadia K, Kothiwal S. Eyelashes trichomegaly: an unusual side effect of gefitinib therapy. Int J Trichol. 2018;10(1):44.
26. Agrawal CR, Talwar V, Babu VP, Jain P, Goyal P. Unusual pattern of whitening of eyebrows following sunitinib therapy: a case report with brief review of literature. Int J Trichol. 2017;9(4):190.
27. Agrawal C, Kapoor R, Saini R. Rare occurrence of bortezomib-induced Sweet's syndrome in multiple myeloma. Int J Health Allied Sci. 2016;5(3):178.
28. Heidary N, Naik H, Burgin S. Chemotherapeutic agents and the skin: an update. J Am Acad Dermatol. 2008;58(4):545–70.
29. Bidoli P, Cortinovis DL, Colombo I, Crippa A, Cicchiello F, Villa F, Cazzaniga ME, Altomare G. Isotretinoin plus clindamycin seem highly effective against severe erlotinib-induced skin rash in advanced non-small cell lung cancer. J Thorac Oncol. 2010;5(10):1662–3.

30. Lacouture ME, Anadkat MJ, Bensadoun RJ, Bryce J, Chan A, Epstein JB, Eaby-Sandy B, Murphy BA. Clinical practice guidelines for the prevention and treatment of EGFR inhibitor-associated dermatologic toxicities. Support Care Cancer. 2011;19(8):1079–95.
31. Roé E, Muret MP, Marcuello E, Capdevila J, Pallarés C, Alomar A. Description and management of cutaneous side effects during cetuximab or erlotinib treatments: a prospective study of 30 patients. J Am Acad Dermatol. 2006;55(3):429–37.
32. Tscharner GG, Bühler S, Borner M, Hunziker T. Grover's disease induced by cetuximab. Dermatology. 2006;213(1):37–9.
33. Jaber SH, Cowen EW, Haworth LR, Booher SL, Berman DM, Rosenberg SA, Hwang ST. Skin reactions in a subset of patients with stage IV melanoma treated with anti–cytotoxic T-lymphocyte antigen 4 monoclonal antibody as a single agent. Arch Dermatol. 2006;142(2):166–72.
34. Lemech C, Arkenau HT. Novel treatments for metastatic cutaneous melanoma and the management of emergent toxicities. Clin Med Insights Oncol. 2012;6:CMO-S5855.
35. Burris HA III, Hurtig J. Radiation recall with anticancer agents. Oncologist. 2010;15(11):1227–37.
36. Cassady JR, Richter MP, Piro AJ, Jaffe N. Radiation-Adriamycin interactions: preliminary clinical observations. Cancer. 1975;36(3):946–9.
37. Yeo W, Leung SF, Johnson PJ. Radiation-recall dermatitis with docetaxel: establishment of a requisite radiation threshold. Eur J Cancer. 1990;33(4):698–9.

Radiotherapy Induced Central Nervous System Toxicity

17

Anusheel Munshi, Biplab Sarkar, Vikas Pandey, and Deepak Raj Sonkar

17.1 Introduction

Along with neurosurgery and chemotherapy, radiation therapy is an essential treatment option for tumours of the central nervous system (CNS) [1]. Radiation therapy is a highly effective treatment that is commonly used for treatment of brain metastases, gliomas, CNS lymphomas, and meningioma, besides other tumours. However, it is also well known that all modalities to treat cancer have their share of side effects and toxicities. While, understanding the consequences of radiation on any normal tissue is essential for the safe radiotherapy delivery, it is especially critical for the nervous system. It is well known that severe and permanent radiation injury to CNS can dramatically impact quality of life (QOL) and daily functioning of the patient. This chapter deals with the side effects related to toxicities related to radiation therapy in CNS malignancies.

17.2 Mechanisms and Radiobiology

Ionizing radiation in all its forms has the potential to produce toxicity in the central nervous system. Radiation toxicity primarily effects (1) Glial oligodendrocytes which are the insulating myelin producing cells and (2) Glial astrocytes (cells responsible for the blood brain barrier). The basic mechanism of injury is the generation of free radicals that cause direct or indirect DNA damage [2]. In the mature CNS where cell division and mitotic potential is limited, it has been suggested that

A. Munshi (✉) · V. Pandey · D. R. Sonkar
Department of Radiation Oncology, Manipal Hospitals, New Delhi, India

B. Sarkar
Apollo Multispeciality Hospitals, Kolkata, West Bengal, India

K. Sood Sharma et al. (eds.), *Complications of Cancer Therapy: Best Practices in Prevention and Management*, https://doi.org/10.1007/978-981-99-0984-1_17

other mechanisms of radiation-induced damage (lipid bilayer oxidation, microvascular permeability, cell junctional rearrangements, and mitochondrial alterations) are likely to be important subcellular targets for ionising radiation [3].

Both the brain and the spinal cord are considered late-reacting tissues with a low alpha/beta ratio. However, in the finer circuitry, brain and spinal cord can be considered as parallel and serial organs respectively, the somewhat parallel circuitry and plasticity of the brain allows for some adaptation in the face of disruption by tumour, surgery, or radiation. On the contrary, the organization of the spinal cord with less redundancy and long fibre tracts is less forgiving. It also means that an extreme injury at one level of the spinal cord can prevent the transmission of neural impulses beyond that point.

Factors contributing to CNS toxicity include fraction size, age, medical comorbidities, psychological and genetic predispositions, characteristics of any underlying malignancy, as well as any additional injuries caused by other treatment modalities such as surgery and chemotherapy. The existing data suggested that, with equivalent volumes, larger fraction sizes produce worse toxicity in the CNS [4].

Emerging data also suggests that there is differential radiation sensitivity exists within various CNS sub compartments. Neurogenesis (a process by which new neurons are produced in the brain), persists throughout life in discrete regions of the adult brain, including the hippocampus. For long, it is known that radiation exposure has a negative impact on neurogenesis· It is believed that these disruptions in neurogenesis and hippocampal function are directly linked to cognitive and mood disruptions [5–7]. However, it is little understood as to what extent and what factors is the spontaneous recovery of neurogenesis and hippocampal function dependent upon. Combination of other agents with radiotherapy too can lead to additive or synergistic effect on CNS toxicity [8]. For these reasons, caution must be observed with a related or unrelated systemic therapy is going on during CNS radiotherapy.

17.3 Acute vs. Late Effects of Radiotherapy

Radiation-induced brain injury is described in three phases: early or acute (within days to weeks after irradiation), early-delayed (within 1–6 months' post irradiation) and late (>6 months' post irradiation)· Both conventional as well as stereotactic radiation treatment have the potential to produce side effects. These include fatigue, cognitive alterations, effects in short-term memory and concentration, pituitary dysfunction resulting in endocrine disruptions and occasionally, dementia [9, 10]. Table 17.1 enumerates the acute and late toxicities after CNS radiotherapy.

Post radiation changes can be observed changes in the entire brain (grey matter, white matter, ventricles) or in some subsections [11, 12]. An important feature of normal tissue toxicity includes vascular injury. Coagulation necrosis of the white matter tracts is an important feature of radiotherapy induced injury. Overproduction of myelin in oligodendrocytes can cause Leukoencephalopathy and is a late toxicity. The process of demyelination can also occur in spinal cord and nerve roots.

Table 17.1 Acute, early delayed and late side effects of CNS radiotherapy

Acute side effects	Early delayed	Late side effects
Fatigue	Persistent fatigue	Pituitary/hypothalamic axis hormonal imbalance
Cognitive alterations	Transient focal neuroprogression	Vascular events
Headache	Pseudoprogression	Memory
Alopecia and radiation dermatitis		Cognition
Nausea and vomiting		Visual pathway (optic nerve, chiasm)
Loss of appetite		Brain stem, spinal cord injury
Worsening of pre-existing symptoms		Radio necrosis, secondary malignancy

17.4 Imaging and Measuring CNS Toxicity

Challenges for assessing CNS toxicity include the usual lack of an accurate pre-treatment baseline, patient noncompliance in neurocognitive testing, attrition due to several reasons, confounding medications (steroids, antiepileptic medications, and chemotherapeutics) and associated depression/anxiety.

Imaging is the most commonly used modality to evaluate the effects of radiation. To be noted, not all radiographic changes have a direct correlation to the functional outcomes and functional toxicities. Radiographic definitions are lacking as conventional magnetic resonance imaging (MRI) has a limited ability to distinguish normal tissue injury from treatment related changes, such radiation necrosis or vascular changes [13]. Structural changes may be present on scans in previously irradiated patients but may have none of the perpetual radiological dilemmas is distinguishing recurrent CNS tumour from radiation necrosis. The classic description on MRI is a "soap bubble" or "Swiss cheese" appearance (Fig. 17.1). However, actually distinguishing radiation necrosis from tumour progression can be extremely challenging at times. On diffusion mapping, radiation necrosis tends to exhibit increased diffusion while tumour progression is associated with diffusion restriction [6]. Magnetic resonance (MR) perfusion can also be used for resolving this dilemma. In general, increased regional cerebral blood volume (rCBV) is associated with tumour recurrence [14, 15]. Magnetic resonance spectroscopy (MRS) using metabolite ratios such as choline/creatine (Cho/Cr) and choline/*N*-acetylaspartate (Cho/NAA) are of some help in this aspect. The use of positron emission tomography (PET), 13C labelled metabolites such as 13C-pyruvate, and cation exchange saturation transfer (CEST) imaging may have some advantages. These imaging modalities allow imaging of altered glucose uptake, energy production, and glutamate neurotransmitter fluctuations. To further complicate issues, post RT changes including necrosis can often coexist with viable/recurrent disease.

Traditionally, for purpose of mental status, the Folstein Mini Mental Status Exam (MMSE) has been used. It is a simple, rapid, and cost effective (albeit crude)

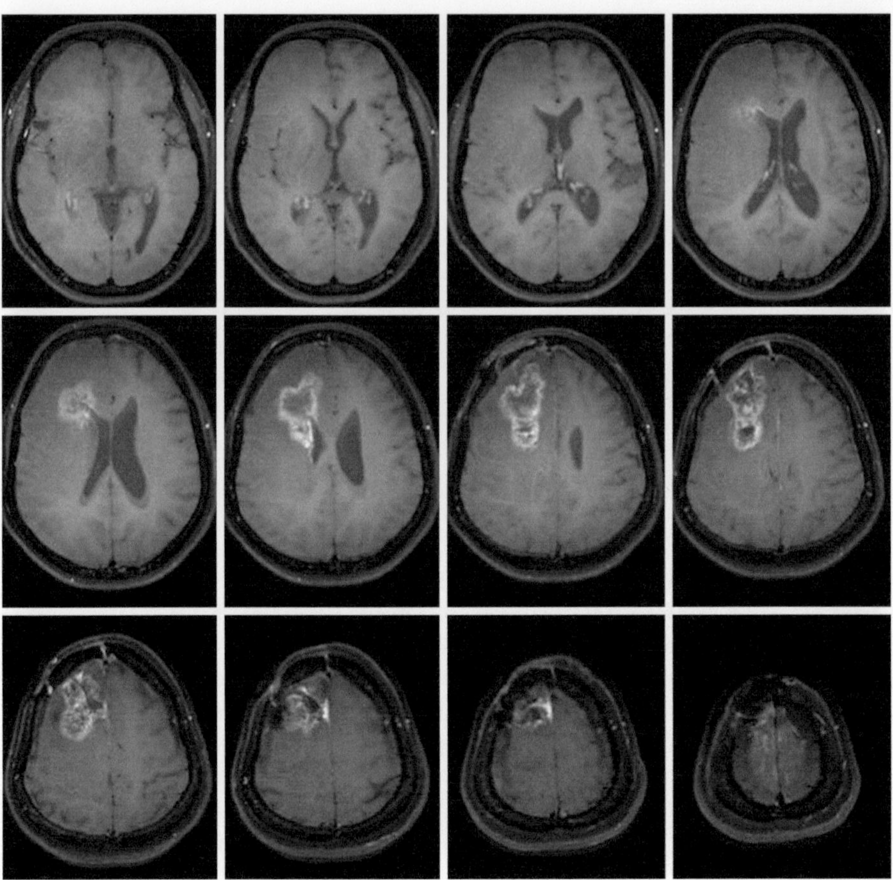

Fig. 17.1 MRI axial sections revealing "soap bubble" or "Swiss cheese" appearance representing radiation necrosis

measure of dementia. Over the years, the tools for neuropsychological testing have evolved further and can detect finer aspects. These are aimed to detect subtle changes in components of various aspects of CNS function such as memory, attention, executive function, processing speed, motor speed and overall sense of well-being The selected neurocognitive function tests include the Hopkins Verbal Learning Tests (HVLT) to evaluate memory, Trail making test (TMT) A and B to measure visual motor speed and executive function, the Grooved Pegboard for fine motor coordination, the Controlled Oral Word Association (COWA) test for verbal fluency and the Barthel Index to evaluate activities of daily living. A challenge in using these scales is to factor the contributions of tumour progression to changes in these measures must also be considered.

17.5 OAR Constraints for CNS

It is critical for radiation oncologist to be cognizant about the tolerance doses of various subsites of the CNS. Over the years, several attempts have been made to objectively quantify the tolerance thresholds of various OAR's. The critical regions typically delineated include optic chiasm, cochlea, hippocampus, brainstem, pituitary gland, circle of Willis, retina, lacrimal gland and lens [16].

An important initial attempt in this direction was that by Emami et al. [17]. The main aim of this publication was to address a clinical need based on available information up to that time. However this attempt had several lacunae including the absence of dose volume histogram (DVH) data. To overcome these lacunae, a group of researchers and clinicians were formed with the name "The Quantitative Analysis of Normal Tissue Effects in the Clinic (QUANTEC)." The goal was to review the available literature of the last 18 years on volumetric/dosimetric information of normal tissue complication. Tables 17.2 and 17.3 lists the dose constraints for important OAR's in CNS for fractionated radiotherapy and single fraction radiosurgery respectively.

Despite these outstanding efforts, many critical questions remain. The subject of normal tissue tolerance is extremely complex issue and multifactorial. As an example, in a particular scenario, even a 5–7% rate of a particular toxicity could be unacceptable. In contrast, there could be situations where a higher risk could be considered acceptable [18]. The need of the hour is to do comprehensive and multi-institutional collaborative research.

Table 17.2 OAR constraints of CNS (fractionated radiotherapy)

Optic chiasma and optic nerves	D_{max} <54 Gy
Cochlea	D_{mean} ≤45 Gy
Hippocampus	D_{max} ≤6 Gy V_{3Gy} ≤20%
Brainstem	D_{max} <54 Gy
Pituitary gland	D_{max} <50 Gy
Retina	D_{max} <45 Gy
Lacrimal gland	$V_{30\ Gy}$ <50%
	D_{max} <40 Gy
Lens	D_{max} <6 Gy

Table 17.3 OAR constraints of CNS (single fraction SRS)

Description	Constraint	1 Fraction	
		Optimal	Mandatory
Optic pathway	D_{max} (0.1 cc)	–	<8 Gy
	<0.2 cc	–	8 Gy
	MPD	–	10 Gy
Brainstem	D_{max} (0.1 cc)	<10 Gy	<15 Gy
	<1 cc	–	10 Gy
	MPD	–	15 Gy
	MPD	12.5 Gy	15–20 Gy
Lens	D_{max} (0.1 cc)	<1.5 Gy	–
Cochlea	Mean	<4 Gy	<9 Gy
	MPD	–	12 Gy
Orbit	D_{max} (0.1 cc)	<8 Gy	–
Normal brain (whole brain-PTV)	$D_{10\,cc}$	<12 Gy	–
	$D_{50\%}$	<5 Gy	–
Spinal canal (including medulla)	D_{max} (0.1 cc)	<10 Gy	<14 Gy
	$D_{1\,cc}$	<7 Gy	–
Spinal cord	<0.25 cc	–	10 Gy
	<1.2 cc	–	7 Gy
	MPD	–	14 Gy
	D_{max} (<0.035 cc)	–	14 Gy
	D_{max} (<0.35 cc)	–	10 Gy
	D_{max} (<1.2 cc) [SBRT only]	–	7 Gy
Cauda equina and sacral plexus	D_{max} (0.1 cc)	–	<16 Gy
	$D_{5\,cc}$	–	<14 Gy
Cauda equina	<5 cc	–	14 Gy
	MPD	–	16 Gy
	D_{max} (<0.035 cc)	–	16 Gy
	D_{max} (<5 cc)	–	14 Gy
Sacral plexus	<3 cc	–	14.4 Gy
	MPD	–	16 Gy
	D_{max} (<0.035 cc)	–	18 Gy
	D_{max} (<5 cc)	–	14.4 Gy

D_{max} is the near-point maximum dose, defined in this case as $D_{0.5\,cc}$, which is the minimum dose to the 0.5 cc volume of the organ receiving the highest doses

$D_{1\,cc}$, $D_{5\,cc}$, $D_{9\,cc}$, $D_{10\,cc}$ and $D_{50\,cc}$ are the minimum doses to the specified volume of the organ (1 cc, 5 cc, etc.) that receive the highest doses

$V_{10\,Gy}$ is the percentage volume of the organ receiving a dose of 10 Gy or higher

<5 cc, <10 cc, <20 cc, 2/third volume refer to the maximum volume which can receive a dose greater than or equal to the dose mentioned against it MPD is the maximum point dose permissible for the concerned organ

17.6 Radiation Fatigue

Radiation fatigue is common after brain radiation therapy (RT) and is likely due to transient demyelination [19]. The reported incidence of radiation fatigue varies widely and is confounded by several factors including prior surgery. Radiation fatigue usually begin by 2 weeks of starting RT and generally peaks 4–8 weeks after treatment and typically recovers from weeks 8 to 12. A severe form of this side effect is somnolence syndrome consisting of fatigue, lethargy, clumsiness, and cognitive decline [20]. There is limited and conflicting evidence for use of modafinil or methylphenidate during RT to counteract fatigue [21].

17.7 Cognitive Decline

Studying, quantifying and identifying risk reduction strategies related to radiation-induced cognitive decline (RICD) is incredibly challenging. Studies in paediatric ALL patients have shown that whole-brain radiation therapy (WBRT) to 24 Gy is associated with significant IQ decline over time in a dose-dependent manner [22]. Risk factors for RICD include younger age at time of irradiation, female gender, NF-1 mutant positive status, use of intrathecal methotrexate, and volume of brain irradiated [23]. The overall picture is even less clear in adults with some studies showing a decline in scores on objective neurocognitive tests compared to pre radiation baseline scores and some studies showing no difference.

17.8 Optic Neuropathy

Certain tumour types treated with radiotherapy, by virtue of their location, expose the optic nerves to high doses of radiation. These primary sites include meningioma, pituitary adenomas, and craniopharyngiomas. Clinically, this may induce a decrease in visual acuity and blindness. In an acute setting, deterioration of vision may be reversible. However, it is more likely to be permanent >6 months after treatment. Optic neuropathy from radiation is usually painless. It can be monocular or binocular. Prominent risk factors for radiation-induced optic neuropathy include absolute doses received, fraction size, length of optic pathway treated and history of prior radiation exposure to the optic pathway. Both prior EBRT and SRS are risk factors for radiation induced optic neuropathy. For SRS, many authors consider <8 Gy to be the upper limit of acceptable tolerability. However single fractions of <12 Gy have been used and validated in recent publications [24, 25]. A large analysis of pooled data considered the risk of radiation induced optic neuropathy to be in the range of 0–2% in patients with no prior irradiation to the optic apparatus and a single fraction <12 Gy [25].

17.9 Hypopituitarism

Hypothalamic–pituitary axis dysfunction may occur in up to 80% of patients treated with RT. The time to onset and severity of symptoms are related to the total dose, dose fraction, the age at time of irradiation and follow up duration. Elective radio sensitivity of the cell populations accounts for different incidence of the hormonal deficits, with the GH axis the most radiosensitive, followed by gonadotropin, ACTH and TSH axes.

Irradiation near or within the hypothalamic–pituitary axis or pituitary can lead to endocrine deficiencies. Prevalence of endocrinopathies is higher with nasopharyngeal cancers compared to intracerebral tumours. Endocrinopathies may include pan hypopituitarism, hypothalamic hypothyroidism, and hypothalamic hypogonadism. The paediatric population, depended critically on these hormones for growth and development, is especially vulnerable. Of importance is the growth hormone deficiency revealing short stature and retarded growth [10]. Usually, endocrine dysfunction is considered a late event. The timelines of onset of hypopituitarism after radiotherapy cannot be predicted. Typically, the vulnerable patients are put on follow up with dynamic serum hormonal value assessments and appropriate hormonal replacements [26].

17.10 Myelopathy

Radiation myelopathy is the term commonly used for radiation related side effects to the spinal cord. This side effects remain a serious concern for all radiation oncologists treating CNS as well as extra-neural tumours close to the neuraxis (lung, certain head and neck, mediastinal tumors). Increasingly SBRT is being considered for limited metastatic disease to the spine, making the spinal cord inside a vulnerable organ at risk (OAR). Myelopathy can have disastrous effects on the life and quality of life of the patient.

Adverse facts of spinal cord irradiation can affect both the central and peripheral nervous system. Akin to the subdivisions in the brain, the spinal cord toxicity can also be sub grouped as early toxicity, early-delayed toxicity, and long term (or late) toxicity. While acute central nervous system (CNS) damage has been reported following acute brain irradiation, there is no clinical or experimental evidence that radiation can also induce acute spinal cord toxicity.

Critical factors associated with risk of neurologic deficit include total dose, length of spinal cord irradiated, fractionation scheme and total duration of treatment. As such, an absolute threshold for development of myelopathy is difficult to state. The usual tolerance doses for the cord can range from 40 to 54 Gy depending on the exact site and the length of cord that is being irradiated. Typically, the risk of myelopathy varies from 0.2 to 5% at 5 years Rock JP et al. The evolving role of stereotactic radiosurgery and stereotactic radiation therapy for patients with spine tumours [27].

Table 17.4 Additional investigations for diagnosing radio necrosis

Modality	Active disease	Radio necrosis
Perfusion weighted MRI	Relative cerebral blood volume (rCBV) increased	rCBV decreased
Diffusion weighted MRI	Restricted	
MRS	NAA/Cho decreases and Cho/Cr ratio increases	Increased lactate
FDG or methionine PET/SPECT	Increased uptake	Decreased uptake

17.11 Radio Necrosis

An important long term side effect of radiation therapy, especially stereotactic radiosurgery (SRS) is radio necrosis. Image based diagnoses can sometimes struggle to distinguish from other phenomena including self-limiting inflammation [28, 29]. The main risk factors of radio necrosis are total dose, maximum tumour diameter and treated volume [30, 31]. The symptoms related to radio necrosis can range from serious neurocognitive deficits to an asymptomatic state. The incidence can range from 2 to 20% as across various studies. Only about one third of patients with radio necrosis present with symptomatic neurologic deficits. Radio necrosis is a diagnostic challenge. Routine contrast enhanced MRI brain is difficult to distinguish active tumor from radio necrosis. Following additional diagnostic investigations can be used in medical dilemmas (Table 17.4).

In occasional cases, biopsy may be needed for confirmation. Management typically involves steroids. In certain situations, surgical resection can be considered. Presently, there is a lack of good certainty evidence to help quantify the risks and benefits of interventions for the treatment of brain radio necrosis after radiotherapy or radiosurgery [31, 32]. In an RCT of 14 patients, bevacizumab showed radiological response which was associated with minimal improvement in cognition or symptom severity [33]. Laser interstitial thermal therapy (LITT) has also been explored [34].

17.12 Migraine-Like Headache Syndrome (SMART)

Rarely, patients after CNS radiotherapy may experience migraine like headaches associated with focal neurological deficits and/or seizures lasting days to weeks, as late effect post radiotherapy. Imaging may show new and prominent gyriform contrast enhancement associated with increased T2 and FLAIR signal. This reversible syndrome is referred as SMART syndrome, often seen many years (even 10–20 years or more) post RT, although cases within 2 years have been described after proton therapy [35]. MRI brain with contrast and perfusion is diagnostic to distinguish it from transient ischemic attack (TIA) or stroke. Treatment includes use of high dose steroids, calcium channel blockers and antiepileptic agents.

17.13 Treatment and Mitigation of RT Induced CNS Toxicity

Efforts for reducing toxicity have focused on sparing of normal tissues by image guidance and intensity modulation.

In recent years, hippocampus has emerged as an important structure for neurocognitive impairment, owing to the presence of neural stem cells [6]. RTOG 0933 used intensity modulated radiation therapy to spare the neural stem cell population in the adult hippocampus in patients receiving whole brain radiation with brain metastases. At 4 months following treatment, a decreased mean relative decline in the HVLT-R delayed recall was observed and was significantly reduced compared to historical controls (7% vs. 30%, $p < 0.001$), demonstrating a limited benefit in memory and quality of life in the short term [36].

Heavy particles with high linear transfer (LET) properties, such as protons, have theoretical advantages in limiting the amount of normal tissue exposed to ionizing radiation. However, randomized data on their use demonstrating reduced CNS toxicities is lacking. Flash radiotherapy, which uses very high dose rates per second has also been found to have promise for sparing CNS related side effects. Long term clinical outcomes in a large patient subset is awaited.

The most common medication in radiotherapy induced CNS toxicity are corticosteroids. These have long been employed to reduce local edema and inflammatory effects of tumor on the CNS. The predominant mechanism of action for corticosteroids is the effects on lymphocyte-mediated inflammation and reduced vascular permeability. However, steroids are to be considered a temporizing measure in view of long term effects of these medications. Investigators have tried neurotransmitter-based pharmacologic therapies borrowed from Alzheimer's treatment in the setting of radiation-induced cognitive decline. Memantine is a NMDA receptor antagonist used in the treatment of Alzheimer's patients and patients with obsessive-compulsive disorder.

RTOG 0614 trial that studied memantine for the prevention of cognitive dysfunction in patients receiving whole-brain radiotherapy [37]. Memantine is a drug that was studied in patients with neurodegenerative disorders, including Alzheimer disease. More recent results on this issue have been provided by Phase III Trial NRG Oncology CC001 trial on hippocampal avoidance during whole-brain radiotherapy plus memantine for patients with brain metastases [38]. Based on these data HA-WBRT plus memantine is better recognised to preserve cognitive function and patient-reported symptoms, with no difference in intracranial PFS and OS. The same should be considered a standard of care for patients with good performance status who plan to receive WBRT for brain metastases with no metastases in the HA region.

A phase III study with donepezil, an acetylcholine esterase inhibitor, was evaluated in patients who had received partial brain irradiation or whole brain irradiation ≥6 months prior to enrolment. With 24 weeks of therapy, donepezil did not significantly improve composite scores for neurocognitive functioning [39].

Certain non-pharmacological strategies, such as exercise-induced stimulation of hippocampal neurogenesis, cognitive therapies and mesenchymal stem cell replacement to prevent or delay onset of normal tissue injury have been under under investigation. The outcomes of these studies are eagerly awaited.

17.14 Future

Over the last three decades, our understanding of brain health and maintenance has revealed that interventions outside the CNS can have durable impacts on brain function, such as the contribution of microbial immunity to brain health and immune function, stem cell biology and the contribution of physical activity. Preventing and treating CNS toxicity will require a multidisciplinary approach. This will include not only the traditional approach of radiation oncologists, dosimetrists and pharmacists, but also physical therapists, nutritionists, and neuropsychologists. Active development of novel strategies is being pursued by investigators to reverse late effects once they have formed. Great improvements in patient functioning and quality of life can be anticipated in near future.

17.15 Summary

Radiation therapy is a highly effective treatment for CNS malignancies. Nevertheless, the limiting step in treatment is the risk of adverse side effects to healthy tissue. Even as the treatment of CNS malignancies advances with novel radiation techniques and high precision technologies, the goal of minimizing treatment side effects remains the same. The radiation oncology community has made significant strides in understanding the mechanisms of brain injury caused by irradiation. As patients continue to live longer, CNS side effects shall become increasingly important to prevent and treat. Increasing and optimizing quality-of-life in addition to overall survival in cancer patients should be the ultimate goal.

Acknowledgments None.

Declarations/Conflict of Interest None.

Funding Received None.

References

1. Munshi A. Central nervous system tumours: spotlight on India. South Asian J Cancer. 2016;5:146–7.
2. Tseng BP, Giedzinski E, Izadi A. Functional consequences of radiation-induced oxidative stress in cultured neural stem cells and the brain exposed to charged particle irradiation. Antioxid Redox Signal. 2014;20:1410–22.

3. Dayal D, Martin S, Owens K. Mitochondrial complex II dysfunction can contribute significantly to genomic instability after exposure to ionizing radiation. Radiat Res. 2009;172:737–45.
4. Kramer S, Henrickson F, Zelen M. Therapeutic trials in the management of metastatic brain tumors by different time/dose fraction schemes of radiation therapy. JNCI. 1977;46:213–21.
5. Andres-Mach M, Rola R, Fike JR. Radiation effects on neural precursor cells in the dentate gyrus. Cell Tissue Res. 2008;331:251–62.
6. Monje M. Cranial radiation therapy and damage to hippocampal neurogenesis. Dev Disabil Res Rev. 2008;14:238–42.
7. Wojtowicz JM. Irradiation as an experimental tool in studies of adult neurogenesis. Hippocampus. 2006;16:261–6.
8. Munshi A. Chloroquine in glioblastoma—new horizons for an old drug. Cancer. 2009;115:2380–3.
9. Baschnagel A, Wolters PL, Camphausen K. Neuropsychological testing and biomarkers in the management of brain metastases. Radiat Oncol. 2008;3:26.
10. Appelman-Dijkstra NM, Kokshoorn NE, Dekkers OM. Pituitary dysfunction in adult patients after cranial radiotherapy: systematic review and meta-analysis. J Clin Endocrinol Metab. 2011;96:2330–40.
11. Robbins ME, Bourland JD, Cline JM. A model for assessing cognitive impairment after fractionated whole-brain irradiation in nonhuman primates. Radiat Res. 2011;175:519–25.
12. Prust MJ, Jafari-Khouzani K, Kalpathy-Cramer J. Standard chemoradiation for glioblastoma results in progressive brain volume loss. Neurology. 2015;85:683–91.
13. Johannesen TB, Lien HH, Hole KH. Radiological and clinical assessment of long-term brain tumour survivors after radiotherapy. Radiother Oncol. 2003;69:169–76.
14. White NS, McDonald C, McDonald CR, et al. Diffusion-weighted imaging in cancer: physical foundations and applications of restriction spectrum imaging. Cancer Res. 2014;74:4638–52.
15. Barajas RF, Chang JS, Sneed PK, et al. Distinguishing recurrent intra-axial metastatic tumor from radiation necrosis following gamma knife radiosurgery using dynamic susceptibility-weighted contrast-enhanced perfusion MR imaging. AJNR Am J Neuroradiol. 2009;30:367–72.
16. Scoccianti S, Detti B, Gadda D, Greto D, Furfaro I, Meacci F, Simontacchi G, Di Brina L, Bonomo P, Giacomelli I, Meattini I, Mangoni M, Cappelli S, Cassani S, Talamonti C, Bordi L, Livi L. Organs at risk in the brain and their dose-constraints in adults and in children: a radiation oncologist's guide for delineation in everyday practice. Radiother Oncol. 2015;114:230–8.
17. Emami B, Lyman J, Brown A, et al. Tolerance of normal tissue to therapeutic irradiation. Int J Radiat Oncol Biol Phys. 1991;21:109–22.
18. Milano MT, Grimm J, Niemierko A, Soltys SG, Moiseenko V, Redmond KJ, Yorke E, Sahgal A, Xue J, Mahadevan A, Muacevic A, Marks LB, Kleinberg LR. Single- and multifraction stereotactic radiosurgery dose/volume tolerances of the brain. Int J Radiat Oncol Biol Phys. 2021;110:68–86.
19. Armstrong TS, Bishof AM, Brown PD, et al. Determining priority signs and symptoms for use as clinical outcomes assessments in trials including patients with malignant gliomas: panel 1 report. Neuro-Oncology. 2016;18(Suppl 2):ii1–ii12.
20. Powell C, Guerrero D, Sardell S, et al. Somnolence syndrome in patients receiving radical radiotherapy for primary brain tumours: a prospective study. Radiother Oncol. 2011;100:131–6.
21. Breitbart W, Alici Y. Psychostimulants for cancer-related fatigue. J Natl Compr Cancer Netw. 2010;8(8):933–42. https://doi.org/10.6004/jnccn.2010.0068.
22. Smibert E, Anderson V, Godber T, Ekert H. Risk factors for intellectual and educational sequelae of cranial irradiation in childhood acute lymphoblastic leukaemia. Br J Cancer. 1996;73:825–30.
23. Wujanto C, Vellayappan B, Chang EL, Chao ST, Sahgal A, Lo SS. Radiotherapy to the brain: what are the consequences of this age-old treatment? Ann Palliat Med. 2021;10:936–52.
24. Stafford SL, Pollock BE, Leavitt JA, Foote RL, Brown PD, Link MJ, Gorman DA, Schomberg PJ. A study on the radiation tolerance of the optic nerves and chiasm after stereotactic radiosurgery. Int J Radiat Oncol Biol Phys. 2003;1(55):1177–81.

25. Milano MT, Grimm J, Soltys SG, Yorke E, Moiseenko V, Tomé WA, Sahgal A, Xue J, Ma L, Solberg TD, Kirkpatrick JP, Constine LS, Flickinger JC, Marks LB, El Naqa I. Single- and multi-fraction stereotactic radiosurgery dose tolerances of the optic pathways. Int J Radiat Oncol Biol Phys. 2021;110:87–99.
26. Toogood AA. Endocrine consequences of brain irradiation. Growth Hormon IGF Res. 2004;14(Suppl A):S118–24.
27. Rock JP, Ryu S, Yin FF, Schreiber F, Abdulhak M. The evolving role of stereotactic radiosurgery and stereotactic radiation therapy for patients with spine tumours. J Neuro-Oncol. 2004;69:319–34.
28. Sahgal A, Chang JH, Ma L, Marks LB, Milano MT, Medin P, Niemierko A, et al. Spinal cord dose tolerance to stereotactic body radiation therapy. Int J Radiat Oncol Biol Phys. 2021;110:124–36.
29. Minniti G, Clarke E, Lanzetta G, Osti MF, Trasimeni G, Bozzao A, Romano A, et al. Stereotactic radiosurgery for brain metastases: analysis of outcome and risk of brain radio necrosis. Radiat Oncol. 2011;6:48.
30. Ahmed KA, Freilich JM, Abuodeh Y, Figura N, Patel N, Sarangkasiri S, et al. Fractionated stereotactic radiotherapy to the post-operative cavity for radio resistant and radiosensitive brain metastases. J Neuro-Oncol. 2014;118:179–86.
31. Kohutek ZA, Yamada Y, Chan TA, Brennan CW, Tabar V, Gutin PH, et al. Long-term risk of radionecrosis and imaging changes after stereotactic radiosurgery for brain metastases. J Neuro-Oncol. 2015;125:149–56.
32. Chung C, Bryant A, Brown PD. Interventions for the treatment of brain radio necrosis after radiotherapy or radiosurgery. Cochrane Database Syst Rev. 2018;9(7):CD011492.
33. Levin VA, Bidaut L, Hou P, Kumar AJ, Wefel JS, Bekele BN, Grewal J, Prabhu S, Loghin M, Gilbert MR, Jackson EF. Randomized double-blind placebo-controlled trial of bevacizumab therapy for radiation necrosis of the central nervous system. Int J Radiat Oncol Biol Phys. 2011;79:1487–95.
34. Palmisciano P, Haider AS, Nwagwu CD, Wahood W, Aoun SG, Abdullah KG, El Ahmadieh TY. Bevacizumab vs laser interstitial thermal therapy in cerebral radiation necrosis from brain metastases: a systematic review and meta-analysis. J Neuro-Oncol. 2021;154(1):13–23.
35. Winter SF, Klein JP, Vaios EJ, Karschnia P, Lee EQ, Shih HA, Loebel F, Dietrich J. Clinical presentation and management of SMART Syndrome. Neurology. 2021;97(3):118–20. https://doi.org/10.1212/WNL.0000000000012150.
36. Gondi V, Pugh SL, Tome WA. Preservation of memory with conformal avoidance of the hippocampal neural stem-cell compartment during whole-brain radiotherapy for brain metastases (RTOG 0933): a phase II multi-institutional trial. J Clin Oncol. 2014;32:3810–6.
37. Brown PD, Pugh S, Laack NN, Wefel JS, Khuntia D, Meyers C, et al. Memantine for the prevention of cognitive dysfunction in patients receiving whole-brain radiotherapy: a randomized, double-blind, placebo-controlled trial. Neuro-Oncology. 2013;15:1429–37.
38. Brown PD, Gondi V, Pugh S, Tome WA, Wefel JS, Armstrong TS, et al. Hippocampal avoidance during whole-brain radiotherapy plus memantine for patients with brain metastases: phase III trial NRG oncology CC001. J Clin Oncol. 2020;38:1019–29.
39. Rapp SR, Case D, Peiffer A. Donepezil for irradiated brain tumor survivors a phase III randomized placebo controlled clinical trial. J Clin Oncol. 2015;33:1653–9.

Determining Risks and Treating of Radiation Pneumonitis After Thoracic Radiation

18

Ashok Kumar

18.1 Introduction

Radiation pneumonitis has been described in various literature since long and dates back to the discovery of X-rays. Patients undergoing radiation to breast, lungs and thoracic cancers in the two dimensional radiation planning era were most affected, however, with the advent of latest technologies the incidence rates have decreased sharply. Radiation pneumonitis and radiation fibrosis are two different terminologies which was described way back in early nineteenth century [1]. Radiation induced thoracic injury can manifest itself as hemoptysis, bronchitis, effusion, dermatitis, esophagitis, pericarditis and in severe cases as pneumothorax. Response of pulmonary epithelium manifests as either histopathologic, biochemical or at molecular levels [2–6]. It can also be complicated by underlying malignancy, infections and associated effusion either due to pleural effusion or pericardial effusion [7]. In this chapter we will describe the risk factors, signs and symptoms, diagnostic work up, management guidelines and management of complications.

18.2 Patho-physiology

Radiation to lungs at molecular level causes breakage of chemical bonds leading to generation of highly reactive free radicals which ultimately affects either directly or indirectly the lipids, DNA due to the property of radiation interaction with water.

Radiation pneumonitis can result either from direct injury to lung parenchyma or due to the development of fibrosis. This will lead to decreased lung functions and

A. Kumar (✉)
Radiation Oncology, Army Hospital R&R, Delhi, India

K. Sood Sharma et al. (eds.), *Complications of Cancer Therapy: Best Practices in Prevention and Management*, https://doi.org/10.1007/978-981-99-0984-1_18

lung capacity. There can be a genetic susceptibility to radiation injury [8–10] and presence of single nucleotide polymorphism in methylene tetrahydrofolate reductase may be associated with increased risk of development of radiation pneumonitis [11]. Ataxia telangiectasia mutated gene has also been seen to associated with development of radiation pneumonitis [12, 13].

Cytokines like TGF-beta which induces fibroblast collagen deposition, TNF alpha, IL6, PDGF and interferon gamma has been studied extensively which has been associated with the development of radiation fibrosis and pneumonitis.

18.3 Pathology

Post irradiation to lungs there are vascular and alveolar changes which manifest as early as within hours and may persists for months to years [14]. There may be reversible or irreversible changes and these changes may or may not manifest clinically [4]. Within hours of radiation to lungs patients are generally asymptomatic however there may be hyperemia and exudative changes leading to increased production of alveolar surfactants. Pulmonary edema may also manifest in some cases. Later in the latent phase there is development of ciliary dysfunction because of thick mucus formation. In the third phase i.e. acute exudative phase when the radiation pneumonitis sets in and develops after 3–12 weeks post radiation there is sloughing of endothelial and epithelial cells causing narrowing of pulmonary capillaries and microvascular thrombosis. These processes may lead to leakage of fibrin rich exudate in the alveoli. In the fourth phase (intermediate phase) there is resolution of the alveolar exudate and dissolution of the hyaline membranes which ultimately leads to thickening of the interstitiam [15, 16]. Lastly fibrosis sets in as early as 6 months and progresses over years which is due to myofibroblasts within the interstitial and alveolar spaces causing increased collagen deposition. Ultimately this causes decreased lung volumes, subintimal fibrosis and loss of capillaries. The entire process may become a harbinger of chronic infections and organizing pneumonia [17–20].

18.4 Risk Factors

There are many risk factors on which radiation induced lung injury depends upon and the major ones being type of radiation, coexisting underlying lung diseases like COPD, interstitial lung disease, method of radiation, the volume of lung irradiated, dose, concurrent chemotherapy use, prior radiation to lungs, history of smoking, history of usage of conventional fuel for cooking and any prior use of endocrine therapy. Age, gender, performance status also have a role to play in the development of radiation pneumonitis. Recently use of immunotherapy has also been implicated in the development of pneumonitis and has been seen with the use of drugs like pemetrexed, erlotinib, geftinib, docetaxel, gemcitabine and crizotinib. There may be a synergistic effect with radiation along with immunotherapy since radiation primes the immune response and can potentiate the effects of immunotherapy. The same has been demonstrated in the PACIFIC trial and KEYNOTE-001 trial [21–27].

Type of surgery is indirectly responsible for development of radiation pneumonitis since it has been shown in some studies that a lesser radical surgery can lead to decreased incidences of radiation pneumonitis [27–29].

As far as the volume of irradiated lung is concerned as seen in patients treated for carcinoma breast where tangential fields are use, the amount of lung volume in the field is directly related to the development of pneumonitis and later fibrosis. Also, in such cases use of concurrent chemotherapy has a well-established data for the development of RP [30–33].

In the QUANTEC series it was concluded that keeping the V20 to <30–35% and mean lung dose (MLD) to less than 20–23 Gy keeps the risk of development of radiation pneumonitis to less than 20% [30].

Use of twice daily radiation to reduce the incidence of RP has also been reported in literature but there was no apparent benefit for the same [34, 35].

Multiple trials have suggested that with the use of advanced radiation techniques like IMRT/IGRT over conventional radiation techniques has reduced the incidences of radiation pneumonitis to a considerable extent as was seen in RTOG 0617 wherein the incidence of radiation pneumonitis was 3.5% with IMRT versus 7.9% with 3D-CRT [36]. With the addition of SBRT the risk of developing radiation pneumonitis has decreased further [37–40]. Addition of proton beam therapy to the armamentarium of radiation techniques may also decrease the incidence of radiation pneumonitis as was seen in a systematic review of patients of breast cancer treated with proton beam therapy wherein only less than 1% patient developed radiation pneumonitis [41–43].

Hence it can be safely deduced that advanced radiation techniques have a distinct advantage over conventional methods in terms of development of radiation pneumonitis and should be used wherever possible.

18.4.1 Role of Chemotherapy in Development of Radiation Pneumonitis

It is well established that some chemotherapeutic agents have a definite role in development of radiation pneumonitis whether they are given in neo-adjuvant form or concurrently with radiation. Taghian et al. assessed the risk of development of radiation pneumonitis in patients of breast cancer treated with paclitaxel and concluded that there was definite risk of increased incidence of radiation pneumonitis along with paclitaxel [44]. Mao et al. in patients treated for esophageal cancer concluded that that patients who received induction chemotherapy had a higher incidence of development of radiation pneumonitis versus those who did not receive induction chemotherapy (49% vs 14%) [45].

Use of chemotherapeutic drugs like doxorubicin, taxanes, dactinomycin, bleomycin, cyclophosphamide, vincristine, mitomycin, gemcitabine, bevacizumab has shown to increase the risk of radiation induced lung injury later developing into pneumonitis.

With the addition of immune check point inhibitors being used for lung cancer there may be a possibility of development of radiation pneumonitis due to its inherent risk of development of pneumonitis of up-to 19% however it still is under evaluation whether when combined with radiation it can have additive effect in the development of radiation pneumonitis [46]. Use of durvalumab has also been associated with increased risk of development of pneumonitis as was seen in the PACIFIC study [47].

Radiation recall phenomenon can occur with certain chemotherapeutic agents like paclitaxel, gemcitabine, doxorubicin and develop cough, dyspnea and radiographic opacities in the prior radiation fields.

Patients of breast cancer on tamoxifen developed lung fibrosis but it is not generally associated with increased incidences of radiation pneumonitis [48].

18.5 Epidemiology

The incidence of radiation pneumonitis depends on the protocol and radiation field used which ultimately manifests in symptomatic pneumonitis and is confirmed in radiology.

Patients with breast cancer develop mild to moderate pneumonia in up to 3% patients and severe pneumonitis may develop in up to 9% patients which again depends upon the type of radiation used and radiation field and use of concurrent chemotherapy [17, 20, 49–51]. Similarly, while using conventional fractionation of 1.8–2 Gy in the management of lung cancer the development of symptomatic lung pneumonitis was 7% where lung volume treated was upto 31% and received more than 20 Gy (V20) and this incidence increased to 13% when V20 was upto 40%. In context to advanced radiation techniques of SBRT in a study where 60 Gy was delivered in three fractions to 80% isodose line almost 9% patients developed symptomatic lung injury [52]. Almost 14% patients developed mild to moderate pneumonitis in patients who were treated for Hodgkin's and non Hodgkin's lymphoma and they presented with cough and dyspnea at rest [53].

18.6 Signs and Symptoms

Symptoms caused by acute radiation pneumonitis usually develop approximately 4–12 weeks following irradiation, whereas symptoms of late or fibrotic radiation pneumonitis develop after 6–12 months.

The symptoms and signs of the two phases are similar, although fever is less likely to occur in the fibrotic phase.

Initially a nonproductive cough, which may occur during therapy as a manifestation of bronchial mucosal injury or later as a manifestation of fibrosis. Dyspnea may only occur with exertion, or may be described as an inability to take a deep breath.

Fever is usually of low grade, but can be more pronounced in severe cases. Chest pain may be pleuritic or substernal and can represent pleuritis, esophageal pathology, or rib fracture. Malaise and weight loss may be observed.

On clinical evaluation there may be crackles or a pleural rub may be heard however in some cases auscultation is normal. Dullness to percussion may be detected as a result of a small pleural effusion and this occurs in about 10% of patients. Effusions often cause no symptoms and may spontaneously remit. In contrast to malignant effusions, radiation-induced effusions do not increase in size after a period of observed stability. Skin erythema may outline the radiation port but it is not predictive of the occurrence or the severity of radiation pneumonitis. Tachypnea, cyanosis, or signs of pulmonary hypertension may be seen in more advanced cases.

18.7 Clinical and Laboratory Evaluation

Radiation pneumonitis should be suspected in any patients who has undergone thoracic radiation and patients presents with dyspnea, cough, mild fever, malaise, crackles and pleural rub. The signs and symptoms may develop after weeks to months after radiation. Other possible causes should be ruled out such as infections, thromboembolic events, drug use, fistulas, COPD, ILD and congestive heart failure. There may be polymorphonuclear leukocytosis, high ESR, high LDH and CRP levels. Procalcitonin levels may be normal or low [54]. Other laboratory parameters such as complete blood counts, differential blood counts cultures, PT/INR, BNP levels must be done. Serum KL6 levels may be expressed and is associated with ILD and post radiation lung injuries. Radiological evaluation includes contrast enhanced computed tomography scans and chest radiography however CECT is much more reliable than chest X-rays. On chest X-rays, a perivascular haziness is an early radiation-induced abnormality on chest radiograph, often progressing to patchy alveolar filling densities. There may be volume loss on chest X-rays during chronic phase of pneumonitis. A distinct feature of straight line effect, which does not conform to anatomical units but rather to the confines of the radiation port, is virtually diagnostic of RILI. Small pleural effusions and rib fractures may be seen, but lymphadenopathy does not occur.

The key step in the evaluation of radiation pneumonitis is comparison of pretreatment CT images, containing irradiation dosimetric information, with diagnostic CT images obtained at the time of symptom presentation by the radiation oncologist. Lung involvement in CT images of radiation pneumonitis typically aligns closely with the irradiated area. Comparisons between pre- and posttreatment images may be difficult due to tumor growth or shrinkage, changes in depth of respiration, and the complexity of the radiation port, but use of specialized software may help [55].

Similar to the plain chest radiograph, the CT scan appearance of radiation pneumonitis correlates with the phase of lung injury, although a given patient may present at any one of the phases [56, 57]. The initial phase, which occurs 3–5 months after completion of radiation therapy, typically shows ground-glass attenuation within the area of irradiated lung. The organizing phase is typically associated with patchy areas of consolidation that coalesce to form a relatively sharp edge that conforms to the radiation therapy portals rather than anatomic structures. These patchy areas sometimes appear nodular. The opacities associated with the organizing phase may resolve with minimal scarring or may evolve into a fibrotic phase, characterized on CT by linear opacities (scarring) or an area of dense consolidation and volume loss. The area of consolidation typically corresponds to the radiation port, although conformal and stereotactic treatment strategies do not yield the classic "straight line" radiographic finding, as described above. SPECT, functional MRI and PET-CT add little to the evaluation and should be done in specific cases.

Pulmonary function tests helps in differentiating whether symptoms are due to a flare of COPD or an interstitial process and to determine the severity of respiratory impairment. Typically, spirometry (before and after bronchodilator), lung volumes, diffusing capacity for carbon monoxide, and a six-minute walk test with oximetry are obtained as a baseline prior to radiation therapy and repeated in response to symptoms. In patients with RILI, PFTs generally demonstrate a reduction in lung volumes (total lung capacity [TLC], forced vital capacity [FVC], residual volume [RV]), diffusing capacity, and lung compliance. Tidal volumes are also decreased, and the respiratory rate may be elevated. As with other causes of interstitial or fibrotic lung disease, resting and ambulatory pulse oxygen saturation (SpO_2) may be reduced. The diffusing capacity for carbon monoxide (DLCO or transfer factor) is usually depressed in patients with radiation-induced lung damage, but this finding is nonspecific, as it can also be reduced in emphysema and interstitial lung disease.

For patients with moderate-to-severe hypoxemia, arterial blood gas analysis may be indicated.

Bronchoscopy is generally done to rule out infection, bleeding, drug hypersensitivity, or spread of the underlying malignancy. Bronchoscopy with bronchoalveolar lavage is performed in the majority of patients. Transbronchial biopsy specimens may be useful for assessment of infection or lymphangitic spread of tumor in cases that are clinically atypical for RILI, but the size of the specimens is usually too small to establish a diagnosis of radiation pneumonitis. Bronchoalveolar lavage fluid findings in radiation pneumonitis are not specific, usually showing an increased number of leukocytes (predominantly lymphocytes).

Diagnosis is based on both clinical, laboratory and radiological findings and at the same time excluding factors leading to infections, heart failure and drug induced, bleeding disorders and progression of malignancy.

18.7.1 Management

There is no specific guidelines to manage radiation pneumonitis however below are the therapeutic modalities used in the management. However some patients may resolve spontaneously without any therapeutic intervention.

Steroids: Glucocorticoids both oral and inhaled has been used in symptomatic cases and there may be no benefit of glucocorticoids where the fibrosis has already established [51, 58].

Oxygen therapy, antitussive medications management of underlying disease such as COPD and heart failure may benefit some cases. Use of dextrometho-rphan and codeine relives cough and symptoms may improve and patient feels better symptomatically. Supplemental oxygen should be used when the oxygen saturation is below 88%. Budesonide 800 mg twice daily for 14 days is useful in symptomatic improvement and can be used for long term for up-to 6–8 months.

Prednisolone approximately 40–60 mg/day is generally given for 2–4 weeks, with a gradual taper over 3–12 weeks, although the guidelines for tapering are poorly defined [51]. Generally speaking, the taper is done with close monitoring of symptoms. If the patient experiences relapse of symptoms we return to full dose for 2 weeks and try again with a slower taper, particularly when the dose is 20 mg/day or less. The recommendation for prednisone use is based upon clinical experience and multiple reports of a prompt response to therapy.

Drugs like azathioprine and cyclosporine has been used by some authors with limited symptomatic benefit [59, 60].

In patients with organizing pneumonia prednisolone at the dose of 0.75–1 mg/kg for 4–8 weeks is to be used and later tapering the dose to 0.5–0.75 mg/kg for next 6 weeks has resulted in clinical benefit [49, 50].

In patients with frank fibrosis there are no specific guidelines and glucocorticoid use should be avoided to prevent long term side effects.

Adjunct therapies like rehabilitation, vaccination for influenzas and pneumococcus should be done.

Pentoxifylline, colchicine, amifostine, penicillamine, interferon gamma, pirfenidone, captopril are other agents which may reduce the incidence and help in prevention of long term side effects of radiation pneumonitis however they are all experimental in nature and more long term data is required to establish their role in prevention and treatment of radiation pneumonitis.

Prognosis: patients may improve after 3–18 months post radiation in terms of ventilation and perfusion however there may not be significant improvement [61, 62].

18.7.2 Prevention Strategies

The only prevention strategies for reducing the risk of radiation pneumonitis are to keep the dose of radiation to lungs as minimum as possible and mean lung doses to be kept below 20 Gy and V 20 to be kept below 35–40% to reduce the risk of clinical radiation pneumonitis to less than 20%. Many drugs mentioned above may be used however the clinical efficacy still remains investigational.

Key Points

- Avoid unnecessary lung doses using advanced radiation techniques.
- Avoid chemotherapeutic drugs known to cause additive effects for causing radiation pneumonitis.
- Keep a check on development of symptoms of radiation pneumonitis like cough, dyspnea, low grade fever after 8–12 weeks post radiation.
- Three monthly follow-up and clinical evaluation for lung functions.
- In cases where symptoms develop do a CECT chest to rule out features of pneumonitis. Chest X-rays may reveal a straight line sign and baseline evaluation pretreatment using CT chest and X-ray chest needs to be done.
- Rule out comorbid conditions and associated effects.
- Optimal treatment still remains elusive however use of prednisolone and antitussive agents may help. Supportive care with use of supplemental oxygen is useful in the management.

References

1. Evans WA, Leucutia T. Intrathoracic changes induced by heavy irradiation. AJR. 1925;13:203.
2. Abratt RP, Morgan GW. Lung toxicity following chest irradiation in patients with lung cancer. Lung Cancer. 2002;35:103–9.
3. Coggle JE, Lambert BE, Moores SR. Radiation effects in the lung. Environ Health Perspect. 1986;70:261–91.
4. McDonald S, Rubin P, Phillips TL, Marks LB. Injury to the lung from cancer therapy: clinical syndromes, measurable endpoints, and potential scoring systems. Int J Radiat Oncol Biol Phys. 1995;31:1187–203.
5. Molls M, Herrmann T, Steinberg F, Feldmann HJ. Radiopathology of the lung: experimental and clinical observations. Recent Results Cancer Res. 1993;130:109.
6. Movsas B, Raffin TA, Epstein AH, Link CJ Jr. Pulmonary radiation injury. Chest. 1997;111:1061–76.
7. Kocak Z, Evans ES, Zhou SM, et al. Challenges in defining radiation pneumonitis in patients with lung cancer. Int J Radiat Oncol Biol Phys. 2005;62:635–8.
8. Haston CK, Begin M, Dorion G, Cory SM. Distinct loci influence radiation-induced alveolitis from fibrosing alveolitis in the mouse. Cancer Res. 2007;67:10796–803.
9. Kelsey CR, Rosenstein BS, Marks LB. Predicting toxicity from radiation therapy—it's genetic, right? Cancer. 2012;118:3450–4.
10. Wen J, Liu H, Wang Q, et al. Genetic variants of the LIN28B gene predict severe radiation pneumonitis in patients with non-small cell lung cancer treated with definitive radiation therapy. Eur J Cancer. 2014;50:1706–16.
11. Mak RH, Alexander BM, Asomaning K, et al. A single-nucleotide polymorphism in the methylene tetrahydrofolate reductase (MTHFR) gene is associated with risk of radiation pneumonitis in lung cancer patients treated with thoracic radiation therapy. Cancer. 2012;118:3654–65.
12. Zhang L, Yang M, Bi N, et al. ATM polymorphisms are associated with risk of radiation-induced pneumonitis. Int J Radiat Oncol Biol Phys. 2010;77:1360–8.
13. Xiong H, Liao Z, Liu Z, et al. ATM polymorphisms predict severe radiation pneumonitis in patients with non-small cell lung cancer treated with definitive radiation therapy. Int J Radiat Oncol Biol Phys. 2013;85:1066–73.
14. Respiratory system. In: Rubin P, Casseratt GW, editors. Clinical radiation pathology. Philadelphia: WB Saunders; 1968. p. 423.

15. Epperly MW, Guo H, Gretton JE, Greenberger JS. Bone marrow origin of myofibroblasts in irradiation pulmonary fibrosis. Am J Respir Cell Mol Biol. 2003;29:213–24.
16. Theise ND, Henegariu O, Grove J, et al. Radiation pneumonitis in mice: a severe injury model for pneumocyte engraftment from bone marrow. Exp Hematol. 2002;30:1333–8.
17. Katayama N, Sato S, Katsui K, et al. Analysis of factors associated with radiation-induced bronchiolitis obliterans organizing pneumonia syndrome after breast-conserving therapy. Int J Radiat Oncol Biol Phys. 2009;73:1049–54.
18. Arbetter KR, Prakash UB, Tazelaar HD, Douglas WW. Radiation-induced pneumonitis in the "nonirradiated" lung. Mayo Clin Proc. 1999;74:27–36.
19. Kwok E, Chan CK. Corticosteroids and azathioprine do not prevent radiation-induced lung injury. Can Respir J. 1998;5:211–4.
20. Takigawa N, Segawa Y, Saeki T, et al. Bronchiolitis obliterans organizing pneumonia syndrome in breast-conserving therapy for early breast cancer: radiation-induced lung toxicity. Int J Radiat Oncol Biol Phys. 2000;48:751–5.
21. Delaunay M, Cadranel J, Lusque A, Meyer N, Gounaut V, Moro-Sibilot D, Michot JM, Raimbourg J, Girard N, Guisier F, et al. Immune-checkpoint inhibitors associated with interstitial lung disease in cancer patients. Eur Respir J. 2017;50:1700050.
22. Nishino M, Giobbie-Hurder A, Hatabu H, Ramaiya NH, Hodi FS. Incidence of programmed cell death 1 inhibitor-related pneumonitis in patients with advanced cancer a systematic review and meta-analysis. JAMA Oncol. 2016;2:1607–16.
23. Crequit P, Wislez M, Fleury Feith J, Rozensztajn N, Jabot L, Friard S, Lavole A, Gounant V, Fillon J, Antoine M, et al. Crizotinib associated with ground-glass opacity predominant pattern interstitial lung disease: a retrospective observational cohort study with a systematic literature review. J Thorac Oncol. 2015;10:1148–55.
24. Liu V, White DA, Zakowski MF, Travis W, Kris MG, Ginsberg MS, Miller VA, Azzoli CG. Pulmonary toxicity associated with erlotinib. Chest. 2007;132:1042–4.
25. Twyman-Saint Victor C, Rech AJ, Maity A, Rengan R, Pauken KE, Stelekati E, Benci JL, Xu B, Dada H, Odorizzi PM, et al. Radiation and dual checkpoint blockade activate non-redundant immune mechanisms in cancer. Nature. 2015;520:373–7.
26. Shaverdian N, Lisberg AE, Bornazyan K, Veruttipong D, Goldman JW, Formenti SC, Garon EB, Lee P. Previous radiotherapy and the clinical activity and toxicity of pembrolizumab in the treatment of non-small-cell lung cancer: a secondary analysis of the KEYNOTE-001 phase I trial. Lancet Oncol. 2017;18:895–903.
27. Kocak Z, Yu X, Zhou SM, D'Amico A, Hollis D, Kahn D, Tisch A, Shafman TD, Marks LB. The impact of pre-radiotherapy surgery on radiation-induced lung injury. Clin Oncol. 2005;17:210–6.
28. Vogelius IR, Bentzen IS. A literature-based meta-analysis of clinical risk factors for development of radiation induced pneumonitis. Acta Oncol. 2013;51:975–83.
29. Albain KS, Swann RS, Rusch VW, Turrisi AT, Shepherd FA, Smith C, Chen Y, Livingston RB, Feins RH, Gandara DR, et al. Radiotherapy plus chemotherapy with or without surgical resection for stage III non-small-cell lung cancer: a phase III randomised controlled trial. Lancet. 2009;374:379–86.
30. Marks LB, Bentzen SM, Deasy JO, et al. Radiation dose-volume effects in the lung. Int J Radiat Oncol Biol Phys. 2010;76:S70–6.
31. Marks LB, Yorke ED, Jackson A, et al. Use of normal tissue complication probability models in the clinic. Int J Radiat Oncol Biol Phys. 2010;76:S10–9.
32. Lind PA, Marks LB, Hardenbergh PH, et al. Technical factors associated with radiation pneumonitis after local +/− regional radiation therapy for breast cancer. Int J Radiat Oncol Biol Phys. 2002;52:137–43.
33. Kimsey FC, Mendenhall NP, Ewald LM, et al. Is radiation treatment volume a predictor for acute or late effect on pulmonary function? A prospective study of patients treated with breast-conserving surgery and postoperative irradiation. Cancer. 1994;73:2549–55.
34. Roach M 3rd, Gandara DR, Yuo HS, et al. Radiation pneumonitis following combined modality therapy for lung cancer: analysis of prognostic factors. J Clin Oncol. 1995;13:2606–12.

35. Kobayashi H, Uno T, Isobe K, et al. Radiation pneumonitis following twice-daily radiotherapy with concurrent carboplatin and paclitaxel in patients with stage III non-small-cell lung cancer. Jpn J Clin Oncol. 2010;40:464–9.
36. Chun SG, Hu C, Choy H, et al. Impact of intensity-modulated radiation therapy technique for locally advanced non-small-cell lung cancer: a secondary analysis of the NRG oncology RTOG 0617 randomized clinical trial. J Clin Oncol. 2017;35:56–62.
37. Okubo K, Gotoh M, Asako M, et al. Efficacy and safety of bilastine in Japanese patients with perennial allergic rhinitis: a multicenter, randomized, double-blind, placebo-controlled, parallel-group phase III study. Allergol Int. 2017;66:97–105.
38. Verma V, Shostrom VK, Zhen W, et al. Influence of fractionation scheme and tumor location on toxicities after stereotactic body radiation therapy for large (≥5 cm) non-small cell lung cancer: a multi-institutional analysis. Int J Radiat Oncol Biol Phys. 2017;97:778–85.
39. Verma V, Simone CB 2nd, Allen PK, et al. Multi-institutional experience of stereotactic ablative radiation therapy for stage I small cell lung cancer. Int J Radiat Oncol Biol Phys. 2017;97:362–71.
40. Zhao J, Yorke ED, Li L, et al. Simple factors associated with radiation-induced lung toxicity after stereotactic body radiation therapy of the thorax: a pooled analysis of 88 studies. Int J Radiat Oncol Biol Phys. 2016;95:1357–66.
41. Verma V, Shah C, Mehta MP. Clinical outcomes and toxicity of proton radiotherapy for breast cancer. Clin Breast Cancer. 2016;16:145–54.
42. Ono T, Hareyama M, Nakamura T, et al. The clinical results of proton beam therapy in patients with idiopathic pulmonary fibrosis: a single center experience. Radiat Oncol. 2016;11:56.
43. Chang JY, Komaki R, Lu C, et al. Phase 2 study of high-dose proton therapy with concurrent chemotherapy for unresectable stage III nonsmall cell lung cancer. Cancer. 2011;117:4707–13.
44. Taghian AG, Assaad SI, Niemierko A, et al. Risk of pneumonitis in breast cancer patients treated with radiation therapy and combination chemotherapy with paclitaxel. J Natl Cancer Inst. 2001;93:1806–11.
45. Mao J, Kocak Z, Zhou S, et al. The impact of induction chemotherapy and the associated tumor response on subsequent radiation-related changes in lung function and tumor response. Int J Radiat Oncol Biol Phys. 2007;67:1360–9.
46. Suresh K, Voong KR, Shankar B, et al. Pneumonitis in non-small cell Lung cancer patients receiving immune checkpoint immunotherapy: incidence and risk factors. J Thorac Oncol. 2018;13:1930–9.
47. Antonia SJ, Villegas A, Daniel D, et al. Durvalumab after chemoradiotherapy in stage III non-small-cell lung cancer. N Engl J Med. 2017;377:1919–29.
48. Varga Z, Cserháti A, Kelemen G, et al. Role of systemic therapy in the development of lung sequelae after conformal radiotherapy in breast cancer patients. Int J Radiat Oncol Biol Phys. 2011;80:1109–16.
49. Ogo E, Komaki R, Abe T, et al. The clinical characteristics and non-steroidal treatment for radiation-induced bronchiolitis obliterans organizing pneumonia syndrome after breast-conserving therapy. Radiother Oncol. 2010;97:95–100.
50. Murofushi KN, Oguchi M, Gosho M, et al. Radiation-induced bronchiolitis obliterans organizing pneumonia (BOOP) syndrome in breast cancer patients is associated with age. Radiat Oncol. 2015;10:103.
51. Bledsoe TJ, Nath SK, Decker RH. Radiation pneumonitis. Clin Chest Med. 2017;38:201–8.
52. Barriger RB, Forquer JA, Brabham JG, et al. A dose-volume analysis of radiation pneumonitis in non-small cell lung cancer patients treated with stereotactic body radiation therapy. Int J Radiat Oncol Biol Phys. 2012;82:457–62.
53. Pinnix CC, Smith GL, Milgrom S, et al. Predictors of radiation pneumonitis in patients receiving intensity modulated radiation therapy for Hodgkin and non-Hodgkin lymphoma. Int J Radiat Oncol Biol Phys. 2015;92:175–82.
54. Wang Z, Huo B, Wu Q, et al. The role of procalcitonin in differential diagnosis between acute radiation pneumonitis and bacterial pneumonia in lung cancer patients receiving thoracic radiotherapy. Sci Rep. 2020;10:2941.

55. Palma DA, Senan S, Haasbeek CJ, et al. Radiological and clinical pneumonitis after stereotactic lung radiotherapy: a matched analysis of three-dimensional conformal and volumetric-modulated arc therapy techniques. Int J Radiat Oncol Biol Phys. 2011;80:506–13.
56. Park KJ, Chung JY, Chun MS, Suh JH. Radiation-induced lung disease and the impact of radiation methods on imaging features. Radiographics. 2000;20:83–98.
57. Choi YW, Munden RF, Erasmus JJ, et al. Effects of radiation therapy on the lung: radiologic appearances and differential diagnosis. Radiographics. 2004;24:985–97.
58. Camus P. Interstitial lung disease from drugs, biologics, and radiation. In: Schwartz MI, King Jr TE, editors. Interstitial lung disease. 5th ed. Shelton: People's Medical Publishing House-USA; 2011. p. 637.
59. Gross NJ, Narine KR, Wade R. Protective effect of corticosteroids on radiation pneumonitis in mice. Radiat Res. 1988;113:112–9.
60. Ozturk B, Egehan I, Atavci S, Kitapci M. Pentoxifylline in prevention of radiation-induced lung toxicity in patients with breast and lung cancer: a double-blind randomized trial. Int J Radiat Oncol Biol Phys. 2004;58:213–9.
61. Borst GR, De Jaeger K, Belderbos JS, et al. Pulmonary function changes after radiotherapy in non-small-cell lung cancer patients with long-term disease-free survival. Int J Radiat Oncol Biol Phys. 2005;62:639–44.
62. Ward WF, Molteni A, Ts'ao CH. Radiation-induced endothelial dysfunction and fibrosis in rat lung: modification by the angiotensin converting enzyme inhibitor CL242817. Radiat Res. 1989;117:342–50.

Prevention and Management of Cardiotoxicity Secondary to Thoracic Radiation

19

Aditi Tanwar, Mohit Rana, and Kanika Sood Sharma

19.1 Introduction

Advancements in clinical sciences and imaging technologies have lead to increase in the detection of cancer at early stages. Patients can therefore benefit with early introduction of anticancer treatment and this has increased the longevity in majority of the sub sites. But owing to exposure to a plethora of new therapies including drugs and radiation, the long term toxicities have become more evident.

Radiation therapy is an integral component of treatment strategies for majority of thoracic malignancies including carcinoma breast, carcinoma lung, carcinoma esophagus, lymphoma etc. wherein radiation can be used in definitive, adjuvant, neoadjuvant or palliative setting. Apart from the tumor, the adjacent organs are also exposed to the effects of radiation and chemotherapy. The heart suffers the major brunt of adverse effects which ranges from pericarditis, pericardial effusion etc. which are common acute side effects appearing within weeks following treatment. Some adverse effects may present months to years after exposure to radiation (as late as 20 years or more) and can be seen in the form of symptomatic coronary artery disease (CAD), valvular heart disease or heart failure [1]. All these side effects combined are classified as RICT (radiation induced cardiotoxicity) [2].

A. Tanwar (✉)
Dharamshila Narayana Superspeciality Hospital, New Delhi, India
e-mail: aditi.tanwar.dr@nhhospitals.onmicrosoft.com

K. Sood Sharma
Department of Radiation Oncology, Dharamshila Narayana Superspeciality Hospital, New Delhi, India

M. Rana
National Heart Institute, New Delhi, India

K. Sood Sharma et al. (eds.), *Complications of Cancer Therapy: Best Practices in Prevention and Management*, https://doi.org/10.1007/978-981-99-0984-1_19

19.2 Pathophysiology

Radiation induces generation of free radicals and pro inflammatory cytokines which react with cellular DNA causing disruption of the strand thereby preventing replication and protein synthesis. Although cardiomyocytes are relatively radiation resistant but still there is 4–16% risk of major cardiac events with each increasing Gray of mean heart dose. Radiation causes endothelial dysfunction of the microvasculature leading to thrombosis and small vessel disease of the myocardium leading to structural changes of the heart as a sequelae of pericardial inflammation, fibrosis of myocardium and electrical conduction system majorly. The inflammation can lead to pericarditis or pericardial effusion. The proinflammatory cytokines can cause intimal reaction and fibrin deposition accelerating the progression of coronary artery disease. Chronic fibrosis of the pericardium can lead to constrictive pericarditis [3]. Diffuse infiltrative fibrosis in the myocardium can impair the ability of the ventricles to relax resulting in a diastolic failure. The conduction system of the heart can also be affected and appear as arrhythmias later in life. The deleterious effects of radiation can be seen even years after wherein the valvular endothelium can be damaged or fibrosed leading to backflow or stenosis [2] (Illustration 19.1).

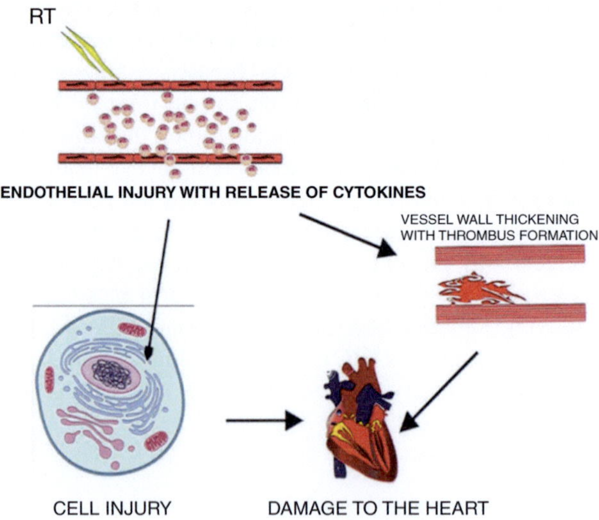

Illustration 19.1 Diagram showing effect of radiation on the vessels

19.3 Risk Factors

The factors predicting the risk of likelihood of cardiac complications after receiving radiation for thoracic malignancies can be classified as:

Patient related—age, preexistence of comorbidities, nature of the underlying malignancy, laterality of the tumor.

The risk for cardiovascular diseases increases with increasing age. The complexity increases due to the presence of confounding factors like diabetes, hypertension, physical inability, obesity, smoking etc. [3]. The female gender is at an increased risk compared with age matched male gender. Cardiovascular events are the major cause of morbidity and death among patients with diabetes mellitus and other comorbidities [4]. The extent of damage to the underlying heart is highly dependent on the thoracic structure harboring the malignancy, the chances are more in carcinoma esophagus and carcinoma lung since these are central structures. Also the risk increases when the tumor lies on the left side like carcinoma left breast, carcinoma left lung [1, 5]. The reason being inclusion of coronary arteries in the field of radiation leading to direct cardiac injury. The main cardiac substructures involved are left anterior descending artery (LAD) and left ventricle. For every 1 Gy increase in mean heart dose, the mean dose to LAD increased by 3.4 Gy [1].

Treatment related—patients receiving cardiotoxic chemotherapy along with radiation therapy are at a relatively higher risk of acquiring a heart disease than those receiving either of them [6]. Dose of radiation is another major factor affecting the damage to the underlying heart, higher the dose more will be the side effects. Similarly older the technique of radiation more are the chances of affecting the underlying structures including heart [7]. Hence the use of brachytherapy is appreciated for giving radiation to the lumpectomy cavity in cases of carcinoma breast undergoing breast conservation treatment, use of APBI (accelerated partial breast irradiation) is practiced at centres equipped with relevant resources [8]. The aim is to minimize the dose received by the underlying organs at risk.

Also the nature of the particle used for imparting radiation contributes to the dose received by the adjacent structures. Use of photons is associated with an increased dose contribution to the underlying structures, this risk is limited with the use of electrons. And this can be further minimized by using proton beam therapy [9]. Proton and heavy ions such as carbon ions majorly contribute to charged particle therapy [10]. They deposit minimal energy at the entrance of the body where their velocity is high and deposit most of the energy at the end of its range (Bragg peak) in the tumor. Intensity modulation is also feasible for these charged particles and therefore present a newer advancement in RT to achieve lower and more targeted dose to tumor and better protect the organs at risk (OAR). But not all the centres are equipped with protons or electrons and majority use photons for delivery of therapeutic radiation (Illustration 19.2).

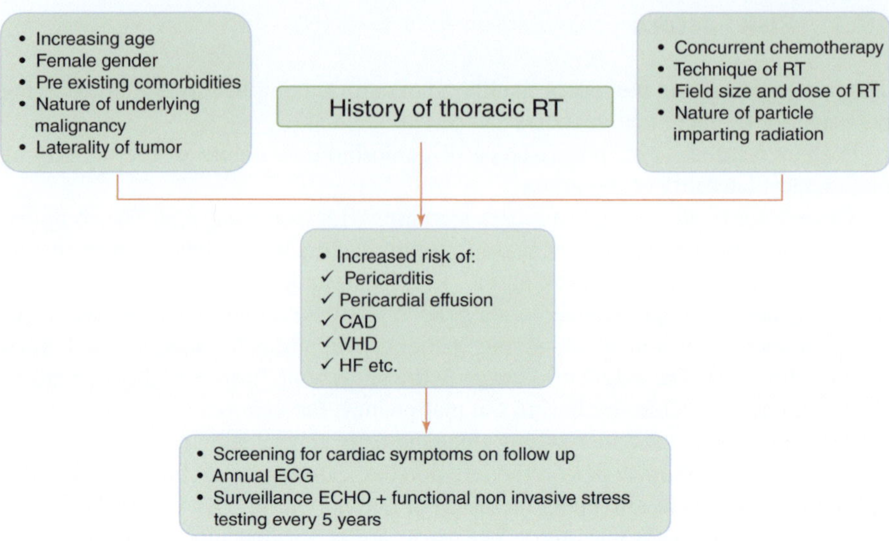

Illustration 19.2 Schematic diagram showing factors affecting cardiotoxicity

19.4 Clinical Features and Diagnostic Work Up

1. **Pericarditis**—it is often defined as a swelling and irritation of the thin membrane surrounding the heart i.e. pericardium [11].

   It presents as sharp stabbing chest pain that usually does not last long. It is frequently found to radiate to left shoulder and increases on cough. The pain is often eased by leaning forward and is worse in the supine position.

   It may be associated with low grade fever, malaise and weight loss in chronic cases.

   Signs include a "pericardial rub"-friction rub on auscultation, often transient.

   Tachycardia is also a common finding in such cases.

   Chest X-ray shows increased cardiac silhouette due to pericardial collection, pleural effusion. In acute pericarditis ECG shows initial diffuse elevated ST segments ± depressed PR segment. The elevation in the ST segment is concave upwards. After 2–5 days isoelectric ST wave is seen with T wave flattening and inversion.

   ECHO shows pericardial collection, thickening of pericardium. Cardiac MRI and CT can be done to see the collection. Blood investigations show increased CRP, ESR. Most of the mild cases are self-resolving. Treatment for acute pericarditis involves NSAIDs like Ibuprofen, Aspirin and proton pump inhibitors.

For severe cases steroids and colchicine may be added. Chronic cases that are unrelieved with medical management may require surgical resection of pericardium (pericardiectomy).

2. **Pericardial effusion**—defined as collection of excess fluid between layers of heart. Patients usually complaint of chest heaviness, pain in the chest, breathing difficulty. In severe cases abdominal distension and leg swelling [12].

   Chest X-ray shows cardiomegaly. The heart's silhouette may be enlarged.

   ECG shows low voltage waves. On auscultation faint cardiac sounds are heard. Echocardiogram shows fluid collection around heart. Treatment involves restriction of fluid, antibiotics, aspirin, steroids and diuretics. Large collection may require surgical drainage in the form of pericardiocentesis (insertion of a needle and drainage of fluid) or pericardiectomy (making a small window in the pericardium).

3. **Coronary artery disease**—Coronary artery disease is the result of deposition of plaque in the arteries that supply oxygen-rich blood to the heart. Plaque causes a narrowing or blockage that could result in a heart attack.

   The proinflammatory effect of radiation can accelerate the damage to the vascular endothelium. This mimics atherosclerosis in the coronary vasculature, leading to fibrin deposition and intimal proliferation fastening the process of coronary artery disease [13].

   Patients present with severe chest pain radiating to jaw, shoulder, back and arm, loss of consciousness, anxiety, sweating. ECG shows ischemic changes, ST elevation or depression. Exercise stress tests, pharmacologic stress tests can be done to evaluate the status of heart. Cardiac enzymes show increased trop T and trop I. Coronary angiogram and conventional angiogram uses CT and contrast dye to view 3 dimensional pictures of the moving heart and detect blockages in the coronary arteries. Management usually involves lifestyle modification along with medical treatment. Majority of the patients require medicines to lower cholesterol levels, such as statins, bile acid sequestrants, niacin and fibrates. Medications to lower blood pressure, such as beta blockers, calcium channel blockers, angiotensin-converting enzyme (ACE) inhibitors or angiotensin II receptor blockers etc. may be needed. Vasodilators such as nitrates/nitroglycerin or ranolazine are effective in relieving the anginal pain. Anticoagulants (including aspirin) and newer generation antiplatelets may have to be considered depending on the clinical manifestations.

   Balloon angioplasty and stenting are the non surgical interventional procedures that may be employed in mild to moderate cases to widen the lumen of the affected arteries. Severe cases may require Coronary artery bypass graft (CABG) surgery which involves surgical creation of new collateral vasculature for the blood to flow when there is a blockage in the coronary arteries.

4. **Valvular heart disease**—after as long as 10–20 years of mediastinal radiation, there can be a risk of heart valve damage characterised by valve fibrosis and calcification [14, 15]. The most commonly observed symptoms are chest pain, shortness of breath, fatigue, pedal edema etc. On examination murmurs can be heard, irregular heart beat can be observed. The findings on a chest X-ray show normal cardiac size in patients with aortic stenosis (AS), with rounding of the left ventricular (LV) border and apex due to the LV hypertrophy. Aortic valve and aortic root calcification can also be appreciated. ECG and echocardiography show abnormal patterns. Computerised tomography and cardiac magnetic resonance imaging can provide a quantitative assessment of the degree of damage. Medical management is usually not found to be of much benefit. Valvular replacement or percutaneous balloon valvotomy may be considered as the treatment option.
5. **Arrythmias**—The persistence of fibrotic changes can also affect the conduction system and lead to a wide spectrum of manifestations from incomplete right bundle branch block to complete AV block. RT has been associated with various nonspecific ECG changes, including QTc interval prolongation, although the most common manifestations are nonspecific T-wave changes and decreased QRS amplitude [16].
6. **Heart failure**—The diffuse infiltrative fibrosis in the myocardium can impair the ability of the ventricles to relax resulting in diastolic failure. Though it is rare but can occur as a late complication [17].

19.5 Screening for Cardiac Symptoms Post Radiation

Patients after receiving mediastinal radiation should be screened for the cardiac symptoms at follow ups. There are various guidelines [4] on what should be the appropriate timing and modality for evaluating cardiac functioning following thoracic radiation as shown in Table 19.1.

Table 19.1 Imaging screening guidelines and consensus recommendations by major societies following chest radiation therapy

Organization(s)	Year	Significant risk factors	Cardiac structure and function screening	Coronary ischemia screening
European Association of Cardiovascular Imaging and American Society of Echocardiography	2013	• Anterior or left chest RT with $\geq$1 risk factor: 1. High cumulative dose (>30 Gy) 2. Younger patients (<50 years) 3. Higher doses of radiation fractions (>2 Gy/day) 4. Presence and extent of tumor in or next to the heart 5. Lack of shielding 6. Concomitant chemotherapy (e.g., anthracyclines) 7. Cardiovascular risk factors 8. Pre-existing cardiovascular disease	• TTE 5 years after RT in patients at high risk • TTE 10 years after RT in patients not at high risk • TTE every 5 years thereafter	• Stress testing 5 years after RT in patients at high risk every 5 years thereafter in patients without previous inducible ischemia
International Late Effects of Childhood Cancer Guideline Harmonization Group	2015	• Surveillance recommended in those with: 1. Chest radiation dose $\geq$35 Gy 2. Moderate to high doses of anthracyclines ($\geq$100 mg/m^2) combined with moderate- to high-dose chest radiation ($\geq$15 Gy) 3. May be reasonable in those with moderate doses of radiation ($\geq$15–<35 Gy)	• TTE no later than 2 years after completion of therapy in high-risk survivors, again at years, and every years thereafter	N/A

(continued)

Table 19.1 (continued)

Organization(s)	Year	Significant risk factors	Cardiac structure and function screening	Coronary ischemia screening
American Society of Clinical Oncology	2017	• High-dose RT (>30 Gy) where the heart is in the treatment field • Lower-dose anthracycline (e.g., 250 mg/m^2 Doxorubicin or 600 mg/m^2 Epirubicin) in combination with lower-dose RT (>30 Gy) where the heart is in the treatment field	• TTE 6–12 months after completion of therapy in patients at increased risk, no specific screening interval recommended thereafter	N/A
Children's Oncology Group	2018	• Increased risk: 1. Any anthracycline exposure or 2. ≥15 Gy radiation • Highest risk: 1. ≥35 Gy or 2. ≥15 Gy in combination with <250 mg/m^2 Doxorubicin (or equivalent) or 3. Any radiation in combination with ≥250 mg/m^2 doxorubicin (or equivalent) • Additional risk factors to consider: <5 years old at treatment, anteriorly weighted radiation field, lack of subcarinal shielding, longer time since treatment	• Annual physical and electrocardiography in patients with ≥15 Gy • Echocardiography every 5 years: 1. 15–35 Gy or 2. <250 mg/m^2 doxorubicin and 0–15 Gy • Echocardiography every 2 years: 1. ≥35 Gy or 2. ≥15 Gy and any anthracyclines or 3. ≥250 mg/m^2 doxorubicin	• Cardiology consultation 5–10 years after radiation in patients at highest risk

European Society of Medical Oncology	2020	• Mediastinal RT ± cardiotoxic chemotherapy, not further specified	• Cardiac biomarkers and potentially cardiac imaging 6–12 months after therapy, 2 years after treatment, and possibly periodically thereafter	• Evaluation for CAD and ischemia starting at 5 years after RT and every 3–5 years thereafter
International Cardio-Oncology Society	2021	• Reasserted previously defined high-risk groups: 1. Mediastinal RT ≥30 Gy with the heart in the treatment field 2. Lower dose RT (<30 Gy) with anthracycline exposure 3. Patients aged <50 years and longer time since RT 4. Higher doses of RT fractions (>2 Gy/day) 5. Presence and extent of tumor in or next to the heart 6. Presence of cardiovascular risk factors 7. Pre-existing cardiovascular disease	• Guided by individual patient risk: TTE as early as 6–12 months after RT in patients at high risk, and all patients should have TTE by 5 years after RT. Additionally TTE and/or NT-proBNP every 5 years can be useful	• Focus on diagnosing early CAD rather than ischemia for initiation of preventive therapy • Review available CT scans for coronary calcifications • In patients without known CAD, screening with stress testing, CAC, or CT angiography every 5 years

Adapted from Carmen Bergom et al. [4]

CAC coronary artery calcium, *CAD* coronary artery disease, *CT* computed tomography, *NT-proBNP* N-terminal pro–B-type natriuretic peptide, *RT* radiation therapy, *TTE* transthoracic echocardiography

19.6 Prevention of Cardiotoxicity Secondary to Thoracic Radiation

- **Risk factor modification**—the risk of acquiring radiation induced cardiotoxicity though is majorly related to radiation exposure but is also dependent on underlying comorbidities. Hence adequate baseline screening of patients for traditional risk factors (smoking, diabetes and hypertension) and imaging risk factors (coronary artery calcifications) is a predictor of future cardiovascular events in survivors of mediastinal radiation. Preexistence of any cardiovascular risk factor increases the risk of acquiring a major coronary event. A history of ischemic heart disease carries almost a six fold higher risk of a future cardiac event in women treated for carcinoma breast. This risk is higher in the first 10 years after cancer diagnosis [1]. Smoking combined with radiation triples the risk of myocardial infarction compared to non smoker patients treated for breast cancer. High cholesterol has been studied as a confounding factor for development of coronary atherosclerosis in Hodgkin lymphoma survivors. The effects of preexisting cardiovascular risk factors have been equally detrimental in patients with advanced carcinoma lung undergoing radiation. Hence smoking cessation, adequate blood sugar control, lowering of blood pressure and cholesterol are the key determinants of the cardiovascular adverse effects following mediastinal radiation.
- **Intensity modulation and daily imaging**—owing to improvements in treatment technology, the cardiac radiation exposure has decreased over time. In the historic era of 2 dimensional radiotherapy, the bony landmarks were used to define borders of the radiation field, hence a documentation of the doses received by the underlying structures was not possible. Overtime the treatment has evolved from 2 to 3 dimension with time now being identified as the fourth dimension which tracks the motion of the tumor. Advancements in radiotherapy techniques such as intensity-modulated radiotherapy (IMRT) may reduce the risk of cardiac toxicity owing to the steep dose gradient limiting the volume of the heart irradiated to a high dose. Image-guided radiotherapy (IGRT) is a further refinement of IMRT delivery with daily imaging, which may further reduce excessive cardiac irradiation. The superiority of IMRT over 3D-CRT (3 dimensional conformal radiotherapy) has been extensively studied in terms of dose reduction to myocardium in patients with left mean heart volume receiving more than 30 Gy were 2.6 and 16.4% for IMRT and 3D-CRT, respectively [7]. The use of image guidance along with IMRT gives the possibility of reduction of set up margins allowing for better sparing of normal tissues and at the same time promoting tumor dose escalation.
- **DIBH**—In an attempt to reduce the dose to underlying heart and lung in patients receiving mediastinal radiation, deep inspiratory breath hold (DIBH) technique has been extensively studied. This technique reduces cardiac exposure by lung expansion physically displacing the heart out of the radiation field as shown in Fig. 19.1. Compared with free breathing, DIBH resulted in a significant reduction in heart V30 (7.1 vs. 2.4%, $P < 0.0001$), mean heart dose (6.9 vs. 3.9 Gy, $P < 0.001$) [18]. In a cohort of breast cancer patients undergoing radiation includ-

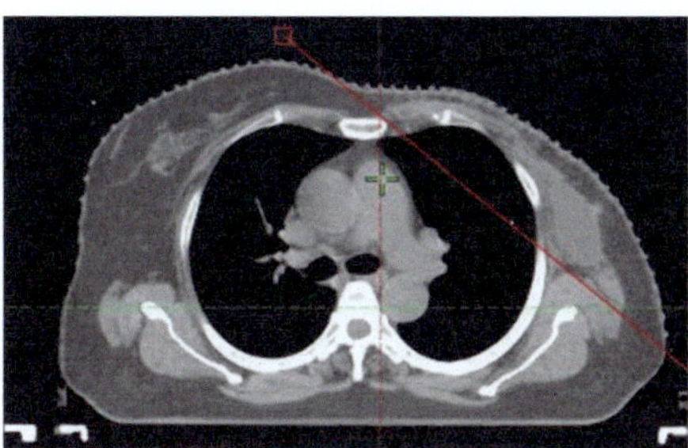
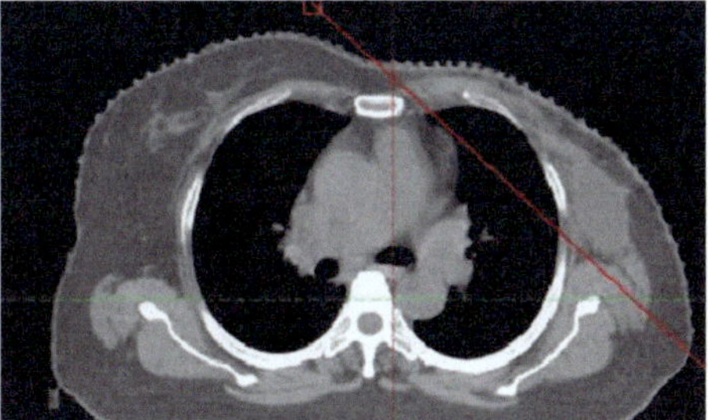

Fig. 19.1 Axial section of CT thorax showing the effect of breath hold and normal breathing

ing regional nodes, DIBH allowed a greater reduction in mean heart dose and LAD (left anterior descending artery) dose compared to free breathing [19]. Tracking of tumor movement with breathing has been successfully exploited for reducing the radiation related cardiac events. ABC (active breathing control) causes moderate to deep inspiratory breath hold, other technique uses respiratory gating with chest wall sensors to trigger delivery of radiation therapy based on respiratory expansion of the thorax can be used. Cardiac mortality can reduce by 4.7% by using Breath hold and respiratory gating techniques compared with free breathing techniques in patients with left sided tumors, with a median cardiac mortality normal tissue complication probability (NTCP) of 0.1% [20, 21]. DIBH combined with IGRT can further reduce the radiation dose to the heart with greater advantage seen in patients with left sided breast cancer. In a study in patients with left-sided breast cancer treated using IGRT, a significant reduction was seen in the percentage of volume of left ventricle irradiation 28% vs 71% for DIBH and free breathing respectively [22].

- **Treatment in prone position**—this technique was developed in an attempt to reduce dose to the underlying structures in patients treated for carcinoma breast. It was found to be of use in patients with large, pendulous breast. It allows the breast to fall away from the chest wall thereby increasing the distance between the heart and the breast tissue being irradiated [23] as shown in Fig. 19.2. An analysis by the New York University on 100 patients (53 with left-sided cancers) comparing prone versus supine treatment found that prone positioning reduced the in-field heart volume by 12 cc in 90% of patients [24]. Mixed data is available regarding use of prone positioning for reducing cardiac dose in patients undergoing breast irradiation majorly due to lack of appropriate reproducibility. In comparison to the supine position, the superior and lateral aspects of the heart typically move anteriorly during prone. This may havc negative consequences in situations in which the target tissues receiving high dose of radiation include the chest wall or deep breast. More long term follow up is needed with cardiac outcomes being evaluated as specific end points.
- **Proton beam therapy**—the beam characteristics of the proton particle allows for a sharp dose fall off beyond the brag peak leading to a dose reduction to critical structures and hence reduction in the acute and late toxicities. Although

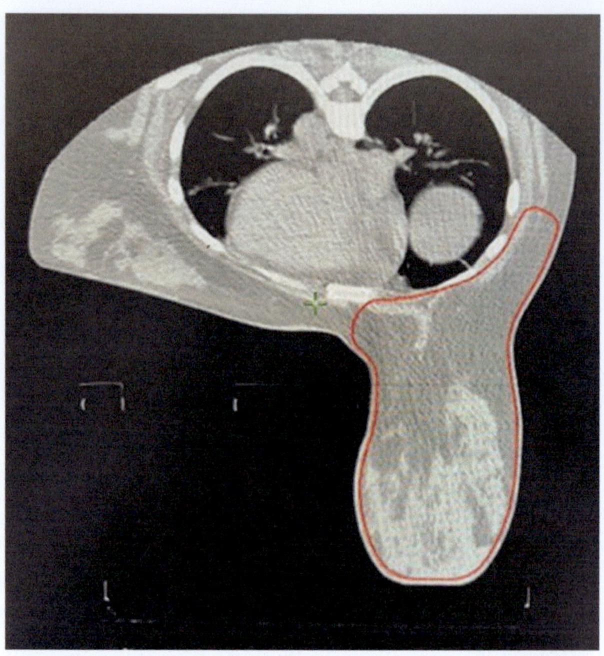

Fig. 19.2 Depiction of prone breast positioning for sparing the heart

it has been majorly utilised in pediatric malignancies, skull base tumors, orbital tumors and reirradiation, is now being employed in other subsites including thoracic malignancies. Use of proton beam therapy (PBT) has been compared with IMRT in treating patients with carcinoma breast and there has been a significant reduction in the heart doses [25]. Single field PBT is now being replaced by intensity modulated proton therapy (IMPT) and has been found to reduce V20Gy and V5Gy of the heart [26]. Despite its promising results the use of PBT is limited due its high cost concerns [27]. Hence in the light of limited data and limited cost effectiveness, proton beam therapy is not one of the choicest modalities for reducing cardiac dose in patients undergoing mediastinal irradiation.

- **Reduction in the field size and dose of radiation**:
  - **Partial breast irradiation**—this technique of irradiating just the lumpectomy cavity with a margin around is being increasingly used in patients with breast cancer. It can be used as an alternative method to reduce cardiac doses since by reducing the volume of tissue being irradiated, the distance between heart and target volume is increased. The only concern is the effect of high dose per fraction on the cardiac tissues which have lower alpha/beta [28]. But a few studies addressing this concern have shown no negative effect on heart [29]. APBI (accelerated partial breast irradiation) is one of the types of partial breast irradiation. APBI can be done with either brachytherapy (interstitial or balloon based) or with external beam therapy [8]. APBI is used in patients with early stage breast cancer who have a long survival post treatment hence every measure should be taken to restore a good quality of life to these

patients. A plethora of dosimetric studies are available on the use of interstitial brachytherapy for APBI. There is a significant reduction not only in the volumes of the lung and heart receiving low doses of radiation (V5 and V10Gy) but also in the maximum dose received by small portions of heart (D 0.1 cc). Taking into account the simplicity of using balloon based catheters, the interstitial brachytherapy is replaced by balloon brachytherapy during the last decade [30]. But the benefit of dose reduction to underlying structures is still maintained.

- **Involved field radiation**—advances in technological aspects and imaging modalities have led to involved field radiation (IFI) being considered over elective nodal irradiation (ENI) in esophageal and lung cancers. The volume of mediastinal structures undergoing radiation reduces significantly with IFI in comparison to ENI. Hence there is a substantial reduction in the side effects of the radiation. A systematic review compared IFI and ENI for definitive chemoradiotherapy for esophageal cancer [31]. The results showed no significant differences in the overall survival and local control rates between the IFI and ENI arms. Stage III and stage IV oligometastatic NSCLC (non small cell lung cancer) patients were compared for ENI and IFI and the differences in 2 year local control, distant control and overall survival were not statistically significant in these two arms [32]. Although cardiac toxicities have not been studied as the primary end point in the above studies but there is a substantial reduction in esophageal and pulmonary toxicities with the use of IFI thereby giving possibilities of reduced cardiac morbidity as well [33].
- The treatment techniques for Hodgkin's lymphoma have evolved dramatically over the past decades. From extended magna fields to involved node radiation (INRT) combined with increasing use of IMRT and proton therapy along with combination chemotherapy [34]. The fields and doses of radiation have reduced over time especially when used with doxorubicin based chemotherapy in order to reduce the adverse effects of combination chemotherapy. Radiation induced heart disease is considered a "late effect" affecting the long term survivors. Among HL survivors, the risk of fatal myocardial infarction has been found to be 2.5 times higher than in the general population. Most of the data related to cardiotoxicity is derived from childhood survivors of HL, a highly curable disease, with toxicities including valvular heart disease (21–41%), coronary heart disease (17–23%), heart failure (8–17%), conduction disorders (12%) and pericardial abnormalities (10%) [35].
- In an attempt to compare the cardiotoxicity as a function of field size, a study was conducted evaluating HL treated with involved-node RT to 30–36 Gy, mantle fields were simulated to a dose of 36 Gy in the same patients. Comparing the mantle RT and involved-node RT, mean doses to the heart were 27.5 Gy versus 7.7 Gy, respectively, and mean doses to the left anterior descending artery (LAD) were 23.1 Gy versus 8.9 Gy. Calculations suggested the 25-year absolute excess risk of cardiovascular disease based on the estimated mean heart dose (MHD) and demonstrated a significant risk reduc-

tion with the use of involved-node versus mantle RT (1.4% vs 9.1%; P < 0.001) [36].
- **Cardiac substructure identification**—the risk of cardiac events is related to the dose and volume of the substructures irradiated. There is a difference in the radiation tolerance of the various cardiac substructures. For proper delineation of these substructures, the University of Michigan cardiac atlas was designed [37]. Anterior myocardial territory (AMT) has been identified to bear the major brunt of dose in mediastinal irradiation. AMT includes the myocardium from the anterior surface of heart to 1 cm from the posterior surface, the major epicardial coronary arteries at the anterior surface such as LAD, left circumflex and left and right main coronary arteries. It is necessary to pay attention to prevent overdosing of these structures in the anterior part of the heart. Strict dose constraints to these structures might be useful in reducing the cardiac events further [38]. Majority of the studies done on the tolerance of various cardiac substructures were conducted in patients of carcinoma lung [39]. Following are the various parameters identified in these studies:
  - Minimum dose to superior vena cava (SVC) and maximum dose to left atrium (LA) is significantly associated with non cancer deaths [40].
  - Higher maximum dose to bilateral ventricles is significantly associated with non cancer deaths [41].
  - There is a decrease in OS if >2.2% of LA wall receives >63 Gy [42].
  - Pericardial V30 >29% is associated with worse overall survival (OS) [43].
  - Dose to base of the heart >8.5 Gy decreases OS [44].
  - The maximum dose received by the combined cardiac region including the right atrium, right coronary artery, and ascending aorta was found to have the greatest effect on patient survival. A maximum dose of 23 Gy was identified as a dose limit for future studies [45]
  - OS decreases if pulmonary artery V40 >80% [46].

19.7 Conclusions

The improvements and advancements in treatment technologies have increased the survival outcome for cancer patients. Hence it is not uncommon to witness long term survivors with late side effects of treatment. Improvement of the quality of life of these patients is the need of the hour. Radiation induced cardiotoxicity is a known complication in patients undergoing mediastinal radiation, hence a better understanding of the underlying pathophysiology is required to improve the screening protocols for identifying preclinical RICT and allow for earlier interventions. Although significant improvement in the techniques of radiation have reduced the incidence of these cardiac events. But still RICT remains a potentially significant toxicity for many patients with thoracic cancers. Improved knowledge about radiation doses limitations to cardiac substructures allows for better personalization of radiation in the times to come. Better application of cardiac contouring atlases in routine clinics and case management is required. Adapting to the protocols of reduced radiation field and dose together with vigorous attempts of using breath

Table 19.2 Depiction of the measures taken to prevent cardiotoxicity

Effort	Effect
Risk factor modification	**Prevents/delays the pathophysiology behind RICT**
Intensity modulated radiation and dally imaging	Conforms the dose to the target Reduces the dose to underlying structures including heart during any mediastinal radiation
Breath hold technique	Inspiration increases the distance of heart from chest wall thereby moving the heart away from field of radiation
Prone position	Used in breast irradiation Breast falls away increasing the distance from heart, hence, putting the heart away from the radiation field
Proton beam therapy	The principle of sharp dose fall off is utilized, hence, better sparing of heart
Reduction in field size and dose of radiation • APBI • Involved field radiation • Limited use of ENI	• Used for carcinoma breast. It limits the field and dose of radiation • Used for Hodgkin lymphoma where radiation fields have evolved from magna fields to involved node radiation • Concept of elective node irradiation is decreasing and only involved nodes are treated in lung and esophageal cancers to decrease toxicity to underlying structures
Cardiac substructure identification	Better understanding of the variation in radiation tolerance by cardiac sub structures helps in refinement of thoracic contours in order to decrease RICT

hold technique, prone positioning and the latest techniques of radiation along with aggressive cardiovascular risk modification (summarized in Table 19.2) can help in further reducing the incidence of radiation induced cardiac disease.

Key Points

1. Radiation is an integral component of the treatment of many thoracic malignancies.
2. Treatment advancements have increased the survival rates so long-term survivors are frequently witnessed in clinical practice. Hence more emphasis needs to be given to chronic side effects of treatment.
3. Radiation induced cardiotoxicity is one such complication of mediastinal irradiation and can be reduced by a variety of efforts.
4. Lifestyle modification remains to be of utmost importance along with other measures taken beginning from the level of simulation to radiation plan execution.
5. Better application of cardiac contouring atlases in routine clinics and case management is required.
6. Adapting to the protocols of reduced radiation field and dose together with vigorous attempts of using breath hold technique, prone positioning and the latest techniques of radiation is the need of the hour.

Acknowledgments I acknowledge Dr. Pankaj Gupta and Dr. Sobhana Vallabhaneni for their contribution towards the illustrations.

References

1. Darby SC, McGale P, Taylor CW, Peto R. Long-term mortality from heart disease and lung cancer after radiotherapy for early breast cancer: prospective cohort study of about 300,000 women in US SEER cancer registries. Lancet Oncol. 2005;6:557–65. https://doi.org/10.1016/S1470-2045(05)70251-5.
2. Banfill K, Giuliani M, Aznar M, et al. Cardiac toxicity of thoracic radiotherapy: existing evidence and future directions. J Thorac Oncol. 2021;16(2):216–27. https://doi.org/10.1016/j.jtho.2020.11.002.
3. Hufnagle JJ, Andersen SN, Maani EV. Radiation therapy induced cardiac toxicity. In: StatPearls. Treasure Island (FL): StatPearls Publishing; 2021. p. 2022.
4. Bergom C, Bradley JA, Ng AK, et al. Past, present, and future of radiation-induced cardiotoxicity: refinements in targeting, surveillance, and risk stratification. JACC Cardio Oncol. 2021;3(3):343–59.
5. Taylor CW, Nisbet A, McGale P, Darby SC. Cardiac exposures in breast cancer radiotherapy: 1950–1990. Int J Radiat Oncol Biol Phys. 2007;69:1484–95. https://doi.org/10.1016/j.ijrobp.2007.05.034.
6. Hardy D, Liu CC, Cormier JN, et al. Cardiac toxicity in association with chemotherapy and radiation therapy in a large cohort of older patients with non small cell lung cancer. Ann Oncol. 2010;21:1825–33.
7. Popescu CC, Olivotto IA, Beckham WA, Ansbacher W, Zavgorodni S, Shaffer R, et al. Volumetric modulated arc therapy improves dosimetry and reduce treatment time compared to conventional intensity-modulated radiotherapy for locoregional therapy of left-sided breast cancer and internal mammary lymph nodes. Int J Radiat Oncol Biol Phys. 2010;76:287–95. https://doi.org/10.1016/j.ijrobp.2009.05.038.
8. Lettmaier S, Kreppner S, Lotter M, et al. Radiation exposure of the heart, lung, and skin by radiation therapy for breast cancer: a dosimetric comparison between partial breast irradiation using multicatheter brachytherapy and whole breast teletherapy. Radiother Oncol. 2011;100:189–94.
9. Akamatsu H, Karasawa K, Omatsu T, Isobe Y, Ogata R, Koba Y. First experience of carbon-ion radiotherapy for early breast cancer. Jpn J Radiol. 2014;32:288–95. https://doi.org/10.1007/s11604-014-0300-6.
10. Moon SH, Shin KH, Kim TH, Yoon M, Park S, Lee DH, et al. Dosimetric comparison of four different external beam partial breast irradiation techniques: three-dimensional conformal radiotherapy, intensity-modulated radiotherapy, helical tomotherapy, and proton beam therapy. Radiother Oncol. 2009;90:66–73. https://doi.org/10.1016/j.radonc.2008.09.027.
11. Imazio M, Gaita F, LeWinter M. Evaluation and treatment of pericarditis: a systematic review. JAMA. 2015;314(14):1498–506.
12. Imazio M, Mayosi BM, Brucato A, Markel G, Trinchero R, Spodick DH, Adler Y. Triage and management of pericardial effusion. J Cardiovasc Med (Hagerstown). 2010;11(12):928–35.
13. Dalen JE, Alpert JS, Goldberg RJ, Weinstein RS. The epidemic of the tweinth century: coronary heart disease. Am J Med. 2014;127(9):807–12.
14. Carlson RG, Mayfield WR, Normann S, Alexander JA. Radiation-associated valvular disease. Chest. 1991;99(3):538–45. https://doi.org/10.1378/chest.99.3.538.
15. Copeland KA, Hosmane VR, Jurkovitz C, Kolm P, Bowen J, Di Sabatino A, Banbury MK, Strasser JF, Weintraub WS, Doorey AJ. Frequency of severe valvular disease caused by mediastinal radiation among patients undergoing valve surgery in a community-based, regional academic medical center. Clin Cardiol. 2013;36(4):217–21. https://doi.org/10.1002/clc.22106.
16. Buza V, Rajagopalan B, Curtis AB, et al. Focus on chemotherapy and targeted therapies. Circ Arrhythm Electrophysiol. 2017;10:e005443.
17. Wang H, Wei J, Zheng Q, Meng L, Xin Y, Yin X, Jiang X. Radiation-induced heart disease: a review of classification, mechanism and prevention. Int J Biol Sci. 2019;15(10):2128–38. https://doi.org/10.7150/ijbs.35460.

18. Hayden AJ, Rains M, Tiver K. Deep inspiration breath hold technique reduces heart dose from radiotherapy for left-sided breast cancer. J Med Imaging Radiat Oncol. 2012;56(4):464–72. https://doi.org/10.1111/j.1754-9485.2012.02405.x.
19. Yeung R, Conroy L, Long K, Walrath D, Li H, Smith W, et al. Cardiac dose reduction with deep inspiration breath hold for left-sided breast cancer radiotherapy patients with and without regional nodal irradiation. Radiat Oncol. 2015;10(1):200. https://doi.org/10.1186/s13014-015-0511-8.
20. Nemoto K, Oguchi M, Nakajima M, et al. Cardiac-sparing radiotherapy for the left breast cancer with deep breath-holding. Jpn J Radiol. 2009;27:259–63.
21. Korreman SS, Pederson AN, Aarup LR, et al. Reduction of cardiac and pulmonary complication probabilities after breathing adapted radiotherapy for breast cancer. Int J Radiat Oncol Biol Phys. 2006;65:1375–80.
22. Borst GR, Sonke JJ, den Hollander S, Betgen A, Remeijer P, van Giersbergen A, et al. Clinical results of image-guided deep inspiration breath hold breast irradiation. Int J Radiat Oncol Biol Phys. 2010;78:1345–51. https://doi.org/10.1016/j.ijrobp.2009.10.006.
23. Chino JP, Marks LB, et al. Prone positioning causes the heart to be displaced anteriorly within the thorax: implications for breast cancer treatment. Int J Radiat Oncol Biol Phys. 2008;70:916–20.
24. Lymberis SC, DeWyngaert JK, Parhar P, et al. Prospective assessment of optimal individual position (prone versus supine) for breast radiotherapy: volumetric and dosimetric correlations in 100 patients. Int J Radiat Oncol Biol Phys. 2012;84:902–9.
25. Ares C, Khan S, Macartain AM, et al. Postoperative proton radiotherapy for localized and locoregional breast cancer: potential for clinically relevant improvements? Int J Radiat Oncol Biol Phys. 2010;76:685–97.
26. Jimenez RB, Goma C, Nyamwanda J, et al. Intensity modulated proton therapy for postmastectomy radiation of bilateral implant reconstructed breasts: a treatment planning study. Radiother Oncol. 2013;107:213–7.
27. Lundkvist J, Ekman M, Ericsson SR, et al. Economic evaluation of proton radiation therapy in the treatment of breast cancer. Radiother Oncol. 2005;75:179–85.
28. Hall EJ, Giaccia AJ. Clinical response of normal tissues. In: Hall EJ, Giaccia AJ, editors. Radiobiology for the radiologists. 6th ed. Philadelphia: Lippincott Williams & Wilkins; 2006. p. 327–48.
29. Badiyan SN, Shah C, Arthur D, et al. Hypofractionated regional nodal irradiation for breast cancer: examining the data and potential for future studies. Radiother Oncol. 2014;110:39–44.
30. Stewart AJ, O'Farrell DA, Cormack RA, et al. Dose volume histogram analysis of normal structures associated with accelerated partial breast irradiation delivered by high dose rate brachytherapy and comparison with whole breast external beam radiotherapy fields. Radiat Oncol. 2008;3:39.
31. Wang X, Miao C, Chen Z, et al. Can involved-field irradiation replace elective nodal irradiation in chemoradiotherapy for esophageal cancer? A systematic review and meta-analysis. Onco Targets Ther. 2017;10:2087–95.
32. Fernandesa AT, Shena J, Finlay J, et al. Elective nodal irradiation (ENI) vs. involved field radiotherapy (IFRT) for locally advanced non-small cell lung cancer (NSCLC): a comparative analysis of toxicities and clinical outcomes. Radiother Oncol. 2010;95(2):178–84.
33. Topkan E, Ozdemir Y, Guler OC, et al. Comparison of involved field radiotherapy versus elective nodal irradiation in stage IIIB/C non-small-cell lung carcinoma patients treated with concurrent chemoradiotherapy: a propensity score matching study. J Oncol. 2020;2020:7083149. https://doi.org/10.1155/2020/7083149.
34. Swerdlow AJ, Higgins CD, Smith P, et al. Myocardial infarction mortality risk after treatment for Hodgkin disease: a collaborative British cohort study. J Natl Cancer Inst. 2007;99(3):206–14.
35. Ratosa I, Pantar MI. Cardiotoxicity of mediastinal radiotherapy. Rep Pract Oncol Radiother. 2019;24(6):629–43.

36. Maraldo MV, Brodin NP, Vogelius IR, et al. Risk of developing cardiovascular disease after involved node radiotherapy versus mantle field for Hodgkin lymphoma. Int J Radiat Oncol Biol Phys. 2012;83:1232–7.
37. Feng M, Moran JM, Koelling T, et al. Development and validation of a heart atlas to study cardiac exposure to radiation following treatment for breast cancer. Int J Radiat Oncol Biol Phys. 2011;79(1):10–8. https://doi.org/10.1016/j.ijrobp.2009.10.058.Epub.
38. Tan W, Liu D, Xu C, et al. Anterior myocardial territory may replace the heart as organ at risk in intensity-modulated radiotherapy for left-sided breast cancer. Int J Radiat Oncol Biol Phys. 2012;82(5):1689–97. https://doi.org/10.1016/j.ijrobp.2011.03.009.Epub.
39. Stam B, Peulen H, Guckenberger M. Dose to heart substructures is associated with non-cancer death after SBRT in stage I–II NSCLC patients. Radiother Oncol. 2017;123:370–5.
40. Hotca A, Thor M, Deasy JO, Rimner A. Dose to the cardio-pulmonary system and treatment-induced electrocardiogram abnormalities in locally advanced non-small cell lung cancer. Clin Transl Radiat Oncol. 2019;19:96–102.
41. Wong OY, Yau V, Kang J. Survival impact of cardiac dose following lung stereotactic body radiotherapy. Clin Lung Cancer. 2018;19:e241–6.
42. Vivekanandan S, Landau DB, Counsell N. The impact of cardiac radiation dosimetry on survival after radiation therapy for non-small cell lung cancer. Int J Radiat Oncol Biol Phys. 2017;99:51–60.
43. Xue J, Han C, Jackson A. Doses of radiation to the pericardium, instead of heart, are significant for survival in patients with non-small cell lung cancer. Radiother Oncol. 2019;133:213–9.
44. McWilliam A, Kennedy J, Hodgson C, Vasquez OE, Faivre-Finn C, van Herk M. Radiation dose to heart base linked with poorer survival in lung cancer patients. Eur J Cancer. 2017;85:106–13.
45. McWilliam A, Khalifa J, Vasquez OE. Novel methodology to investigate the effect of radiation dose to heart substructures on overall survival. Int J Radiat Oncol Biol Phys. 2020;108:1073–81.
46. Ma JT, Sun L, Sun X. Is pulmonary artery a dose-limiting organ at risk in non-small cell lung cancer patients treated with definitive radiotherapy? Radiat Oncol. 2017;12:34.

20 Prevention and Management of Cardiotoxicity Caused by Chemotherapeutic Agents

Nikhil Himthani

20.1 Introduction

Recent advances in cancer therapy have significantly improved cure rates in the last few decades. With prolonged survival, more cancer patients are developing cardiovascular problems, therefore it is important to be familiar with cardiovascular complications of cancer therapy. Cardiac complications have a marked effect on the quality of life and may often be life-threatening. They manifest in the form of arrhythmia, QT prolongation, pericarditis, myocarditis, cardiomyopathy, and acute coronary syndrome.

20.2 Definition of Cardiotoxicity

Cardiotoxicity caused by chemotherapy is the evidence of cardiac injury that is thought to be primarily related to cancer chemotherapy or radiotherapy as shown by any of the following indications [1]:

- Elevation of serum Troponin I or Troponin T levels above the normal range
- Transient or persistent decrease in left ventricular ejection fraction of ≥10% from pretreatment baseline or to <55% (or less than the lower limit of normal value for the laboratory)
- New myocardial fibrosis and scar as detected by the late enhancement of gadolinium in cardiac MRI
- New onset or worsening of diastolic dysfunction as detccted by echocardiography or cardiac MRI

N. Himthani (✉)
Batra Hospital, Delhi, India

K. Sood Sharma et al. (eds.), *Complications of Cancer Therapy: Best Practices in Prevention and Management*, https://doi.org/10.1007/978-981-99-0984-1_20

- Evidence of new or unstable myocardial ischemia
- Pericarditis
- Symptomatic or asymptomatic arrhythmias
- Symptomatic or asymptomatic cardiac conduction system abnormalities
- Symptomatic or asymptomatic abnormal valve structure and/or function

20.3 Etiology

The following table enlists the chemotherapeutic agents associated with cardiac toxicity (Table 20.1):

Table 20.1 Chemotherapeutic drugs associated with cardiovascular complications

Category of drugs	Chemotherapeutic agents	Incidence of cardiotoxicity	Cardiovascular complications
Anthracycline	Doxorubicin, daunorubicin, epirubicin, mitoxantrone	Depends upon cumulative dose	Myocarditis, pericarditis arrhythmia, nonischemic cardiomyopathy, CHF
Antimicrotubules	Paclitaxel Docetaxel	Asymptomatic sinus bradycardia-30% [2] Others-<5% [2]	Asymptomatic sinus bradycardia, arrhythmia, heart block, myocardial infarction, hypertension, hypotension [2, 3]
Alkylating agents	Cyclophosphamide Ifosfamide Busulfan Cisplatin	1.5–3% [4–7]	Myopericarditis, arrhythmia, thromboembolism, cardiomyopathy [4–7]
Antimetabolites	5 Fluorouracil Capecitabine	Continuous infusional-6.3% [8] Short term infusional-2.2% [8] Bolus-1.6–3% [9] Capecitabine-5.5% [8]	Myocardial infarction, angina, arrhythmia [8, 9]
Her 2 neu blockers	Trastuzumab Pertuzumab Adotrastuzumab emtansine Lapatinib	2.5–4% [10–12]	Left ventricular dysfunction, CHF [10–12]
Proteasome inhibitor	Bortezomib Carfilzomib	2% [13] 7% [14]	CHF, hypotension, myocardial infarction, venous thromboembolism [13, 14]
Tyrosine kinase inhibitor	Imatinib, Dasatinib, Nilotinib, Ponatinib, Sunitinib, Lenvatinib, Pazopanib, Sorafenib, Vandetanib	Ponatinib-7% [15] Other BCR-ABL inhibitors-2% [16, 17]	CHF arrhythmia, hypertension, QT prolongation, myocardial infarction, LV dysfunction, venous thromboembolism [15–17]

Table 20.1 (continued)

Category of drugs	Chemotherapeutic agents	Incidence of cardiotoxicity	Cardiovascular complications
Antiandrogens	Abiraterone, enzalutamide, Degarelix	3–5%	Hypertension, arrhythmia, hyperlipidemia, myocardial infarction
Antiestrogens	Tamoxifen, Letrozole	<5%	Thromboembolism, hyperlipidemia, hypertension, myocardial infarction
Miscellaneous	Bleomycin	<3% [18]	Myopericarditis
	Arsenic trioxide	40%	QT prolongation
	All-transretinoic acid	3%	Thromboembolism, myocardial infarction, hyperlipidemia

20.4 Cardiotoxicity Induced by Anthracyclines

Anthracyclines are an essential class of chemotherapeutic agents and are used in a wide range of cancers including leukaemia, lymphomas, sarcomas, and breast cancer. It may cause acute or chronic cardiotoxicity.

Acute toxicity manifests as myopericarditis, which is often self-limiting and reversible, however, it may rarely proceed to non-ischemic cardiomyopathy.

Chronic cardiotoxicity is delayed in onset and irreversible. It manifests as dilated cardiomyopathy leading to LV dysfunction and heart failure.

20.4.1 Mechanism of Cardiotoxicity Caused by Anthracyclines

- Reactive oxygen species formation and site-specific DNA damage. Oxidative stress induction can induce DNA and sarcomere damage, and mitochondrial dysfunction mediating the death of cardiomyocytes [19].
- Binds to Cardiac Top 2 enzyme to form cleavage complex leading to double strand DNA break and cell death [20].

Table 20.2 highlights the comparative lifetime cumulative intravenous anthracycline dose.

The risk of heart failure against cumulative dose of doxorubicin is elaborated in Table 20.3.

Risk factors for anthracycline-induced cardiomyopathy are:

- Prior mediastinal radiation
- Age >60 years
- Young patients <15 years

Table 20.2 Recommended Lifetime Cumulative Dose of Anthracyclines

Anthracycline	Conversion factor	Maximum recommended cumulative dose
Doxorubicin[a]	1	550 mg/m^2
Daunorubicin	1	550 mg/m^2 (no cardiotoxic risk factors)
	0.7	400 mg/m^2 (chest irradiation or risk factors
Epirubicin	1.6	900 mg/m^2
Idarubicin[b]	0.3	≥150 mg/m^2
Mitoxantrone[c]	0.25	140 mg/m^2

Source: Wolters Kluwer. LexiComp. www.wolterskluwercdi.com/lexicomp-online. Accessed November 3, 2018. (Access by paid subscription)

[a]Patient-specific cumulative dose may be decreased if the patient was previously treated with anthracycline, had previous exposure to or concurrent administration of cardiotoxic agents, or has a history of mediastinal radiation. The manufacturer only provides maximum recommended doses as 550 mg/m^2, and no guidelines provide clear recommendations for patient-specific modifications

[b]The maximum cumulative dose remains unclear. Variable reports support a maximum cumulative dose of 150 mg/m^2, but other investigators did not observe an increased risk in anthracycline-induced cardiotoxicity with cumulative doses of idarubicin up to 540 mg/m^2

[c]Maximum recommended dose for multiple sclerosis

Table 20.3 Risk of Heart Failure Associated with Doxorubicin

The cumulative dose of doxorubicin	Risk of heart failure [21] (%)
400 mg/m^2	3–5
550 mg/m^2	7–26
700 mg/m^2	18–48

- Multiple cardiovascular risk factors—smoking, hypertension, diabetes dyslipidemia, and obesity.
- Compromised cardiac function—history of myocardial infarction, moderate valvular heart disease, borderline low LVEF-50-55%.
- Concomitant cardiotoxic therapy e.g.—trastuzumab, taxanes.

Patients with anthracycline-induced cardiotoxicity present with symptoms of dyspnoea, orthopnoea, Paroxysmal Nocturnal Dyspnoea, fatigue, pedal oedema, weight loss, raised JVP, hypotension and tachycardia.

20.5 Evaluation of Anthracycline-Induced Cardiotoxicity

Even though the diagnosis of anthracycline-induced cardiotoxicity is primarily clinical, the following tests are available for evaluation:

- ECG—shows nonspecific changes such as sinus tachycardia, low voltage QRS complex, poor R wave progression, and T wave changes.
- Cardiac biomarkers:

- pro-BNP—it is a peptide released by the myocardium and its elevated values are suggestive of the risk of heart failure.
- Troponin I and highly sensitive Troponin I-identify patients at risk of developing LV dysfunction. Negative troponin I strongly predict the likelihood that LV dysfunction would not deteriorate [22].

- Serial determination of left ventricular dysfunction:
- It can be determined by MUGA (multigated acquisition scan), transthoracic echocardiogram, and cardiac MRI. Most commonly 2D echocardiogram are used to assess left ventricular dysfunction.

20.5.1 Prevention of Anthracycline Induced Cardiotoxicity

1. Monitoring and limiting total cumulative dose of anthracyclines.
2. Use of adjunctive cardioprotective agents:

   Dexrazoxane is an iron chelating agent that prevents the formation of anthracycline iron complexes and the generation of free radicals and binds to topoisomerase IIB which inhibits doxorubicin-induced DNA breakdown. It is not routinely used in clinical practice and is recommended as a cardio protectant by the American Society of Clinical Oncology (ASCO) only for patients with metastatic breast cancer who have already received more than 300 mg/m^2 of doxorubicin.
3. The use of a modified infusional regimen decreases peak dose delivery and hence decreases the incidence of cardiotoxicity. Pegylated regimens are also associated with lower cardiotoxicity due to increased overall cumulative dose.
4. Early detection strategies—the rationale for early detection of subclinical cardiotoxicity and timely intervention can decrease the risk of progression to heart failure.

20.6 Identification of Patients at Increased Risk

As described by ASCO expert consensus guidelines, the following criteria are used to identify patients at increased risk of cardiotoxicity from anthracycline use [23]:

Treatment that includes any of the following:

- High dose of anthracycline (e.g. doxorubicin ≥250 mg/m^2, epirubicin <600 mg/m^2)
- High dose of radiotherapy (RT ≥30 Gy) where the heart is in the treatment field.
- Lower dose of anthracycline (e.g., doxorubicin <250 mg/m^2, epirubicin <600 mg/m^2) in combination with lower dose RT (30 Gy), where the heart is in the radiation field.
- Treatment with lower dose of anthracyclines (e.g., doxorubicin <250 mg/m^2, epirubicin <600 mg/m^2) or trastuzumab alone and the presence of any one of the following risk factors:

  - Multiple cardiovascular risk factors (≥2 risk factors) like smoking, diabetes, dyslipidemia, and obesity, during or after completing therapy.
  - Older age (≥60 years) at cancer treatment.
  - Compromised cardiac function (e.g., history of myocardial infarction, borderline low left ventricular ejection fraction (50–55%), moderate or greater valvular heart disease at any time before or during treatment.
- Treatment with lower dose of anthracyclines (e.g., doxorubicin <250 mg/m^2, Epirubicin <600 mg/m^2) followed by trastuzumab.

Early detection strategies include measuring serum troponin levels, it detects anthracycline-induced cardiotoxicity in its earliest phase, and is a highly sensitive and specific tool for its monitoring [22].

Periodic measurement of LVEF by echocardiography should be performed during treatment and 6–12 months after completion of chemotherapy in asymptomatic patients at increased risk of cardiac dysfunction as per ASCO guidelines [23].

20.7 Management of Anthracycline Induced Cardiotoxicity

20.7.1 General Management

For all patients planning to receive anthracycline chemotherapy, cardiovascular risk factors such as hypertension, pre-existing heart failure, angina, etc. should be optimally managed before starting treatment. Patients should be counselled regarding smoking cessation, weight loss, and physical activity when possible.

Management of heart failure includes initiation of ACE (angiotensin converting enzyme) inhibitors, ARBs (angiotensin receptor blocker), beta blockers, and mineralocorticoid receptor antagonists as appropriate.

For patients who develop HF with LVEF <50%, or a decline in LVEF to under 40%, or a significant decline in EF (15 absolute percentage points) to <50%, anthracyclines are withheld, and treatment with an ACE inhibitor (or ARB) plus beta-blocker is started as per standard evidence-based guidelines for Heart Failure with reduced Ejection Fraction. For such patients, non-anthracycline-based regimens should be utilized for future treatment cycles.

20.7.2 Taxanes

20.7.2.1 Paclitaxel

Bradycardia and heart block are the most commonly described side effects of paclitaxel although these usually are asymptomatic [2]. The overall incidence of these cardiac events is low, therefore routine cardiac monitoring is not required for patients without any risk factors. Most serious cardiac side effects such as atrioventricular conduction block, ventricular tachycardia, and cardiac ischemia are seen in 5% of cases [2]. Cardiomyopathy is reported when paclitaxel is combined with doxorubicin. Heart failure may develop in up to 20% of patients when treated with paclitaxel and doxorubicin [24]. The development of heart failure may occur at cumulative doxorubicin doses that are much lower than would be expected with doxorubicin alone. Nab-paclitaxel has the same cardiac toxicity profile as the non-albumin-bound formulation.

20.7.2.2 Docetaxel

Conduction abnormalities, angina, and cardiovascular collapse have been reported in patients with Docetaxel. Like paclitaxel, docetaxel also potentiates the cardiotoxicity of anthracyclines.

20.7.2.3 Fluropyrimidines

Cardiotoxicity due to Fluropyrimidines most commonly presents as chest pain which may be nonspecific or anginal and is often associated with ECG changes; serum biomarkers of cardiac injury may or may not be elevated. Patients may also present with palpitations, dyspnea, supraventricular arrhythmias such as atrial fibrillation and hypotension. In rare cases, myocardial infarction, ventricular fibrillation, myocarditis, and sudden death have been reported. Mortality rates range from 2 to 13% [8, 9]. Cardiotoxicity in these patients is due to vascular spasm in reaction to the drug and its metabolites and occurs most commonly during the first cycle of administration.

20.7.2.4 Fluorouracil

The reported incidence of 5FU-related cardiotoxicity ranges from 1 to 19% [8, 9]. Risk factors for its increased incidence include the presence of underlying CAD (15% vs 1.5%), old age, use of concurrent radiation therapy or anthracyclines method of 5FU administration being 2–18% for continuous infusion and 1.6–3% for bolus infusion [8, 9].

20.7.2.5 Capecitabine

The incidence of cardiac toxicity of capecitabine is 3–9% [8, 9].

20.7.3 Prevention of Fluropyrimidines Induced Cardiotoxicity

There are no known prophylactic regimens to avert cardiotoxicity in these patients.

20.7.4 Management of Fluropyrimidines Induced Cardiotoxicity

Discontinue 5FU infusion, administer antianginal treatment-nitrates, calcium channel blockers. Cardiotoxicity appears to be completely reversible after cessation of therapy.

Rechallenge should be avoided as recurrence rates are as high as 90%. If a rechallenge is attempted, prophylactic aspirin, calcium channel blockers, and long-acting nitrates should be considered at least 72 h prior.

20.7.5 Alkylating Agents

20.7.5.1 Cyclophosphamide

Classical cardiac toxicity is acute myopericarditis which is associated with high dose protocols, develops early, and is not related to cumulative dose. Acute cardiotoxicity is rare and is reversible and self-limiting.

20.7.5.2 Ifosfamide

It has been associated with arrhythmias, ST-T changes, and heart failure in a dose-related manner. These cardiac complications are generally reversible with medical management.

20.7.6 Her-2 Target Agents

20.7.6.1 Trastuzumab

Trastuzumab-related cardiotoxicity is most often manifested by an asymptomatic decrease in LVEF and less often by clinical heart failure. It is not related to cumulative dose and is often reversible with treatment discontinuation and rechallenge is usually tolerated well after recovery [10–12]. Risk factors for a higher likelihood of trastuzumab-related cardiotoxicity are age >50 years, previous or concurrent anthracycline use, pre-existing cardiac dysfunction, and high BMI. Assessment of LVEF should be done after completion of anthracycline, prior to initiation of trastuzumab. In the adjuvant setting cardiac function is assessed every 3 months. Patients with normal baseline LVEF and no signs of heart failure may proceed to trastuzumab chemotherapy.

20.7.7 Prevention

Concurrent extended administration of anthracycline and trastuzumab should be avoided due to an increased risk of cardiotoxicity. Based upon NOAH trial trastuzumab concurrent with limited anthracycline (≤3 cycles or ≤180 mg/m^2 of doxorubicin is a potentially safe option) [25].

20.8 Dose Adjustment for Cardiotoxicity

As per the NSABP B-31 and NCCTG N9831 trial, trastuzumab dose modification is done [26].

If the LVEF declines by more than >15% from baseline or 10–15% from baseline to below the lower limit of normal, trastuzumab is withheld for 4 weeks at which time the LVEF is reassessed. If the LVEF remains below these levels trastuzumab should be discontinued. If the patient has symptomatic heart failure while receiving trastuzumab, it should be discontinued. Symptomatic heart failure is defined by (a) the presence of symptoms (dyspnoea, orthopnoea, pedal edema), (b) objective findings (elevated JVP, sinus tachycardia, S3 gallop, crackles, etc.) (c) LVEF decline or chest X-ray findings of pulmonary oedema.

For treatment, standard medical therapy for heart failure including ACE inhibitors and B blockers should be initiated.

20.8.1 Lapatinib

Unlike trastuzumab, lapatinib has a more favorable cardiac safety profile even among patients who have previously received anthracycline. Normal LVEF should be confirmed prior to starting treatment with lapatinib. Discontinuation of lapatinib is recommended for a drop in LVEF to less than 50% or patients who develop clinical heart failure. Dose reduction is recommended if LVEF returns to normal.

20.8.2 Pertuzumab

Combined therapy with pertuzumab and trastuzumab was not associated with significantly worse cardiotoxicity as seen in CLEOPATRA trial [10–12].

20.8.3 Adotrastuzumab Emtansine

Incidence of cardiac toxicity is around 3–4% mostly involving asymptomatic LVEF drop [10–12].

20.9 Conclusion

Adequate preventive measures and timely management of cardiotoxicity secondary to chemotherapeutic agents can improve the quality of life and prevent cardiovascular morbidity in cancer patients.

References

1. Niederhuber JE, Armitage JO, Doroshow JH, Kastan MB, Tepper JE. Abeloff's clinical oncology E-book. Elsevier Health Sciences; 2013.
2. Rowinsky EK, McGuire WP, Guarnieri T, et al. Cardiac disturbances during the administration of taxol. J Clin Oncol. 1991;9:1704–12.

3. Mandel EM, Lewinski U, Djaldetti M. Vincristine-induced myocardial infarction. Cancer. 1975;36:1979–82.
4. Ishida S, Doki N, Shingai N, et al. The clinical features of fatal cyclophosphamide-induced cardiotoxicity in a conditioning regimen for allogeneic hematopoietic stem cell transplantation (Allo-HSCT). Ann Hematol. 2016;95:1145–50.
5. Quezado ZM, Wilson WH, Cunnion RE, et al. High-dose ifosfamide is associated with severe, reversible cardiac dysfunction. Ann Intern Med. 1993;118:31–6.
6. Tomirotti M, Riundi R, Pulici S, et al. Ischemic cardiopathy from *cis*-diamminedichloroplatinum (CDDP). Tumori. 1984;70:235–6.
7. Perry MC. Effects of chemotherapy on the heart. In: Kapoor AS, editor. Cancer and the heart. New York: Springer; 1986. p. 223.
8. Kosmas C, Kallistratos MS, Kopterides P, et al. Cardiotoxicity of fluoropyrimidines in different schedules of administration: a prospective study. J Cancer Res Clin Oncol. 2008;134:75–82.
9. Anand AJ. Fluorouracil cardiotoxicity. Ann Pharmacother. 1994;28:374–8.
10. Dang C, Guo H, Najita J, et al. Cardiac outcomes of patients receiving adjuvant weekly paclitaxel and trastuzumab for node-negative, ERBB2-positive breast cancer. JAMA Oncol. 2016;2:29.
11. Swain SM, Ewer MS, Cortés J, et al. Cardiac tolerability of pertuzumab plus trastuzumab plus docetaxel in patients with HER2-positive metastatic breast cancer in CLEOPATRA: a randomized, double-blind, placebo-controlled phase III study. Oncologist. 2013;18:257–64.
12. Pondé N, Ameye L, Lambertini M, et al. Trastuzumab emtansine (T-DM1)-associated cardiotoxicity: pooled analysis in advanced HER2-positive breast cancer. Eur J Cancer. 2020;126:65–73.
13. Richardson PG, Sonneveld P, Schuster MW, et al. Bortezomib or high-dose dexamethasone for relapsed multiple myeloma. N Engl J Med. 2005;352:2487–98.
14. Carfilzomib for injection. United States Prescribing Information. US National Library of Medicine. http://www.accessdata.fda.gov/drugsatfda_docs/label/2012/202714lbl.pdf?et_cid=29661884&et_rid=463638624&linkid=http%3a%2f%2fwww.accessdata.fda.gov%2fdrugsatfda_docs%2flabel%2f2012%2f202714lbl.pdf.
15. Cortes JE, Kim DW, Pinilla-Ibarz J, et al. A phase 2 trial of ponatinib in Philadelphia chromosome-positive leukemias. N Engl J Med. 2013;369:1783–96.
16. Atallah E, Durand JB, Kantarjian H, Cortes J. Congestive heart failure is a rare event in patients receiving imatinib therapy. Blood. 2007;110:1233–7.
17. Abu Rmilah AA, Lin G, Begna KH, et al. Risk of QTc prolongation among cancer patients treated with tyrosine kinase inhibitors. Int J Cancer. 2020;147:3160–7.
18. Durkin WJ, Pugh RP, Solomon J, et al. Treatment of advanced lymphomas with bleomycin (NSC-125066). Oncology. 1976;33:140–5.
19. Adderley SR, Fitzgerald DJ. Oxidative damage of cardiomyocytes is limited by extracellular regulated kinases 1/2-mediated induction of cyclooxygenase-2. J Biol Chem. 1999;274:5038–46.
20. Lyu YL, Kerrigan JE, Lin CP, et al. Topoisomerase IIbeta mediated DNA double-strand breaks: implications in doxorubicin cardiotoxicity and prevention by dexrazoxane. Cancer Res. 2007;67:8839–46.
21. Von Hoff DD, Layard MW, Basa P, Davis HL Jr, Von Hoff AL, Rozencweig M, Muggia FM. Risk factors for doxorubicin-induced congestive heart failure. Ann Intern Med. 1979;91(5):710–7. https://doi.org/10.7326/0003-4819-91-5-710.
22. Cardinale D, Sandri MT, Colombo A, et al. Prognostic value of troponin I in cardiac risk stratification of cancer patients undergoing high-dose chemotherapy. Circulation. 2004;109:2749–54.
23. Armenian SH, Lacchetti C, Barac A, et al. Prevention and monitoring of cardiac dysfunction in survivors of adult cancers: American Society of Clinical Oncology clinical practice guideline. J Clin Oncol. 2017;35:893–911.
24. Gianni L, Munzone E, Capri G, et al. Paclitaxel by 3-hour infusion in combination with bolus doxorubicin in women with untreated metastatic breast cancer: high antitumor efficacy and cardiac effects in a dose-finding and sequence-finding study. J Clin Oncol. 1995;13:2688–99.

25. Gianni L, Eiermann W, Semiglazov V, et al. Neoadjuvant chemotherapy with trastuzumab followed by adjuvant trastuzumab versus neoadjuvant chemotherapy alone, in patients with HER2-positive locally advanced breast cancer (the NOAH trial): a randomised controlled superiority trial with a parallel HER2-negative cohort. Lancet. 2010;375:377–84.
26. Romond EH, Perez EA, Bryant J, et al. Trastuzumab plus adjuvant chemotherapy for operable HER2-positive breast cancer. N Engl J Med. 2005;353:1673–84.

Risk Identification and Treatment of Hormone Therapy Related Adverse Events in Patients of Carcinoma Breast

21

Deni Gupta and Sachin Sekhar Biswal

21.1 Introduction

Care for patients with breast cancer tends toward more selective interventions to minimize acute and late toxicity without compromising efficacy. Recent improvements in the survival of hormone-responsive breast cancer are strongly associated with therapeutic advances, particularly with the advancement of adjuvant endocrine therapy. Despite the fact that metastatic breast cancer would not be cured, the development of more efficient systemic medicines, such as endocrine therapy (ET) for the treatment of hormone-sensitive illness, has resulted in appreciable survival gains. Initial adjuvant endocrine therapy is advised to be administered for a minimum of 5 years, while some individuals have benefited from further 3–5 years of adjuvant therapy. Adverse events (AEs) that occur while undergoing treatment must be handled because they are more than just a temporary inconvenience for patients with such a lengthy course of treatment. Endocrine therapy is nevertheless associated with side effects that affect quality of life, social interaction, and treatment compliance.

D. Gupta (✉)
Dharamshila Narayana Hospital, (DNSH), Delhi, India
e-mail: deni.gupta.dr@narayanahealth.org

S. S. Biswal
Department of Medical Oncology, DNSH, Delhi, India

K. Sood Sharma et al. (eds.), *Complications of Cancer Therapy: Best Practices in Prevention and Management*, https://doi.org/10.1007/978-981-99-0984-1_21

21.2 Agents

There are several types of ETs. These can be characterized as strategies to deplete estrogen and strategies to directly target the estrogen receptor (ER). Strategies to deplete estrogen consists of surgical oophorectomy and luteinizing hormone-releasing hormone agonists and antagonists. In post-menopausal women, where the main source of estrogen is by peripheral conversion by aromatase, AIs (aromatase inhibitors) are the mainstay of treatment. Anastrozole and letrozole, two of these, are azoles, and exemestane is a 17-hydroxy steroid. Clinical activity, side effects, and toxicity of these three aromatase inhibitors have been shown to be almost equivalent in prospective randomised clinical trials conducted in the adjuvant and metastatic settings.

Targeting the ERs is mainly by selective modulation or receptor downregulation. The use of selective ER modulators such as tamoxifen or raloxifene, or selective ER down-regulators. Fulvestrant is the only available agent that down-regulates ER.

Estrogen depletion	Surgical oophorectomy
	LHRH agonist: leuprolide, goserelin
	AIs: anastrozole, letrozole and exemestane
ER modulation	SERMs: tamoxifen, raloxifene
	SERDs: fulvestrant

21.3 Tamoxifen, AIs and SERD

Therapies that result in oestrogen deprivation have the potential to cause widespread toxicity, including effects on the reproductive system, including vaginal and urothelial irritation, dryness and atrophy; on the musculoskeletal system, including arthralgia, osteopenia, osteoporosis, and bone fractures; on the cardiovascular system, including hypercholesterolemia, angina, myocardial and cerebrovascular ischemia; and on the central nervous system including fatigue, headache to depression and cognitive dysfunction [1]. Since most of the symptoms overlap with menopausal symptoms and since most of the breast cancer patients are peri-menopausal or post-menopausal, the symptom burden may be quite high.

Patients on AIs have a higher incidence of vaginal dryness and dyspareunia and typically patients on tamoxifen experience more vaginal bleeding and vaginal discharge [2]. Patients on AIs have a higher incidence of musculoskeletal disorders, which typically include arthralgia and increase of osteoporosis and fractures. Tamoxifen leads to an increase of endometrial cancer and venous thromboembolic events [3].

Extension of ET up to 10 years, implies a prolonged duration of side effects, such as vasomotor, gynaecological and musculoskeletal symptoms and an increased prevalence of the rare but serious side effects reported. For example, in the MA.17R trial, the fracture incidence was significantly higher in the extended 10 years letrozole arm when compared with 5 years arm (14% vs. 9%, respectively) [4]. Similarly, in the ATLAS trial, the risk of pulmonary embolism and endometrial cancer were higher in the extended 10 years of treatment with tamoxifen arm vs. 5 years of treatment (0.9% vs. 0.5% and 3.1% vs. 1.6%respectively) [5]. The same trend was observed in the aTTom trial [6].

Addition of ovarian function suppression (OFS) with LHRH agonist is also associated with an increase of symptoms. For example, in the SOFT trial, patients undergoing OFS + tamoxifen vs. patients on tamoxifen monotherapy experienced more vasomotor symptoms (hot flashes, night sweats) and vulvo-vaginal symptoms when compared with those only treated with tamoxifen (any grade: hot flashes, 93.4% vs. 79.8%; sweating, 61.8% vs. 48.3%; vaginal dryness, 49.8% vs. 41.8%; dyspareunia 26.1% vs. 23.7% respectively) [7].

Side effects of ET can have an impact on patients' quality of life, social functions (e.g., ability to return to work, partner relationship). They also often lead to poor adherence to ET, which can impact on outcomes. In the ATLAS trial, 2 years after study entry, only 84% of patients allocated to continue treatment (tamoxifen up to 10 years) were still on treatment. Some studies show discontinuation rates of up to 25% before completion of the first year of adjuvant therapy [8].

Fulvestrant is the only drug in the SERD (Selective Estrogen Receptor Down regulator) approved in advanced breast cancer to be used either as monotherapy or in combination. The adverse event profile of Fulvestrant is similar to AIs. As it has only parenteral administration, it is associated with significant local site reactions (up to 10%).

21.4 Management of Adverse Events

The management of the adverse events associated with ETs need anticipation and prompt management. The treatment should be individualized to improve adherence and to reduce discontinuation rates. The symptoms and management strategies are discussed in a systematic manner in the following text.

- **Vasomotor symptoms**:

  A. **Pharmacologic management**:

    1. **Hormonal strategies**: Theoretically, the most effective therapy to treat vasomotor symptom seems to be estrogen replacement, nevertheless it is contraindicated among BC survivors given concerns of its negative impact on BC recurrence. The women health initiative (WHI) trial randomized 16,608 postmenopausal women, aged 50–79 years, to receive combined conjugated equine estrogen plus medroxyprogesterone acetate or placebo for 5 years. This trial revealed that the conjugated oestrogen and progestin medication compared to placebo was associated with an increase in the overall number of BC (hazard ratio 1.24), as well as invasive BC (hazard ratio 1.24) [9].

       The evidence regarding the use of progestogens in breast cancer (BC) survivors is mixed. Evidence suggests that tibolone, a selective tissue estrogenic activity regulator, is more effective than placebo in reducing vasomotor symptoms [10]. Nevertheless, there are safety concerns regarding its use among breast cancer survivors given the concern of increase risk of breast cancer recurrence with its use.

2. **Non-hormonal strategies**:
   (a) **Anti-depressants (SSRIs/SNRIs)**: The efficacy of serotonin–norepinephrine reuptake inhibitor, venlafaxine has been demonstrated in several trials. In one trial 229 participants were assigned to placebo or venlafaxine at 3 different dosages (37.5 mg daily, 75 mg daily, 150 mg daily). After 4 weeks of treatment, median hot flash scores decreased by 27%, 37% and 61% respectively [11].

   Several other Selective Serotonin reuptake inhibitors (SSRIs) and SNRIs have been tested and found effective in reducing the vasomotor symptoms. The efficacy of different SSRI (citalopram, escitalopram, fluoxetine, paroxetine, sertraline) was evaluated in a systematic review of 11 randomized controlled trials, enrolling 2069 healthy menopausal and post-menopausal women, treated with a SSRI versus placebo or another SSRI. The endpoint was the improvement of vasomotor symptoms (daily hot flash frequency or improvement in vasomotor scores). Compared with placebo, SSRIs were associated with a statistically significant decrease in hot flash frequency without significantly higher side effects [12]. SSRIs are to be used with caution in patients receiving Tamoxifen as SSRIs are potent inhibitors of the cytochrome P450 (CYP2D6).

   (b) **Anticonvulsants**: Gabapentin and pregabalin were both tested for the treatment of hot flashes demonstrating efficacy.

   (c) **Clonidine**: Clonidine, a centrally active α-adrenergic agonist antihypertensive, has been tested against vasomotor symptoms with inconsistent results. In a meta-analysis of 10 trials comparing clonidine with placebo, only 4 trials reported reduced frequency of hot flashes with clonidine compared with placebo [13].

   (d) **Other agents**: Agents such as vitamin E, omega 3, black cohosh, magnesium, soy products, adenosyl-methionine, flaxseed, aprepitant were tested but overall do not seem to be effective in the treatment of hot flashes.

B. **Non-pharmacologic management**:
   1. **Cognitive Behavioural Therapy (CBT)**: CBT has been shown to be significantly improving the symptoms. A randomized controlled trial randomly assigned 96 participants to receive usual care or usual care plus CBT. In this trial, CBT consisted of 90 min session a week for 6 weeks of: psycho-education, paced breathing, cognitive and behavioural strategies to manage hot flashes and night sweats. Two assessments were planned at 9 and 26 weeks after randomization, and at both time points CBT significantly reduced symptoms' rating compared with usual care (mean difference −1.67, $P < 0.0001$, −1.76, $P < 0.0001$; respectively) [14].

2. **Weight control**: Recommending women to lose weight to reduce hot flashes may be useful, as suggested by a cross-sectional study of 300 BC patients receiving AIs therapy. In this trial, weight gain was independently associated with hot flashes occurrence (odds ratio 2.1, 95% CI 1.1–4.4) and hot flash severity (OR 2.6, 95% CI 1.3–5.0) [15].
3. **Physical Activity**: Physical activity seem to be ineffective to treat vasomotor symptoms, although it may be associated with other benefits, such as improvement of sleep [16].
4. **Acupuncture**: Recently, Acupuncture has been shown to be an effective alternative.

- **Musculoskeletal symptoms**:

  A. **Pharmacologic management**:

  1. **Switching of AI**: In clinical practice is common to switch from an AI to another, trying to reduce the intensity of the symptoms and maintain adherence to treatment. This attitude has been evaluated in clinical trials that reported variable persistence rates of symptoms after the switch. One study that looked at this question was the ATOLL trial, in which patients who had discontinued anastrozole due to musculoskeletal symptoms, after 1 month of wash-out, were assigned to letrozole for 6 months. At the end of the study, 71.5% of patients were still on letrozole while 28.5% discontinued treatment due to joint symptoms. Nevertheless, a substantial proportion of patients continued to experience musculoskeletal symptoms including 73.9% of patients complaining of arthralgia, 21.0% Accepted Manuscript myalgia, 15.9% arthritis, 14.0% tendinitis, 12.7% polyalgic syndrome, after the sixth month of letrozole [17].
  2. **Duloxetine**: In the recently presented SWOG S1202 trial, 299 patients were randomized to duloxetine or placebo for 12 weeks. After 12 the treatment, improvements in the duloxetine arm in terms of general pain, joint pain, pain interference, knee/hip/hand arthritis scales, stiffness and quality of life were documented [18].
  3. **Vitamin D**: There are mixed results regarding the efficacy of vitamin D supplementation to treat musculoskeletal symptoms associated with ET.
  4. **Non-steroidal anti-inflammatory drugs (NSAIDs)**: NSAIDs are commonly used as first line strategy to treat musculoskeletal symptoms, although little evidence of their efficacy exists, therefore their beneficial pain relief effect should be balanced with their adverse effects that include gastrointestinal, renal and cardiovascular effects.
  5. **Omega-3 fatty acids**: The SWOG S0927 trial randomized 262 patients to receive omega-3 fatty acids 3.3 g or placebo daily for 24 weeks, finding a similar improvement in AIs arthralgia with both strategies [19].

  B. **Non-pharmacologic management**:

  1. **Physical activity**: It has been shown that physical activity reduces the musculo-skeletal pain symptoms significantly. The HOPE trial randomly allocated 121 patients to exercise (150 min per week of aerobic exercise and supervised strength training twice per week) or usual care. At

12 months, there was a 29% reduction in worst joint pain scores among women assigned to exercise vs. a 3% increment among the women assigned to usual care ($P < 0.0010$). In addition, at 12 months, in the experimental group, pain severity, pain interference and other codified pain scores, decreased significantly while increased among the usual care group (all $P < 0.0010$) [20].
2. **Acupuncture**: It has shown improvement in pain scores, in pain severity and pain interference with activities of daily living.

- **Vulvo-vaginal symptoms**:
  A. **Pharmacologic management**:
    1. **Hormonal approaches**: Since AIs act by lowering estrogen levels and tamoxifen acts by selectively modulating the estrogen receptor, the safety concerns surrounding the use of local HRT are higher among patients treated with AIs, being generally accepted that among women treated with tamoxifen can use vaginal hormonal therapy. As an example, in a recent randomized controlled trial of 76 patients receiving AIs treated with intravaginal testosterone cream or an estradiol-releasing vaginal ring, there was no evidence that estradiol releasing vaginal ring was associated with higher rates of estradiol elevation compared with testosterone.
    2. Non-hormonal approaches:
      (a) **Moisturizers and lubricants**: Non-hormonal options of moisturizers and lubricants are safe although less effective. Moisturizers should be administrated 2 or more times a week at bedtime; lubricants should be used immediately before sexual activity. Typically, recommended lubricants are either water-based or silicone-based. Petroleum or oil-based lubricants should be avoided since they increase the risk of vaginal infection and can damage latex condoms.
      (b) **Lidocaine**: A prospective study suggested that use of lidocaine was associated with 90% of patients reporting comfortable penetration (37/41) and 85% (17/20) of abstainers from intercourse being able to resumed comfortable intercourse [21].
      (c) **Ospemifene**: Ospemifene is a SERM approved to treat dyspareunia; nevertheless, its safety and efficacy in BC survivors is yet to be established [22].

  B. **Non-pharmacologic management**:
  For situations associated with atrophy, stenosis, pelvic weakness, recurring to a specialized clinic and exploring options as physical therapy should be considered. If associated there are reports of decreased libido, treatment options include counselling or even inclusion of an SNRI.

- **Bone health and endocrine therapy**:
  A. **Pharmacologic management**:
  Selection of women based on fracture risk, as indicated by a combination of bone mineral density (BMD) (osteoporosis i.e., T-Score −2.5 or worse)

and clinical risk factors, or with higher risk of fracture as measured by clinical assessment tools (e.g., FRAX tool) is therefore necessary since those women who have the highest risk of fracture are also the ones who are most likely to benefit from pharmacological therapy.

1. **Bisphosphonates**: Bisphosphonates are the favoured initial therapy because of their efficacy, long term data and cost. In several randomized trials, bisphosphonates prevented or reduced bone loss in women receiving AIs. In a meta-analysis of six trials evaluating bisphosphonates in women with breast cancer receiving AIs, bisphosphonates did not significantly decrease the number of fractures compared with placebo or no treatment (odds ratio [OR] 0.79, 95% CI 0.53–1.17) [23]. None of the trials were designed or powered to assess fractures as a primary outcome. Either oral or intravenous (IV) bisphosphonates are acceptable options, depending upon patient preference, availability of drugs, and potential cost issues. Risedronate and Alendronate are preferred oral bisphosphonates and among IV agents Zoledronate and Pamidronate are preferred agents.
2. **Denosumab**: Denosumab is a humanized monoclonal antibody against receptor activator of nuclear factor kappa B ligand (RANKL) that reduces osteoclastogenesis. The dose of denosumab is 60 mg administered as a subcutaneous injection (upper arm, thigh, or abdomen) once every 6 months. It is not renally excreted, and therefore, dose adjustments for chronic kidney disease are not necessary.

B. **Non-pharmacologic management**:

1. **Lifestyle interventions**: weight reduction, regular physical activity, stopping smoking and reducing alcohol intake have positive impact on bone health.
2. **Vitamin D and calcium**: Adequate calcium and vitamin D intake can result in positive calcium balance and a reduction in the rate of loss of bone. Most of the guidelines for cancer treatment-induced bone loss include supplementation with calcium and vitamin D. Recommended doses are 1200 mg of elemental calcium (total diet plus supplement) and 800 international units of vitamin D daily for women receiving aromatase inhibitors (AIs) [24].

- **Cardiovascular and metabolic adverse events**:

  Numerous studies have shown that using tamoxifen is linked to a higher frequency of venous thromboembolic events. When compared to women not taking tamoxifen, the relative risks (RRs) of VTE are increased by two to three times. The RR decreases with time after initiation of therapy, with the first 2 years being the most hazardous [25]. The data on arterial ischemic events is conflicting. Any increased risk of stroke may be counterbalanced by favourable effects on ischemic heart disease. This was shown in the most recent overview analysis of randomized trials of adjuvant tamoxifen from the Early Breast Cancer Trialists' Collaborative Group (EBCTCG). The nonsignificant excess of stroke deaths (three extra per 1000 women during the first 15 years) in women treated with tamoxifen was exactly balanced by a nonsignificant reduction in cardiac deaths (three fewer per 1000 women during the first 15 years). Thus, there was little net effect of tamoxifen on overall vascular mortality [26]. Risk factors for tamoxifen-induced VTE include prior surgery, fracture, obesity, and immobilization. Atherosclerotic risk factors, including older age, elevated blood pressure, high total cholesterol, smoking, and a family history of coronary heart disease (CHD), also have been shown to increase the risk of VTE among tamoxifen users [27]. In addition, there is evidence that patients receiving tamoxifen who harbour a heterozygous Factor V Leiden mutation have a nearly fivefold risk of thromboembolism relative to those taking tamoxifen who do not have a mutation [28].

It is important to educate patients regarding the importance of modifying risk factors for deep vein thrombosis (DVT)/PE, including obesity, cigarette smoking, and hypertension. It is also important to educate patients about venous thromboembolic disease so that they can seek medical evaluation promptly if they develop signs and symptoms concerning for DVT/PE. For patients with a family history of clots, a workup prior to initiating tamoxifen should be undertaken, to exclude known genetic causes of hypercoagulability. If a genetic cause of hypercoagulability is found, tamoxifen should not be used. Additionally, for those with a personal history of DVT, tamoxifen should be avoided.

21.5 Conclusion

Endocrine manipulations are generally well tolerated, although several types of side effects should be taken into account when evaluating the risk–benefit ratio of given alternatives, as well as considering the risk of relapse, endocrine responsiveness of the disease, and expectations of the patient. For endocrine responsive early breast cancer, endocrine therapy has greatly contributed to the improved survival in early breast cancer. Nevertheless, endocrine therapy is also associated with substantial toxicity that can impact overall quality of life, social function and adherence to treatment. Implementation of strategies to mitigate endocrine treatments' side effects is of significant importance; assessment of symptoms and patients' education and counselling is mandatory to significantly improve care of early breast cancer survivors.

References

1. Clemons M, Goss P. Estrogen and the risk of breast cancer. N Engl J Med. 2001;344(4):276–85.
2. Cuzick J, Sestak I, Baum M, Buzdar A, Howell A, Dowsett M, et al. Effect of anastrozole and tamoxifen as adjuvant treatment for early-stage breast cancer: 10-year analysis of the ATAC trial. Lancet Oncol. 2010;11(12):1135–41.
3. Ganz PA, Petersen L, Bower JE, Crespi CM. Impact of adjuvant endocrine therapy on quality of life and symptoms: observational data over 12 months from the mind-body study. JCO. 2016;34(8):816–24.

4. Goss PE, Ingle JN, Pritchard KI, Robert NJ, Muss H, Gralow J, et al. Extending aromatase-inhibitor adjuvant therapy to 10 years. N Engl J Med. 2016;375(3):209–19.
5. Davies C, Pan H, Godwin J, Gray R, Arriagada R, Raina V, et al. Long-term effects of continuing adjuvant tamoxifen to 10 years versus stopping at 5 years after diagnosis of oestrogen receptor-positive breast cancer: ATLAS, a randomised trial. Lancet. 2013;381(9869):805–16.
6. Gray RG, Rea D, Handley K, Bowden SJ, Perry P, Earl HM, et al. aTTom: long-term effects of continuing adjuvant tamoxifen to 10 years versus stopping at 5 years in 6953 women with early breast cancer. JCO. 2013;31(18_suppl):5.
7. Ribi K, Luo W, Bernhard J, Francis PA, Burstein HJ, Ciruelos E, et al. Adjuvant tamoxifen plus ovarian function suppression versus tamoxifen alone in premenopausal women with early breast cancer: patient-reported outcomes in the suppression of ovarian function trial. J Clin Oncol. 2016;34(14):1601–10.
8. Aiello Bowles EJ, Boudreau DM, Chubak J, Yu O, Fujii M, Chestnut J, et al. Patient-reported discontinuation of endocrine therapy and related adverse effects among women with early-stage breast cancer. JOP. 2012;8(6):e149–57.
9. Chlebowski RT, Hendrix SL, Langer RD, Stefanick ML, Gass M, Lane D, et al. Influence of estrogen plus progestin on breast cancer and mammography in healthy postmenopausal women: the women's health initiative randomized trial. JAMA. 2003;289(24):3243–53.
10. Formoso G, Perrone E, Maltoni S, Balduzzi S, Wilkinson J, Basevi V, et al. Short-term and long-term effects of tibolone in postmenopausal women. Cochrane Database Syst Rev. 2016;10:CD008536.
11. Loprinzi CL, Kugler JW, Sloan JA, Mailliard JA, LaVasseur BI, Barton DL, et al. Venlafaxine in management of hot flashes in survivors of breast cancer: a randomised controlled trial. Lancet. 2000;356(9247):2059–63.
12. Shams T, Firwana B, Habib F, Alshahrani A, AlNouh B, Murad MH, et al. SSRIs for hot flashes: a systematic review and meta-analysis of randomized trials. J Gen Intern Med. 2014;29(1):204–13.
13. Nelson HD, Vesco KK, Haney E, Fu R, Nedrow A, Miller J, et al. Nonhormonal therapies for menopausal hot flashes: systematic review and meta-analysis. JAMA. 2006;295(17):2057.
14. Mann E, Smith MJ, Hellier J, Balabanovic JA, Hamed H, Grunfeld EA, et al. Cognitive behavioural treatment for women who have menopausal symptoms after breast cancer treatment (MENOS 1): a randomised controlled trial. Lancet Oncol. 2012;13(3):309–18.
15. Su HI, Sammel MD, Springer E, Freeman EW, DeMichele A, Mao JJ. Weight gain is associated with increased risk of hot flashes in breast cancer survivors on aromatase inhibitors. Breast Cancer Res Treat. 2010;124(1):205–11.
16. Daley A, Stokes-Lampard H, Thomas A, MacArthur C, Cochrane Collaboration. Exercise for vasomotor menopausal symptoms. Cochrane Database Syst Rev. 2014;2014(11):CD006108.
17. Briot K, Tubiana-Hulin M, Bastit L, Kloos I, Roux C. Effect of a switch of aromatase inhibitors on musculoskeletal symptoms in postmenopausal women with hormone receptor-positive breast cancer: the ATOLL (articular tolerance of letrozole) study. Breast Cancer Res Treat. 2010;120(1):127–34.
18. Henry N, Unger J, Schott A, Fehrenbacher L, Flynn P, Prow D, et al. Abstract S5-06: randomized, placebo-controlled trial of duloxetine for aromatase inhibitor (AI)—associated musculoskeletal symptoms (AIMSS) in early-stage breast cancer (SWOG S1202). Cancer Res. 2017;77(4 Supplement):S5–06.
19. Hershman DL, Unger JM, Crew KD, Awad D, Dakhil SR, Gralow J, et al. Randomized multicentre placebo-controlled trial of omega-3 fatty acids for the control of aromatase inhibitor induced musculoskeletal pain: SWOG S0927. J Clin Oncol. 2015;33(17):1910–7.
20. Irwin ML, Cartmel B, Gross CP, Ercolano E, Li F, Yao X, et al. Randomized exercise trial of aromatase inhibitor–induced arthralgia in breast cancer survivors. J Clin Oncol. 2015;33(10):1104–11.
21. Goetsch MF, Lim JY, Caughey AB. A practical solution for dyspareunia in breast cancer survivors: a randomized controlled trial. J Clin Oncol. 2015;33(30):3394–400.

22. Simon JA, Lin VH, Radovich C, Bachmann GA, Ospemifene Study Group. One-year long-term safety extension study of ospemifene for the treatment of vulvar and vaginal atrophy in postmenopausal women with a uterus. Menopause N Y N. 2013;20(4):418–27.
23. Valachis A, Polyzos NP, Georgoulias V, Mavroudis D, Mauri D. Lack of evidence for fracture prevention in early breast cancer bisphosphonate trials: a meta-analysis. Gynecol Oncol. 2010;117(1):139–45.
24. Gralow JR, Biermann JS, Farooki A, Fornier MN, Gagel RF, Kumar R, et al. NCCN task force report: bone health in cancer care. J Natl Compr Cancer Netw. 2013;11(Suppl 3):S1–50.
25. Hernandez RK, Sørensen HT, Pedersen L, Jacobsen J, Lash TL. Tamoxifen treatment and risk of deep venous thrombosis and pulmonary embolism: a Danish population-based cohort study. Cancer. 2009;115(19):4442–9.
26. Davies C, Godwin J, Gray R, Clarke M, Cutter D, Darby S, et al. Relevance of breast cancer hormone receptors and other factors to the efficacy of adjuvant tamoxifen: patient-level meta-analysis of randomised trials. Lancet. 2011;378(9793):771–84.
27. Decensi A, Maisonneuve P, Rotmensz N, Bettega D, Costa A, Sacchini V, et al. Effect of tamoxifen on venous thromboembolic events in a breast cancer prevention trial. Circulation. 2005;111(5):650–6.
28. Garber JE, Halabi S, Tolaney SM, Kaplan E, Archer L, Atkins JN, et al. Factor V Leiden mutation and thromboembolism risk in women receiving adjuvant tamoxifen for breast cancer. J Natl Cancer Inst. 2010;102(13):942–9.

Prevention and Management of Complications of Androgen Deprivation Therapy for Treatment of Cancers of Prostate

22

Deni Gupta and Ashutosh

22.1 Introduction

Prostate cancer is one of the leading causes of cancer and cancer related death among men both worldwide and in India [1]. Prostate gland is heavily dependent on androgens for growth, differentiation, and maintenance of homeostasis [2]. This forms the basis of Androgen Deprivation Therapy (ADT) in prostate cancer. ADT is indicated in metastatic prostate cancer, in intermediate or high-risk localized prostate cancer or in cases of biochemical recurrence in disseminated disease. Androgen deprivation can be offered to patients in the form of surgical or medical castration. With trials showing survival benefit of adding ADT to other modalities of treatment, it has become very important to recognize and manage complications of ADT to improve compliance and outcome of the therapy.

22.2 Androgen Deprivation Therapy

There are several modalities to render patient of prostate cancer androgen deprived. However, these modalities work either by depleting the level of testosterone or by androgen receptor blockade. Depletion of male androgen, most importantly testosterone and dihydro testosterone can be achieved surgically or by medical castration. In hormone sensitive prostate cancer ADT can be given surgically by bilateral orchiectomy or medically by GnRH analogues, GnRH antagonists or first-generation antiandrogens. Patient who become castrate resistant administration of ADT can be

D. Gupta (✉) · Ashutosh
Dharamshila Narayana Superspeciality Hospital, DNSH, Delhi, India
e-mail: deni.gupta.dr@narayanahealth.org

K. Sood Sharma et al. (eds.), *Complications of Cancer Therapy: Best Practices in Prevention and Management*, https://doi.org/10.1007/978-981-99-0984-1_22

done by use of second-generation androgen receptor blockade, androgen metabolism inhibitor or by use of other agents like corticosteroid, ketoconazole, antiandrogen withdrawal or first-generation antiandrogens.

22.3 Surgical Castration

Surgical removal of both testes is called bilateral orchiectomy. This procedure reduces serum level of testosterone which is necessary for growth of prostatic tissue. Orchiectomy is especially useful in situations where rapid decrease in levels of serum testosterone is required, for example impending cord compression although a very safe surgery but can rarely lead to intraoperative hemorrhage [3]. Most wound complication resolve spontaneously with only few requiring aspiration and re-exploration. Long term psychosocial complication due to absence of testes can be mitigated through testicular prosthesis [4, 5].

Medical castration—Objective of medical castration is to achieve similar level of serum testosterone achieved by surgical castration. This can be accomplished through use of either GnRH Analogues, GnRH antagonists and anti androgens.

GnRH analogues—GnRH analogues approved for parenteral administration include leuprolide, goserelin, triptorelin, buserelin, and histrelin. These are synthetic version of naturally occurring Gonadotropin releasing hormone and are less susceptible to enzymatic degradation and more potent than their natural counterpart [6]. These agent act by binding to GnRH receptors on pituitary gland and cause initial increase in LH and FSH secretion which in turn leads to increase in serum testosterone level. After about a week there is downregulation of GnRH receptors in pituitary cells due to continuous stimulation. This in turn leads to decrease in level of LH and FSH and subsequently decrease in level of serum testosterone [7].

Complication of GnRH Analogue—Flare phenomenon—The initial transient increase in testosterone level with use of GnRH Analogue may stimulate growth in prostate cancer tissue. Although rare, but this 'Flare up' of testosterone may lead to worsening of symptoms [8]. Hence, initial treatment of prostate cancer with only GnRH analogue in severe urinary tract obstruction or painful bone metastasis is contraindicated. The flare phenomenon can be effectively managed with short course of antiandrogen therapy (combined Androgen Blockade) [9].

As compared to orchiectomy which is irreversible procedure castration with GnRH analogue is reversible and avoid psychosocial issues associated with bilateral orchiectomy. Besides studies have found equal survival, progression free survival and time to treatment failure [10].

GnRH Antagonist—Pure GnRH antagonists bind to GnRH receptors on pituitary cells without stimulating them initially. This prevents flare phenomenon seen with GnRH analogue but there is more injection site reaction with GnRH Antagonist [11]. GnRH antagonists are used in situation where rapid decrease in serum levels of testosterone is needed such as impending cord compression or obstruction of urinary tract. Commonly Used GnRH Antagonists are Degarelix and Relugolix.

Abufaraj et al. [12] in a meta-analyses of eight clinical trials reported lower rate of cardiovascular events with GnRH antagonist whereas side effects like loss of libido, erectile dysfunction, injection site reaction lower with GnRH analogue.

22.4 Androgen Receptor Blockers

Androgen receptor blockers are often used in combination with GnRH Analogues for the management of prostate cancer. Androgen receptor blockers, commonly called antiandrogens, are divided into first generation and second generation antiandrogen. First generation antiandrogen i.e. bicalutamide, flutamide, nilutamide are used mainly to prevent flare reaction with GnRH analogues (called "combined androgen blockade" [CAB]). Beyond this there is no established role of first generation antiandrogens except in resource limited setting where they can be offered in combination with GnRH analogues to the patient having nonmetastatic, locally advanced prostate cancer [13].

Out of three first generation anti androgen Bicalutamide is most commonly used owing to its better toxicity and side effect profile. Nilutamide is associated with light dark adaptation [14] and pulmonary toxicity where as Flutamide is associated significant liver toxicity [15].

Second generation antiandrogens Enzalutamide and apalutamide have shown significant activity in castrate resistant prostate cancer. In Enzamet trial The enzalutamide group had a higher incidence of seizures (seven patients [1%] versus none with standard care) and other toxic effects, especially among those treated with early docetaxel [16].

22.5 Abiraterone

It is an androgen metabolism inhibitor used in CRPC. LATITUDE trial which compared GnRH analogue and Abiraterone vs GnRH analogue showed increase in the rates of grade 3 or higher hypertension (21 versus 10%) and hypokalemia (12 versus 2%) [17]. To minimize hormonal side effects of Abiraterone, it is prescribed with prednisolone.

22.5.1 Intermittent ADT

In selected patient with biochemical recurrence after first or second line local therapy Intermittent ADT can be given to attempt for minimizing acute and chronic side effect of prolonged exposure to castrate level of serum testosterone [18]. Other rationale is that continuous ADT may facilitate progression from androgen dependence to androgen independence.

22.5.2 Chronic Complications and Management of ADT

Sexual Dysfunction A large proportion of male receiving ADT develop loss of libido in first few month of commencement of treatment followed by erectile dysfunction [19]. However, loss of libido is common with ADT but it is not universal. Due to complex interplay between emotional wellbeing, psychological issues and physiological responses, management of sexual dysfunction requires multidisciplinary approach including couple's counselling and management of their expectation post initiation of ADT. Interventions like phosphodiesterase 5 inhibitors [20], vacuum therapy to promote quality erections [21], transdermal estradiol for desire etc. can also be prescribed. Erectile dysfunction may recover after cessation of ADT but may not become completely normal [19].

Osteoporosis ADT is known to cause increase in bone turnover and decrease in bone mineral density [22]. The longer the duration of ADT the higher is the risk of osteoporosis [23]. Osteoporosis associated fractures occur in up to 1 in 5 males within 5 years of starting ADT. Before starting ADT a baseline Dual X-ray absorptiometry (DXA) should be done to assess for bone marrow density and to recognise individual at higher risk of osteoporotic fractures [24, 25]. However few studies have suggested quantitative CT to be better than DXA for evaluation of osteoporotic fracture risk in males on ADT [26].

Patients starting ADT should follow lifestyle modification as a preventive measure. Regular weight bearing and resistance exercises, smoking cessation, and moderation of alcohol consumption are beneficial. Along with this dietary supplementation of vitamin D 800–1000 IU daily and calcium 1000–1200 mg daily as per ASCO guidelines [24, 25].

On the basis of findings of DXA scan or by use of WHO FRAX algorithms patients at high risk of osteoporotic fractures are offered osteoclast inhibitors i.e. bisphosphonates or Denosumnab. Although these agents are offered when DXA scan suggest T score lower than −2.5 or FRAX algorithm predict 10 year probability of hip fracture to be ≥3%, ASCO guidelines also suggest to use them at higher T scores on DXA scan or lower probability of hip fracture on FRAX algorithm as ADT may cause rapid bone turnover and accelerated osteoporosis.

When an osteoclast inhibitor is indicated, most guidelines suggest use of Denosumab 60 mg q6 monthly [27]. However, due to issues related to logistics or denosumab being contraindicated bisphosphonates are also reasonable choice. Optimal duration of treatment is not uniform with studies showing data of up to 3 years.

22.5.3 Falls and Fractures

Second generation Androgen receptor blockers have shown in studies for increase propensity for fall and fractures in trials. This risk is especially frequent with apalutamide. However, the cause of this increased risk is not clear [28]. Physicians are advised to use fall-risk assessment tool while prescribing these agents to elderly patients.

22.5.4 Vasomotor Symptoms

Approximately 80% patient using GnRH analogues report vasomotor symptoms as intense feeling of warmth over face and upper chest. Few patients acclimatize over time to low testosterone state and their symptoms improve with time. However many patient require intervention to ameliorate their symptoms. Medroxyprogesterone (20 mg/day), cyproterone (100 mg/day), or the serotonin uptake inhibitor venlafaxine (75 mg/day) have been reported to improve symptoms [29]. Megestrol acetate also improves symptoms of hot flashes but there are reports suggesting that it may cause rapid progression of carcinoma prostate [30]. Besides these, high dose Gabapentin to the dose of 900 mg PO per day and oxybutynin has also been shown effective [31]. In an study acupuncture has also been found effective in management of hot flashes.

22.5.5 Cardiovascular Side Effects

Cardiovascular diseases are most common cause of non-cancer related death in patient of carcinoma prostate. There are no specific study designed to assess CVD risk in patients of carcinoma prostate on ADT. However, there is enough observational data to suggest that ADT may increase risk of CVD morbidity and mortality [32]. Metabolic changes associated with ADT also significantly increases risk of cardiovascular disease. Risk of CVD complication is more in patients having prior history of CVD. These patients should be managed by a multidisciplinary team and should be aggressively screened for major CVD risk factors like hypertension, diabetes, dyslipidemia and appropriately managed. Patients should be encouraged to maintain a healthy lifestyle and follow regular exercise regime along with smoking cessation counselling [33].

22.5.6 Thromboembolic Disease

Thromboembolic events like DVT, pulmonary embolism and arterial embolism are more frequently seen in patients taking ADT. Patients with known CVD and are at increase risk of thromboembolic events should take aspirin (generally 81 mg/day) unless contraindicated [33].

22.5.7 Renal Complications

There is data to suggest an association between use od ADT and acute kidney injury. However, studies on which this observation is based on have large numbers of confounders and additional studies might be needed to confirm the strength of association [34].

22.5.8 Hepatic Complication

When compared to men who are not receiving ADT, patients with prostate cancer on ADT may have a higher chance of developing liver disorders. Especially patients on Abiraterone are increased risk of toxicity since hepatic impairment reduces its excretion [35].

22.5.9 Gynecomastia

Gynecomastia can develop when oestrogen action is unopposed and this condition can be painful or upsetting for cosmetic reasons. It may happen with ADT, but anti-androgens are more problematic because of the accumulation of androgens and their peripheral conversion to oestrogen in breast tissue. Gynecomastia also causes significant body image problems. Tamoxifen and prophylactic breast irradiation are two therapeutic choices; these modalities however are more effective in prevention and have limited role after development of gynecomastia [22].

22.5.10 Metabolic Changes

Patient treated with ADT experience increased deposition of body fat mostly in subcutaneous tissue, loss of lean body mass, decreased insulin sensitivity leading to hyperglycemia and sarcopenia [36, 37]. These patients also experience increase in serum level of cholesterol and triglycerides. FDA has issued class labeling for GnRH analogues suggesting that this class of drug may produce hyperglycemia and there is risk of developing diabetes [38]. In light of above-mentioned complications patient who are started on ADT should be aggressively screened for diabetes and dyslipidemia. They should also be counselled for life style modification and follow a regular exercise regime.

22.5.11 Anemia

Anemia develops in approximately 90% of patient receiving ADT and is usually normochromic and normocytic [22, 39]. Some studies have shown ADT associated anemia to be highly responsive to erythropoietin (EPO) but EPO is rarely necessary and is reserved for severe cases.

22.5.12 Neurocognitive

There is continuous decline in levels of serum testosterone associated with normal aging. Various retrospective studies have suggested association of cognitive decline as suggested by performance on MMSE [40]. Apart from this, increased risk of developing Alzheimer's disease [41], depression and anxiety have also been reported in patients on ADT. However, major confounder in these studies was increased age. International Society of Geriatric Oncology (SIOP) suggest that clinicians discuss the risk of neurocognitive dysfunction with older patients with prostate cancer who are considering use of ADT [42].

22.5.13 Fatigue

Fatigue is a highly prevalent and troublesome side effect of ADT. In one study, fatigue was severe in 14% of males after only 3 months of therapy [43]. Before diagnosing as ADT associated fatigue other causes such as diabetes, hypothyroidism, anemia etc. should be ruled out. Life style modification in the form of regular exercise appears to be beneficial in improving the fatigue associated with ADT [44].

To conclude ADT is an important cornerstone in the management of prostate cancer. With growing data, the complications associated with use of androgen deprivation and their management have become more evidence based. Data support role of structured exercise regimen in improving lean mass, cardiorespiratory fitness and fatigue. Multidisciplinary approach improves outcome of sexual dysfunction, fractures and cognitive dysfunction associated with ADT. Various societies have provided criteria for use of drugs like denosumab and bisphosphonate for the prevention of osteoporotic fractures. Apart from this aggressive screening and management of metabolic disorders and cardiovascular risk factors like diabetes hypertension and dyslipidemia prevents cardiovascular complications.

References

1. Sung H, Ferlay J, Siegel RL, Laversanne M, Soerjomataram I, Jemal A, Bray F. Global cancer statistics 2020: GLOBOCAN estimates of incidence and mortality worldwide for 36 cancers in 185 countries. CA Cancer J Clin. 2021;71(3):209–49. https://doi.org/10.3322/caac.21660. Epub 2021 Feb 4.
2. Denmeade SR, Lin XS, Isaacs JT. Role of programmed (apoptotic) cell death during the progression and therapy for prostate cancer [Erratum in: Prostate 1996 Jun;28(6):414.]. Prostate. 1996;28(4):251–65. https://doi.org/10.1002/(SICI)1097-0045(199604)28:4<251::AID-PROS6>3.0.CO;2-G.
3. Oefelein MG, Feng A, Scolieri MJ, Ricchiutti D, Resnick MI. Reassessment of the definition of castrate levels of testosterone: implications for clinical decision making. Urology. 2000;56(6):1021–4. https://doi.org/10.1016/s0090-4295(00)00793-7.
4. Zhang XZ, Donovan MP, Williams BT, Mohler JL. Comparison of subcapsular and total orchiectomy for treatment of metastatic prostate cancer. Urology. 1996;47(3):402–4. https://doi.org/10.1016/S0090-4295(99)80460-9.
5. Chapman JP. Comparison of testosterone and LH values in subcapsular vs total orchiectomy patients. Urology. 1987;30(1):27–8. https://doi.org/10.1016/0090-4295(87)90565-6. PMID: 3603905.
6. Schally AV, Coy DH, Arimura A. LH–RH agonists and antagonists. Int J Gynaecol Obstet. 1980;18(5):318–24. https://doi.org/10.1002/j.1879-3479.1980.tb00507.x.

7. Conn PM, Crowley WF Jr. Gonadotropin-releasing hormone and its analogues. N Engl J Med. 1991;324(2):93–103. https://doi.org/10.1056/NEJM199101103240205.
8. Waxman J, Man A, Hendry WF, Whitfield HN, Besser GM, Tiptaft RC, Paris AM, Oliver RT. Importance of early tumour exacerbation in patients treated with long acting analogues of gonadotrophin releasing hormone for advanced prostatic cancer. Br Med J (Clin Res Ed). 1985;291(6506):1387–8. https://doi.org/10.1136/bmj.291.6506.1387.
9. Loblaw DA, Mendelson DS, Talcott JA, Virgo KS, Somerfield MR, Ben-Josef E, Middleton R, Porterfield H, Sharp SA, Smith TJ, Taplin ME, Vogelzang NJ, Wade JL Jr, Bennett CL, Scher HI, American Society of Clinical Oncology. American Society of Clinical Oncology recommendations for the initial hormonal management of androgen-sensitive metastatic, recurrent, or progressive prostate cancer [Erratum in: J Clin Oncol 2004 Nov 1;22(21):4435.]. J Clin Oncol. 2004;22(14):2927–41. https://doi.org/10.1200/JCO.2004.04.579. Epub 2004 Jun 7.
10. Seidenfeld J, Samson DJ, Hasselblad V, Aronson N, Albertsen PC, Bennett CL, Wilt TJ. Single-therapy androgen suppression in men with advanced prostate cancer: a systematic review and meta-analysis [Erratum in: Ann Intern Med 2005 Nov 15;143(10):764–5.]. Ann Intern Med. 2000;132(7):566–77. https://doi.org/10.7326/0003-4819-132-7-200004040-00009.
11. Smith MR, Klotz L, Persson BE, Olesen TK, Wilde AA. Cardiovascular safety of degarelix: results from a 12-month, comparative, randomized, open label, parallel group phase III trial in patients with prostate cancer. J Urol. 2010;184(6):2313–9. https://doi.org/10.1016/j.juro.2010.08.012. Epub 2010 Oct 16. PMID: 20952020; PMCID: PMC3047399.
12. Abufaraj M, Iwata T, Kimura S, Haddad A, Al-Ani H, Abusubaih L, Moschini M, Briganti A, Karakiewicz PI, Shariat SF. Differential impact of gonadotropin-releasing hormone antagonist versus agonist on clinical safety and oncologic outcomes on patients with metastatic prostate cancer: a meta-analysis of randomized controlled trials. Eur Urol. 2021;79(1):44–53. https://doi.org/10.1016/j.eururo.2020.06.002. Epub 2020 Jun 27.
13. Virgo KS, Rumble RB, de Wit R, Mendelson DS, Smith TJ, Taplin ME, Wade JL 3rd, Bennett CL, Scher HI, Nguyen PL, Gleave M, Morgan SC, Loblaw A, Sachdev S, Graham DL, Vapiwala N, Sion AM, Simons VH, Talcott J. Initial management of noncastrate advanced, recurrent, or metastatic prostate cancer: ASCO guideline update. J Clin Oncol. 2021;39(11):1274–305. https://doi.org/10.1200/JCO.20.03256. Epub 2021 Jan 26.
14. Decensi AU, Boccardo F, Guarneri D, Positano N, Paoletti MC, Costantini M, Martorana G, Giuliani L, The Italian Prostatic Cancer Project. Monotherapy with nilutamide, a pure nonsteroidal antiandrogen, in untreated patients with metastatic carcinoma of the prostate. J Urol. 1991;146(2):377–81. https://doi.org/10.1016/s0022-5347(17)37799-6.
15. Wysowski DK, Fourcroy JL. Flutamide hepatotoxicity [Erratum in: J Urol 1996 Apr;155(4):1396.]. J Urol. 1996;155(1):209–12.
16. Davis ID, Martin AJ, Stockler MR, Begbie S, Chi KN, Chowdhury S, Coskinas X, Frydenberg M, Hague WE, Horvath LG, Joshua AM, Lawrence NJ, Marx G, McCaffrey J, McDermott R, McJannett M, North SA, Parnis F, Parulekar W, Pook DW, Reaume MN, Sandhu SK, Tan A, Tan TH, Thomson A, Tu E, Vera-Badillo F, Williams SG, Yip S, Zhang AY, Zielinski RR, Sweeney CJ, ENZAMET Trial Investigators and the Australian and New Zealand Urogenital and Prostate Cancer Trials Group. Enzalutamide with standard first-line therapy in metastatic prostate cancer. N Engl J Med. 2019;381(2):121–31. https://doi.org/10.1056/NEJMoa1903835. Epub 2019 Jun 2.
17. Chi KN, Protheroe A, Rodríguez-Antolín A, Facchini G, Suttman H, Matsubara N, Ye Z, Keam B, Damião R, Li T, McQuarrie K, Jia B, De Porre P, Martin J, Todd MB, Fizazi K. Patient-reported outcomes following abiraterone acetate plus prednisone added to androgen deprivation therapy in patients with newly diagnosed metastatic castration-naive prostate cancer (LATITUDE): an international, randomised phase 3 trial. Lancet Oncol. 2018;19(2):194–206. https://doi.org/10.1016/S1470-2045(17)30911-7. Epub 2018 Jan 8.
18. Hussain M, Tangen CM, Berry DL, Higano CS, Crawford ED, Liu G, Wilding G, Prescott S, Kanaga Sundaram S, Small EJ, Dawson NA, Donnelly BJ, Venner PM, Vaishampayan UN, Schellhammer PF, Quinn DI, Raghavan D, Ely B, Moinpour CM, Vogelzang NJ, Thompson

IM Jr. Intermittent versus continuous androgen deprivation in prostate cancer. N Engl J Med. 2013;368(14):1314–25. https://doi.org/10.1056/NEJMoa1212299.

19. Gay HA, Sanda MG, Liu J, Wu N, Hamstra DA, Wei JT, Dunn RL, Klein EA, Sandler HM, Saigal CS, Litwin MS, Kuban DA, Hembroff L, Regan MM, Chang P, Prostate Cancer Outcomes and Satisfaction with Treatment Quality Assessment Consortium, Michalski JM. External beam radiation therapy or brachytherapy with or without short-course neoadjuvant androgen deprivation therapy: results of a multicenter, prospective study of quality of life. Int J Radiat Oncol Biol Phys. 2017;98(2):304–17. https://doi.org/10.1016/j.ijrobp.2017.02.019. Epub 2017 Feb 22. PMID: 28463150; PMCID: PMC5493021.
20. Tsertsvadze A, Fink HA, Yazdi F, MacDonald R, Bella AJ, Ansari MT, Garritty C, Soares-Weiser K, Daniel R, Sampson M, Fox S, Moher D, Wilt TJ. Oral phosphodiesterase-5 inhibitors and hormonal treatments for erectile dysfunction: a systematic review and meta-analysis. Ann Intern Med. 2009;151(9):650–61. https://doi.org/10.7326/0003-4819-151-9-200911030-00150.
21. Medina-Polo J, García-Gómez B, Alonso-Isa M, Romero-Otero J. Clinical guidelines on erectile dysfunction surgery: EAU–AUA perspectives. Actas Urol Esp (Engl Ed). 2020;44(5):289–93. https://doi.org/10.1016/j.acuro.2019.10.008. Epub 2020 Mar 12.
22. Nguyen PL, Alibhai SM, Basaria S, D'Amico AV, Kantoff PW, Keating NL, Penson DF, Rosario DJ, Tombal B, Smith MR. Adverse effects of androgen deprivation therapy and strategies to mitigate them. Eur Urol. 2015;67(5):825–36. https://doi.org/10.1016/j.eururo.2014.07.010. Epub 2014 Aug 2.
23. Smith MR, Lee WC, Brandman J, Wang Q, Botteman M, Pashos CL. Gonadotropin-releasing hormone agonists and fracture risk: a claims-based cohort study of men with nonmetastatic prostate cancer. J Clin Oncol. 2005;23(31):7897–903. https://doi.org/10.1200/JCO.2004.00.6908.
24. NCCN Guidelines. https://www.nccn.org/professionals/physician_gls/.
25. Shapiro CL, Van Poznak C, Lacchetti C, Kirshner J, Eastell R, Gagel R, Smith S, Edwards BJ, Frank E, Lyman GH, Smith MR, Mhaskar R, Henderson T, Neuner J. Management of osteoporosis in survivors of adult cancers with nonmetastatic disease: ASCO clinical practice guideline. J Clin Oncol. 2019;37(31):2916–46. https://doi.org/10.1200/JCO.19.01696. Epub 2019 Sep 18.
26. Yamada M, Ito M, Hayashi K, Ohki M, Nakamura T. Dual energy X-ray absorptiometry of the calcaneus: comparison with other techniques to assess bone density and value in predicting risk of spine fracture. AJR Am J Roentgenol. 1994;163(6):1435–40. https://doi.org/10.2214/ajr.163.6.7992742.
27. Smith MR, Egerdie B, Hernández Toriz N, Feldman R, Tammela TL, Saad F, Heracek J, Szwedowski M, Ke C, Kupic A, Leder BZ, Goessl C, Denosumab HALT Prostate Cancer Study Group. Denosumab in men receiving androgen-deprivation therapy for prostate cancer. N Engl J Med. 2009;361(8):745–55. https://doi.org/10.1056/NEJMoa0809003. Epub 2009 Aug 11. PMID: 19671656; PMCID: PMC3038121.
28. Myint ZW, Momo HD, Otto DE, Yan D, Wang P, Kolesar JM. Evaluation of fall and fracture risk among men with prostate cancer treated with androgen receptor inhibitors: a systematic review and meta-analysis. JAMA Netw Open. 2020;3(11):e2025826. https://doi.org/10.1001/jamanetworkopen.2020.25826.
29. Irani J, Salomon L, Oba R, Bouchard P, Mottet N. Efficacy of venlafaxine, medroxyprogesterone acetate, and cyproterone acetate for the treatment of vasomotor hot flushes in men taking gonadotropin-releasing hormone analogues for prostate cancer: a double-blind, randomised trial. Lancet Oncol. 2010;11(2):147–54. https://doi.org/10.1016/S1470-2045(09)70338-9. Epub 2009 Dec 4.
30. Sartor O, Eastham JA. Progressive prostate cancer associated with use of megestrol acetate administered for control of hot flashes. South Med J. 1999;92(4):415–6. https://doi.org/10.1097/00007611-199904000-00013.
31. Loprinzi CL, Dueck AC, Khoyratty BS, Barton DL, Jafar S, Rowland KM Jr, Atherton PJ, Marsa GW, Knutson WH, Bearden JD 3rd, Kottschade L, Fitch TR. A phase III randomized, double-blind, placebo-controlled trial of gabapentin in the management of hot flashes in men

(N00CB). Ann Oncol. 2009;20(3):542–9. https://doi.org/10.1093/annonc/mdn644. Epub 2009 Jan 6. PMID: 19129205; PMCID: PMC2733071.

32. Levine GN, D'Amico AV, Berger P, et al. Androgen-deprivation therapy in prostate cancer and cardiovascular risk: a science advisory from the American Heart Association, American Cancer Society, and American urological association: endorsed by the American Society for Radiation Oncology. Circulation. 2010;121:833–40.
33. Kenk M, Grégoire JC, Coté MA, Connelly KA, Davis MK, Dresser G, Ghosh N, Goodman S, Johnson C, Fleshner N. Optimizing screening and management of cardiovascular health in prostate cancer: a review. Can Urol Assoc J. 2020;14(9):E458–64. https://doi.org/10.5489/cuaj.6685.
34. Lapi F, Azoulay L, Niazi MT, Yin H, Benayoun S, Suissa S. Androgen deprivation therapy and risk of acute kidney injury in patients with prostate cancer. JAMA. 2013;310(3):289–96. https://doi.org/10.1001/jama.2013.8638.
35. Marbury T, Lawitz E, Stonerock R, et al. Single-dose pharmacokinetic studies of abiraterone acetate in men with hepatic or renal impairment. J Clin Pharmacol. 2014;54:732–41.
36. Smith MR, Finkelstein JS, McGovern FJ, Zietman AL, Fallon MA, Schoenfeld DA, Kantoff PW. Changes in body composition during androgen deprivation therapy for prostate cancer. J Clin Endocrinol Metab. 2002;87(2):599–603. https://doi.org/10.1210/jcem.87.2.8299.
37. Smith MR, Lee H, Fallon MA, Nathan DM. Adipocytokines, obesity, and insulin resistance during combined androgen blockade for prostate cancer. Urology. 2008;71(2):318–22. https://doi.org/10.1016/j.urology.2007.08.035.
38. Keating NL, Liu PH, O'Malley AJ, Freedland SJ, Smith MR. Androgen-deprivation therapy and diabetes control among diabetic men with prostate cancer. Eur Urol. 2014;65(4):816–24. https://doi.org/10.1016/j.eururo.2013.02.023. Epub 2013 Feb 22. PMID: 23453420; PMCID: PMC3779484.
39. Beer TM, Tangen CM, Bland LB, Hussain M, Goldman BH, DeLoughery TG, Crawford ED, Southwest Oncology Group Study. The prognostic value of hemoglobin change after initiating androgen-deprivation therapy for newly diagnosed metastatic prostate cancer: a multivariate analysis of southwest oncology group study 8894. Cancer. 2006;107(3):489–96. https://doi.org/10.1002/cncr.22029.
40. Nead KT, Gaskin G, Chester C, Swisher-McClure S, Leeper NJ, Shah NH. Association between androgen deprivation therapy and risk of dementia. JAMA Oncol. 2017;3(1):49–55. https://doi.org/10.1001/jamaoncol.2016.3662.
41. Baik SH, Kury FSP, McDonald CJ. Risk of Alzheimer's disease among senior medicare beneficiaries treated with androgen deprivation therapy for prostate cancer. J Clin Oncol. 2017;35(30):3401–9. https://doi.org/10.1200/JCO.2017.72.6109. Epub 2017 Aug 25. PMID: 28841388; PMCID: PMC5648173.
42. Boyle HJ, Alibhai S, Decoster L, Efstathiou E, Fizazi K, Mottet N, Oudard S, Payne H, Prentice M, Puts M, Aapro M, Droz JP. Updated recommendations of the International Society of Geriatric Oncology on prostate cancer management in older patients. Eur J Cancer. 2019;116:116–36. https://doi.org/10.1016/j.ejca.2019.04.031. Epub 2019 Jun 10.
43. Stone P, Hardy J, Huddart R, A'Hern R, Richards M. Fatigue in patients with prostate cancer receiving hormone therapy. Eur J Cancer. 2000;36(9):1134–41. https://doi.org/10.1016/s0959-8049(00)00084-8.
44. Taaffe DR, Newton RU, Spry N, Joseph D, Chambers SK, Gardiner RA, Wall BA, Cormie P, Bolam KA, Galvão DA. Effects of different exercise modalities on fatigue in prostate cancer patients undergoing androgen deprivation therapy: a year-long randomised controlled Trial. Eur Urol. 2017;72(2):293–9. https://doi.org/10.1016/j.eururo.2017.02.019. Epub 2017 Feb 27.

Secondary Infertility After Cancer Treatment

23

Tara Chand Gupta and Snehpreet Kaur

23.1 Introduction

With the advancement in therapeutics lead to improvement in cure rates and survival thus making the long term side effects like infertility an issue of discussion. Currently, most of the childhood malignancies has 5 year survival rate of 80% or more and 10 year survival rate of more than 75%. Overall, since mid-1970s there is improvement, when the 5-year survival rate was about 58% [1]. These improvements in survival have come with many issues like the long-term treatment sequelae, infertility is among the most important in these cancer survivors. The definition of "cancer survivor" includes patients from the confirmation of diagnosis and identifying and managing the survivorship issues, even those arising a long time even years after treatment, must start at diagnosis. Fertility is the major survivorship issue that needs to be addressed and discussed with the patient before initiating any therapy to allow for informed decision-making regarding treatment options, family planning, and fertility preservation strategies [2].

23.2 Biology of Male Fertility

The testis consists of the seminiferous tubules and endocrine components (testosterone-producing Leydig cells) in the interstitial region between the tubules. The seminiferous tubules contain the germ cells, which consist of stem and differentiating spermatogonia, spermatocytes, spermatids, sperm, and the Sertoli cells, support and regulate the germ cell differentiation. The vasculature of testcs is

T. C. Gupta (✉) · S. Kaur
Bhagwan Mahaveer Cancer Hospital and Research Centre (BMCHRC), Jaipur, India

K. Sood Sharma et al. (eds.), *Complications of Cancer Therapy: Best Practices in Prevention and Management*, https://doi.org/10.1007/978-981-99-0984-1_23

permeable, and drugs can freely reach the outer part of the tubules that is Leydig and Sertoli cells and the spermatogonia. There are chemotherapeutic drugs which may penetrate the blood testes barrier, but the penetration is very low, and can damage damage germ cells in later stages. Differentiating spermatogonia are more susceptible to cytotoxic agents because these are active dividing cells. In contrast to these cells, less actively dividing cells like the Leydig and Sertoli cells, are relatively resistant to the cytotoxic therapies. However, these may suffer some functional damage. Secondary effects of the loss of germ cells are on the hypothalamic–pituitary–gonadal axis. Secretion of inhibin by the Sertoli cells decreases which in turn leading to secretion of follicle-stimulating hormone (FSH) secretion by the pituitary, thus causing rise in serum FSH levels. As inhibin limits the secretion of FSH by pituitary [3].

23.3 Biology of Female Fertility

In women, the germ cells are nonproliferative, whereas the somatic cells proliferate. In females, the germ cells proliferate during prenatal period, and by birth, these germ cells are arrested in the oocyte stage. There are one million oocytes at the time of birth, which are reduced to 300,000 at puberty and to fewer than 1000 oocytes when menopause occurs at the age 50 years. Before the start of process ovulation, these oocytes are found in primordial follicles with few pre granulosa cells, surrounded by theca cells of the ovarian stroma. Once maturation starts, this follicle develops until it either degenerates or ovulates. In follicular maturation, there is proliferation of granulosa cells and the development of steroidogenic potential of both the theca and granulosa cells. Production of estrogen involves the stimulation of both these cell types by LH and FSH and causes the LH surge that triggers ovulation. The cyclic variations in FSH, LH, and estradiol are essential for menstrual cycles and reproduction. Whenever there is destruction of oocytes results in loss of follicles, causing estrogen insufficiency. Radiation and chemotherapy cause the destruction of oocytes by direct apoptotic action in mouse models. Although the direct action is the dominant mechanism in the most of the chemotherapeutic agents, other mechanisms also exists like effects on granulosa cells, surrounding stroma, and blood vessels which may indirectly affect the oocyte. When maturing follicles are destroyed by cytotoxic therapy, the result is oligomenorrhea or temporary amenorrhea [4].

23.4 Pre Treatment Evaluation of Fertility

23.4.1 Males

A sexual and reproductive history should be taken, which includes information on developmental factors such as age at testicular descent and puberty; any history of surgery or injury to the genitals; diseases that might affect reproduction; drug, chemical, or heat exposure; and pretreatment fertility and libido status.

A physical examination should consist of an examination of the testicles and secondary sexual characteristics such as beard and hair distribution pattern. If there are indications, a semen analysis and a hormone profile should be done and results should be compared with normal values.

23.4.2 Females

Menstrual and obstetric histories are important in assessing the effects of cytotoxic therapy on ovarian function. Pre chemotherapy sexual function and menstrual histories is particularly useful. Pretherapy ovarian function should be evaluated from the history of menarche, menses, pregnancies, and oral contraceptive use.

Laboratory measurements of hormone levels are most definitive in the diagnosis of primary ovarian failure. FSH level is the most sensitive, but LH and estradiol levels are also useful. But these are the late markers of ovarian aging. Antimüllerian hormone (AMH), a hormone produced by growing follicles from the primary to antral stage, is hormone that can be used to determine ovarian reserve by inferring the number of primordial follicles present. It is an earlier predictor of decreased ovarian reserve. AMH is evaluable in both pre- and postmenarchal females [5–7].

23.5 Risk Factor

1. Location of tumor
2. Type of cancer
3. Stage of tumor
4. Systemic therapy
5. Radiotherapy
6. Surgery

23.5.1 Risk Categorization

Based on the above factors, they are further grouped into three risk categories

1. Low risk (<25% decrease in likelihood of pregnancy)
2. Intermediate risk (25–75% decrease in likelihood of pregnancy)
3. High risk (>75% decrease in likelihood of pregnancy)

23.5.2 Chemotherapy Associated with Infertility

The most common agent causing infertility in both males and females is alkylating agents. The cumulative dose is more important predictor of chemotherapy induced infertility. Multiple reports from the Childhood Cancer Survivor Study (CCSS) found correlation with the risk of infertility with summed alkylating dose or cyclophosphamide equivalent dose (CED). According to 2016 report, it was found that alkylating agents are associated with decreased likelihood of pregnancy only at the highest quartile of CED exposure (>11.3 g/m^2, hazard ratio [HR] = 0.85, 95% CI = 0.74–0.98). This report suggesting that the treatment in most survivors with various chemotherapy regimens alone are not at high risk of infertility [8].

Other sterilizing agents are procarbazine and cisplatin in high doses (>600 mg/m^2). Busulfan when given with cyclophosphamide has an additive effect on the sterility [9]. The ifosfamide in high doses (46 g/m^2) added to cisplatin-containing chemotherapy regimens significantly reduced the recovery of spermatogenic function. Carboplatin, as compared to cisplatin produce less sterility [10]. The treatment with carmustine (BCNU) and lomustine (CCNU) produced prolonged azoospermia in young boys than in adults.

Chemotherapy with low risk of infertility was observed with 5-fluorouracil, methotrexate, vincristine, etoposide (5 g), or cisplatin (<450 mg/m^2) plus doxorubicin (<400 mg/m^2) in women aged 15–35 years. Doxorubicin (300 mg/m^2), bleomycin, vincristine, and dacarbazine (ABVD) regimen used in Hodgkin lymphoma do not appear to cause ovarian failure because in studies none was observed after this treatment of women up to age 41 years [11].

Combination protocols that include procarbazine and other alkylating agents (mechlorethamin, vincristine, procarbazine, prednisone [MOPP]; CHOP; mechlorethamine, vinblastine, procarbazine, and prednisone [MVPP]; and chlorambucil, vinblastine, procarbazine, and prednisone [ChlVPP]) induce gonadal failure in almost all patients treated in Hodgkin lymphoma more in adult age group than young patients [12].

23.5.3 Infertility After Oncosurgery

Testicular cancer: In testicular cancer, although unilateral orchiectomy spares the unaffected testis, but the sperm concentration decreases. The incidence of bilateral testicular cancer is very rare accounting for only 1% of testicular cancers and the majority are present as metachronous rather than synchronous malignancy [13, 14].

In non seminoma germ cell tumors treated with retroperitoneal lymph node dissection associated with retrograde ejaculation was a frequent complication, but the incidence is now decreasing with the use of nerve sparing techniques [15].

Studies suggesting that testicular cancer survivors are as likely to sire a pregnancy as age-matched control subjects, although adjuvant therapy for testicular cancer affects fertility in some patients [16]. A dose-dependent effect was demonstrated in men receiving adjuvant chemotherapy, with post-treatment paternity rates among men receiving two, three, and four cycles was 100%, 83%, and 76%, respectively. Mean sperm counts recover as early as 12 months following two or fewer cycles and by 24 months following more than two cycles, and more men who receive high-dose cisplatin experience prolonged azoospermia [17].

23.5.3.1 Prostate Cancer

In localized non metastatic prostate cancer, radical prostatectomy is one of the treatment options. Surgery removes the prostate gland and leaves men with no semen production. In prostate surgery the removal of prostate can damage the nerves that allow a man to get an erection, causing erectile dysfunction (ED).

Although this cancer usually occurs in elderly group but in western world, erectile dysfunction and infertility remains an issue.

In metastatic setting, castration is done either by medical or via surgical removal of both testes.

23.5.3.2 Bladder Cancer Surgery

Radical cystectomy removes bladder, prostate gland and lymph nodes for treatment of nonmetastatic localized bladder cancer.

23.5.3.3 Gynaecological Malignancies

In early stages of cervical cancer, the treatment includes surgery i.e. modified radical hysterectomy or fertility sparing surgeries. The risk of infertility with hysterectomy is 100%, but pregnancies with success have occurred with oocyte retrieval and use of a surrogate [18]. Fertility-sparing procedures, includes vaginal or abdominal radical trachelectomy in which the cervix and upper vagina are removed, are now options for highly selected patients [19]. Pregnancy rates among women estimates above 40%. Miscarriage rates range from 9 to 42% and rates of pregnancies with gestation beyond 37 weeks range from 14 to 55% [20]. A recent systematic review compared pregnancy rates associated with vaginal radical trachelectomy (57%) vs laparotomic abdominal radical trachelectomy (44%) [21]. In selected patients, neoadjuvant chemotherapy (cisplatin plus ifosfamide in squamous cell carcinoma or cisplatin plus doxorubicin in adenocarcinoma) has been used to downstage in patients who were not candidates for upfront fertility-sparing surgery and this resulted in fertility preservation in 20 of 28 patients (71%), 10 of whom (50%) became pregnant in one series [22].

In endometrial cancer, the treatment is hysterectomy with bilateral salpingo-oophorectomy and lymph node dissection. But in selected patients with endometrial hyperplasia or stage IA endometrial adenocarcinoma, continuous progestin therapy is a fertility-sparing option [23].

In ovarian cancer also the treatment includes total hysterectomy with bilateral salpingo-oophorectomy with omentectomy and lymph node dissection is the standard approach. But for highly selected women, depending on extent and type of disease, fertility-sparing procedures with unilateral salpingo-oophorectomy and complete surgical staging may be performed and complete surgery may be performed after family completion. Pregnancy rates in women trying to conceive after unilateral salpingo-oophorectomy for EOC have ranged from 27 to 53% [24].

23.6 Radiotherapy

23.6.1 Pelvic Radiation

23.6.1.1 In Males

The effects of radiation on the testes depend on the fractionation regimen. When radiation doses given in 3–7-weeks of fractionated course causes more gonadal damage than single doses. Doses required to produce any reduction in sperm count, are above 0.15 Gy with usual fractionation courses. Doses between 0.15 and 0.5 Gy cause oligospermia. Above 0.6 Gy, azoospermia occurs [25]. The duration of azoospermia is dose dependent, and recovery can begin within 1 year after doses of less than 1 Gy, but not until more than 2 years after delivery of 2 Gy. More than 2.5 Gy of cumulative doses of fractionated radiotherapy result in prolonged and more likely permanent azoospermia. However, as seen in retrospective data, a single dose of 8 Gy or fractionated doses of 10–13 Gy, given as total body irradiation in preparation for bone marrow transplantation, and sometimes also given with cyclophosphamide (4.5 g/m^2), spermatogenesis eventually recovers in 15% of the patients [26].

23.6.1.2 In Females

Permanent ovarian failure occurred after cumulative dose of radiation of 20 Gy, 7 Gy, 3 Gy, <2 Gy in prepubertal age, 20, 35 and 45 years of age respectively. Doses of radiation up to 7 Gy do not cause ovarian failure or inhibit puberty [27].

Due to the normal decline in ovarian reserve and an increase in radiosensitivity of oocytes in growing follicles relative to primordial oocytes, the exposure required to induce ovarian failure decreases with age [28].

23.6.2 Cranial Irradiation

Cranial irradiation results in the development of endocrinopathies involving the hypothalamic–pituitary–gonadal axis thus causing infertility. Prophylactic cranial irradiation done in ALL patients (18–24 Gy) is associated with a lower birth rate than chemotherapy alone. Among adult male survivors of childhood ALL, decreased fertility is associated with high-dose PCI (>24 Gy) [29]. Another analysis demonstrated the effect of high dose PCI on fertility in survivors treated at ages less than 10 years (RR = 0.09, 95% CI = 0.01–0.82) and 10 years or older (RR = 0.54, 95% CI = 0.25–1.28). Within the CCSS, a statistically non significant trend was identified following 0–40 Gy of hypothalamic/pituitary radiation (HR = 0.52, 95% CI = 0.13–2.16) and more than 40 Gy (HR = 0.29, 95% CI = 0.06–1.28) [30]. Now modern protocols tailor dose of PCI in CNS leukemia, slower early responders and uses lower doses of 12–18 Gy, which do not appear to affect spermatogenesis [31].

23.6.3 Radio-Iodine Ablation

In males, no data about effect of ^{131}I on spermatogenesis or fertility are available as it is associated with a testicular radiation exposure of about 0.10 Gy.

In 20% of female patients treated with ^{131}I leads to transient amenorrhea and the average age of menopause is slightly lower following ^{131}I (49.5 vs 51.0 years), but there is no statistically significant difference in birth rate and ^{131}I does not appear to have long-term effects on fertility [32, 33].

23.6.4 Hematopoietic Cell Transplant

Survivors who undergo HCT are at high risk for ovarian failure and infertility because of treatment with the conditioning regimen, which generally includes chemotherapy regimens having high risk of gonadotoxic potential with or without radiation [34].

Combination of radiation and conditioning chemotherapy frequently lead to severe decline in male fertility. Nearly one third patients that is less than 30% of men recover normal spermatogenesis and testicular function after HCT, but when the exposure to cytotoxic agent is greater lead to the lower rates of recovery. Older age, total body irradiation and development of chronic GVHD have been associated with high risk of impaired spermatogenesis [35].

23.6.5 Type and Location of Tumor

Location of tumor—Pelvic malignancies with direct involvement of reproductive organs, abdominal masses compressing the nerves leading to erectile dysfunction and ejaculation problems in males, colorectal cancers due to their location and treatment via surgery and radiation lead to infertility issues, testicular tumors, brain tumors specially pituitary tumors causing endocrinopathies.

Type of tumor—Osteosarcoma, Ewing sarcoma, rhabdomyosarcoma, Wilm's tumor, medulloblastoma are treated with chemotherapy regimens with high risk of developing infertility.

Hodgkin lymphoma treated with procarbazine and other alkylating agents.

Breast cancer treated with alkylating agents are at high risk of developing treatment related amenorrhea with rates of 0–15%, 30–50%, and about 70% among women age younger than 35 years, 36–40 years, and older than 40 years, respectively, and younger women in which TRA develops are more likely to resume menses. In a randomized trial comparing the efficacy of a doxorubicin/docetaxel to regimens combining cyclophosphamide, doxorubicin, and a taxane, either sequentially (AC-T) or concurrently (TAC), in which 70% of participants were older than 40 years old, rates of TRA were lower with doxorubicin/docetaxel (38%) relative to AC-T (70%) and TAC (58%) ($P < 0.001$) [36].

Platinum agents are increasingly being explored for triple negative breast cancer and it will be important to characterize their impact on TRA [37]. Tamoxifen use following adjuvant chemotherapy is associated with a twofold increase in risk of TRA [38], though no women age 40 years or younger treated with tamoxifen alone developed amenorrhea within a large prospective cohort study [39]. Tamoxifen does not appear to have permanent effects on menstrual function or fertility but is teratogenic and must be held before and during pregnancy; thus, the need to delay childbearing can pose a risk to fertility through ovarian aging.

23.7 Management

Prevention is the key for management of cancer treatment related infertility.

There are various methods that are incorporated in treatment design to reduce or eliminate the chances of infertility.

1. Choose chemotherapy regimens with low risk

   In Hodgkin lymphoma, ABVD regimen is associated with low rates of treatment related amenorrhea (3–7%) and it is effective as other regimens with high rate of infertility.
2. Surgery

   In testicular germ cell tumor, nerve sparing retroperitoneal lymph node dissection leads to decreased chances of erectile dysfunction.
3. Prevention in patients undergoing radiotherapy

   In both males and females of adult and prepubertal age group, shielding of the gonadal area is the recommended procedure for reducing the scatter radiation to the reproductive organs and thus reducing the risk of infertility. Clamshell or other shields and beam blocking devices are used which can reduce the testicular doses two- to fivefold to 2–3 Gy for the inverted Y field used for Hodgkin's lymphoma and to 0.2–0.8 Gy for the hemipelvic field used for seminoma.

   To reduce ovarian dose, an oophoropexy is done which is a surgical procedure in which ovaries are surgically translocated away from the area of radiation beam. That region where translocated ovaries are present is further shielded using lead blocks. In some studies, investigator reports reduction in cumulative dose to ovaries upto 4–5 Gy during total nodal irradiation, which helps in preserving the fertility in younger women. With advancement in the field of surgery, these procedures are now be performed laparoscopically or robotically, thus decreasing the hospital stay, earlier mobilization, and earlier return to normal activity
4. Fertility preservation methods in males

   Preemptiveness of physicians in assessing during the diagnostic process that the patient will most likely need to receive potentially sterilizing cytotoxic therapy, before the exact diagnosis and stage. The time between the diagnostic procedures and final diagnosis and this time should be used to initiate and complete the cryopreservation procedure.

5. Sperm banking prior to chemotherapy
6. Testicular cryopreservation and future transplantation

   Mature spermatozoa can be found at Tanner III stage with a testis volume above 5 mL; nevertheless, production of spermatozoa is generally effective only at the age of 13–14 years. Cryopreservation of at least three semen samples with an abstinence period of at least 48 h in between samples is recommended for male patients interested in preserving fertility.
7. Fertility preservation methods in females

   Cryopreservation of embryos or oocytes for females.

   Cryopreservation of gonadal tissue: assisted reproductive technology includes embryo banking and oocyte banking.

23.8 Conclusion

1. Improved survival in cancer patients comes at the cost of some cancer related long term sequelae.
2. Treatment related infertility in young cancer patients is a major concern which leads to social and mental trauma to survivors.
3. Fertility sparing surgeries are the attractive option for patients undergoing surgeries but these are possible in only a small fraction of patients with early stage disease.
4. Newer techniques of radiotherapy like IMRT, IGRT and now proton beam therapy are helpful to some extent in avoiding infertility if the treatment field is not big especially in early disease.
5. Sperm cryopreservation, oocyte preservation and zygote preservations are major instrument in preserving the fertility of patients undergoing systemic therapy for cancer especially cytotoxic chemotherapy
6. There is some benefit of Gonadotropin releasing hormone agonist during chemotherapy has been observed in female patients.
7. With the availability of newer targeted drugs and monoclonal antibodies along with newer immunotherapies cancer related infertility incidence has come down.
8. However, before planning fertility preservation methods risk benefit ration must be calculated.
9. Health care practitioner must discuss the fertility related issues with patient before starting treatment.
10. Although above measures are helpful in fertility preservation but still there is a long way to go for infertility management.

References

1. American Cancer Society. Cancer facts and figures 2022. Atlanta: American Cancer Society; 2021.
2. Ethics Committee of the American Society of Reproductive Medicine. Fertility preservation and reproduction in patients facing gonadotoxic therapies: an ethics committee opinion. Fertil Steril. 2018;110(6):380–6.

3. Bart J, Groen HJ, van der Graaf WT, et al. An oncological view on the blood testis barrier. Lancet Oncol. 2002;3:357–63.
4. Tilly JL, Kolesnick RN. Sphingolipids, apoptosis, cancer treatments and the ovary: investigating a crime against female fertility. Biochim Biophys Acta. 2002;1585:135–8.
5. Burger HG, Dudley EC, Hopper JL, et al. Prospectively measured levels of serum follicle-stimulating hormone, estradiol, and the dimeric inhibins during the menopausal transition in a population-based cohort of women. J Clin Endocrinol Metab. 1999;84(11):4025–30.
6. Fanchin R. Serum anti-Mullerian hormone is more strongly related to ovarian follicular status than serum inhibin B, estradiol, FSH and LH on day 3. Hum Reprod. 2003;18(2):323–7.
7. Kevenaar ME, Meerasahib MF, Kramer P, et al. Serum anti-Mullerian hormone levels reflect the size of the primordial follicle pool in mice. Endocrinology. 2006;147(7):3228–34.
8. Chow EJ, Stratton KL, Leisenring WM, et al. Pregnancy after chemotherapy in male and female survivors of childhood cancer treated between 1970 and 1999: a report from the childhood cancer survivor study cohort. Lancet Oncol. 2016;17(5):567–76.
9. Buchanan JD, Fairley KF, Barrie JU. Return of spermatogenesis after stopping cyclophosphamide therapy. Lancet. 1975;2:156–7.
10. Hansen PV, Trykker H, Helkjoer PE, et al. Testicular function in patients with testicular cancer treated with orchiectomy alone or orchiectomy plus cisplatin-based chemotherapy. J Natl Cancer Inst. 1989;81:1246–50.
11. Koyama H, Wada T, Nishizawa Y, et al. Cyclophosphamide-induced ovarian failure and its therapeutic significance in patients with breast cancer. Cancer. 1977;39:1403–9.
12. Kreuser ED, Xiros N, Hetzel WD, et al. Reproductive and endocrine gonadal capacity in patients treated with COPP chemotherapy for Hodgkin's disease. J Cancer Res Clin Oncol. 1987;113:260–6.
13. Petersen PM, Skakkebaek NE, Rorth M, Giwercman A. Semen quality and reproductive hormones before and after orchiectomy in men with testicular cancer. J Urol. 1999;161(3):822–6.
14. Che M, Tamboli P, Ro JY, et al. Bilateral testicular germ cell tumors: 20-year experience at M. D. Anderson Cancer Center. Cancer. 2002;95(6):1228–33.
15. Nijman JM, Schraffordt Koops H, Oldhoff J, Kremer J, Jager S. Sexual function after bilateral retroperitoneal lymph node dissection for nonseminomatous testicular cancer. Arch Androl. 1987;18(3):255–67.
16. Brydoy M, Fossa SD, Klepp O, et al. Paternity and testicular function among testicular cancer survivors treated with two to four cycles of cisplatin-based chemotherapy. Eur Urol. 2010;58(1):134–40.
17. Bujan L, Walschaerts M, Moinard N, et al. Impact of chemotherapy and radiotherapy for testicular germ cell tumors on spermatogenesis and sperm DNA: a multicenter prospective study from the CECOS network. Fertil Steril. 2013;100(3):673–80.
18. Giacalone P, Laffargue F, Benos P, Dechaud H, Hedon B. Successful in vitro fertilization-surrogate pregnancy in a patient with ovarian transposition who had undergone chemotherapy and pelvic radiation. Fertil Steril. 2001;76(2):388–9.
19. Cervical Cancer Version 1. 2017. https://www.nccn.org/professionals/physician_gls/pdf/cervical.pdf. Accessed 29 Dec 2016.
20. Shepherd JH, Spencer C, Herod J, Ind TE. Radical vaginal trachelectomy as a fertility-sparing procedure in women with early-stage cervical cancer-cumulative pregnancy rate in a series of 123 women. BJOG Int J O&G. 2006;113(6):719–24.
21. Bentivegna E, Maulard A, Pautier P, Chargari C, Gouy S, Morice P. Fertility results and pregnancy outcomes after conservative treatment of cervical cancer: a systematic review of the literature. Fertil Steril. 2016;106(5):1195–1211.e5.
22. Robova H, Halaska MJ, Pluta M, et al. Oncological and pregnancy outcomes after high-dose density neoadjuvant chemotherapy and fertility-sparing surgery in cervical cancer. Gynecol Oncol. 2014;135(2):213–6.
23. Uterine Neoplasms Version 1. 2017. https://www.nccn.org/professionals/physician_gls/pdf/uterine.pdf. Accessed 29 Dec 2016.

24. Satoh T, Hatae M, Watanabe Y, et al. Outcomes of fertility-sparing surgery for stage I epithelial ovarian cancer: a proposal for patient selection. J Clin Oncol. 2010;28(10):1727–32.
25. Meistrich ML, van Beek MEAB. Radiation sensitivity of the human testis. Adv Radiat Biol. 1990;14:227–68.
26. Anserini P, Chiodi S, Spinelli S, et al. Semen analysis following allogeneic bone marrow transplantation. Additional data for evidence-based counselling. Bone Marrow Transplant. 2002;30:447–51.
27. Wallace WHB, Thomson AB, Kelsey TW. The radiosensitivity of the human oocyte. Hum Reprod. 2003;18(1):117–21.
28. Morice P, Juncker L, Rey A, et al. Ovarian transposition for patients with cervical carcinoma treated by radiosurgical combination. Fertil Steril. 2000;74:743–8.
29. Byrne J, Fears TR, Mills JL, et al. Fertility of long-term male survivors of acute lymphoblastic leukemia diagnosed during childhood. Pediatr Blood Cancer. 2004;42(4):364–72.
30. Green DM, Kawashima T, Stovall M, et al. Fertility of male survivors of childhood cancer: a report from the childhood cancer survivor study. J Clin Oncol. 2010;28(2):332–9.
31. Green DM, Zhu L, Wang M, et al. Effect of cranial irradiation on sperm concentration of adult survivors of childhood acute lymphoblastic leukemia: a report from the St. Jude Lifetime Cohort Study. Hum Reprod. 2017;32(6):1192–201.
32. Vini L, Hyer S, Al-Saadi A, Pratt B, Harmer C. Prognosis for fertility and ovarian function after treatment with radioiodine for thyroid cancer. Postgrad Med J. 2002;78(916):92–3.
33. Ceccarelli C, Bencivelli W, Morciano D, Pinchera A, Pacini F. ^{131}I therapy for differentiated thyroid cancer leads to an earlier onset of menopause: results of a retrospective study. J Clin Endocrinol Metab. 2001;86(8):3512–5.
34. Sanders JE, Hawley J, Levy W, et al. Pregnancies following high-dose cyclophosphamide with or without high-dose busulfan or total-body irradiation and bone marrow transplantation. Blood. 1996;87(7):3045–52.
35. Socie G, Salooja N, Cohen A, et al. Nonmalignant late effects after allogeneic stem cell transplantation. Blood. 2003;101(9):3373–85.
36. Ganz PA, Land SR, Geyer CE Jr, et al. Menstrual history and quality-of-life outcomes in women with node-positive breast cancer treated with adjuvant therapy on the NSABP B-30 trial. J Clin Oncol. 2011;29(9):1110–6.
37. Sharma P, Rock L, Kimler BF, et al. Chemotherapy-induced amenorrhea (CIA) risk associated with taxane/platinum-based chemotherapy in young (≤45 years) breast cancer patients. J Clin Oncol. 2014;32:9592.
38. Petrek JA, Naughton MJ, Case LD, et al. Incidence, time course, and determinants of menstrual bleeding after breast cancer treatment: a prospective study. J Clin Oncol. 2006;24(7):1045–51.
39. Poorvu PD, Gelber SI, Rosenberg SM, et al. Treatment-related amenorrhea among young women 1 year following diagnosis of early-stage breast cancer. J Clin Oncol. 2015;33(15):9523.

Part II

Cancer Surgery Related Complications

Prevention and Management of Complications of Surgery for Brain Tumour

24

Ashish Kumar Shrivastav

24.1 Introduction

The word "complications" as pertaining to surgical outcome is yet undefined. The characteristics included to call something as a complication include unwanted, undesirable, unexpected/expected and above all unintended. However, they are inadequate, leaving many lacunae in the strictest sense. Differences of perception among surgeons, patients and elements of subjectivity preclude a universal definition. Neurosurgical decompression or excision for brain tumour is done with the goals of establishing a tissue diagnosis, improving neurological symptoms and prolonging survival. All adverse effects are not complications and all complications are certainly not due to negligence.

24.2 Classification of Neurosurgical Complications

A. **Neurological complications**—adverse events that directly impair motor, sensory, language, or visual functions (e.g., hematoma, vascular injury, oedema).
B. **Regional complications**—adverse events related either to the wound (e.g., infection, pseudo-meningocele) or to the brain (e.g., seizures, hydrocephalus), but they are not associated with any neurologic deficit.
C. **Systemic complication**—Generalised medical conditions.

Incidence—Overall, about a quarter to a third of neurosurgical procedures will have a "complication", adverse events regardless of severity. Complications in

A. K. Shrivastav (✉)
Dharamshila Narayana Superspeciality Hospital, Delhi, India
e-mail: ashish.kumarshrivastav.dr@narayanahealth.org

K. Sood Sharma et al. (eds.), *Complications of Cancer Therapy: Best Practices in Prevention and Management*, https://doi.org/10.1007/978-981-99-0984-1_24

neurosurgical intervention in brain tumour, can be patient specific, pathology specific (nature of tumour and site of tumour), technique specific and surgeon specific.

24.3 Systemic Complication

While systemic complications are not directly related to the neurosurgical procedure, they have an adverse influence on the neurosurgical outcome contributing to morbidity and mortality.

1. **Thromboembolic events**—Deep venous thrombosis and pulmonary embolism, usually develop after the first week of neurosurgery. While most DVTs may be asymptomatic, 15% of silent DVT can lead to pulmonary embolism.

   Common risk factors include prolonged surgery and immobilization, previous DVT, malignancy, ischemic stroke, direct lower extremity trauma, limb weakness, seizure disorder, chronic smoking, use of oral contraceptive, pregnancy and puerperium, obesity, gram-negative sepsis, advance age, pregnancy and congestive heart failure. Patients with deficiencies in antithrombin III protein C, or protein S and with various genetic clotting factors abnormalities, such as factor V Leiden, not routinely screened during preoperative assessment, are also at risk for venous thromboembolism.

   Prevention and detection—Doppler ultrasonography, pulmonary CT angiogram and impedance plethysmography are used to diagnose thromboembolic events. Pneumatic leg compression devices for DVT and transvenous greenfield filter placement to prevent pulmonary embolism. Anticoagulant agents are generally not preferred as they increase haemorrhagic complication in the immediate post operative period.
2. **Nosocomial infection**—Especially meningitis, in the post op neurosurgical patient should be aggressively diagnosed and treated with antibiotics. Strict glycaemic control, stopping steroids (if feasible), implementation of strict aseptic protocols while dealing with drains and other catheters like EVD should be followed.
3. **Cardiac complications** occur in the post operative period in about 1% of patients undergoing neurosurgery. Hypo or hypertension, arrhythmias and cardiac failure should be treated appropriately.
4. **Renal complications** like acute renal failure in post op period may occur in about 1–1.5% patients undergoing glioma or meningioma surgeries. Nephrotoxic medication, dehydration and septicaemia are other factors leading to renal complications.
5. **Gastrointestinal complications** such as stress ulcers, gastritis or diarrhea/constipations can complicate patients undergoing neurosurgery for brain tumours.
6. **Endocrinological disturbances**—These may be sometimes associated with tumour surgery in the vicinity of anterior circulation, hypothalamic and sellar—suprasellar region. Fluid and electrolyte abnormalities, diabetes insipidus(DI),syndrome of inappropriate antidiuretic hormone secretion

(SIADH) or cerebral salt wasting (CSW) in neurosurgery for pituitary tumour, craniopharyngioma and hypothalamic hamartoma are common, if not routine. Fluid volume differentiates between SIADH and cerebral salt wasting.

Maintenance of normal volume and serum sodium with adequate water and sodium replacement is the mainstay of treatment in cerebral salt wasting. On the contrary, SIADH is treated with fluid restriction. Replacement of fluid with hypotonic solutions is done for diabetes insipidus initially. Replacement of antidiuretic hormone, either orally or by nasal route, is done for long term treatment.

7. **Air embolism**—Absorption of air through open venous channels, venous sinuses or diploic veins can lead to catastrophic results. Patient position during surgery in which the non-collapsible/open veins or sinuses are above the level of the heart, most commonly sitting, are the main culprits.

   Diagnosed by a sudden fall in end-tidal CO_2 level, hypotension and with transoesophageal echocardiography, this air embolism needs aggressive measures consisting of sealing of venous channels, administration of pure oxygen. Stopping nitrous oxide and rapid aspiration of air through the right atrial catheter. All this with hemodynamic stabilization prevents serious consequences.
8. **Excessive bleeding**—It can cause haemorrhage related complications viz., disseminated intravascular coagulation (DIC) and thrombocytopenia. DIC causes consumptive coagulopathy leading to further bleeding.
9. **Psychiatric complications**—Such as acute delirium or psychosis, especially in the elderly population and in prolonged ICU, are usually self-limiting once the patient comes out of the ICU, steroids or certain pain medications (tramadol in particular) are stopped.
10. **Pulmonary complications**—Last but not least, severe infection causing acute respiratory distress syndrome (ARDS) and septicaemia, may culminate in multi organ failure syndrome which entails very high mortality.

24.4 Patient Specific Complications

Extremes of age are known to be associated higher neurosurgical risk for myriad reasons.

From hypothermia, limited tolerance to blood loss (rapid or excessive), clinically asymptomatic and hence undetected congenital malformations or variations in the paediatric age group, to critically compensated degenerative changes in the elderly, age of the patient has an important bearing the development of complications.

Limitations of positioning and surgical approach, use of rigid implants, patent fontanelles and unfused cranial sutures in infants, dura adherent to skull bones in the elderly, labile blood pressure, and fragile skin pose restrictions during neurosurgery for brain.

Delicate balance and equilibrium of fluid and electrolytes, with higher susceptibility to dyselectrolytemia, dehydration or fluid overload, can result in seizures or cardiac complications.

Maintaining body temperature during long neurosurgical operations for tumours is essential.

Preoperative medical comorbidities are common and may adversely affect the perioperative period in neurosurgery for brain tumours.

Diabetes mellitus, hypertension, ischaemic heart disease, renal disease, obstructive or restrictive pulmonary conditions, primary malignancy (in neurosurgical interventions for intracranial metastatic tumours), chronic smoking, excessive alcohol consumption and poor performance scale grade, all have important bearing on the perioperative course.

Maintaining blood glucose levels less than 180 mg/dL (140 mg/dL is better) in the perioperative period mitigates hyperglycaemia related complications to large extent.

Systolic blood pressure of less than 160 mmHg (preferably 140 mmHg, if feasible) in the post operative period prevents postoperative haemorrhage and haematoma formation.

Blood pressure is prone to shoot very high during the reversal of general anaesthesia or extubation. Premature administration of drugs before adequate spontaneous respiration is restored or delay in extubation causing the patient to struggle and fight the tube or wretch, can raise both the intracranial pressure and the systemic blood pressure.

Anatomical variations can change the planning, course and results of neurosurgery for brain tumours. Complications are liable to occur if provision is not made for them.

Rare conditions not investigated during preoperative workup can cause vascular complications in brain tumour surgery. Deficiencies in antithrombin III, protein C or protein S and genetic clotting factor anomalies such as factor V Leiden, can induce venous thromboembolism.

Rupture of a emphysematous bulla during ventilation may cause intraoperative pneumothorax especially if positive end expiratory pressure is high, seriously threatening the course of the procedure.

24.5 Site Specific Complications

Skull base neurosurgery for brain tumours is, an ever-widening horizon. Microscopic and endoscopic skull base neurosurgery, involve long learning curves [1]. Previously "inoperable" areas and tumours are now being treated with better results, lesser rates of morbidity and mortality.

Skull base approaches demand critical decisions in selection of patients, and the most appropriate approach according to the pathology. Detailed imaging, micro neurosurgical anatomy knowledge, liberal use of technical gadgets and the neurosurgeon's skills honed with experience.

Vascular injuries are the most dreaded complications. Major vessels of the circle of Willis and their branches are at risk because of inadequate preoperative imaging or utilization of interventions like tumour embolization, unidentified or unattended tumour infiltration/adherence to major vessels, and direct inadvertent injury.

Neuronavigation (especially with barrier techniques in which alarms are set to prevent dangerous advance towards vascular or neural structures), intraoperative micro-Doppler or ultrasound to localize and preserve vasculature or intraoperative MRI, are well-nigh essential for safe skull base neurosurgery.

Cranial nerve palsies, partial or complete, transient or permanent are common after skull base neurosurgery for brain tumours. Oculomotor and facial palsies are the commonest. Abducens is another martyr in some cases. Lower cranial nerves are at risk in posterior fossa surgeries.

In depth analysis of the pathological anatomy, application of microneursurgical anatomy in planning the neurosurgical trajectory, gentle handling and meticulous dissection after identifying the nerve and avoiding traction or heat injury by cauterization or drilling in the vicinity of cranial nerves are essential skills in skull base approaches for brain tumours.

CSF leaks are more common in skull base neurosurgical approaches [2].

Endoscopic skull base approaches for tumour (or other indications) do not allow formal dural stitching.

Dura closure in skull bae neurosurgery is more often done by using autologous fascial grafts, fat or muscle patches, artificial dura substitutes, and neurovascular pedicled flaps. Hadad-Bassagasteguy is the mainstay in endonasal cranial base surgery [3]. It is based on the nasoseptal artery. Use of fibrin glue after such dura closure is of doubtful value at best.

Bone resection can lead to the cerebellar hanging if the posterior fossa craniectomy is more than 3 cm in size, particularly with excision of the rim of the foramen magnum, more in the paediatric age group.

Fluid and electrolyte and endocrine disturbances may appear after microscopic or endoscopic approaches for sellar-suprasellar tumours if the normal pituitary descends from the bony defect in the sellar floor. Pituitary stalk traction or ischaemia is an unusual complication in this "herniation".

Neurosurgery for tumours in the anterior cranial fossa requires the frontal lobes to be displaced to reach various entry point to cisterns. This used to be achieved by fixed retractors applied for long durations leading to "retraction haematomas", cerebral oedema or contusions [4, 5]. Such insult to the frontal lobes occasionally required re-exploration for evacuation in the early postoperative period. Late consequences of these complications were encephalomalacia, seizures, dysphasia/aphasia, cognitive and intellectual deterioration. Dynamic retraction by suction tube is safer and more efficient.

Fixed long duration retraction has been replaced by making the frontal lobes fall back by better positioning, skull base approaches to minimize retraction in select situations, CSF drainage for brain relaxation by early opening of cisterns to facilitate CSF drainage, lumbar drainage, and neuroanaesthetic techniques.

CSF leaks or fistulas (rhinorrhoea) are common more so if the tumour erodes the floor of the anterior cranial fossa. If CSF diversion, by any standard, appropriate method is not effective, formal repair may be required.

24.5.1 Pneumocephalus

Sources of infection in close proximity, the frontal, ethmoid and sphenoid sinuses, direct communication with the nasal cavity after some types of tumour excision, may increase chances of infection.

24.5.2 Cerebrovascular

Vasospasm during neurosurgery for brain tumours is treated with local application of papaverine soaked neuro cotton patties. Pseudoaneurysm formation may occur rarely if traction or rough handling of an artery causes intimal disruption. Preserving at least on olfactory nerve is desirable. Sacrifice of one or both olfactory nerves, is quite common. Other cranial nerves at risk are the optic, oculomotor, trochlear and the abducens. Unless the optic nerves are compromised preoperatively, loss of visual acuity is uncommon.

24.5.3 Cosmetic

Ptosis resulting from injury to orbital branches of the facial nerve, poor bony alignment following orbitozygomatic approach, or removal orbital roof/floor can lead to orbital deformity and may cause enophthalmos.

Depressions in the forehead due to underlying burr holes after anterior fossa approaches are particularly unsightly frontal approaches and should be meticulously repaired.

Middle cranial fossa approaches can cause traction or injury to the greater superficial petrosal nerve leading to facial nerve injury. Internal carotid artery within the petrous bone may be injured in skull base route for petrous—petroclival meningiomas. Bony dehiscence over the ICA, a normal congenital variation, increases the risk. Drilling around various foramens in this approach can cause heat induced cranial nerve damage, best prevented by copious irrigation. Using this route for small intracanalicular vestibular schwannomas, while providing higher chance of hearing preservation, places the facial nerve between the surgeon and the tumour increasing risk facial nerve damage.

CSF leak may develop in middle cranial fossa neurosurgery due to a damaged tegmen tympani and overlying dura, space around the ICA left open, open mastoid air cells or vestibular apparatus. Meticulous bone wax packing and water tight dural closure prevents CSF leak from these sites.

Temporalis muscle ischaemia and atrophy can lead to headaches, difficulty in mastication and unsightly depression in the temporal region.

Posterior fossa is unique due to the dense and compact position of a large number of vital neural structures like the brain stem and cranial nerves VI–XII, the three arteries (superior cerebellar, anterior inferior cerebellar and post inferior cerebellar) and the vertebral arteries joining to form the basilar artery, the fourth ventricle and boundaries of major sinuses (transverse, sigmoid, occipital and the marginal). Inadvertent injury to a single perforating artery supplying the brain stem or the draining veins can lead to brain stem infarcts [6]. Vasospasm of the arteries can cause damage even without obvious injury. Anatomic variations in the course of the vertebral arteries or the basilar artery are common making them susceptible to injury. Operating in narrow trajectories in the midst of the cranial nerves, blood vessels and sinuses can be daunting and risk of injury high.

From making the surgeon miserable during surgery, converting a routine procedure hazardous, to complete inability to achieve the tumour exposure or its decompression or excision, positioning influences the outcome.

This is particularly important in prone or park bench positions for posterior fossa tumours. Retrosigmoid exposure is a workhorse approach for cerebellopontine angle tumours. Minor nuances in exposing the sigmoid sinus' medial edge or angulation and rotation of the head can preclude smooth exposure of the trigeminal nerve or the vestibulocochlear-facial nerve complex.

Undue flexion or rotation neck can cause venous congestion due to obstruction of jugular veins. In the elderly with cervical spine degenerative changes or other patients with borderline asymptomatic and undetected disc pathologies can precipitate cervical cord or nerve root injuries.

Eye injury during prone position, occasionally leading to loss of vision, brachial plexus injury due to excessive traction on the shoulder or not protecting it by padding of the axilla in the lateral or park-bench position, ulnar at the elbow, common peroneal nerve at the fibular head, and the lateral femoral cutaneous nerve at the iliac crest or shoulder dislocations caused by hyperabduction of arms, are consequences of poor positioning.

Tumour manipulations, especially cystic tumours, or lack definite plains of cleavage between the tumour and adjacent is known to cause traction injuries to the brain stem, nerves and arteries and veins.

Incomplete tumour resection may be forced on the surgeon in any of these situations with consequent problems.

24.5.4 Pineal Tumours

Site specific—nestled in between the deep venous channels, cerebellum, collicular plate, and pulvinars, these tumours pose the highest degree of neurosurgical challenge, not to be embarked on lightly or by the tenderfoot.

Parinaud syndrome, pupillary changes, impaired focusing, accommodation, and extraocular movements, due to tumour dissection off the quadrigeminal plate, are usually temporary but slow to recover [7, 8].

Hydrocephalus if present before surgery should be treated with CSF diversion by ventriculoperitoneal shunt (VPS) or endoscopic third ventriculostomy (ETV). Peritoneal seeding is sometimes considered as a contraindication for VPS and ETV preferred. For some benign non-progressing tumours, treating the hydrocephalus may be sufficient. Acute hydrocephalus due to blood or tumour debris blocking a pre-existing VPS or ETV, requires urgent revision of the VPS/ETV or an urgent EVD.

Many varied types of tumours, benign and malignant. Complete removal, though desirable, may not be possible at all times. Haemorrhage in the residual tumour is the dreaded complication, more so in the malignant tumours.

In pineal region tumours, more than any other, it is very important to tailor the treatment strategy in each case. From masterly inactivity and serial scans in pineal cyst or low grade gliomas, to just CSF drainage for benign lesions associated with hydrocephalus and no significant growth potential, to highly radiosensitive germ cell tumours and metastatic malignant lesions, strategy should be individualized.

24.6 Surgical Complications in Neurosurgery for Brain Tumours

24.6.1 Oedema

Neurosurgical intervention of any kind and complexity will produce oedema. Clinically silent and limited oedema seen on only on scans may produce an acceptable lag in recovery of sensorium and normal neurological function, not requiring any treatment over and above the routine. Severe oedema is associated with altered or worsening sensorium, neurological deficits and seizures. Oedema out of proportion to the neurosurgical intervention and usually unresponsive to standard treatment measures is termed “malignant cerebral oedema”.

All the three pathophysiological causes contribute to postoperative oedema.

Venous flow retarded by surgically damaged or sacrificed veins or thrombosis of veins lead to haemodynamically induced oedema. Venous obstruction may also be caused by incorrect positioning. Venous thrombosis may occur intraoperatively due to hypotension or in the postoperative period due to dehydration.

Direct damage of neural tissue or ischaemia produced in the parenchyma either due to prolonged retraction or arterial compromise, cause cytotoxic oedema.

“Flooding” of brain with blood may be induced by nitrous oxide and isoflurane. Halothane and enflurane can impair CSF absorption. Minor oedema does not require any intervention other than maintaining normal blood pressure and hydration, elevation of head above the level of heart and unobstructed respiration. Flexion of neck can impair jugular venous outflow from the brain and is better avoided.

Moderate oedema is treated by intravenous mannitol, hypertonic saline or frusemide. Hypertonic saline is preferred in situations where fluid volume is to be maintained and in paediatric patients. Hypertonic saline as an agent to reduce intracranial pressure is given rapidly unlike its slow infusion to correct hyponatremia. Urinary catheterization, preventing cough and constipation are measures to prevent raised intrabdominal/intrathoracic pressures which impair venous return and increase intracranial pressure. Malignant cerebral oedema usually does not resolve by routine measures. Such oedema, especially if caused by and associated with residual tumour or postoperative haematoma, requires surgical intervention by way of removal of bone flap (decompressive craniectomy).

24.6.2 Haemorrhage

While 10–50% of postoperative scans following brain tumour neurosurgery may reveal haemorrhage in the operative site, only about a tenth of these will require active intervention, and approximately 1–2% require reoperation [9]. Postoperative haematomas are usually at the primary operative site. A very small number of postoperative haematomas may develop at a remote site. They can be intraparenchymal, subdural, subarachnoid or extradural and in ipsilateral or contralateral compartments.

Not all are due to inadequate haemostasis. Dural penetration/injury to dural or subdural blood vessels by pins of the head holding clamps can lead to such a situation, particularly overzealous application in the paediatric patients. Operating with lower blood pressure may reduce blood loss but at the time of haemostasis and before dural closure, blood pressure ought to be normal. Rise in blood pressure after haemostasis and dural closure can cause haemorrhage and haematoma formation later. Blood pressure is particularly prone to shoot very high during reversal of general anaesthesia or extubation. Premature reversal agents before adequate establishment of spontaneous respiration or delay in extubation which causes the patient to struggle can raise both intracranial pressure and systemic blood pressure. During suturing of dura after tumour excision, an unidentified injury to surface veins is a known cause for subdural haematoma formation. Even excessive bleeding from scalp vessels may seep in through bone cuts or burr hole sites and lead to an extradural haematoma. If the dura closure is not watertight, this can actually cause intraparenchymal blood collection. Rapid decompression of ventricles by uncontrolled release of CSF during a tumour surgery or excessive use of antioedema agents like mannitol causing undue brain shrinkage are situations in which remote subdural veins may bleed leading to remote site haemorrhage.

Evacuation of haematomas after brain tumour surgery reduces mortality rates but may not result in improving morbidity. Residual neurological deficits can be significant, hence, attention to meticulous surgical technique at all times during the operation, during reversal of anaesthesia and early postoperative period is mandatory. Normotension, euvolemia and high degree of alertness to intraoperative development of disseminated intravascular coagulopathy or fall in platelet count in surgeries involving excessive blood loss prevents postoperative haematoma formation. An unexplained brain swelling with a clean operative field usually implies a remote site haematoma formation.

24.6.3 Infarction

Direct injury to arteries adjacent to the tumour, arteries encased by tumours, manipulation or traction on arteries causing vasospasm and delayed compression of arteries from oedema or post operative haematoma [10], lead to infarcts. Hypotension compounds the deleterious effects of such infarcts. Infarcts can produce neurological deficits by direct ischaemia which may improve depending on the degree of collateral supply—the "umbra" and "penumbra" phenomenon. Oedema is usually produced by these infarcts, adding increased intracranial pressure to the pathophysiology.

To a very large extent, arterial misadventures are directly surgeon and technique dependent com.

Exposed brain parenchyma and surface during a brain tumour neurosurgery should be kept wet and frequently irrigated with normal saline. Dry cortical surface can lead to thrombosis of cortical veins. Unduly aggressive coagulation of veins may retard venous outflow. Tumours near the major venous sinuses are associated with sinus thrombosis. It is of great help to see the venous anatomy prior to embarking on brain tumour surgery, a step invariably neglected. Neurosurgical trajectory is influenced by venous anatomy. Sacrifice of veins should be avoided at all cost.

Venous infarcts, acute or chronic, lead to cerebral oedema which may be associated with venous haematoma. They are progressive and produce more oedema and mass effect than comparable arterial infarcts, and require removal of bone flap. Attempts to decompress the infarcts particularly those with haemorrhage meet with little success. Resolution of venous infarct leads to lesser neurological deficits than arterial infarcts.

24.6.4 Seizures

Seizures occurring in the first 24 h after neurosurgery for brain tumours in the supratentorial compartment harbingers of serious complications—haemorrhage or infarction. Prophylactic anticonvulsant medication, though not supported by evidence, is widely used. Dyselectrolytemia (hyponatremia, hypocalcaemia, hypomagnesemia) and hypoxia are other culprits. Past history of seizures lowers the threshold in postoperative period and prophylactic or ongoing anticonvulsants are given.

24.6.5 Neurological Deficits

From minor or undetected cognitive deficits to dense motor and cranial nerve deficits, neurosurgery for brain tumours can lead to these site specific deficits. The initial dismal picture usually improves as the deficits get confined to the directly and more completely injured neuronal structures and oedema subsides. Late appearing deficits are the consequence of ischaemia. The extent of deficits also depends on the neural "density" and plasticity of the affected brain. Deeper the structure injured, denser the deficit. Brain tumours in the insular region and thalamus, most commonly gliomas, are a case in point.

Hydrocephalus—Acute hydrocephalus, a life threatening condition, may develop almost immediately in the postoperative period, Intraoperative causes (haemorrhage, tumour tissue and debris) may acutely block CSF pathways. Acute hydrocephalus is more dangerous in patients without prior ventricular enlargement. Preoperatively enlarged ventricles compensate to some extent. Oedema or haematoma adjacent to ventricles or CSF pathways and procedures around the third and fourth ventricles leads to hydrocephalus by pressure from outside. Acute hydrocephalus can be fatal and should be treated with external ventricular drain, some of which may need a ventriculoperitoneal shunt permanently.

CSF Leaks—Acute CSF leaks are common but chronic fistulas, rare. They are due to faulty closure technique, dural tears, thinned out dura in the posterior fossa, increased CSF pressure, wound complications and sepsis. Inability to identify the possibility and underlying cause are both surgeon specific and technique specific complications.

If CSF can come out, infection can march in—meningitis or ventriculitis are serious consequences of such leaks.

Pneumocephalus—Pneumocephalus, acute or delayed, develops due to trapping of air during closure, suction of air from lumbar drain or basal dura after skull base neurosurgery [11].

Most cases can be managed by placing the patient in 30° Fowler's position, giving 100% oxygen by mask and preventing Valsalva manoeuvre. Rarely it may require reopening the craniotomy or a frontal burr hole to release air compressing brain parenchyma.

Osteomyelitis, empyema or abscess formation are almost always treated surgically with appropriate antibiotics.

24.7 Technique Specific Complications

These complications are dependent on the neurosurgical approach, the neurosurgical technique and the neurosurgeon her/himself.

- Strict adherence to fundamentals of neurosurgical technique, regular upgradation of the neurosurgical repertoire by training and apprenticeship leads to enhanced skills. Of utmost importance is to progressively become a safer neurosurgeon. And in the current medicolegal context, safer not only for the patient but also for oneself.
- The medical status of the patient decides whether surgery is needed at all. The safety of general anaesthesia, preoperative radiological and special investigations to create the most comprehensive road map—the best trajectory and approach, need for preoperative embolization of vascular lesions, the strategies for complication avoidance and intraoperative/postoperative management of

complications, involvement of colleagues from otorhinolaryngology or maxillofacial departments etc., should be established.

- A critical assessment of one's own skills and capability, and of the neurosurgical setup is essential to prevent complications. Neurosurgery is arachnoid surgery, approaches are cistern based and dissection is sharp.***"RES IPSA LOQUITOR" Every possible safeguard should be taken to avoid wrong side craniotomy.***

24.7.1 Tips for Surgical Approach

1. Successful technique starts with proper positioning which allows adequate exposure without retraction or manipulation of brain, venous drainage, prevents pressure points and injury to eyes and allows the surgeon to operate for long hours.
2. The best approach to a brain tumour is the one which is shortest, whose trajectory does not violate vital neurological structures like the motor cortex, cross cranial nerves or major vessels, requires the least possible or no brain retraction at all and allows for maximum resection. An approach which allows devascularization of a tumour at the earliest is preferred.
3. The approach should be the best for that particular patient, for that particular tumour and for that particular neurosurgeon and his skill and experience.
   - Respecting the veins is a fundamental of neurosurgical technique which prevents oedema (including malignant oedema), infarction, and seizures. Anatomical variations in the venous architecture are common. This variation can be the cause of direct venous injury if not examined preoperatively.
   - The importance of injury to major dural sinuses (parasagittal/falcine meningiomas), deep cerebral veins (pineal region tumours), superficial veins (vein of Labbe, vein of Trolard) and the superior petrosal vein (cerebellopontine), is usually associated with sinister results and neurological deficits.
   - Bridging veins are the usual cause of remote site haematomas due to rapid decompression release of CSF. If necessary, bridging veins should be sacrificed as close to the dura as possible. Cortical veins are at risk if the exposed cortical surface is not irrigated frequently.
   - Prolonged retraction especially with fixed retractors, was associated with venous oedema, infarction and late venous thrombosis. Dynamic retraction is the technique to avoid such problems. Excessive coagulation of veins can be avoided by using neuro-cotton patties, surgical and some patience.
   - Direct intraoperative arterial injury is invariably due to poor surgical technique. If the artery is encased or adherent to the tumour, injury may be avoided by preoperative planning, exercising sound surgical judgement and respecting fundamental rules and principles of neurosurgical technique. Electronic barriers utilized during neuronavigation and use of intraoperative vascular micro Doppler or angiogram, aid in preserving arteries during delicate dissections. Discretion being the better part of valour, leaving a part of tumour is wiser than "extirpating "it with the artery.

- Primary watertight dural closure is best. Primary duraplasty with autologous fascia or dural substitutes is next best. CSF leaks may still occur after adequate dural closure if CSF pressure is high or in the face of infection.

24.8 Tumour Specific Complications

24.8.1 Gliomas

Aggressive safe surgical decompression followed by radiotherapy remains the mainstay of glioma treatment. The amount of tumour remaining (Residual tumour Volume, ROL) and Degree of resection (Extent of Resection, EOR), remain the main prognostic factors. Even in low grade gliomas a high EOR correlates with higher survival.

Gliomas spread without respect to anatomical structures. While gray matter damage produces obvious deficits depending on the location of the tumour, increasing attention is being paid to white matter involvement and techniques to reduce neurological deficits. Intratumoral decompression prevent direct injury to adjacent normal tissue. Preoperative imaging with diffusion tensor imaging (DTI or tractography) delineates white matter architecture and helps plan a three-dimensional surgical roadmap. Intraoperative tools such as intraoperative MRI (MRI suite, iMRI), ultrasound especially in tumours with cystic component, 5 aminolevulinic acid fluorescence (5-ALA) and conventional neuronavigation with or without barrier technique increase the EOR, reduce ROL and generally lead to better surgical result and improved overall prognosis. Intraoperative mapping of critical structures and awake craniotomy further increase the safety in resection.

24.8.2 Meningiomas

An higher risk of seizures and thromboembolic complications is associated with meningiomas.

24.8.3 Craniopharyngiomas

Aseptic meningitis from the fluid released peroperatively from the cystic part of craniopharyngioma, can be troublesome.

Traction injuries to adjacent vessels and neural structures are more common in total removal of craniopharyngiomas due to adherence of the tumour to these structures.

24.8.4 Epidermoid

Aseptic meningitis due the spillage of contents of a epidermoid may be the forerunner of secondary bacterial meningitis or persistent CSF leaks.

24.8.5 Pituitary Tumours

While trans sphenoidal approaches revolutionized the surgery for sellar and suprasellar tumours, there are situations where transcranial approach may be preferred.

Indications for the transcranial route

Rudimentary sphenoid sinus
"Kissing" carotids
Extensions not accessible by endoscope (parasellar, retrosellar, retroclival, subfrontal, sometimes suprasellar)
Constriction of diaphragma sellae in "dumbbell" tumours
Fibrotic tumour due to prior radiotherapy or surgery
Cavernous sinus invasion
Brain invasion, cerebral oedema
Involvement or encasement of major vessels of the circle of Willis
Coexistent adjacent aneurysm

Transcranial route is associated with higher incidence of diabetes insipidus, visual deterioration and endocrine disturbances. Hypothalamic injury though rare, is known when the pial boundaries are breached as evident by oedema in preoperative scans.

Major vessels and their perforators, optic apparatus proximity especially prefixed optic chiasm, cavernous sinus on either side, hypothalamus and pituitary stalk are vulnerable to operative trauma. Large tumours distorting normal vasculature and optic apparatus, obliterating cisterns and those associated with perilesional oedema should serve as warning for the surgeon in planning the surgery. If the tumour shares the blood supply with the optic structures, visual impairment may occur due to devascularization during decompression or haemostasis. Preoperative hormone profile done before surgery guides postoperative hormone replacement in the particularly replacement of thyroxine for free T4, and hydrocortisone for cortisol deficiency. Injury to the anterior pituitary or the pituitary stalk lead to partial or complete hypopituitarism. Central adrenal insufficiency, a potentially life-threatening condition manifesting clinically as lethargy, altered sensorium, dyselectrolytemia, volume depletion sufficient to produce hypotension and tachycardia. This develops due to mineralocorticoid and glucocorticoid underproduction.

Diabetes insipidus is common and managed along standard protocols for the triphasic course of the condition. Pituitary apoplexy is an emergency. Acute haemorrhage within the pituitary macroadenoma can cause sudden loss of vision. This loss of vision can be reversed if the surgical intervention is in time.

24.8.6 Ependymomas/Medulloblastomas/Pilocytic Astrocytomas

One third of medulloblastomas invade the floor of the fourth ventricle. Dissecting this part of the tumour can cause ipsilateral nuclear palsy of the abducens and facial nerves and contralateral hemiparesis. While majority of the juvenile pilocytic astrocytomas arise within cerebellar parenchyma, a small fraction grows exophytically from the brain stem in to the fourth ventricle. Pulling on this subgroup puts the brain stem in jeopardy. Ependymomas get their blood supply from perforators from the brain stem. Unless formally coagulated and cut, they can retract and bleed within the brain stem. Those ependymomas which grow out from the foramen of Luschka and grow towards the cerebellopontine angle place the lower cranial nerves and the vertebrobasilar complex in danger.

References

1. Mazzoni A, Krengli M. Historical development of the treatment of skull base tumours. Rep Pract Oncol Radiother. 2016;21(4):319–24. https://doi.org/10.1016/j.rpor.2014.12.001. Epub 2015 Jan 16. PMID: 27330417; PMCID: PMC4899480.
2. Sokoya M, Mourad M, Ducic Y. Complications of skull base surgery. Semin Plast Surg. 2017;31(4):227–30. https://doi.org/10.1055/s-0037-1607203. Epub 2017 Oct 25. PMID: 29075162; PMCID: PMC5656445.
3. Wardas P, Tymowski M, Piotrowska-Seweryn A, Markowski J, Ładziński P. Hadad-Bassagasteguy flap in skull base reconstruction—current reconstructive techniques and evaluation of criteria used for qualification for harvesting the flap. Wideochir Inne Tech Maloinwazyjne. 2019;14(2):340–7. https://doi.org/10.5114/wiitm.2018.79633. Epub 2018 Nov 15. PMID: 31119003; PMCID: PMC6528130.
4. Fujimoto S, Kuyama H, Nishimoto K, Akioka T, Nagao S, Nishimoto A. Effect of local brain retraction on local cerebral blood flow and neural function. Experimental study. Neurol Med Chir (Tokyo). 1982;22:893–900. (in Japanese).
5. Kageyama Y, Fukuda K, Kobayashi S, Odaki M, Nakamura H, Satoh A, Watanabe Y. Cerebral vein disorders and postoperative brain damage associated with the pterional approach in aneurysm surgery. Neurol Medico-chir. 1992;32(10):733–8. https://doi.org/10.2176/nmc.32.733. https://www.jstage.jst.go.jp/article/nmc1959/32/10/32_10_733/_article/-char/en.
6. Dubey A, Sung WS, Shaya M, Patwardhan R, Willis B, Smith D, Nanda A. Complications of posterior cranial fossa surgery—an institutional experience of 500 patients. Surg Neurol. 2009;72(4):369–75. https://doi.org/10.1016/j.surneu.2009.04.001. Epub 2009 Jul 14. PMID: 19604553.
7. Kennedy BC, Bruce JN. Surgical approaches to the pineal region. Neurosurg Clin N Am. 2011;22(03):367–80.
8. Murphy M, Gilder H, McCutcheon BA, et al. Increased operative time for benign cranial nerve tumor resection correlates with increased morbidity postoperatively. J Neurol Surg B Skull Base. 2016;77(04):350–7.
9. De la Garza-Ramos R, Kerezoudis P, Tamargo RJ, Brem H, Huang J, Bydon M. Surgical complications following malignant brain tumor surgery: an analysis of 2002–2011 data. Clin Neurol Neurosurg. 2016;140:6–10. https://doi.org/10.1016/j.clineuro.2015.11.005. Epub 2015 Nov 12. PMID: 26615463; PMCID: PMC4750489.

10. Ko SB. Perioperative stroke: pathophysiology and management. Korean J Anesthesiol. 2018;71(1):3–11. https://doi.org/10.4097/kjae.2018.71.1.3. Epub 2018 Feb 1. PMID: 29441169; PMCID: PMC5809704.
11. Dabdoub CB, Salas G, Silveira Edo N, Dabdoub CF. Review of the management of pneumocephalus. Surg Neurol Int. 2015;6:155. https://doi.org/10.4103/2152-7806.166195.

Complications of Oral Cancer Surgery Reconstruction

25

Ashish Goel and Vikash Nayak

25.1 Introduction

Composite oral resection and neck dissection including marginal/segmental mandibulectomy, hemi/subtotal or total glossectomy, neck dissection and reconstruction of defect by loco-regional flaps or free flaps are the main treatment modality for oral cancers. The complication rates for oral cavity carcinoma surgery may be as high as 20–50%. Comorbidities such as cardiac, respiratory or hepatic diseases, diabetes and malnutrition and other surgical factors contribute to higher risk of complications. Cancer-related risk factors such as advanced stage at presentation and critical tumor location may result in more extensive resections with more consequential sequelae and rehabilitation needs. Risk of surgical complications can be higher in patients who have a history of prior radiotherapy or require adjuvant radiation therapy.

Complications of Oral Cancer Surgery may be classified as local or systemic, minor or major and immediate, intermediate or late (Table 25.1). Surgical complications will depend on extent of resection, type of neck dissection, choice of reconstruction and duration of surgery.

A. Goel (✉) · V. Nayak
Department of Surgical Oncology, Jaypee Hospital, Noida, Uttar Pradesh, India

K. Sood Sharma et al. (eds.), *Complications of Cancer Therapy: Best Practices in Prevention and Management*, https://doi.org/10.1007/978-981-99-0984-1_25

Table 25.1 Complications of oral resection & reconstruction

Immediate local complications
1. Bleeding
2. Raised intracranial tension
3. Intracranial thrombosis
4. Carotid sinus syndrome
5. Airway obstruction
6. Nerve injury
Intermediate local complications
1. Wound healing and infection
2. Flap Failure
3. Oro-cutaneous fistula
4. Seroma
5. Chyle fistula
Late complications
1. Functional deficits
2. Recurrence
3. Hypertrophic scars

25.2 Complications of Oral Resection & Neck Dissection

25.2.1 Bleeding

Potential sources of bleeding in oral resections & neck dissection include injury to major blood vessels, bleeding from suture line and anastomotic sites and from skin flaps. The most common sources of bleed are small anterior cervical veins, branches of maxillary artery, pterygoid plexus, external carotid artery, thyrocervical trunk and occasionally lingual artery. Patients may present with bleeding into oral cavity/pharynx, hematoma under flap or increased drain collection during early post operative period. It is very important to identify warning bleeds to avoid catastrophic sequelae. General steps of management include adequate resuscitation and early treatment of cause. Pressure over neck rarely controls the bleed. In case of warning bleeds, patient should be taken up for re-exploration as soon as possible and tracheostomy should be performed with cuffed tube to avoid aspiration.

25.2.2 Air Embolism

Another major complication of neck dissection is air embolism due to injury to internal jugular vein which may present as hypotension, cardiovascular collapse and arrest. Surgical management includes initial tamponade, surgical exploration to identify, skeletonize, clamp and ligate the major vascular site in order to reduce chances of air embolism. Bleeding from carotid artery directly is very rare but has life threatening consequences. Long term prognosis is poor and patients who survive often have neurological deficits. Predisposing factors include direct involvement by tumor, atheromatous disease, stripping of adventitia during surgery with thrombosis of vasa vasorum leading to gangrene of vessel wall. It is most commonly seen in post radiation neck dissections.

25.2.3 Carotid Blowout

Carotid blowout occurs in patients undergoing post radiation surgery or those with salivary oro-cutaneous fistulae. Patients should be explored at the earliest in order to ligate and transfix the bleeding site and cover with vascularized flaps. Most patients may have long term sequelae in the form of hemiplegia, aphasia, dysarthria. This needs immediate intervention in the form vein patch or an inter-positional vessel graft along with adequate coverage of vessel with well-vascularized flaps to prevent further blowouts. A second free flap or the pedicled pectoralis major muscle flap is ideal for this purpose.

25.2.4 Raised Intracranial Tension

It commonly occurs after division of internal jugular vein during radical neck dissection (RND). The risk is threefold with unilateral IJV ligation versus fivefold risk with bilateral ligation. Patients present with headache and restlessness, bradycardia, hypertension, swelling and cyanosis of face. Risk of raised ICT can be decreased by avoiding hyperextension of neck during surgery, avoiding tight dressings around the neck and safeguard at least one IJV. Sequential ligation should be done if bilateral RND is indicated. Medical management includes administration of dexamethasone and mannitol injection.

25.2.5 Intracranial Thrombosis

Post-operative imaging may demonstrate intracranial thrombosis in up to 30% cases after RND, most frequently in sigmoid and transverse sinus. Lateralized headache in post operative patients should not be ignored and patients should be subjected to MRI Brain for early diagnosis.

25.2.6 Carotid Sinus Syndrome

It usually occurs if there is extensive post-operative scarring and recurrent tumor over the carotid bulb. Careful dissection should be done over the carotid bulb and the anaesthetist should be informed while dissecting in the area. Local lignocaine spray may be used if intraoperative bradycardia occurs.

25.2.7 Airway Obstruction

Airway obstruction occurs during extensive oropharyngeal resections and bilateral neck dissection, especially during post radiation salvage surgery. Elective tracheostomy is indicated, when performing extensive oropharyngeal or craniofacial resections, central arch mandibulectomies, total/subtotal glossectomies and during post radiation salvage surgery.

25.2.8 Nerve Injury

The nerves at risk for iatrogenic injury during oral cancer surgery include spinal accessory nerve, marginal mandibular nerve, phrenic nerve, vagus, hypoglossal and lingual nerve. These nerve are at risk due to their anatomic proximity to the surgical field. Operating surgeon should have a good working knowledge of these nerves in order to avoid injury by transaction or traction during neck dissection.

Injury to **spinal accessory nerve** (SAN) during neck dissection leads to long term sequelae. In most cases SAN can be safely preserved without jeopardising completeness of resection as long as it not grossly involved by disease. Care should be taken when elevating skin flaps in posterior triangle of neck where SAN is surprisingly superficial. Consistent and rapid identification of SAN in upper neck during dissection can be facilitated by identification of Erb's points. SAN nerve injury may result into drooping of shoulder and limitation of range of movement of shoulder joint due to subluxation. Patients usually present with shoulder pain, stiffness, discomfort & flattening of shoulder. It is important to realize that nerve preservation is not synonymous with nerve function preservation as above symptoms may develop even when the spinal accessory nerve is not sacrificed. Careful dissection around the vicinity of nerve with limited use of electrocautery, and early identification based on known anatomical landmarks, may help to reduce chances of SAN injury.

Although the **ansa cervicalis** is frequently sacrificed during neck dissection; vagus, lingual, hypoglossal and marginal mandibular nerves should be identified and preserved. Identification of **marginal mandibular nerve** is at risk of injury during incision and elevation of skin flap for standard neck dissections, and access to oral cavity for composite resection. It runs on under surface of platysma & superficial to facial vein in submandibular gland region. If the nerve cannot be identified by visual inspection through the layers of the deep cervical fascia; its integrity should be preserved by dividing the facial vessels approximately 1 cm below the lower border of mandible and then retracting the divided ends upwards, in order to lift it away from the surgical field. Injury to this nerve leads to altered mobility of corner of the mouth due to disruption of innervation to orbicularis oris and depressor anguli oris muscles along with cosmetic appeal. Careful planning of neck incisions, taking into consideration the route of the nerve and identification early during flap elevation, are the best ways to prevent inadvertent iatrogenic injury.

Hypoglossal nerve is responsible for motor innervation to ipsilateral tongue while lingual nerve provides sensation and taste innervation, via chorda tympani branch of facial nerve to anterior two thirds of oral tongue. Both nerves may be injured during neck dissection & during glossectomy and excision of floor of mouth. Unless there is gross neural invasion by cancer, or the path of the nerve runs directly through the tumour, both should be preserved. Hypoglossal nerve can be identified crossing the external carotid artery and emerging from underneath the posterior belly of digastric on hyoglossus muscle. It may be inadvertently damaged at both these points. Hypoglossal nerve dysfunction presents with deviation of tongue to ipsilateral side of injury (wheel barrow sign), accidental tongue biting and dysarthria. Some patients may also experience difficulty with mastication and deglutition.

Lingual nerve injury may occur from traction or dissection during excision of submandibular gland or resection of floor of mouth. Sometimes the effects of injury may not be recognized until later in postoperative period. Patients present with loss of sensation in ipsilateral tongue resulting into difficulty with mastication speech and swallowing.

Injury to **phrenic nerve** may lead to paralysis of ipsilateral diaphragm as it is the only motor innervation to it. Diaphragm is responsible for 70% of respiratory movements and injury to phrenic nerve may have long-term pulmonary sequelae. Transient neuropraxia often manifest sub-clinically in post-operative period with changes identified only on plain chest X Ray. In severe cases respiration may be compromised especially when pectoralis major muscle flaps are used for oral cavity reconstruction. Surgical dissection should be limited to a layer superficial to prevertebral fascia to prevent iatrogenic injury.

The **brachial plexus** lies between scalenus anterior and medius muscles in posterior triangle. It is not usually encountered other than in the extended radical neck dissection but knowledge of its location is important in preventing further readily avoidable complications. Intentional transection of **vagus nerve** may result in intraoperative cardiac problems of for which the anaesthetist needs to be alert and responsive.

25.2.9 Wound Infection and Healing

Local complications such as wound healing and infection are common to all surgical procedures. In oral cancer surgery wound complications may result from surgical site infections, skin flap and soft tissue necrosis with resultant dehiscence and locoregional/microvascular flap failures. Risk factors include wound infection, poor choice of incisions, closure of skin flaps under tension and presence of hematoma or seroma. Patients with anaemia, diabetes and poor nutrition have more wound healing problems. The age old principles of proper preop skin preparation and adherence to good surgical techniques should be followed in oral cancer surgery and neck dissection to allow for good wound healing and prevent surgical site infections. Skin flaps should be elevated in sub-platysmal planes and three point junction sutures should be avoided during skin closure. Skin flaps should be kept moist and should not be allowed to dry out during surgery. Careful tissue approximation should be done avoiding any dead spaces as well as preventing marginal skin necrosis by tight sutures. If necessary margins should be freshened for 2–3 mm prior to skin approximation. Tracheostomy and drain catheters should not be placed through main incision to avoid wound contamination. Prophylactic antibiotics should be administered for 5–7 days to all patients undergoing composite resection of upper aerodigestive tract and those undergoing revision surgery or post radiation salvage surgery.

25.2.10 Oro-cutaneous Fistula

Oro – cutaneous fistula are most commonly seen after composite resections of tongue, floor of mouth and mandible combined with neck dissection. The incidence and extent depends on amount of tissue resected and completeness of reconstruction. All patients presenting with delayed fluid collection under skin flaps in neck and reconstructed flaps in oral cavity and cheek should be aspirated and oral cavity carefully examined to look for any dehiscence. In case OCF is identified skin wound should be enlarged to allow adequate drainage of collection and wound irrigation should be performed 2–3 times a day. All necrotic tissue should be excised in staged manner and Ryles' tube feeding should be maintained. The key principle of management is to reduce oral contamination into fistula from above and facilitate egress from neck wound inferiorly. Patients require clinical vigilance and early recognition in order to facilitate early wound healing and commencement of adjuvant therapy. Most wounds gradually granulate from deeper aspects and finally skin closes on its own in 2–3 weeks. Closure of wound with secondary flaps is indicated only if there is major tissue loss and only when a clean granulating recipient bed is available. Rarely non-healing of oro-cutaneous fistula may be due to recurrent tumour, presence of distal obstruction of pharynx and metabolic abnormalities such as hypothyroidism and malnutrition.

25.2.11 Seroma

Fluid mostly collects in supraclavicular fossa especially in patients with high BMI. All dead spaces should be obliterated after neck dissection and drains should be kept in place until skin flaps adhere to underlying fascia. Repeated aspiration of seroma and pressure dressings should be done if seroma collects after drain removal. Prophylactic antibiotics may be administered if there is haemorrhagic or purulent collection. It is important to differentiate simple seroma collection from oro-cutaneous fistulae.

25.2.12 Chylous Fistula

Chyle leaks are more common with comprehensive neck dissection as against patients undergoing supra-omohyoid dissection. The thoracic duct arises from the cysterna chyli at level of second lumbar vertebra in abdomen and crosses the thorax before terminating in left IJV. If the undamaged chyle duct is identified during neck dissection, it should be left undisturbed. Intraoperative identification may be done by performing forced Valsalva manoeuvre with patient in Trendelenburg position. If damaged duct is identified; repair should be done with 4-0 or 5-0 prolene sutures buttressed with muscle patch. Sometimes inadvertent thoracic duct damage may remain unrecognized during surgery and may present later with chylous discharge in neck drain. Such patients should be put to bed rest with head elevation and strict input/output and weight charting. Local wound care should be done with regular pressure dressings in supraclavicular fossa and collections should be aspirated if not adequately drained. Patients should be managed with enteral feeds low in long chained triglycerides (LCTs) & high in medium chained triglycerides (MCTs) or with Total Parenteral Nutrition. Low output leaks may be managed conservatively, however chyle leaks >400 ml should be reexplored for suturing and repair of damaged ducts. Selected cases may require thoracoscopic ligation.

25.3 Complications of Flap Reconstruction

Head and neck reconstruction forms an integral part of surgical management of head and neck cancer. The goals of reconstructive surgery mainly focusses on restoring form, function and aesthetics with application of proper and safe surgical techniques. Considering whether integrity, function, and form should be the goals of the reconstruction alone or in combination will depend on the patient's state of health, comorbidities, and wishes. Using reconstructive ladder as guide for reconstruction helps in formulating appropriate plan. Smaller defect could be managed with local flaps or grafts, whereas larger and complex defect require regional or free flaps (Fig. 25.1).

Postoperative complications arising from reconstructive flap failure, tend to increase the patient's health and financial burden, delay in initiating adjuvant treatment and reduce short-term and long-term quality of life resulting into overall poorer prognosis. Overall post operative complications after oral reconstruction ranges from 15% to 62%. The incidence was 32.4% with locoregional flaps including donor and recipient sites; with total flap loss in only 1–4%. Donor site complications range from 1% to 5.3% while recipient site complications from 9.5% to 29.7% patients.

Recipient site problems include vascular thrombosis, hematoma or flap failure. Donor site problems include hematoma, wound dehiscence, delayed healing or seroma.

CLINICAL PARAMETER	NORMAL CIRCULATION	VENOUS OCCLUSION	ARTERIAL OCCLUSION
COLOUR	PINK	BLUE/PURPLE HUE CYANOTIC	PALE, MOTTLED BLUE
CAPILLARY REFILL TIME	1-2 SEC	INCREASED, FAST<1S	DECREASED, SLOW>2SEC
TEMPERATURE	WARM	WARM-COLD	COOLER
TISSUE TURGOR	FULL	DISTENDED, SWOL LEN, TENSE	HOLLOW, PRUNE LIKE
DERMAL BLEEDING	BRIGHT RED COLOUR	BLOOD CHANGES FROM DARK RED OR BLUISH HUE TO EVENYUALLY PINK. BLEEDS BRISKLY. BLEEDS FOR ALONG TIME	MINIMAL BLEEDING TO ABSENCE OF BLEEDING. ONLY SERUM=DEAD TISSUE

Fig. 25.1 Clinical assessment of flap circulation

25.4 Risk Factors for Flap Complications

These can be largely subdivided into three categories preoperative factors, tumor characteristics & perioperative factors such as operation time, blood transfusion and antibiotic prophylaxis.

Although anatomic site of tumor and flap donor site may vary with age but various studies have established no adverse outcome in surgical complications in older age. It however does correlate with other medical complications.

ACE-27 comorbidity index is a widely accepted comorbidity evaluation system for oncology patients. It consists of 12 categories and 27 subcategories, each of which quantifies a specific disease within the circulatory, respiratory, digestive or nervous system and its severity. Various studies have shown 2 or more comorbidities or a severe comorbidity can be a high-risk factor for poor short-term outcomes. The most significant factor for flap failure is presence of uncontrolled diabetes mellitus. Microvascular angiopathy could be a contributing factor in these patients. ACE-27 index can be useful when deciding which treatment option is more suitable for advanced-stage oral cancer patients.

Several studies have demonstrated increased risk for surgical complications, including flap failure, haematoma, wound dehiscence and impaired wound healing in smokers after head and neck reconstructive surgery.

Poor preoperative nutritional status may be an important factor affecting surgical tolerance and increasing the risk of complications. Preoperative weight loss may be more common in oral cancer because eating function is affected. Preventing a decline in the nutritional status prior to surgery could be a means to reduce these negative consequences.

Preoperative or previous radiotherapy is reported to be associated with a higher risk of free flap failure and complications as it produces macro and microscopic alterations on vascular structures.

Post operative flap complications have been seen to be higher in patients with locally advanced tumors both T & N Stage. Advanced tumor invades many important surrounding anatomical structures making complete excision and hemostasis difficult, leading to higher risk complications. Extensive tumor resection may also result in larger surgical dead space with increased risk for hematoma, seroma and postoperative infections. Tumors with advanced nodal disease have extensive lymphatic metastasis or extranodal extension both of these are strongly associated with a poor prognosis.

It is well known that prolonged operative time is accompanied by prolonged anaesthesia time, more blood loss and may lead to many adverse events such as surgical site infection, wound dehiscence, higher reoperation rates or need for blood transfusion. Long operation time increases wound exposure and decreases the effects of sterilization and antibacterial measures.

Tracheostomy is a useful method to prevent asphyxia caused by airway obstruction after surgery. Direct exposure of respiratory tract caused by tracheostomy may result in contamination, leading to adverse events such as pulmonary infection. Tracheostomy tends to be used during tongue, floor of mouth or mandible resection, indicating a high risk of post operative complications.

Use of blood transfusion may be considered as an important indicator for adverse short-term outcomes in patients undergoing oncological surgery, mainly for flap related complications mainly for free flap rather than pedicled flap reconstructions.

Most clinicians agree that antibiotic prophylaxis is the most effective means to prevent infective complications (Table 25.2).

Table 25.2 How to prevent flap failure?

• Plan flap of appropriate size
• Strict adherence to territory of supply
• During transfer avoid sharp bending or kinking
• Avoid pressure dressing over pedicle
• Avoid tension in suture line
• Early evacuation of seroma or hematoma
• Watch for signs of poor flap viability

25.5 Complications of Loco Regional Flaps

Mostly results into loss of viability of a small portion of flap with marginal dehiscence and salvage is successful. Most of these are obvious clinically and do not require any imaging. Ischaemia to a greater percentage of flap may result from vascular thrombosis. Complete flap failure occurs when venous thrombosis outnumbers arterial thrombosis. Majority of these occur within three days of surgery. As a quick guide to learners clinically, if the flap is pale, or does not blanch with local pressure, flap viability is questionable.

25.6 Complications of Microvascular Flaps

The common causes of microvascular flap failure include arterial and venous thrombosis, infection, anatomic variations, and flap dissection errors.

Arterial Failure: These are common causes of flap failure in head and neck region' mostly due to thrombosis in the arterial supply. Bleeding can occur along the anastomotic site due to poor vessel apposition or hemodilution. Any form of hematoma around the vessel anastomosis can lead to extrinsic compression or vessel spasm. Kinking of the pedicle because of redundant vessel length or improper lie may also lead to arterial insufficiency. Avulsion of the anastomosis from uncontrolled physical movement or coughing bouts has also been incriminated in some cases. Compression of the pedicle may also occur due to narrow tunnelling of pedicle or pressure against bony edges.

Venous Failure: Flap failure because of venous insufficiency are common as veins are low-pressure systems and more susceptible to compression, twisting, and kinking. Venous spasm is uncommon. Venous congestion may cause retrograde propagation of clots within the fine radicals of the venous network leading to complete failure of flap.

25.7 Other Complications of Flaps

25.7.1 Infection

Poor adherence to asepsis is one of the common causes of infection as the head and neck is a potential source of bacterial contamination. Flap failure if unrecognized and left unattended may lead to partial or complete flap necrosis. This in turn becomes a nidus for infection further aggravating flap failure. Frequently such infective foci need debridement to prevent the emergence of sepsis. The defect arising from it may be either managed conservatively with secondary healing or may need new tissue cover from a new flap.

25.7.2 Hardware Exposure

Plates, screws, and titanium meshes are commonly used hardware in head and neck reconstruction. Common causes of early hardware exposure are wound dehiscence due to tension, infection, or flap necrosis while late exposure of implant is usually due to skin thinning over the implant, most commonly as a result of radiation therapy. Intraorally, plates exposure above the salivary line needs minimal intervention while those below the salivary line, heals poorly because of constant exposure to saliva necessitating fresh soft tissue to close the defect. Implant extrusion over critical areas such as the cranium and base of skull, may become a portal of infection to the brain and meninges.

25.7.3 Skull Base Reconstruction

The common complications of base of skull reconstructions are cerebrospinal fluid leak due to incomplete dural closure and infection. Later complications include diplopia caused by a lack of bony support for the globe, facial deformity secondary to soft tissue atrophy, and trismus due to postoperative radiotherapy fibrosis.

25.7.4 Midface Reconstruction

The common complications arising from reconstruction of maxillary defects are enophthalmos and diplopia, speech, swallowing and occlusal derangements, and facial asymmetry and deformity. Oronasal fistulas occurs commonly from hard and soft palates defects causing passage of food into the nasal cavity and hypernasal speech.

25.7.5 Mandible Reconstruction

Mandibular reconstruction need focus on dentition and occlusal relationships but the common complications arising from its reconstruction are jaw asymmetry and malocclusion. Such errors can result in retrognathia, prognathism, or a midline shift. Late presentation of above complications usually relates to radiotherapy resulting into tissue fibrosis.

Non-union is the next common complication resulting from failure to consolidate after 4 months, with clinical and radiologic evidence of impaired healing. Irradiated jaw takes longer to heal. These typically manifest as pain, instability, or plate fractures.

25.8 Summary

Although some early complications of oral cancer surgery are similar to other surgical procedures; potential long-term complications are quite challenging for the oncologic team as well as the patient. It is very important for the oncology team to discuss all possible complications in great detail with family and appropriately prepare the patient for surgery. It is of even greater importance to recognize and avoid these potential complications adhering to basic surgical principles and in depth knowledge of the complex regional anatomy.

Suggested Reading

Harvey C, et al. Principles of head and neck reconstruction: an algorithm to guide flap selection. Semin Plast Surg. 2010;24(2)

Kerawala CJ, Heliotos M. Prevention of complications in neck dissection. Head Neck Oncol. 2009;1:35. https://doi.org/10.1186/1758-3284-1-35.

Kolokythas A. Long-term surgical complications in the oral cancer patient: a comprehensive review. Part I. J Oral Maxillofac Res. 2010a;1(3):e1. https://doi.org/10.5037/jomr.2010.1301.

Kolokythas A. Long-term surgical complications in the oral cancer patient: a comprehensive review. Part II. J Oral Maxillofac Res. 2010b;1(3):e2. https://doi.org/10.5037/jomr.2010.1302.

Singh B, Cordeiro PG, Santamaria E, et al. Factors associated with complications in microvascular reconstruction of head and neck defects. Plast Reconstr Surg. 1999;103:403–11.

Tan, et al. Complications of head and neck reconstruction and their treatment. Semin Plast Surg. 2010;24(3)

Tenkos, et al. Complications of myocutaneous and local flaps. Complications Otolaryngol Head Neck Surg. 2013; https://doi.org/10.1055/b-0034-79226.

Chemoport (TIVADs—Totally Implantable Venous Access Devices): Complications and Management

26

Vedant Kabra

26.1 Introduction

The administration of chemotherapy was revolutionized by introduction of chemoport (also called TIVAD—Totally Implantable Venous Access Devices or Portacath or simply "Ports") by John Niederhuber from MD Anderson Cancer Centre in 1982 [1]. They have since proven to be effective and safe for administration of infusional drugs including chemotherapy, parenteral nutrition, blood products and for repeated blood sampling. Chemoport consists of a subcutaneously placed reservoir chamber with a self-sealing septum and a catheter. The chamber is accessed percutaneously using a special non-coring (Huber) needle which is inserted in a sterile manner through the septum. The reservoir is connected to one end of a catheter whose tip (the other end) is placed in a central vein that facilitates delivery of hyperosmolar solutions, extreme pH drugs or vesicant chemotherapeutic agents directly into a large bore vein thus avoiding endothelial damage which happens when they are administered in a peripheral vein.

Inspite of being the safest way of long term central venous access, chemoports do have their share of adverse events. They are broadly classified as early and late complications each of which could arise either due to catheter or the reservoir. There is no clear cut-off defined between early and late but aetiopathologically, the early complications mainly arise as a result of injury to adjacent structures while inserting the catheter or implanting the reservoir whereas the late complications happen due to long term use (or misuse), maintenance, trauma and wear and tear of the implanted system. With nearly 1.5 million new cancer patients every year in

V. Kabra (✉)
Department of Surgical Oncology, Fortis Memorial Research Institute, Gurugram, Haryana, India

Surgical Oncology, Fortis Healthcare, Delhi NCR, India

K. Sood Sharma et al. (eds.), *Complications of Cancer Therapy: Best Practices in Prevention and Management*, https://doi.org/10.1007/978-981-99-0984-1_26

India, there is a large potential of chemoport use and surgeons should be well versed not only with insertion techniques but also how to prevent complications, recognize them early and manage effectively.

26.2 Chemoport Related Complications

Chemoport related complications can be divided into early or peri-procedural (most people use a cut off limit of ≤30 days while a few keep a cut-off of only upto the first use of chemoport) and late complications (occurring after 30 days). Table 26.1 summarizes the complications according to chronology and the part of chemoport that causes it or is affected by it.

26.2.1 Complications Related to Port Insertion

There are various approaches for venous access [1]—surgical cut-down using cephalic vein or less commonly external jugular vein and a percutaneous approach by Seldinger technique using either the anatomical landmarks or ultrasound (USG) guidance [2] to locate internal jugular vein (IJV) or Subclavian vein (SV). Both IJV and SV approaches have been found to be safe in experienced hands [3–5]. Author's preference is to use subclavian approach as it avoids acute bending of catheter over the clavicle, no scar in neck, avoids visible skin hump in neck due to catheter in thin patients.

26.2.1.1 Malposition

What is the normal placement/appearance of catheter on imaging?

There is no universally accepted ideal position of the catheter tip. Nonetheless, it is recommended to place the tip at the junction of superior vena cava (SVC) and

Table 26.1 Early and late complications of chemoport

Early complications		Late complications	
Catheter Insertion	Reservoir Implantation	Catheter related	Reservoir related
Malposition	Wound infection	Catheter Blockage	Infection
Pneumothorax	Seroma	Catheter pinch-off	Reservoir rotation
Hemothorax	Hematoma	Catheter fracture with or without migration	Reservoir -Catheter disconnection
Arterial puncture/ hematoma	Wound dehiscence	Thrombosis/ thromboembolism	Extravasation
Arrhythmia	Reservoir rotation	Infection	Membrane disruption
Air Embolism			
Thoracic duct injury (left side)			

right atrium (RA). As per European Society for Clinical Nutrition and Metabolism (ESPEN) guidelines based on grade A level of evidence it can be placed anywhere between lower third of SVC to upper part of RA [6].

To add to the woes, precise localization of the junction of SVC and RA may be difficult to ascertain on a plain radiograph. Furthermore, Intra-thoracic tumors and mediastinal shift may obscure these structures and some thin catheters may not be easily seen specially in obese patients. Inspite of these limitations, a post op chest radiograph (CXR) is recommended (preferably two views in supine position) to confirm appropriate placement which is considered to be one of the following—6th thoracic vertebra, just below the right bronchus, notch at the right cardio-mediastinal contour (Fig. 26.1a–c). Since a malposition would mean another surgical procedure with its associated cost, it is also recommended to insert the port under fluoroscopic guidance to minimize the chance of malpositioning. Another method of intraop assessment of catheter tip is based on intravenous electrocardiography technique to find the junction of SVC and RA [7].

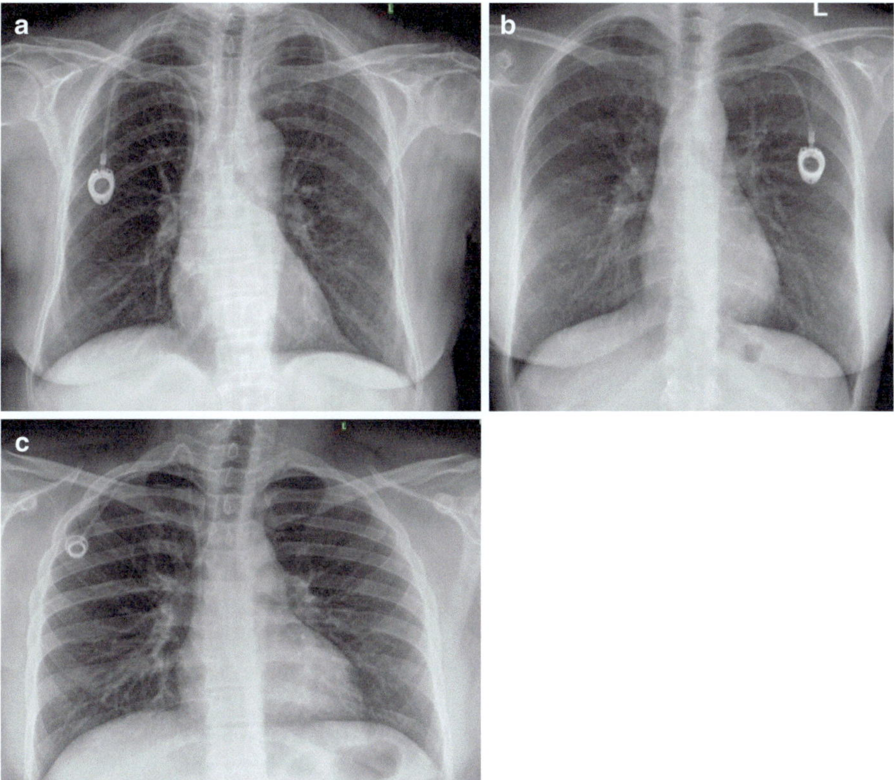

Fig. 26.1 (**a–c**) Normal catheter tip placement through various routes—Right subclavian (**a**), Left subclavian (**b**) and Right internal jugular vein (**c**)

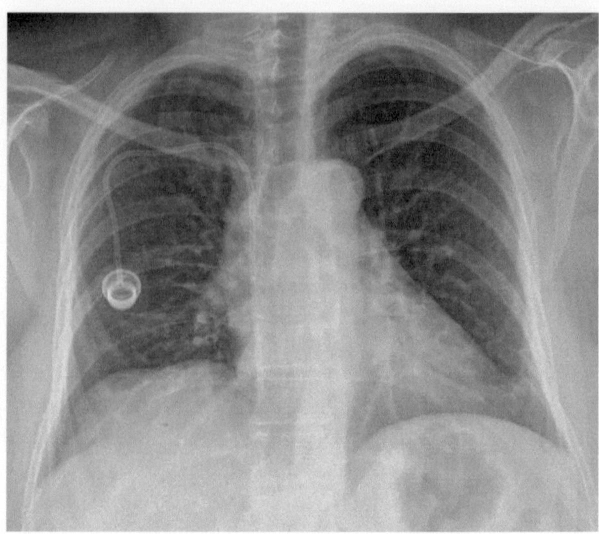

Fig. 26.2 Malpositioning of catheter tip in right ventricle

Sites of malposition and diagnosis: Catheter may commonly be malpositioned from subclavian vein (SV) to ipsilateral internal jugular vein (IJV) or vice versa, to azygous vein, internal mammary vein and left superior intercostal vein, from SV to opposite subclavian or IJV or into the heart (Fig. 26.2). This may lead to turbulence in blood flow, trauma to vessel or cardiac wall which in turn increases the incidence of catheter related thrombosis. It may be accidentally inserted intra-arterially, or in extravascular space. Arterial puncture is usually detected easily and immediately and does not cause complications. However, if artery is dilated it can result into arterial dissection, thromboembolism, stroke, pseudoaneurysm or arterio-venous fistula. Subclavian or common carotid arteries are the commonly punctured arteries.

Treatment: Correct the position of the catheter tip by maneuvering under fluoroscopic guidance which has been possible almost all the time in author's experience. If re-positioning in this way is not possible then re-insert through another site which offers a more straight route to SVC. Accidental arterial puncture needs withdrawal of the needle and application of pressure for a few minutes to prevent hematoma or continuing hemorrhage from the puncture site.

Prevention tips: Several studies have reported that arterial puncture can be avoided by use of USG guidance during venous puncture [8]. An arterial puncture should be recognized before the dilator is introduced to avoid complications related to it.

26.2.1.2 Pneumothorax

The incidence of pneumothorax various between 0.5% to 8.3% [7–9] in different series and differs according to the technique most commonly seen with unguided subclavian cannulation due to its proximity to the pleura. It is caused by unintended puncture of pleura during insertion which leads to air escaping into the pleural cavity.

Diagnosis: A post-operative chest (CXR) is recommended to document its absence. A few studies have raised a doubt on the utility and cost-effectiveness of

CXR because of a low complication rate, especially in a seemingly uncomplicated procedure which was done under fluoroscopy guidance. However, intra-op fluoroscopy with its limited resolution cannot reliably exclude pneumo/hemothorax and in countries with low cost of CXR, it should routinely be done. We must remember though a possibility of delayed development of significant pneumothorax.

Treatment: An asymptomatic patient with a small pneumothorax (<3 cm from Apex to Cupola or <15% of hemithorax) which has not increased in a follow-up X-ray taken a few hours later can be discharged. Those with large pneumothorax causing symptoms, unstable patients and those with high risk features like emphysema or expected to require mechanical ventilation would need chest tube drainage either a small or a large bore depending upon the condition.

Prevention tips: Properly following the anatomical landmarks, using ultrasound guidance for needle insertion, avoiding sudden coughing by patient will minimize the chances of Pneumothorax.

26.2.1.3 Hemothorax

Although a rare occurrence, this complication could prove fatal if not diagnosed or treated timely in patients with large amount of blood loss.

Causes: It can result due to inadvertent arterial puncture of intrathoracic arteries or extension of venous laceration intrathoracically.

Diagnosis: A sudden onset hypotension and breathlessness soon after the procedure is suggestive of a significant hemothorax. A CXR can detect a significant hemothorax but can easily miss up to 200–300 ml of blood in hemithorax, USG being more sensitive.

Treatment: Initial treatment of a symptomatic patient is by resuscitation and wide bore chest tube placement. If the initial drainage is more than 1.5 L or there is a continuing drainage of 200–300 ml per hour for 3 h, exploration and surgical repair is needed. Arterial puncture incidence can vary from 2% to 4.5% and is more commonly encountered with IJV cannulation as compared to subclavian. In an Indian series of 98 patients, inadvertent arterial puncture occurred in 3 patients (3.06%) none requiring any additional treatment [10].

Prevention tips: Arterial puncture/hemothorax can be avoided by proper attention to anatomic landmark, having a high index of suspicion in detecting arterial puncture and application of pressure for 10 min at the puncture site. USG guided procedure is preferable for IJV especially in obese individuals. Though subclavian artery puncture is less common than carotid puncture, it can lead to hematoma or hemothorax more commonly as it is located deep to clavicle and pressure cannot be applied easily over it. Gentle handling of vein during puncture, careful dilatation of vein and meticulous peeling off of the sheath will prevent venous laceration.

26.2.1.4 Air Embolism

This is an extremely rare complication and the amount of air required to cause cardiovascular collapse is 3–5 ml/kg. However, it would take only 2–3 s for this amount of air to enter through a 14 G needle with a pressure gradient of as small as −3.5 mm of Hg being present [9].

Diagnosis: Symptoms may range from low oxygen saturation to sudden onset breathlessness to circulatory collapse and death.

Treatment: Once suspected, supplemental 100% oxygen should be started, patient should be positioned in head low with left lateral tilt in order to keep the air bubble away from right ventricular outlet. Cardiopulmonary support and resuscitation may be needed in case of collapse.

Prevention tips: It can be prevented by using Trendelenberg position (head low), preop fluid loading to keep the veins full, use of Valsalva maneuver and by not keeping the needle or sheath open to air.

26.2.1.5 Arrhythmias

Arrhythmias happen when the guidewire or catheter is inserted too deep into the heart and they irritate the endocardium. Most of the time it's a temporary phenomenon and reverses on withdrawal of the guidewire/catheter. However, cases of life-threatening complete heart block have been reported [9]. Special care is needed in patients with pre-existing rhythm disturbance and in those with uremia or electrolyte imbalance that may lower the threshold for causing arrhythmia.

26.2.2 Reservoir Insertion and Indwelling Reservoir Related Complications

26.2.2.1 Wound Dehiscence

Causes: It may happen as a result of improper suturing technique, poor healing due to malnutrition, immunocompromised state, irradiated skin, thin skin flap, use of bevacizumab within a fortnight.

Treatment: It is managed by controlling the underlying factor and repositioning or removal of the port.

Prevention tips: Adequate thickness of subcutaenousl fat must be left in the flap in malnourished patients or those who are likely to become cachectic while on therapy to prevent delayed skin necrosis and exposure of the device.

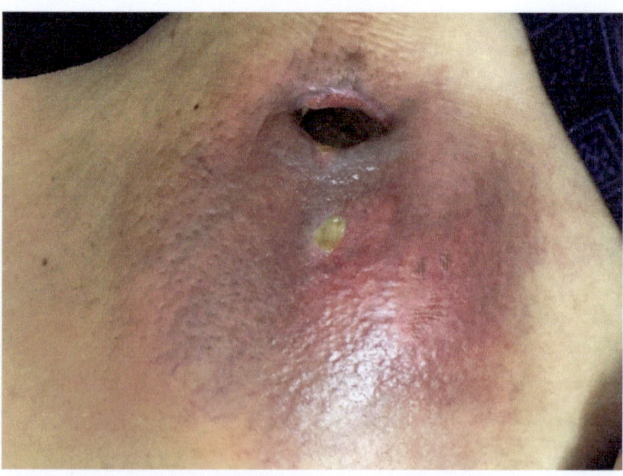

Fig. 26.3 Post extravasation extensive inflammation, necrosis and wound dehiscence around the pocket. This required extensive debridement and full thickness flap cover

26.2.2.2 Extravasation

It has been reported to range from 0.1% to 6% in various series with the Indian series reporting 2% [10].

Causes: It can happen because of inappropriate placement of non-coring needle, disconnection or fracture of catheter, disintegration of the reservoir septum due to improper use (e.g. use of ordinary needle instead of Huber needle) or unrecognized reservoir rotation.

Diagnosis: Symptoms are related to the amount of leaked fluid and the toxicity of the medication. Irritant drugs would result in inflammation whereas the vesicant ones can cause severe necrosis and ulceration involving a large area which could progress slowly over weeks (Fig. 26.3).

Treatment: Early recognition, termination of infusion and aspiration of the drug already infused are keys to minimize the damage. Local heat is applied to increase local circulation except in case of anthracycline extravasation which requires cold compress. Hyaluronidase or placental extract injections decrease tissue concentrations of vinca alkaloids; intravenous dexrazoxane as an antidote to anthracyclines; topical application of 99% dimethyl sulfoxide for cisplatin, mitomycin C and anthracyclines. Surgical excision of dead tissue with reconstruction using full thickness cover is reserved for those cases that do not respond to above measures.

Prevention tips: Appropriate training of staff, meticulous needle insertion, confirmation of backward and forward flow and watching for any local swelling in the initial phase of the infusion will prevent or diagnose it early thus preventing the damage to the surrounding tissues. Even in absence of backflow, most of the time the needle is in place and the port can be safely used. However, it is recommended to confirm it by contrast study before starting any irritant or vesicant drug.

26.2.2.3 Hematoma and Seroma

Hematoma around the catheter may form if hemostasis is not take care of during insertion. Seroma formation occurs after port removal due to fluid collection in the pseudocapsule that forms around the reservoir in the long term. This capsule should either be plicated or excised while port removal to avoid seroma formation.

Infection of the port site and port malfunction will be described along with catheter related issues in the next section.

26.2.3 Complications Related to the Indwelling Catheter

26.2.3.1 Infection

Although chemoport related infection has become less common due to technical improvement in insertion techniques (moving from open cut-down to percutaneous technique) and better antiseptic practices, it continues to be the most common reason for port removal and has been reported to be in a very wide range of 0.5–27% [11] but usually in the range of 5–8% at a rate of 0.2–0.67/1000 catheter days [9, 12].

Risk Factors & Causative Agents: It is higher with open cut-down technique (10.8% for open technique vs 2.8% in USG guided percutaneous technique in a prospectively collected data of 796 patients [7] and in those having hematolymphoid malignancies due to higher immunocompromised status. Gram positive bacteria are the predominant causative agents in early infections while gram negative bacteria are more commonly involved in later infections [12]. The common agents overall are species of Staphylococci, Streptococci, Enterobacteriacae, Klebsiella, Pseudomonas and Candida. Frequent port access, chemotherapy induced neutropenia, parenteral nutrition, hematologic malignancy, prolonged steroid use, thrombosis and metastatic disease are the risk factors [9]. Infection of the pocket is the most frequent late complication, is the main cause of port removal and occurrs most often after 20 weeks (related mainly to its use) and after 60 weeks (lack of maintenance) suggestive that post-operative port site infections are rare [13].

Diagnosis: Catheter related blood stream infection usually presents with fever and confirmation of diagnosis can be reliably done by differential quantitative blood cultures and differential time to positivity (DTTP). Paired blood culture samples for aerobic and anerobic cultures are drawn from the port and a peripheral vein in an aseptic manner. It is important to document either a more than thrice the colony count or earlier time to culture positivity (≥2 h) in the port sample as compared to the peripheral sample. Infection of the port pocket presents with local signs of infection and distal 5 cm of the catheter and the reservoir septum have the highest chance of culture positivity by quantitative techniques [9].

Treatment: Initial management is with intravenous empirical antibiotics having broad spectrum which are modified or de-escalated once the sensitivity is available. Antifungal should be added in suspected parenteral nutrition related infection. Caspofungin is preferred over Fluconazole [9]. Most of the time port does not need removal. However, in severe sepsis with organ failure, complications like endocarditis, osteomyelitis, suppurative thrombophlebitis etc., and fungal infection port should be removed and long term antimicrobial therapy instituted. Antibiotic lock therapy has shown promising results and they can be administered at doses that are 1000 times higher than the MIC as they remain inside the port chamber and do not enter systemic circulation. They contain high concentration of antibiotics with anticoagulants like Citrate or EDTA (ethylene diamine tetraacetic acid) and should be used for >12 h with re-installation time not exceeding 48 h [14].

Infection or abscess of the pocket/tunnel mostly needs removal of the port with debridement of non-viable adjacent tissue. A superficial infection at the needle entry or catheter entry can usually be controlled by antibiotics. Figure 26.4 shows a needle entry site infection due to neglected needle left in-situ after first chemotherapy administration. This was managed conservatively and port could be saved.

Prevention tips: Most effective preventive measure is strict observation of aseptic techniques during implantation and every subsequent use. Multicentric prospective study in over a hundred ICUs proved the effectiveness of adoption of a bundle of evidence based interventions like hand washing, barrier precautions during insertion, skin antisepsis with chlorhexidine, avoiding femoral route and removing unnecessary catheters at the earliest opportunity—it decreased up to 66% reduction in Catheter related blood stream infection for central lines [15]. Appropriate training and education of staff and patient is recommended as one of the most important evidence based strategies to prevent infection [14].

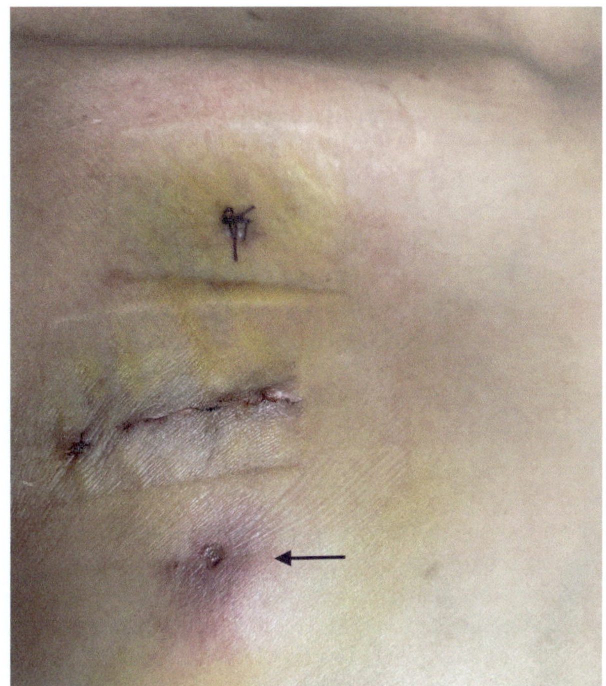

Fig. 26.4 The needle was accidentally left in-situ after administration of first chemotherapy cycle and caused localized infection (arrow). Impression of needle prick point can be seen at 10–11 o'clock position of the inflamed area

26.2.3.2 Thrombosis

Risk Factors: Catheter related thrombosis is more relevant in cancer patients due to markedly increased incidence of venous thromboembolism due to cancer related hypercoagulability or as an indirect consequence of cancer therapy, venous stasis, vessel trauma, catheter related infection. Malposition of catheter in a smaller, low flow vein can also lead to thrombosis. It can take two forms—stenosis of the host vein due to venous wall trauma or thrombus around the catheter tip [7, 8]. The peri-catheter thrombus formation is caused by pro-coagulant state and a fibrin sheath is formed around the catheter leading to increased resistance to flow during infusions. Around 5% of ports are associated with upper limb deep vein thrombosis (DVT) and, if not treated, will cause venous thromboembolism in around 5% cases [9].

Diagnosis: Presence of ipsilateral pitting edema, pain and prominence of superficial veins strongly indicated upper limb DVT in a patient with chemoport. However, these symptoms are non-specific and many patients remain asymptomatic until late stages. Color Doppler USG can diagnose DVT but is neither specific nor sensitive. If Color doppler is normal in a patient with suspicion of DVT then MR venography or CT angiography is indicated and serum D-dimer would also be helpful.

Treatment: It is possible to continue using the port in most situations while treating the thrombosis for at least 3–6 months with low molecular weight heparin (LMWH) or newer direct oral anticoagulants (DOACs) e.g. Rivoroxaban that have more predictable anticolagulation and lesser risk of bleeding as compared to warfarin. Port removal should be in done in patients with severe pain, upper limb cellulitis, malposition of the catheter tip and irreversible occlusion of the catheter lumen [14].

Thrombolytics (streptokinase, urokinase) have high success rate in acute symptomatic cases diagnosed within 24 h of symptoms and in fibrin sheath formation.

USG guided insertion technique requires lesser number of punctures thus causing minimal damage to venous wall with subsequent lower rate of thrombotic events.

Prevention tips: Catheter made of silicone and second or third generation polyurethane have been shown to cause lower rate of thrombosis as compared to more rigid materials like PVC, tetrafluoroethylene and polyethylene. Role of prophylactic use of anticoagulants is debatable and recent RCTs as well as meta-analyses have not shown clinically significant benefit of using either LMWH or DOACs. More studies are needed to identify the subset of cancer patients who may be at a higher risk of catheter related thrombosis and may be the ideal candidates for prophylaxis

26.2.3.3 Mechanical Factors Causing Chemoport Malfunction

Causes: Fibrin sheath around the catheter tip (it can form as early as first 24 h) and thombotic blockage is the most common cause of port malfunction and have been discussed earlier. Catheter kinking, pinch-off between first rib and clavicle in case of subclavian insertion and subsequent fracture of the catheter, rotation of the reservoir, rolling up of catheter into the pocket (Fig. 26.5a, b) can also lead to port malfunction. An incompatible drug combination or lipid component in TPN can precipitate inside the catheter lumen causing obstruction [8].

Diagnosis: Accurate diagnosis of the underlying cause of mechanical obstruction is the key to appropriate management of this complication. Initial imaging should be a CXR; contrast injection through the port may be needed to confirm the integrity or otherwise of the port system.

Treatment: A pinch-off syndrome is usually relieved on abduction of the arm so a CXR should be obtained with arms on the sides instead of the usual abducted position. Once a diagnosis of pinch-off syndrome is made, the port needs to be reimplanted at another site because it can lead to potentially disastrous complication of catheter fracture and embolization. Author has had two catheter fractures in last 600 port implantations in patients who had completed their therapy and it was diagnosed during port maintenance. One had gone into the IVC and the other one was in the right atrium—both were removed by interventional cardiologist using the femoral vein route (Fig. 26.6a–d). Catheter fracture can also be caused by external forces

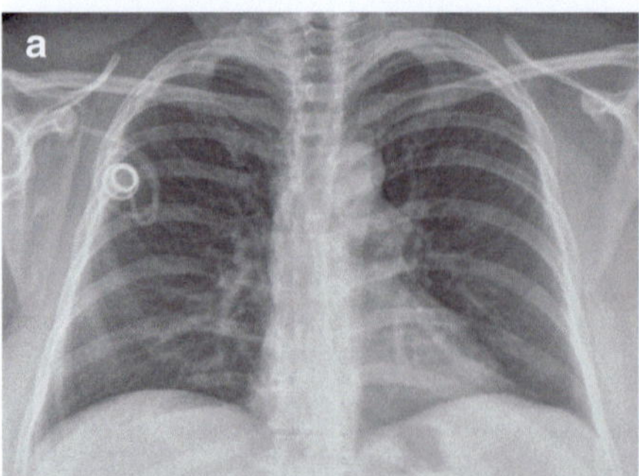

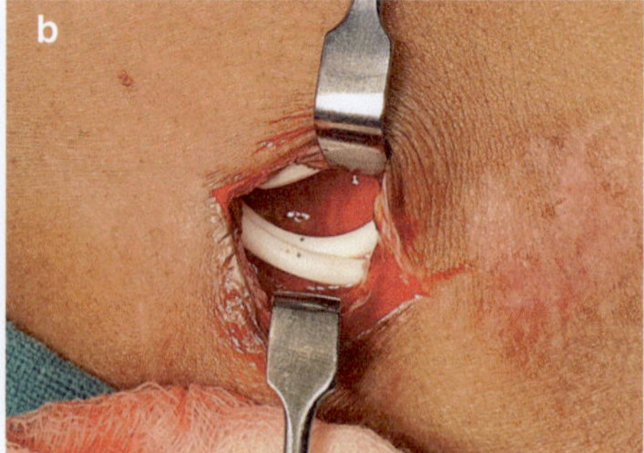

Fig. 26.5 (**a**, **b**) CXR done prior to port removal showed rolled up catheter near the port pocket (**a**) in an asymptomatic patient. Intraoperative appearance (**b**)

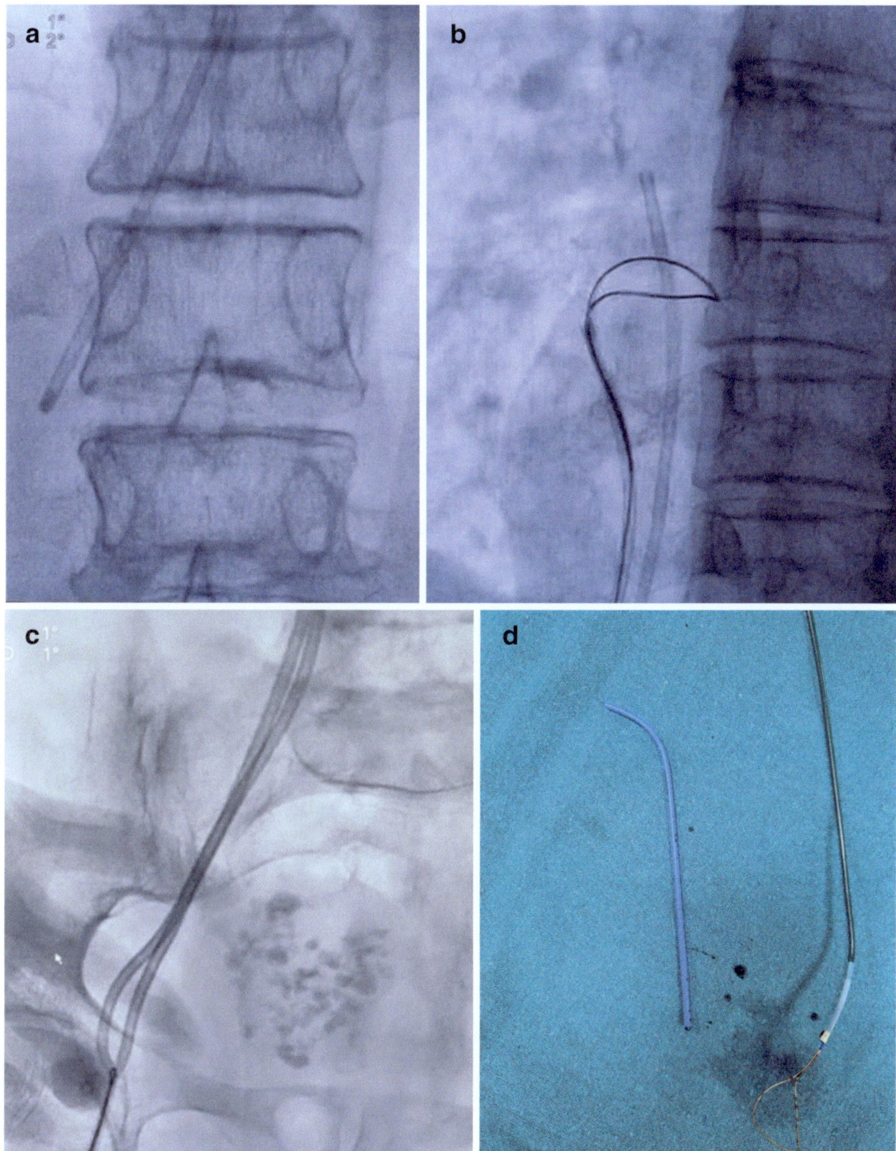

Fig. 26.6 (**a–d**) Catheter inserted through right subclavian route got fractured and migrated to inferior vena cava (**a**). Interventional cardiologist hooked the catheter (**b**) through femoral route and pulled it out after hooking the catheter (**c**). Fractured catheter after removal (**d**). Chemoport was removed separately. Photograph courtesy Dr Viveka Kumar, Director, Interventional Cardiology, Max Superspeciality Hospital, Saket, Delhi

like rapid deceleration against the seatbelt, friction against tight clothing or flushing using high pressure with syringes smaller than 10 ml capacity.

Drug precipitation can be relieved by using appropriate agent depending upon the cause; 70% ethanol for TPN, 0.1 mol/L of hydrochloric acid for calcium phosphate crystals or acidic drug particles and sodium hydroxide (0.1 mol/L) or sodium bicarbonate (1 mol/L) for alkaline drug precipitate [8].

26.3 Conclusions

Chemoport plays an important role in treatment of patients requiring long term intravenous therapy particularly chemotherapy. Inspite of being the safest mode of chemotherapy administration, they are associated with a number of potentially serious but preventable complications. Appropriate training, careful technique of insertion using appropriate guidance and meticulous after-care of the port are the ways to minimize the complications. Future research needs to focus on finding better material, safe and effective agents for thromboprophylaxis and infection prevention.

Key Points

- Chemoport is an important tool for safe administration of chemotherapy or medications over a long time period.
- It appears to be a simple procedure but can have potentially life-threatening complications.
- Percutaneous USG guided technique using SV or IJV under fluoroscopic monitoring is the safest and most effective way of implanting a chemoport.
- Post-op two-view Check X-ray is recommended to diagnose procedure related complications.
- Clinical monitoring should continue even in a seemingly easy implantation and a normal post-op CXR because a few procedure related complications may appear later e.g. pneumothorax
- Appropriate training of staff/patient for meticulous port handling at all times will prevent infection to a large extent
- Early diagnosis and appropriate treatment of complications may avoid life threatening situations (e.g. air embolism, hemothorax, etc.) or long term morbidity (e.g. extravasation related tissue necrosis)
- New research should focus on finding more bio-compatible materials, identifying high risk patients and safe and effective agents for thromboprophylaxis and infection prevention

Acknowledgements To my colleagues Dr Pushipinder Gulia, Dr Jaiprakash Gurawalia and Dr Amit Sahni for their help in clinical care of the patients and our specialty nurse Mr Dinakaran Unnikrishnan for helping me with compiling the photographs.

References

1. Niederbuber JE, Ensminger W, Gyves JW, et al. Totally implanted venous and arterial access system to replace external catheters in cancer treatment. Surgery. 1982;92:706–12.
2. Brass P, Hellmich M, Kolodziej L, et al. Ultrasound guidance versus anatomical landmarks for internal jugular vein catheterization. Cochrane Database Syst Rev. 2015;1:Cd006962.
3. Matsushima H, Adachi T, Iwata T, et al. Analysis of the outcomes in central venous access port implantation performed by residents via the internal jugular vein and subclavian vein. J Surg Educ. 2016; (Epub ahead of the print)
4. Biffi R, Orsi F, Pozzi S, et al. Best choice of central venous intersion site for the prevention of catheter-related complications in adult patients who need cancer therapy: a randomized trial. Ann Oncol. 2009;20:935–40.
5. Nagasawa Y, Shimizu T, Sonoda H, et al. A comparison of outcomes and complications of totally implantable access port through the internal jugular vein versus the subclavian vein. Int Surg. 2014;99:182–8.
6. Pittiruti M, Hamilton H, Biffi R, et al. ESPEN guidelines on parenteral nutrition: central venous catheters (access, care, diagnosis and therapy of complications). Clin Nutr. 2009;28:365–77.
7. Biffi R, Toro A, Pozzi S, et al. Totally implantable vascular access devices 30 years after the first procedure. What has changed and what is still unsolved. Supp Care Cancer. 2014;22:1705–14.
8. Machat S, Eisenhuber E, Pfarl G, et al. Complications of central venous port systems: a pictorial review. Insights Into Imaging. 2019;10:86–98.
9. Tabatabaie O, Kasumova G, Eskander M, et al. Totally implantable venous access devices: a review of complications and management strategies. Am J Clin Oncol. 2017;40:94–105.
10. Vinchurkar K, Maste P, Togale M, et al. Chemoport-associated complications and its management. Ind J Surg Oncol. 2020;11:394–7.
11. Yildizeli B, Lacin T, Batirel HF, et al. Complications and management of long-term central venous access catheters and ports. J Vasc Access. 2004;5:174–8.
12. Aparna S, Ramesh S, Appaji L, et al. Complications of chemoport in children with cancer: Experience of 54,100 catheter days from a tertiary cancer center of Southern India. South Asian J Cancer. 2015;4:143–5.
13. Granziera E, Scarpa M, Ciccarese A, et al. Totally implantable venous access devices: Retrospective analysis of different insertion techniques and predictors of complications in 796 devices implanted in a single institution. BMC Surg. 2014;14:27–35.
14. Sousa B, Furlanetto J, Hutka M, et al. Central venous access in oncology: ESMO clinical practice guidelines. Ann Oncol. 2015;26:v152–68.
15. Provonost P, Needham D, Berenholtz S, et al. An intervention to decrease catheter-related bloodstream infections in the ICU. N Engl J Med. 2006;355:2725–32.

27 Prevention and Treatment of Arm Lymphedema After Axillary Lymph Node Dissection

Geeta Kadayaprath and Shreya Sardana

27.1 Introduction

Breast cancer has become the most common cancer amongst women. There has been a de-escalation in the surgical management of breast cancer over the past couple of decades. However, axillary dissection continues to be performed for node positive disease and is fraught with the possibility of lymphedema. Lymphedema continues to be a major cause of morbidity in breast cancer patients and is often referred to as Breast Cancer Related Lymphedema (BCRL) it is defined as abnormal limb swelling caused by the accumulation of increased amounts of high protein in the interstitial fluid secondary to defective lymphatic drainage in the presence of near normal net capillary filtration. Lymphedema may set in as early as 3 months of breast cancer surgery. Most lymphedema manifests by 3 years and may continue over a lifetime. It is going to be an even more significant determinant of quality of life with increasing life span of breast cancer survivors. The advances in breast oncology are not only aimed at improving survival but also to ensure that the morbidity associated with its treatment is minimised. Prevention of lymphedema, which is a distressing sequelae of treatment, needs to be addressed appropriately . Prospective surveillance to identify the onset of lymphedema, early and prompt institution of lymphedema preventive measures are crucial elements of care. With the advent of sentinel lymph node biopsy to stage the axilla, it is fortunate that the incidence of lymphedema has diminished significantly. Once lymphedema sets in, then one has to resort to systematic measures in the form of manual lymphatic

G. Kadayaprath (✉)
Max Institute of Cancer Care, Max Healthcare, Delhi, India

S. Sardana
Breast Unit, Max Institute of Cancer Care, Max Healthcare, Delhi, India

K. Sood Sharma et al. (eds.), *Complications of Cancer Therapy: Best Practices in Prevention and Management*, https://doi.org/10.1007/978-981-99-0984-1_27

drainage, multilayer compression bandaging, gentle massage, compression sleeve, etc. In non-responsive Grade 3 lymphedema, one may have to resort to surgical measures to address this condition.

27.2 Incidence

The incidence of BCRL has been variably cited between 0–77% in literature owing to the non-standardized definition and classification [1]. McLaughlin et al reported an incidence of 40% [2] while, Shaitelman et al cited lymphedema risk post axillary lymph node dissection (ALND) averaging 28% with a range from 11% to 57% in larger trials [3]. Lymphedema after Sentinel lymph node biopsy (SLNB) averages 6.3% with a range between 0% to 23%. In Axillary Lymphatic Mapping Against Nodal Axillary Clearance (ALMANAC) trial, the lymphedema rate was 5% after SLNB [4] while in (ACOSOG), trial Z0010, it was in about 7% of patients [5]. To overcome this wide variation in literature, Common Terminology Criteria for Adverse Events v5.0 Criteria for Limb Edema was used.

Grade	Descriptor
1.	5–10% inter-limb discrepancy in volume or circumference at point of greatest visible difference, or swelling or obscuration of anatomic architecture on close inspection
2.	>10–30% inter-limb discrepancy in volume or circumference at point of greatest visible difference, or readily apparent obscuration of anatomic architecture, or obliteration of skin folds, or readily apparent deviation from normal anatomic contour, or limiting instrumental ADL
3.	>30% inter-limb discrepancy in volume, or gross deviation from normal anatomic contour, or limiting self-care ADL (activity of daily living) [6]

Using this terminology, the incidence of lymphedema was found to be 16.8% after SLNB and 47.1% after ALND. After SLNB, acute lymphedema of severity level I developed in 65% and severity level II in 35%. In the ALND group, severity level II lymphedema reached 60% [7].

27.3 Pathophysiology of Lymphedema: Lymphostasis and Lymphotension

Lymphedema, unlike all other types of edema, is confined to the epifascial space, while deep muscle compartments remain non-edematous. Lymphedema results from either obliteration of lymphatic system continuity by neoplastic, infective or inflammatory processes or congenital absence. This leads to lymphatic hypertension and distension, resulting in secondary impairment of contractility and valvular competence. Lymphostasis and lymphotension lead to the accumulation of fluid, proteins, growth factors and other active peptide moieties, glycosaminoglycans and particulate matter, including bacteria in the interstitial tissue spaces. As a consequence, there is increased collagen production by fibroblasts, an accumulation of inflammatory cells (predominantly macrophages and lymphocytes) and activation of keratinocytes. The end result is protein-rich edema fluid, increased deposition of ground substance, subdermal fibrosis and dermal thickening and proliferation. Lymphedema, unlike all other types of edema, is confined to the epifascial space. Although muscle compartments may be hypertrophied because of the increased work involved in limb movement, they are characteristically free of edema. Further, neurologic deficit with loss of sympathetic vasoconstrictor control causes increased blood flow accentuating the lymphedema [8].

27.3.1 Classification of Lymphedema

Lymphedema may be classified into subclinical, mild, moderate and severe according to several staging systems, ISL and Campisi are the most commonly followed systems.

1. **ISL (International Society of Lymphology) staging**
   (a) Stage 0: This stage is also known as latent or subclinical. Swelling is not clinically evident despite impaired lymph transport. It may exist months or years before overt edema occurs.
   (b) Stage I: This stage represents an early accumulation of fluid relatively high in protein content and subsides with limb elevation. Pitting may occur.
   (c) Stage II: IIa: Limb elevation alone rarely reduces tissue swelling, and pitting is manifest. IIb: Late in stage II, the limb may or may not pit as tissue fibrosis supervenes.
   (d) Stage III: This stage encompasses lymphostatic elephantiasis, where pitting is absent and trophic skin changes such as acanthosis, fat deposits, and warty overgrowths develop.

Within each stage, severity based on limb volume difference can be assessed as minimal (<20% increase), moderate (20–40% increase), or severe (>40% increase) [9].

2. **Campisi staging system is another useful classification which divides lymphedema into 5 stages:**
   (a) Ia No overt swelling despite impaired lymph drainage
   (b) Ib Reversible swelling with limb elevation
   (c) II Mild persistence of swelling with elevation
   (d) IIb Loss of pitting owing to progression of dermal fibrosis. Sometimes called spontaneously irreversible lymphedema.
   (e) III Persistent swelling with recurrent lymphangitis
   (f) IV Fibrotic changes with columnlike limb
   (g) V Elephantiasis with limb deformation including widespread lymphostatic warts [10].

3. **Clinical classification (Brunners classification)**
   (a) Subclinical (latent): There is excess interstitial fluid and histological abnormalities in lymphatics and lymph nodes, but no clinically apparent lymphoedema
   (b) I: Oedema pits on pressure and swelling largely or completely disappears on elevation and bed rest
   (c) II: Oedema does not pit and does not significantly reduce upon elevation, positive Stemmer's sign
   (d) III: Oedema is associated with irreversible skin changes, i.e. fibrosis, papillae

27.3.2 Diagnosis

A careful history and physical examination at every surveillance visit is the most important measure to diagnose and treat lymphedema. The commonest symptom reported is heaviness or fullness of arms. It is followed by decreased function of the extremity eventually to the extent of debilitating edema due to deposition of protein rich fluid in the tissues and resulting fibrosis of tendinous and ligamentous structures. Symptoms questionnaire: (FACT B+4) Functional Assessment of Cancer Therapy for Breast cancer and arm function is a useful tool.

An objective assessment can be done by limb size and volume measurements, photographs especially in afternoon when maximum edema manifests. The techniques used to assess lymphedema include measurement of arm circumference, ultrasound, water displacement technique, tonometry, optoelectric perometry, bioimpedance, and combined optoelectric perometry, 3D stereophotogrammetry and bioimpedance [3].

Limb circumference measurement with reference to fixed anatomical bony landmarks is one of the simplest methods and the most economical tool. A limb circumference discrepancy of more than 10 cm or a 2 cm change represents lymphedema [10].

Water displacement techniques are the most accurate method and are considered the gold standard. A water displacement measurement of 15 cm above epicondyles is most sensitive test. A value of 200 ml is the most validated cutoff [11].

Tonometry is a method of assessing the degree of compressibility which indirectly correlates with the circumference and the extent of lymphedema. The electronic tonometer also called lymphometer has two plungers: an outer one that is compressed fully when applied to the area being measured and an inner one that moves freely and is located in the center of the inner plunger [12]. The indurometer is a tool designed to replace the tissue tonometer and measures the resistance to an applied force to quantitate the amount of fibrosis present in the extremity [13].

These methods are fraught with the inaccuracy of measurement of the whole limb size and volume, while lymphedema is an increased extracellular deposition of protein rich fluid as well as alteration of the resistance of the tissues. A direct measure of lymph fluid volume can be estimated by Bioimpedance spectroscopy. An electrical current is passed through a body segment, and impedance to flow is measured which is inversely related to fluid content. It has been claimed to be the most sensitive test reaching 100% while circumference techniques claim 77% sensitivity. It helps in early institution of preventive measures [14].

A 10% change in limb volume measured by perometry or a 2-cm change in arm circumference are the commonly applied criteria [14]. Perometry is a noninvasive optoelectronic device that uses infrared light to quantify limb volume.

Radiologic studies such as lymphoscintigraphy, magnetic resonance imaging (MRI), and computed tomography (CT) have also been employed. They become necessary when surgical therapy is contemplated.

Lymphoscintigraphy is the gold standard to assess the caliber and anatomic location of lymphatic vessels, functional status, and disease severity. Radionuclide dye is injected intradermally via the interdigital space and taken up by the lymphatic system to visualize dynamic flow, areas of blockage, and dermal backflow [3].

Near-infrared fluorescence (NIRF) uses indocyanine green (ICG) as an optical contrast agent and provides immediate, high resolution, dynamic images [3].

27.3.3 Prevention of Lymphedema

27.3.3.1 Primary Prevention

1. Prevention of lymphedema should begin from the day the diagnosis of Breast cancer is established. Measures to preserve lymphatic as well as venous drainage of the respective upper limb should be instituted which include avoidance of intravenous or subcutaneous injections, avoiding measurement of blood pressure, preventing skin infections and trauma. Arm exercises like swimming, biking, and other isometric exercises augment the lymph and blood flow [15].
2. Sentinel Lymph Node biopsy (SLNB)

   Sentinel Lymph Node biopsy is undoubtedly one of the best measures to reduce the incidence of lymphedema as discussed previously. This was best demonstrated in the multicenter trial NSABP 32 which enrolled 5611 women with invasive breast cancer randomized to receive immediate ALND or SLND only if the sentinel node was negative. The SLN was identified in level I and II of the axilla in 98.6% of cases. The overall accuracy was 97.1%, with a false-negative rate of 9.8%. After mean follow-up of 95.6 months, overall survival, disease-free survival, and regional control were equivalent between treatment arms. The trial showed significant arm volume differences at 36 months between the SLNB group (8%) and the ALND group (14%) by volume displacement [16].

   ALMANAC trial also showed lymphedema rates of 5% after SLNB versus 13% for ALND at 1 year [4]. Similar results have been reported in Sentinella/GIVOM trial as well.
3. Radiation to axilla

   Substitution of axillary lymph node dissection by axillary radiation has been an active area of research. Initial studies by Greco, Veronsi and Galper led the way to AMAROS trial (After Mapping of the Axilla: Radiotherapy or Surgery Trial). It is a prospective randomized phase III noninferiority trial with 1425 women with clinical T1-2N0 invasive breast cancer with a positive SLN randomized to axillary radiation versus ALND. Axillary recurrence was low in both arms (0.43% in the ALND vs. 1.19% in the axillary radiation arm) with no differences in disease-free and overall survival. Lymphedema was significantly higher in the ALND arm (23%) compared with the axillary radiation arm (11%) at 5 years ($p < .0001$) [17].

4. Observation after axillary Ultrasound

   The SOUND (Sentinel node vs. Observation after axillary UltrasouND) trial is an ongoing prospective randomized trial of SLNB versus no axillary staging of clinical negative axilla by ultrasound. It utilised Quick-DASH assessment to measure physical function and symptoms. In the preliminary report of the first 180 patients recruited there was significant higher morbidity in the SLNB group versus the nonoperative arm [18].

5. ARM Axillary reverse mapping

   In ARM, technetium sulfur colloid is injected in the subareolar plexus, and blue dye is injected subcutaneously in the ipsilateral upper extremity (split mapping). A volume of 2–5 mL of isosulfan blue is injected subcutaneously into the volar aspect of the upper arm in the medial bicipital sulcus before incision. Use of ARM has been shown to reduce the lymphedema rates in multiple studies (33% vs. a range of 4–9% in ARM groups) [19–23]. There are chances of crossover (where the ARM node was identified as the SLN) in 3.8% of patients. These nodes should be removed and preferably the afferent and efferent limbs of any crossover node should be reanastomosed or reapproximated because they are SLNs.

6. LYMPHA technique of lymphovascular anastomosis (Lymphedema Microsurgical Preventive Healing Approach):

   Alongwith preservation of arm lymphatics, performing a lymphatic-venous anastomoses at the time of ALND has shown a statistically significant reduction in the development of lymphedema at 18 months (30% vs. 4.05%; $P < .01$) by Boccardo et al. [24] During axillary dissection , ARM allows identification of blue afferent lymphatics which are clipped near insertion into the node. After dissection, these are directly anastomosed into a collateral tributary of axillary vein under microscopy.

27.3.3.2 Secondary Prevention

1. Physiotherapy. Complex decongestive therapy is the standard of care in management of lymphedema. It consists of massage, compression bandages, and physiotherapy of the limb in different phases.

   Phase I includes four components which are skin care, manual lymphatic drainage, compression bandages and specialised physical therapy followed by massage.

   (a) Skin care to maintain skin integrity and decrease infections.
   (b) Manual lymphatic drainage to remove excess lymphatic fluid from the affected regions and open collateral lymphatics through the unaffected regions.

(c) Compression bandaging to maintain and increase compartment pressure and prevent retrograde flow of lymphatic fluid.
(d) Specialised physical therapy followed by massage. The massage begins by emptying the lymphatics of the trunk, followed by areas adjacent to the affected limb, concentrating on central portions of the limbs gradually working towards distal portions of the extremity (Foldi technique) [9].

Phase II of CDT includes low resistance short stretch multi-layer compressive bandages, which help in lymphatic pumping. It needs skilled personnel while graduated compression garments can be worn by the patients themselves. Australian studies have shown a benefit of 65% using this techniques [25].

2. Exercises: Isometric exercises like swimming, biking increase circulation in the affected limb. Weight training improves range of motion, strength and even quality of life. NCCN is in support of women with lymphedema participating in supervised exercise programs while wearing a compression sleeve starting with low weights and low repetitions with gradual increases [15].
3. Hyperbaric oxygen has also been found beneficial in arm lymphedema in several non randomised studies [26].
4. Medical therapy: Coumarin (Venalot), a benzopyrene, breaks down large protein molecules, facilitating absorption of the proteins into the vascular system at the level of the capillaries. Pentoxifylline (Trental) has been used in ameliorating postradiation fibrosis and may be used in refractory cases of lymphedema associated with radiation fibrosis to ameliorate the swelling and fibrosis.
5. Surgical therapy

   Surgeries for lymphedema can be divided into physiologic and reductive procedures. Physiologic procedures aim to increase the lymphatic flow and circulation in the affected limb, thereby being effective in fluid predominant earl disease with early pitting edema. Reductive procedures, on the other hand are aimed at decreasing the size of the extremity, and are employed in solid predominant disease with non-pitting edema. However a combination of physiological and reductive procedures is more effective.

   (a) Lymphaticovenous Anastomosis (LVA) first described by Campisi and colleagues, is a microsurgical procedure providing direct drainage from afferent lymphatics into the venous system. The lymphatics being small require serial anastomoses with the subdermal venules along the entirety of upper extremity. It is indicated after failure of conservative therapy and ISL stage II disease. Contraindication includes absolute occlusion of the lymphatics as seen in late stages of disease. Peri-operative lymphoscintigraphy improves the success rates [27].

Technique: Suitable venules and lymphatic vessels should be identified, which should be ideally similar diameter, preferably less than 0.8 mm, in close proximity to one another, and with minimal to no venous backflow after division. Larger veins have higher intraluminal pressure and greater risk of venous reflux into the lymphatics. There is no consensus on the number and location of anastomoses required. Stepped anastomosis creates multiple bypasses at various levels of the affected extremity (i.e., wrist, forearm, and arm in the upper extremity).

Any configuration including end-to-end, end-to-side, or side-to-end anastomoses can be used without significant difference in outcomes.

LVA is an efficacious treatment option for early stage disease. Chang and colleagues found that, after LVA, stage I and II patients experienced a 61% volumetric reduction compared with 17% volumetric reduction in stage III patients after 1 year of follow-up. It is a safe and feasible procedure with complication rates of 5.9% which includes infection, lymphatic fistula, partial skin ulceration, and wound dehiscence [28].

(b) Vascularised Lymph Node Transfer (VLNT)

VLNT is a recently popularized method, which involves microsurgical reconstruction with a soft tissue flap containing lymphatic tissue and its associated arteriovenous supply, relocated into the axilla. The transferred lymph nodes absorb lymphatic fluid and redistribute into the lymphovascular system. It also promotes lymphangiogenesis by vascular endothelial growth factor secretion [29].

VLNT is indicated in stage II to V lymphedema, complete lymphatic occlusion, fibrosis precluding lymphaticovenous bypass, brachial plexus neuropathy, chronic infections, and failed conservative management. Some authors advocate its role in early lymphedema as well.

Technique: Preoperative lymphodynamic evaluation is required which is best done by indocyanine green (ICG). Tc99 lymphoscintigraphy can be used to confirm the obstruction, but it does not provide spatial and temporal resolution. MRI and dynamic magnetic lymphangiography has high sensitivity and specificity for anatomic delineation of lymphatics.

Axilla is the most commonly selected recipient site. It entails wide removal of all axillary scar tissue during the axillary dissection with careful identification of the thoracodorsal vessels. A neuroma if identified should be removed by external neurolysis. The axillary dissection is more challenging in those who have undergone prior radiotherapy. Alternative recipient sites include wrist and elbow. Wrist is less cosmetically appealing but more suitable for function, however the elbow is more aesthetic.

Most common donor site is the inguinal region, based on branches of superficial circumflex iliac or superficial inferior epigastric vessels. It is defined by 3 borders: caudally inguinal ligament, muscular aponeurosis as deep and cribriform fascia as superficial margin. Other potential donor sites include the submental, supraclavicular, thoracic and omental tissues.

VLNT can be performed as an isolated VLNT or in combination with microvascular breast reconstruction based on deep inferior epigastric vessels. The recipient vessels can be either thoracodorsal or internal mammary vessels. VLNT can be ipsilateral or contralateral depending upon whether bilateral breast reconstruction is required and/or previous midline incision is present.

VLNT has shown promising results in terms of absolute reduction in limb size as well as limb functionality. Despite this, it is not a curative measure and conservative therapies need to be continued lifelong.

Complications include donor site seroma, lymphocele, infection, delayed wound closure, and the most dreaded donor site lymphedema.

(c) SAPL(Suction Assisted Protein Lipectomy)

SAPL is a method to remove fat and fibrosis with suction technique, and is indicated in stage II and III disease. However, it is only indicated in pitting edema. SAPL begins with application of tourniquet to drain the fluid from the affected limb. Liposuction is started distal to the tourniquet, circumferentially and in longitudinal direction using suction cannulas through multiple 3mm incisions. Compression sleeve and gloves are applied at all times post procedure. SAPL provides significant volume reduction and improved quality of life, without altering the underlying pathophysiology [30].

(d) Surgical Excision/Radical Debulking/Charles Procedure

Surgical excision is indicated in severe lymphedema. It involves circumferential excision of skin and subcutaneous tissue down to the level of the deep fascia using longitudinal skin incision. Split skin grafts are harvested from the excised skin and are implanted onto the deep fascial layer. Indications include advanced lymphedema, recurrent cellulitis, inability to exclude sarcoma, severe disfigurement or dysfunction.

(e) Combination Procedures

Physiologic procedures combined with reductive surgery are the best treatment of lymphedema. Examples include VLNT with SAPL, VLNT with microvascular breast reconstruction and LVA and VLNT with maximum limb volume reductions reported in VLNT and SAPL [31].

LV shunt: interposition autologous lymphatic-venous-lymphatic anastomoses Fig. 27.1

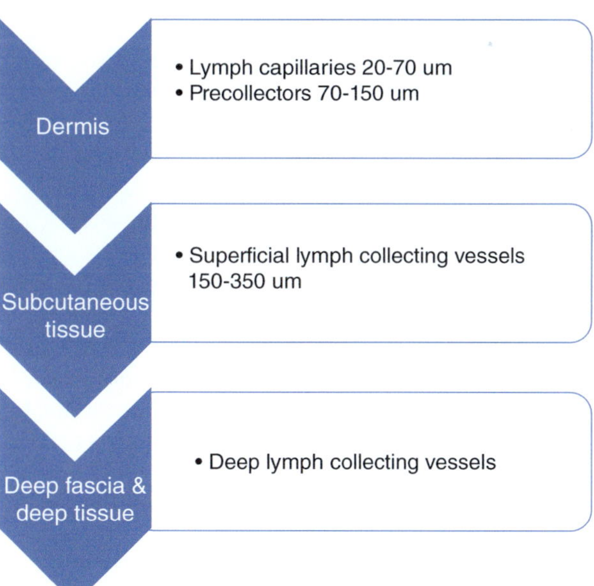

Fig. 27.1 Lymphatic pathway of skin and subcutaneous tissues

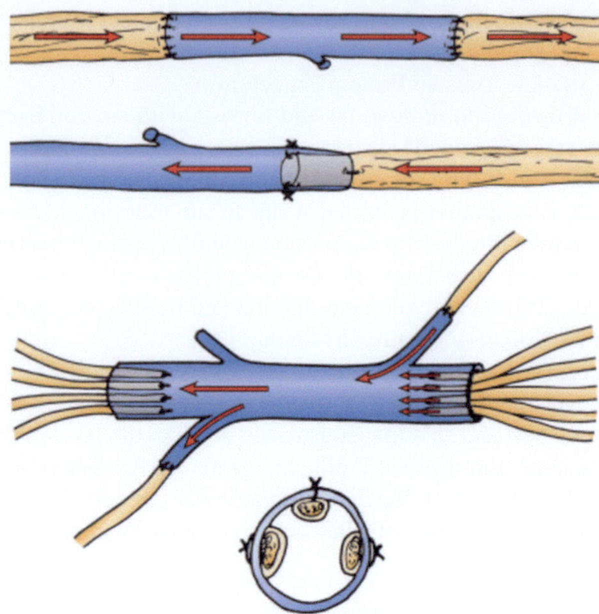

Schematic drawing of the derivative multiple lymphatic venous anastomoses and the reconstructive multiple lymphatic venous lymphatic anastomoses technique with the interposition of an autologous vein graft between lymphatics above and below the obstacle to the lymph flow
(From Campisi CC, Ryan M, Boccardo F, Campisi C. A single-site technique of multiple lymphatic-venous anastomoses for the treatment of peripheral lymphedema: long-term clinical outcome. J Reconstr Microsurg. 2016;32:42–49.)

Key Points

- Lymphedema is best prevented, as once it sets in, it is tough to restore normalcy. Precautions to prevent injury or infection in the arm on the operated side sand lifestyle modifications should be followed diligently.
- Sentinel lymph node biopsy should be performed in all suitable cases to reduce the incidence of lymphedema.
- To treat it well, identification and diagnosis of lymphedema at the earliest offers better treatment options.
- A proper objective assessment of the grade of lymphedema allows for assigning appropriate treatment.
- Conservative measures in the form of complex decongestive therapy and exercises, contribute to good results if done diligently.
- In women with a high BMI, extensive nodal involvement, it may be worthwhile to offer prophylactic lymphovenous anastomosis by an experienced microvascular surgeon.
- In progressive lymphedema with fibrosis, various surgical techniques have been offered with varying degrees of success.

References

1. Sackey H, Magnuson A, Sandelin K, et al. Arm lymphoedema after axillary surgery in women with invasive breast cancer. Br J Surg. 2014;101:390–7.
2. McLaughlin SA, Bagaria S, Gibson T, Arnold M, Diehl N, Crook J, Parker A, Nguyen J. Trends in risk reduction practices for the prevention of lymphedema in the first 12 months after breast cancer surgery. J Am Coll Surg. 2013;216:380–9. quiz 380-389
3. Shaitelman SF, Cromwell KD, Rasmussen JC, et al. Recent progress in the treatment and prevention of cancer-related lymphedema. CA Cancer. 2015;65:55–81.
4. Mansel RE, Fallowfield L, Kissin M, et al. Randomized multicenter trial of sentinel node biopsy versus standard axillary treatment in operable breast cancer: The ALMANAC Trial. J Natl Cancer Inst. 2006;98:599–609.
5. Wilke LG, McCall LM, Posther KE, et al. Surgical complications associated with sentinel lymph node biopsy: results from a prospective international cooperative group trial. Ann Surg Oncol. 2006;13:491–500.
6. Douglass J, Kelly-Hope L. Comparison of staging systems to assess lymphedema caused by cancer therapies, lymphatic filariasis, and podoconiosis. Lymphatic Research and Biology. 2019;17(5):550–6. https://doi.org/10.1089/lrb.2018.0063.
7. Francis WP, Abghari P, Du W, et al. Improving surgical outcomes: standardizing the reporting of incidence and severity of acute lymphedema after sentinel lymph node biopsy and axillary lymph node dissection. Am J Surg. 2006;192:636–9.
8. Svensson W, Mortimer PS, Tohno E, Cosgrove DO. Increased arterial flow demonstrated by Doppler ultrasound in arm swelling following breast cancer treatment. Eur J Cancer. 1994;30A:661–4.
9. Földi E. The treatment of lymphedema. Cancer. 1998;83:2833–4.
10. Armer JM, Stewart BR. A comparison of four diagnostic criteria for lymphedema in a post-breast cancer population. Lymphat Res Biol. 2005;3(4):208–17.
11. Kissin M, Querci Della Rovere G, Easton D, et al. Risk of lymphedema following treatment of breast cancer. Br J Surg. 1986;73:580–4.
12. Bagheri S, Ohlin K. Tissue tonometry before and after liposuction of arm lymphedema following breast cancer. Lymphat Res Biol. 2005;3(2):66–80.
13. Vanderstelt S, Pallotta OJ, McEwen M, et al. Inurometer vs tonometer: is the inurometer currently able to replace and improve upon the tonometer? Lymphat Res Biol. 2015;13:131–6.
14. Cornish BH, Chapman M, Hirst C, et al. Early diagnosis of lymphedema using multiple frequency bioimpedance. Lymphology. 2001;34:2–11.
15. Denlinger CS, Ligibel JA, Are M, et al. Survivorship: healthy lifestyles, version 2.2014. J Natl Compr Canc Netw. 2014;12:1222–37.
16. Krag DN, Anderson SJ, Julian TB, et al. Sentinel-lymph-node resection compared with conventional axillary-lymph-node dissection in clinically node-negative patients with breast cancer: overall survival findings from the NSABP B-32 randomised phase 3 trial. Lancet Oncol. 2010;11:927–33.
17. Donker M, van Tienhoven G, Straver ME, et al. Radiotherapy or surgery of the axilla after a positive sentinel node in breast cancer (EORTC 10981-22023 AMAROS): a randomised, multicentre, open-label, phase 3 non-inferiority trial. Lancet Oncol. 2014;15:1303–10.
18. Gentilini O, Botteri E, Dadda P, et al. Physical function of the upper limb after breast cancer surgery. Results from the SOUND (Sentinel node vs. Observation after axillary Ultra-souND) trial. Eur J Surg Oncol. 2016;42:685–9.
19. Thompson M, Korourian S, Henry-Tillman R, et al. Axillary Reverse Mapping (ARM): a new concept to identify and enhance lymphatic preservation. Ann Surg Oncol. 2007;14(6):1890–5.
20. Nos C, Kaufmann G, Clough KB, et al. Combined axillary reverse mapping (ARM) technique for breast cancer patients requiring axillary dissection. Ann Surg Oncol. 2008;15(9):2550–5.

21. Gennaro M, Maccauro M, Sigari C, et al. Selective axillary dissection after axillary reverse mapping to prevent breast-cancer-related lymphoedema. Eur J Surg Oncol. 2013;39(12):1341–5.
22. Han JW, Seo YJ, Choi JE, et al. The efficacy of arm node preserving surgery using axillary reverse mapping for preventing lymphedema in patients with breast cancer. J Breast Cancer. 2012;15(1):91–7.
23. Boneti C, Korourian S, Bland K, et al. Axillary reverse mapping: mapping and preserving arm lymphatics may be important in preventing lymphedema during sentinel lymph node biopsy. J Am Coll Surg. 2008;206(5):1038–42.
24. Feldman S, Bansil H, Ascherman J, et al. Single institution experience with lymphatic microsurgical preventive healing approach (LYMPHA) for the primary prevention of lymphedema. Ann Surg Oncol. 2015;22(10):3296–301.
25. Zeissler RH, Rose GB, Nelson PA. Post mastectomy lymphedema: late results of treatment in 385 patients. Arch Phys Med Rehabil. 1972;53:159.
26. Gothard L, Stanton A, MacLaren J, et al. Non-randomised phase II trial of hyperbaric oxygen therapy in patients with chronic arm lymphoedema and tissue fibrosis after radiotherapy for early breast cancer. Radiother Oncol. 2004;70:217–24.
27. Campisi C, Boccardo F, Zilli A, Macciò A, Napoli F. Long-term results after lymphatic-venous anastomoses for the treatment of obstructive lymphedema. Microsurgery. 2001;21(4):135–9.
28. Suami H, Chang DW. Overview of surgical treatments for breast cancer-related lymphedema. Plast Reconstr Surg. 2010;126(6):1853–63.
29. Nguyen AT, Chang EI, Suami H, et al. An algorithmic approach to simultaneous vascularized lymph node transfer with microvascular breast reconstruction. Ann Surg Oncol. 2015;22(9):2919–24.
30. Brorson H, Svensson B, Ohlin K. Suction-assisted lipectomy. In: Greene AK, Slavin SA, Brorson H, editors. Lymphedema. Cham, Switzerland: Springer International Publishing; 2015. p. 313–24.
31. Nicoli F, Constantinides J, Ciudad P, et al. Free lymph node flap transfer and laser-assisted liposuction: a combined technique for the treatment of moderate upper limb lymphedema. Lasers Med Sci. 2015;30(4):1377–85.

Stoma Complications and Management 28

Aseem Jindal and Neeraj Goel

28.1 Introduction

Intestinal stoma (usually ileostomy or colostomy) creation is an indispensable part of the surgical management of various emergency and elective surgeries of the gastrointestinal tract.

Patients with a well-functioning stoma can lead a normal life with limited lifestyle restrictions. In contrast, when a patient develops complications related to their stoma, the trauma on their physical and mental health can be quite significant.

Stoma creation can be either temporary or permanent, which can be either end or loop stoma. The most performed stomas are ileostomy and colostomy.

28.2 Classification of Stoma

The intestinal stomas can be classified on the basis of

(a) Bowel loop used: Ileostomy or Colostomy
(b) Function required: Diversion or defunctioning stoma
(c) Conformation: End or loop or double barrel type or end -loop stomas

A. Jindal · N. Goel (✉)
Department of Surgical Gastroenterology, Dharamshila Narayana Superspeciality Hospital, Delhi, India
e-mail: neeraj.goel.dr@narayanahealth.org

K. Sood Sharma et al. (eds.), *Complications of Cancer Therapy: Best Practices in Prevention and Management*, https://doi.org/10.1007/978-981-99-0984-1_28

28.2.1 Indications of Stoma

End ileostomy would be required when there is requirement of total colectomy or as a part of complete diversion in different settings like perforation, etc.

Total colectomy for hereditary bowel cancer—FAPC/HNPCC.
Total colectomy for fulminant ulcerative colitis refractory to medical therapy.
Total colectomy for Crohn's disease.

28.2.2 Defunctioning Loop Ileostomy

Protection of a distal rectal anastomosis (e.g., low anterior resection).

Relieve distal obstruction (e.g., malignant/inflammatory stricture).

Emergency management of anastomotic leak.

To defunction an intestinal fistula.

To defunction in the presence of severe perianal sepsis (e.g., Crohn's, Fournier's gangrene/necrotizing fasciitis).

Rectal trauma/sphincteric injury.

Fecal incontinence.

28.2.3 Indications for Colostomy

28.2.3.1 End Colostomy

Low rectal or anal cancer where sphincter complex excision is necessary.

Hartmann's procedure.

Faecal incontinence.

Radiation proctitis.

28.2.3.2 Defunctioning Loop Colostomy

Relieve distal obstruction (e.g., malignant/inflammatory stricture).

Fecal incontinence.

Emergency management of anastomotic leak.

To defunction an intestinal fistula or peri anal complex fistulae.

28.2.4 Stoma Complications and Management

The reported incidence of stoma-related complications ranges from 20% to 70% [1].

The complications recorded are generally classified as early and late complications.

28.2.5 Early Complications

28.2.5.1 Inappropriate Site

An inappropriate site leads to leakage, skin irritation and skin breakdown around the stoma.

It should be a practice to site the stoma before surgery and mark on the skin preoperatively. The stoma should not be in a skin crease and should be visible to the patient in all positions.

28.3 Electrolyte Imbalance

Significant diarrhea and dehydration occur in up to 20% of ileostomy patients [2]. It all depends on the length of the bowel remaining before the stoma as to get the maximum absorptive surface area. Electrolyte imbalances are more common with jejunostomies than ileostomies and uncommon with colostomies.

For management of a high output stoma, high-fiber diet, low sugar, salt, and fat is important. Drugs like anticholinergics(loperamide), PPIs, Rececadrotil (antisecretory) are required. Food materials which are absorbed in early part of the intestine are important. These include simple sugars, predigested foods (which are commercially available). If the imbalance becomes severe patient may require IV fluids and electrolyte replacement.

28.3.1 Cutaneous

The contents of stoma especially Ileostomy contains proteolytic enzymes and high alkaline content which can damage the epidermal structure. Skin complications include.

Peristomal dermatitis is majorly a problem for the ileostomy patients. Peristomal dermatitis is reported in 5–25% of patients [3]. The best method of prevention is to fashion a protrubent spout to the ileostomy of 2–3 cm in length which prevents the direct contact of the fluid with the skin.

Some less common but troublesome skin problems include **parastomal ulceration (PSU)** and **pyoderma gangrenosum (PG).**

Topical, oral, or intralesional steroids are used for management depending on the severity of ulceration. The aim of therapy is to keep the affected area dry and allow an appliance to be placed. Application of stoma or antibiotic powder covered by a hydrocolloid usually serves the purpose.

In case of severe pyoderma is severe, resisting the ostomy is done, but frequently pyoderma recurs at the new ostomy site. If possible, the best management of peristomal pyoderma is to close the ostomy.

In general, to prevent the cutaneous complications it is important to make a good stoma and to use a well-fitting stoma appliance.

28.3.2 Retraction

Retraction is the inversion of the mucocutaneous junction toward the abdominal wall, The commonest underlying cause for stoma retraction is tension on the bowel. It is more commonly seen in patients with a higher body mass index.

To prevent tension on the bowel wall for stomas adequate mobilization is mandatory.

A stoma rod has traditionally been used to prevent retraction; however, a recent systematic review and meta-analysis showed that a stoma rod for loop stoma construction did not prevent stoma retraction.

28.4 Ischemia or Necrosis

Various studies have reported different incidence rates for stoma necrosis ranging from 1% to 10% in colostomies and 1–5% for ileostomies [4].

The commonest causes of ischemia are tension on the mesentery or too much trimming of the mesentery at the time of stoma formation. This more commonly seen in patients with high BMI and after emergency stoma formation. Another cause is tight stoma that is there is pressure on to the stomal mesentery because of small opening being made in the sheath. This leads to hampered vascularity and consequent stomal ischemia.

If the necrosis involves only the superficial few millimeters of the spout, then a 'wait and watch' policy is used. If required that very involved part may be resected and stoma skin sutures can be retaken. However, if the necrosis extends deep to the fascial planes, then an urgent refashioning of the stoma is warranted.

28.4.1 Intestinal Obstruction

Bowel obstruction after ileostomy creation is relatively common, affecting up to 25% of ileostomies during their lifetime [5].

Small bowel obstruction in the early postoperative period can be due to Twisting of the stoma. The 'twist' may be because of failure to orientate the stoma appropriately at the time of surgery or could be related to a volvulus of small bowel around the ileostomy. Volvulus can be potentially avoided by suturing the cut edge of mesentery to the peritoneum, closing any lateral space.

CT is the imaging modality of choice when a mechanical small bowel obstruction is suspected. Surgical exploration is required for the management of twisting or volvulus.

Simple adhesions can also lead to the intestinal obstruction. Most of the times the condition is relieved conservatively, but surgery may also be required.

28.4.2 Late Complications

28.4.2.1 Stenosis

Stomal stenosis is reported in 2–15% of the stomas [6].

The majority of stenoses develop within the first 5 years of stoma formation. It is more common in Crohn's patients.

If the underlying problem is narrowing of the skin trephine it can be treated with a local procedure.

If the underlying problem is IBD or ischemic stricturing of the stoma, then refashioning of the stoma may be required. Beraldo et al. have described a novel W-plasty technique for dealing with the stenotic stomas.

28.4.2.2 Parastomal Hernia

The most common complication associated with a stoma is parastomal herniation (PSH) (Diagram 28.1).

They occur in approximately 30% of stomas and in up to 50% of colostomies [7].

Symptoms of PSH include peristomal discomfort, pain, appliance leakage, difficulty in fitting appliances, bowel obstruction, and incarceration Table 28.1.

The incidence of parastomal hernias can be reduced by using an extra-peritoneal technique, limiting the size of the trephine, or by strengthening with a mesh.

Management of PSH can be surgical or non- surgical. The nonsurgical treatment includes the use of a hernia support belt and flexible appliance. An elective surgery may be indicated depending on the patient's comorbidities and symptoms, after a risk-benefit analysis.

Emergency surgery is required for non-resolving bowel obstruction and incarcerated PSH.

Diagram 28.1 Parastomal Hernia. Small bowel herniating in the subcutaneous region by the side of the stoma

Parastomal hernia-

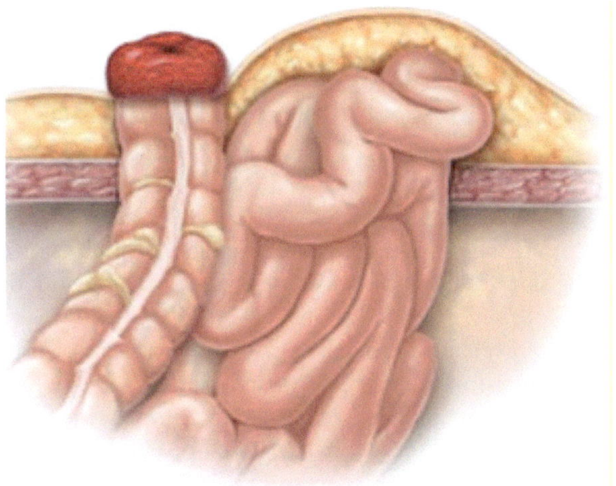

Table 28.1 Risk factors for parastomal hernia

Patient factors
• Obesity
• Malnutrition
• Advanced age
• Smoking
• Collagen abnormalities
• Corticosteroid use
• Postoperative wound sepsis
• Ascites
• Abdominal distention
• Chronic constipation
• Obstructive uropathy
• Chronic obstructive lung disease.
Surgical technical factors
• Inappropriate stoma site selection
• Oversized fascial trephine
• xcessive splitting and stretching of abdominal rectus muscle.
• Epigastric nerve denervation
• Emergency stoma creation

28.5 Surgical Repair of Parastomal Hernia

28.5.1 Indications of Surgical Repair

Absolute: Obstruction, Incarceration with strangulation.

Relative: Incarceration, Prolapse, Stenosis, Intractable dermatitis, Difficulty with appliance management, Large size, Cosmesis, Pain.

28.5.2 Local Repair (Direct Suture Repair)

Local repair includes a local exploration around the stoma site, with primary closure of the defect with either absorbable or nonabsorbable sutures. The advantages of this approach are avoidance of formal laparotomy and the ability to maintain stoma in the same location. Local repair is generally avoided due to high recurrence rates (75%) [8].

Stoma relocation can be performed with a peristomal incision. Benefits of peristomal incision include less postoperative pain, reduced operative time and lower incidence of incisional hernia. A laparotomy is generally required in patients who have had multiple previous surgeries or if the hernia is very large. The recurrence rate associated with this technique varies from 0% to 76% [8].

Mesh repair is considered as the standard treatment of PSH.

Repairs including onlay, sublay, and open intraperitoneal mesh placement, with recurrence rates of 17%, 6.9%, and 9.2%, respectively.

In the laparoscopic approach, the Sugarbaker technique has a lower recurrence rate than the Keyhole technique (12% vs. 35%) [9].

28.5.2.1 Prolapse

Stoma prolapse is full-thickness protrusion of bowel through the stoma. It can occur in up to that occurs in 3% of ileostomies, 2% of colostomies, and 1% of urostomies [10] (Diagram 28.2).

Prolapse can occur with any stoma and a highest incidence of approximately 7–25% is reported with loop transverse colostomy [11].

28.5.3 Classification

Sliding: It occurs intermittently with a increase in intra-abdominal pressure.

Fixed: It is present constantly.

Prolapse occurs more commonly with loop stomas and more commonly involves the efferent limb.

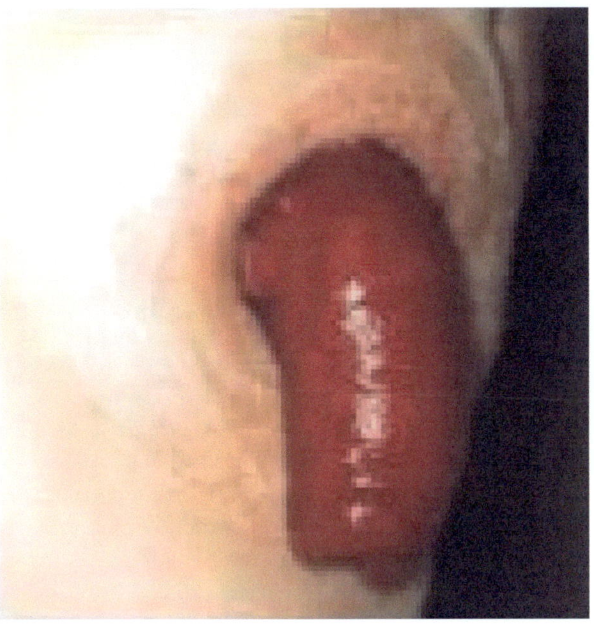

Diagram 28.2 Stoma prolapse

28.5.4 Risk Factors

(a) Patient Factors: Age, obesity, increased intra-abdominal pressure, chronic obstructive pulmonary disease, bowel redundancy, and weak fascia
(b) Surgical factors: improper stoma site (outside the rectal muscle), oversized aperture, redundancy of the bowel at the stoma site, and the space between the abdominal wall and the stoma.

Mesenteric fixation does not reduce the incidence of stomal prolapse.

28.5.5 Complications

Bowel obstruction,

Incarceration.

Strangulation.

28.5.6 Symptoms

Include pain, difficulty in fitting the appliance, skin excoriation.

28.5.7 Management

Acute: Can often be reduced. Sometimes hygroscopic agents like sugars, glycerine may be required to reduce the oedema before the reduction of stoma. It can convert an emergency situation to elective one.

28.5.8 Surgical Management

In most cases it requires local procedures only.

The surgical procedures include Fixation or resection of prolapsed bowel. Altemier's procedure or Delorme's procedure.

Rarely stoma needs to be resited. Minimally invasive techniques have also been described using linear stapler.

In conclusion stoma formation is an important surgical procedure. It is associated with its own complications which can majority of the times be dealt with by conservative methods but may require surgery in few cases.

References

1. Bafford A, Irani J. Management and complications of stomas. Surg Clin N Am. 2013;93(1):145–66.
2. Wexner S, Taranow D, Johansen O, Itzkowitz F, Daniel N, Nogueras J, et al. Loop ileostomy is a safe option for fecal diversion. Dis Colon Rectum. 1993;36(4):349–54.
3. Leong A, Londono-Schimmer E, Phillips R. Life-table analysis of stomal complications following ileostomy. Br J Surg. 1994;81(5):727–9.
4. Salvadalena G. Incidence of complications of the stoma and peristomal skin among individuals with colostomy, ileostomy, and urostomy. J Wound Ostomy Continence Nurs. 2008;35(6):596–607.
5. Marcello P, Roberts P, Schoetz D, Coller J, Murray J, Veidenheimer M. Obstruction after ileal pouch-anal anastomosis. Dis Colon Rectum. 1993;36(12):1105–11.
6. Beraldo S, Titley G, Allan A. Use of W-plasty in stenotic stoma: a new solution for an old problem. Color Dis. 2006;8(8):715–6.
7. Saunders R, Hemingway D. Intestinal stomas. Surgery (Oxford). 2008;26(8):347–51.
8. Rubin M. Parastomal hernia. Arch Surg. 1994;129(4):413.
9. Hansson B, Slater N, van der Velden A, Groenewoud H, Buyne O, de Hingh I, et al. Surgical techniques for parastomal hernia repair. Ann Surg. 2012;255(4):685–95.
10. Fleshman J, Lewis M. Complications and quality of life after stoma surgery: a review of 16,470 patients in the UOA Data Registry. Semin Colon Rectal Surg. 2007;18(1):19–24.
11. Renzulli C. Der künstliche Darmausgang—Indikationen, Stomaformen, chirurgische Technik. Ther Umsch. 2007;64(9):517–27.

Prevention and Management of Anastomotic Leaks and Fistulae

29

Neeraj Goel and Aseem Jindal

29.1 Introduction

Anastomosis is an integral part of any gastrointestinal surgical procedure be it esophago-gastric anastomosis or colorectal anastomosis or pancreatic or biliary anastomosis. Whenever an anastomosis leaks it is associated with significant morbidity, reoperations, and mortality.

Anastomotic leak is defined as the communication between lumen of anastomosis and the peritoneal cavity at the anastomotic level.

Overall, the incidence of anastomotic leak ranges from 2% to 10% in people undergoing Gastrointestinal surgery.

The anastomotic leak is associated with major morbidity, mortality, and poor long-term outcomes. The rate of morbidity lies between range of 20–30% and rate of mortality lies between 7–12%.

The major leaks encountered include esophago-gastric anastomosis, colorectal anastomosis, and Pancreatic Fistula. Any of these anastomotic leaks lead to significant morbidity.

A. Jindal · N. Goel (✉)
Department of Surgical Gastroenterology, Dharamshila Narayana Superspeciality Hospital, Delhi, India
e-mail: neeraj.goel.dr@narayanahealth.org

K. Sood Sharma et al. (eds.), *Complications of Cancer Therapy: Best Practices in Prevention and Management*, https://doi.org/10.1007/978-981-99-0984-1_29

29.2 Colorectal Anastomotic Leak

Anastomosis leak (AL) is still the most serious complication of colorectal surgery. The overall incidence ranges from 2.8% to 8.4% [1]. AL was documented to occur in 8.1% of patients after right hemicolectomy according to the 2015 ESCP snapshot audit. It was 6.4% after colonic cancer surgery according to a nationwide Danish study which included 9333 patients. A systematic review and meta-analysis pooling 84 studies reported the leak rate to be 11% after rectal cancer surgery [2]. Anastomosis done lower down in the pelvis have an increased propensity to leak.

It is important to note that in cancer surgery, along with septic complications, AL is associated with increased local recurrences and reduced overall survival.

It is grouped as: Grade A (no management), Grade B (non-operative management), Grade C (operative management)

29.2.1 Risk Factors

The risk factors can be divided into three broad categories

29.2.1.1 Pre-operative

Statistically speaking male gender, smoking, obesity, alcohol, steroid, and non- steroidal anti-inflammatory drugs; all have been incriminated as risk factors for the AL. Various studies have shown that poor nutrition status as indicated by Albumin <3.5 g/dL is associated with increased chances of anastomotic dehiscence. Preoperative radiotherapy and chemotherapy especially if surgery occurred within an interval of 11–17 d after intervention has also been documented as risk factor for anastomotic leak [3].

29.2.1.2 Operative

Major risk factor is the ischemia at the anastomotic level. To achieve a well vascularized bowel end, strict adherence to the anatomic blood supply pattern is utmost important. Taking wide resection to healthy uninvolved bowel reduces the risk of AL.

Prolonged operative time, transfusion, contamination of the operative field and emergency surgery are other factors associated with AL.

Distance of the tumor from the anal verge is also recognized as a risk factor for AL. In a study comprising of 35 patients demonstrated that resection of rectal tumors which are located within 12 cm of anal verge have an increased incidence of anastomotic dehiscence when compared with tumor resection more than 12 cm away (7.4% vs. 3.0%) (OR, 4.5) [4].

29.2.2 Surgical Technique

It is important to understand that the mode of surgery be it open, laparoscopic, or robotic does not have significant differences in leak rates. A systematic review and meta-analysis including 7780 patients undergoing right colectomies found no difference in terms of AL between the laparoscopic and robotic approaches. Similarly, a Cochrane systematic review and meta-analysis of RCTs for elective and emergency sigmoidectomy for diverticulitis, did not show any difference in terms of reoperation due to AL between patients with who underwent laparoscopic colectomy or open colectomy. Also, in the intermediate analysis of the ROLARR trial there was no difference in AL rate between surgical approaches for rectal cancer [5].

29.2.3 Anastomotic Technique

There was no difference in incidence of ALs in patients undergoing hand sewn or stapled anastomosis in a Cochrane systematic review and meta-analysis of 1233 patients from 9 RCTs [6]. A study from Austria showed that if three or more cartridges are used to transect rectum (double stapling technique (transection with linear stapler and anastomosis with circular stapler), the chances of AL increase (19.4% AL in this subgroup). Also, the number of intersections of staple lines also correlated to the rate of AL in colorectal anastomosis using a double stapling technique [7].

29.2.3.1 Postoperative

Post operative hypotension and use of inotropic support has also been implicated as risk for AL.

29.2.4 Prevention of Anastomosis Leak

29.2.4.1 Preoperative Measures

(a) It is imperative to improve onto the modifiable risk factors such as nutrition if the time permits before surgery. This correction can lead to decrease in AL. Implementation of Enhanced Recovery After Surgery, ERAS, protocols have revolutionized the postoperative management and have led to decreased postoperative morbidity and length of stay. However, their effect on the rate of AL is yet to be demonstrated.
(b) Oral antibiotics and mechanical bowel preparation: The American college of surgeon's national surgical quality improvement program database showed that use of mechanical bowel preparation alone or the use of oral antibiotics alone have no role in prevention of AL. But it also demonstrated that the use of oral antibiotic with mechanical bowel preparation can decrease the risk of AL from 5.7% to 2.8% [8].
(c) Microbiome study: It is a recent and upcoming field of research in colorectal surgery. The unfavorable microbiome, which comprises of pathogens with high collagenase activity, if minimized can lead to decrease AL rate. This can be done by using appropriate antibiotic regimen (per os, intravenous or by enema) and/or fecal transplantation if required. For instance, in an experimental study

by Shogan *et al* in a rat model, it was seen that *Enterococcus faecalis* leads to the degradation of collagen IV at the anastomotic level by activating of MMP9.

29.2.5 Management of AL

Anastomotic leaks once occurred is a nightmare for the surgeon and the patients both. Management involves both operative and non-operative measures.

(a) Non-Operative Measures

The patient with Colorectal AL needs to be assessed for the signs of sepsis. The antibiotics usually needs to be escalated. If drain is present, it may assist in assessing the magnitude of leak.

Non operative management is usually acceptable in patients who have a diversion ileostomy in place or having a minimal amount of leak and minimal pelvic sepsis.

A CT scan requires to be done to assess the amount of free fluid present. If significant amount is present it may require to be drained by radiologic placements of drains.

A patient with diversion ileostomy in place usually would not require operative management and leak heals on its own.

But the patients who have no diversion stoma and severe spillage and sepsis would require surgical intervention.

(b) Operative Measures

Prevention is the key.

1. **Assessment of blood supply to the anastomosis**: Doppler ultrasound, light spectroscopy and Fluorescence perfusion angiography are various methods for assessment of blood supply. Fluorescence perfusion angiography with use of ICG has showed to reduce the AL. Jafari et al. reported that fluorescence perfusion angiography allowed to reduce AL from 18% to 6% after robotic–assisted anterior resection [9].
2. **Intraoperative assessment of the anastomosis:**

   Various methods include. Air leak test and intraoperative endoscopy.

   We routinely use Air leak test at our Institute. Endoscopy is employed on as required basis. Endoscopy in addition can help identify the bleeding site.
3. **Diverting stoma**: A Cochrane systematic review and meta-analysis including RCT assessing the use of prophylactic stoma versus no stoma in patients with low anterior resection for rectal cancer described the use of covering stoma to lower the incidence of AL (RR 0.33) [10]. The results are controversial, but diversion stomas do decrease the morbidity and mortality in patient with low anastomosis. Also, diverting stoma expose the patients to the risk of dehydration or to stoma closure-related complications. We at our Institute routinely make stomas for low pelvic anastomosis.

4. **Prophylactic intra-abdominal drainage**: The GRECCAR 5 trial, systematic review, and meta-analysis pooling 760 patients from 4 RCT and A Cochrane systematic review found that there is no role of intraabdominal drainage for prevention of anastomosis leak but again it helps in reducing the morbidity by draining the collections [11].
5. **Prophylactic trans anal tube decompression**: A systematic review and meta-analysis pooling 1772 patients undergoing anterior resection described trans anal tube decompression to lower the risk of AL (RR 0.44) [12].

   In patients who do not have covering ileostomies surgical intervention may be required which involves doing a thorough lavage, putting drains, and making the covering stomas. The surgery can be done both open and laparoscopic. Such patients are usually sick and would require ICU management and prolonged hospital stays.

29.2.6 Pancreatic Fistula

Postoperative pancreatic fistula (POPF) is the most serious complication after pancreaticoduodenectomy (PD). The incidence range is quite variable ranging from 2% to 51% in different series [13].

The International Study Group on Pancreatic Surgery (ISGPS) recently defined the PF as any measurable volume of fluid (more than 30–50 ml/day) on or after post- operative day 3, with amylase content greater than three times the reference serum amylase activity.

With advances in surgical techniques and perioperative management, the mortality caused by PD decreased to less than 5% in high-volume centers, while the rate of postoperative complications remained as high as 50%, especially postoperative pancreatic fistulas (POPF) and delayed gastric emptying (DGE) [14]

ISGPS classifies fistulas as:

Grade A (patient is stable and asymptomatic, has a transient fistula and no collections in computed tomography)

Grade B (symptomatic fistula, patient needs parenteral nutrition, antibiotics and somatostatin and has peripancreatic collections that can be percutaneously drained)

Grade C (severe fistula, patient needs to be under intensive care, have percutaneous drainage of the collections or surgery to repair the leakage, to change from PJ to PG or to do a total pancreatectomy)

29.2.7 Risk Factors

These include

Pancreas risk factors (pancreatic texture, pancreatic duct size, blood supply to the stump, volume of pancreatic juice output, and pathologic features)

Patient risk factors (age, sex, bilirubin level, and comorbid illness)

Operation risk factors (operating time, blood loss, type of anastomosis, and stent use).

Among these risk factors, pancreatic texture (soft pancreas), pancreatic duct size (< 3mm), blood supply to the stump, and volume of pancreatic juice output have been considered the most significant [15].

Reconstruction Methods: Always a contentious issue whether Pancreaticogastrostomy (PG) or Pancreatojejunostomy (PJ) is superior. There is no clear-cut winner in terms of ALs, but PJ is more physiologic. It is matter of surgeon's preference.

Anastomotic Techniques: Duct to mucosa anastomosis (Baumgart's or Berger's) is the primary method of reconstruction. But sometimes the duct is not dilated in such a scenario we find the Invagination method is good.

Multiple meta-analysis has found no difference in the incidence of POPF with different types of anastomoses. The search for the best one continues [16].

Similarly pancreatic stents, Glue application at anastomosis and somatostatin use are all controversial.

At our center we prefer Duct to mucosa anastomosis for dilated ducts and invagination method for non-dilated ducts. We use pancreatic stents and somatostatin during the anastomosis and continue it in the post operative period.

29.2.8 Management

It would not be wrong to say that POPF is the Achilles Heel of all the complications after PD.

The management depends upon the grade of the fistula. Grade A and B fistulae usually heal with conservative methods. A good clinical care is required for these POPF patients. All the undrained collections should be drained by putting image guided catheters. Patient's may need higher antibiotics. Somatostatin has limited role in the management of the POPF

It is the Grade C type of fistulas which are particularly serious ones. Patient may be in sepsis; again, good critical care is required along with image guided catheters. But the patients who don't improve with measures and have other sequelae like fever and bleeding would require surgery.

During surgery the PJ may be converted to PG or in rare cases total pancreatectomy may be employed. The surgical interventions in such a scenario is associated with high morbidity and mortality and prolonged ICU stays.

29.2.9 Esophagogastric Anastomosis Leak

According to the recent Esophagectomy Complications Consensus Group (ECCG) consensus definition, anastomotic leakage is defined as a "full thickness gastrointestinal defect involving esophagus, anastomosis, staple line, or conduit irrespective of presentation or method of identification"

The incidence of esophagogastric anastomosis, ranges between 5% to 30% of patients, anastomosis leak is major cause of morbidity and mortality.

29.2.9.1 Classification of Anastomotic Leakage Severity According to the ECCG [17]

Leakage severity

Grade I: Local defect requiring no change in therapy or treated medically or with dietary modification
Grade II: Localized defect which needs some intervention like Pigtail insertion, stent, or bedside drainage but not surgical therapy.
Grade III: Localized defect which needs surgical therapy

29.2.10 Risk Factors

Patient factors includes Hypoalbuminemia, Older age, Alcohol abuse Obesity (BMI >30 kg/m^2) and Comorbidities including diabetes, hypertension, COPD can contribute to ALs. Celiac artery calcifications and systemic atherosclerosis can lead to impaired blood supply to anastomosis resulting in leaks. Steroid, immunosuppressant use and Anti-angiogenic therapy can delay healing of anastomosis. Preoperative Radiation therapy especially radiation of gastric fundus or in field anastomosis have major implication in anastomosis leak [18].

Perioperative including Gastric distention and delayed gastric emptying can also contribute to Leaks.

29.2.11 Prevention of Anastomosis Leak

This goes without saying that maintenance of a well vascularized gastric conduit is utmost important. The stomach should be mobilized well preserving the Right Gastric and Right Gastro-epiploic arteries. Sometimes a good Kocher's maneuver may also be required.

Cervical anastomosis is believed to be associated with higher chances of anastomosis leak than thoracic anastomosis, but thoracic anastomosis leaks results in mediastinal and thoracic manifestation leading to increased morbidity and mortality. **In addition, cervical ALs are easier to manage. Majority of the esophageal surgeons prefer cervical anastomosis because of said reasons. But which anastomosis to apply depends upon the approach.**

29.2.12 Omentoplasty

Role of omentoplasty is reduction of leaks is not supported by recent meta-analysis.

29.2.13 Ongoing Research

Ischemic preconditioning of the stomach -This approach includes selective ligation or occlusion of left gastric artery by either laparoscopic or radiofrequency ablation. This is done 2 weeks prior to surgery. This is thought to improve gastric perfusion prior to resection. This technique is also known as "supercharging". The role of this technique in under evaluation [19].

Intra-operative assessment of conduit- The most recent method for intraoperative assessment of perfusion of conduit is fluorescent imaging using indocyanine green (ICG). A recent meta-analysis reported that the use of ICG fluorescence imaging leads to a change in management in about 25% of cases [20].

Stem cell therapy is another theoretic approach for the treatment of anastomotic leakage. A higher healing rate and decreased wound infection rate was seen in a study from China when of a mixture of autologous mesenchymal stem cells in a fibrin solution was injected around a cervical anastomotic leak in an animal model and compared to fibrin injection alone [21].

29.2.14 Management

29.2.14.1 Non-invasive Treatment

Conservative non-invasive management includes use of antibiotics, placement of a nasogastric tube, and nutritional support.

29.2.14.2 Endoscopic Management

Collections which cannot be drained using a chest tube or percutaneous Endoscopic drain, the endoscopic drain placement through the anastomotic defect may be used for drainage of fluid cavities. Endoscopy may also aid in placement of a fully covered self-expanding stent, to prevent further leakage in patients with limited contamination.

Endoluminal vacuum assisted closure devices (E-VAC or EsoSponge) is most recent advancement. These devices act by combining effective drainage with stimulation of anastomotic healing [22].

29.2.14.3 Surgical Management

Surgical treatment of anastomotic leakage includes bedside chest tube placement, reoperation for drainage, re-anastomosis or taking down the anastomosis in combination with esophageal diversion. Reoperations can be performed by either an open or minimally invasive approach.

29.2.14.4 Surgical Drainage

A "three-tube" strategy, in which nasogastric decompression tube, nasojejunal feeding tube and chest tube placement was performed. With this technique the healing time of the leak was shorter, and this strategy was effective in patients with both contained intrathoracic leaks and patients with uncontained leaks, when compared with patients who underwent surgical re-exploration [23].

29.2.14.5 Surgical Repair and Diversion

Surgical treatment is used in a failed non operative management. Surgical repair options may range from suture repair to Re-anastomosis.

A muscle flap repair using either diaphragm, latissimus dorsi, serratus anterior or pectoralis muscle flaps can be performed as primary treatment or secondary treatment depending on the location of the leak [24].

In fulminant cases with increasing sepsis and gastric necrosis, Excision and diversion is done. A common technique for diverting the esophagus is performing an end-esophagostomy or a double-barrel esophago-gastrostomy [25].

References

1. Park J, Huh J, Park Y, Cho Y, Yun S, Kim H, et al. Risk factors of anastomotic leakage and long-term survival after colorectal surgery. Medicine. 2016;95(8):e2890.
2. 2015 European Society of Coloproctology Collaborating Group. The impact of stapling technique and surgeon specialism on anastomotic failure after right-sided colorectal resection: an international multicentre, prospective audit. Colorectal Dis. 2018;20(11):1028–40.
3. Choudhuri A, Uppal R, Kumar M. Influence of non-surgical risk factors on anastomotic leakage after major gastrointestinal surgery: audit from a tertiary care teaching institute. Int J Crit Illn Inj Sci. 2022;
4. Mäkelä J, Kiviniemi H, Laitinen S. Risk factors for anastomotic leakage after left-sided colorectal resection with rectal anastomosis. Dis Colon Rectum. 2003;46(5):653–60.
5. Solaini L, Bazzocchi F, Cavaliere D, Avanzolini A, Cucchetti A, Ercolani G. Robotic versus laparoscopic right colectomy: an updated systematic review and meta-analysis. Surg Endosc. 2017;32(3):1104–10.
6. Neutzling C, Lustosa S, Proenca I, da Silva E, Matos D. Stapled versus handsewn methods for colorectal anastomosis surgery. Cochrane Database Syst Rev. 2012;2
7. Braunschmid T, Hartig N, Baumann L, Dauser B, Herbst F. Influence of multiple stapler firings used for rectal division on colorectal anastomotic leak rate. Surg Endosc. 2017;31(12):5318–26.
8. Scarborough J, Mantyh C, Sun Z, Migaly J. Combined mechanical and oral antibiotic bowel preparation reduces incisional surgical site infection and anastomotic leak rates after elective colorectal resection. Ann Surg. 2015;262(2):331–7.
9. Jafari M, Lee K, Halabi W, Mills S, Carmichael J, Stamos M, et al. The use of indocyanine green fluorescence to assess anastomotic perfusion during robotic assisted laparoscopic rectal surgery. Surg Endosc. 2013;27(8):3003–8.
10. Montedori A, Cirocchi R, Farinella E, Sciannameo F, Abraha I. Covering ileo- or colostomy in anterior resection for rectal carcinoma. Cochrane Database Syst Rev. 2010;(5):CD006878. https://doi.org/10.1002/14651858.CD006878.pub2.
11. Denost Q, Rouanet P, Faucheron J, Panis Y, Meunier B, Cotte E, et al. Impact of early biochemical diagnosis of anastomotic leakage after rectal cancer surgery: long-term results from GRECCAR 5 trial. Br J Surg. 2017;108(6):605–8.

12. Yang Y, Shu Y, Su F, Xia L, Duan B, Wu X. Prophylactic transanal decompression tube versus non-prophylactic transanal decompression tube for anastomotic leakage prevention in low anterior resection for rectal cancer: a meta-analysis. Surg Endosc. 2016;31(4):1513–23.
13. Büchler M. Changes in morbidity after pancreatic resection. Arch Surg. 2003;138(12):1310.
14. Kitahata Y, Hirono S, Kawai M, Okada K, Miyazawa M, Shimizu A, et al. Intensive perioperative rehabilitation improves surgical outcomes after pancreaticoduodenectomy. Langenbeck's Arch Surg. 2018;403(6):711–8.
15. Poon R, Lo S, Fong D, Fan S, Wong J. Prevention of pancreatic anastomotic leakage after pancreaticoduodenectomy. Am J Surg. 2002;183(1):42–52.
16. Langrehr J, Bahra M, Jacob D, Glanemann M, Neuhaus P. Prospective randomized comparison between a new mattress technique and Cattell (duct-to-mucosa) pancreaticojejunostomy for pancreatic resection. World J Surg. 2005;29(9):1111–9.
17. Low D, Alderson D, Cecconello I, Chang A, Darling G, D'Journo X, et al. International consensus on standardization of data collection for complications associated with esophagectomy. Ann Surg. 2015;262(2):286–94.
18. Kamarajah S, Lin A, Tharmaraja T, Bharwada Y, Bundred J, Nepogodiev D, et al. Risk factors and outcomes associated with anastomotic leaks following esophagectomy: a systematic review and meta-analysis. Dis Esophagus. 2020;33(3):doz089.
19. Yetasook A, Leung D, Howington J, Talamonti M, Zhao J, Carbray J, et al. Laparoscopic ischemic conditioning of the stomach prior to esophagectomy. Dis Esophagus. 2012;26(5):479–86.
20. Slooter M, Eshuis W, Cuesta M, Gisbertz S, van Berge HM. Fluorescent imaging using indocyanine green during esophagectomy to prevent surgical morbidity: a systematic review and meta-analysis. J Thorac Dis. 2019;11(S5):S755–65.
21. Xue X, Yan Y, Ma Y, Yuan Y, Li C, Lang X, et al. Stem-cell therapy for esophageal anastomotic leakage by autografting stromal cells in fibrin scaffold. Stem Cells Transl Med. 2019;8(6):548–56.
22. Bludau M, Hölscher A, Herbold T, Leers J, Gutschow C, Fuchs H, et al. Management of upper intestinal leaks using an endoscopic vacuum-assisted closure system (E-VAC). Surg Endosc. 2013;28(3):896–901.
23. Guo J, Chu X, Liu Y, Zhou N, Ma Y, Liang C. Choice of therapeutic strategies in intrathoracic anastomotic leak following esophagectomy. World J Surg Oncol. 2014;12(1)
24. Kotzampassakis N, Christodoulou M, Krueger T, Demartines N, Vuillemier H, Cheng C, et al. Esophageal leaks repaired by a muscle onlay approach in the presence of mediastinal sepsis. Ann Thorac Surg. 2009;88(3):966–72.
25. Manghelli J, Ceppa D, Greenberg J, Blitzer D, Hicks A, Rieger K, et al. Management of anastomotic leaks following esophagectomy: when to intervene? J Thorac Dis. 2019;11(1):131–7.

Prevention and Management of Chylothorax Post Esophagectomy in Carcinoma Oesophagus

30

Sandeep K. Mohan, Ashwani Sharma, and Surender Dabas

Chylothorax is by definition a collection of chyle in the pleural cavity resulting from leakage from the lymphatic vessels, usually from the thoracic duct. Any lesions of the thoracic duct can quickly lead to the formation of large fluid collections, as the duct transports around 2–4 L of fluid a day. Esophagectomy being a complicated and technically demanding surgery has its inherent complications, chylothorax being uncommon albiet one of the most debilitating and potentially life threatening, with a reported incidence of 0.4–4% [1, 2].

30.1 Anatomy and Pathophysiology

The thoracic duct drains the cisterna chyli, in which the lymph from the lower half of the body and the abdominal cavity joins the chyle coming from the intestinal trunk, forming a mixture also referred to as chyle. Its close spatial relationships with other structures explain why it is at risk of injury during surgery especially esophagectomy along the course of this lymph drainage pathway. When the thoracic duct (or a large communicating lymph vessel) is leaky or damaged, due a traumatic or a non traumatic cause, the fluid that leaks out either collects locally and later breaks through into the pleural cavity, or it flows directly into the latter via existing pleural defects (e.g., caused by surgery). Rarely, chylothorax may occur due to transdiaphragmatic flow in a patient with chylous ascites. Presently the most common traumatic cause is chest surgery [1], e.g., esophageal resection, which leads to chylothorax in about 3% of cases.

S. K. Mohan · A. Sharma (✉) · S. Dabas
Department of Surgical Oncology and Robotic Surgery, BLK MAX Superspeciality Hospital, New Delhi, India

K. Sood Sharma et al. (eds.), *Complications of Cancer Therapy: Best Practices in Prevention and Management*, https://doi.org/10.1007/978-981-99-0984-1_30

30.2 Clinical Presentation

The most common clinical presentation in the postoperative period is with excessive external drainage via a chest thoracostomy in the early postoperative period or a large effusion (chylothorax) where no drain is present. Since enteral nutrition via a feeding jejunostomy or nasojejunally is commonly begun on the first or second postoperative day, the drainage of cream like effluent is the most common observation that establishes a clinical diagnosis [3]. This may be confirmed with laboratory evidence of a triglyceride levels >110 mg/dL (6.1 mmol/L) or less commonly via the confirmation of chylomicrons in the effluent. The volume of drainage is important, particularly if over 1 L in 24 h that may suggest complete disruption of the thoracic duct. A patient who persistently loses chyle will be losing considerable amounts of fat and fat-soluble vitamins, proteins (chyle contains 12–60 g/L, depending on nutritional intake), electrolytes, immunoglobulins, and T-lymphocytes, with resulting malnutrition, weight loss, and an impaired immune system [4, 5]. After only 8 days of T-cell depletion due to external chyle drainage, patients are already at risk of septicemia [6]. About 50% of patients with untreated chylothorax die from the resulting complications with 30-day mortality going up to fivefold [7, 8].

30.3 Prevention and Management

The anatomy of the thoracic duct varies considerably. This can make it difficult to assess during surgery. Techniques have been described in literature including administering cream orally before primary oesophageal surgery to aid in the identification of the thoracic duct. The duct along with other lymphatic channels can then be ligated as appropriate, helping reduce the incidence of post-operative chylothorax [8]. Prophylactic ligation of the thoracic duct has been described as an efficacious method to prevent chylothorax after oesophagectomy, but there are few relevant studies available that attest to the effectiveness of this surgical technique characterized by contradictory results [9, 10]. Meta-analysis on the prophylactic ligation of the thoracic duct during oesophagectomy reports a slight and statistically significant clinical advantage in performing prophylactic ligation of thoracic duct to prevent chylothorax [11].

30.4 Therapeutic Options

Because of the rarity of this complication, there are no prospective or even randomized studies that give a clear answer to questions about how best to treat chylothorax and for how long. In general, conservative treatment is attempted first, usually for a limited time, before more invasive measures are embarked on [7, 12].

30.4.1 Conservative Treatment

The cornerstones of treatment are adequate fluid and electrolyte replacement along with appropriate nutrition. Repeated thoracocentesis is usually not performed and in patients with high-volume or, especially, symptomatic chylothorax, continuous drainage is put in place to allow the lung to re-expand and to optimize pulmonary function [13].

As part of initial conservative treatment, an attempt is made to reduce the flow of lymph through the thoracic duct to the point that the lymph leak will close up and the chytothorax eventually heal itself. The patient can be given a diet containing medium-chain triglycerides (MCT), which are absorbed directly into the portal venous system without going through the intestinal lymph vessels and the thoracic duct. It is rare, however, that these measures alone will suffice, so although it is more expensive and is associated with more problems, complete parenteral nutrition has in many places become established as the first step [14]. In addition to diet, it is possible to reduce lymph low by means of medication using somatostatin or its analog octreotide. Neither chylothorax as an indication nor the dose, method, and duration of drug administration have been confirmed or standardized in prospective studies. Mediastinal irradiation has been tried in as an adjuvant therapy in chylothorax but its role remains unclear.

Generally, the success rate of conservative treatment ranges from 16% to more than 75% but at output rates of more than 1000 mL/day, the success rate of conservative treatment is low [7, 12]. If the drain output reduces markedly under conservative treatment, it is advisable to consolidate the therapeutic outcome with a strict MCT diet for a few weeks.

Locating the exact site of a lymph leak is worthwhile only if the result is going to affect therapeutic management. Basically, a leak can be located non-invasively using radionuclides or magnetic resonance imaging [15, 16]. Diagnostic MRI uses so-called fluid-sensitive sequences (analogous to magnetic resonance cholangiopancreatography, MRCP). Its accuracy in terms of locating the leak site is superior to that of radionuclide imaging, and it can be helpful in the planning of an interventional procedure. Lymphography can also demonstrate a leak, but as the only invasive procedure is rarely indicated nowadays [17].

30.4.2 Surgical Treatment

When conservative treatment fails over a period of time, the only remaining treatment method is surgery, which if used early, can reduce the mortality rate associated with chylothorax from 50% to 10% [18–20].

Operative treatment was and is regarded as indicated when, for example:

- More than (1000–)1500 mL chyle is being drained every day (in children the threshold is >100 mL/kg body weight [BW])

- For 5 treatment days drain output is up to 1000 mL/day, or, in children, 100 mL/year of age.
- A leak persists for more than 2 weeks (100 mL/day >2 weeks)
- The drain output remains unchanged over 1–2 weeks
- Clinical deterioration occurs, e.g., malnutrition or metabolic problems

In patients with postoperative chylothorax, it must be remembered that early reoperation can put anastomoses at risk, so quite long attempts at conservative treatment are recommended, e.g., 2–4 weeks after esophagectomy. Early surgical treatment is recommended in young patients, those with a high-volume chyle leak, and those with a very lean body weight and poor physiological reserve.

Ligation of the thoracic duct is usually carried out above the right diaphragm between T8 and T12; after ligation, the lymph drains via lymphatic collaterals and lymphovenous anastomoses [21]. In general, the main difficulty in surgical treatment is identifying the thoracic duct or the leak. This becomes easier if cream is administered (e.g., intraoperatively via a stomach probe) [8]. If the duct is still not identifiable, mass ligation of the tissue in the presumed course of the thoracic duct can help [12]. Other problems that can lead to failure of surgery are failure to identify accessory lymphatic pathways, technically inadequate ligation, and surgical injury of the fragile duct during manipulation [22, 23].

If an operation has failed, or if thoracic duct ligation does not appear feasible or worthwhile, pleurodesis may heal the chylothorax [7, 12, 23]. Pleurodesis also offers a treatment option when a malignant tumor is the cause of the chylothorax. It is employed when treatment of the tumor has not resulted in sufficient improvement, or in situations where interrupting the thoracic duct is regarded as not feasible or worthwhile. It must be borne in mind that pleurodesis can only be successful in patients with expandable lungs (i.e., nontrapped lungs) [24]. Creation of lymphovenous anastomoses may be considered though it has not become established as a therapy. As a surgical last resort, creation of a pleuroperitoneal shunt or external intermittent permanent drainage through placement of a suitable catheter system may be considered [25].

Surgical treatment is successful in about 90% of cases, although some 10% of patients have to undergo several procedures [23]. For thoracic duct ligation, which is usually carried out in severely ill patients, high complication rates and mortality rates have been reported [16, 22] which have improved over a period of time owing to surgery being performed earlier, is less traumatic and better supportive measures being available.

30.5 Intervention Radiology

Today there are several radiology guided treatments that can be used in the management of chylothorax, although availability of these procedures is an issue.

Lymphography has been one such described procedure. After lymphography, healing of the chylothorax has been observed in about 6–50% of cases [26, 27].

However, the therapeutic success of lymphography cannot be assessed, so given the existence of other, more effective measures, this procedure has not become an established therapy. Direct occlusion of the lymph leak site can be tried using targeted CT-guided injection of tissue adhesive near the leak. Overall, there has not been much experience with these procedures.

However much more experience is available for percutaneous embolization of the thoracic duct, which can be performed as an alternative to thoracic duct ligation and can be performed in both adults and children [18, 20, 21, 28].

For thoracic duct embolization, first the abdominal lymph vessels, including the thoracic duct, are imaged lymphographically. After fine-needle puncture (21G) of a suitable lymph vessel, the thoracic duct is accessed with a thin guidewire (0.018 in.), and a microcatheter (F3) is introduced and placed below an identifiable leak [20, 28]. This technically demanding procedure cannot, however, always be performed as described, because the existence of anatomic variants -means that up to 30% of patients do not have a cisterna chyli or lymph vessel that is suitable for puncture [18, 20]. In these cases, the attempt may be made to "scratch" any prevertebral small lymph pathways identified lymphographically with a puncture needle ("needle disruption") and to reduce the flow of lymph by this means [20, 28]. In about one third of patients treated in this way, this leads to healing of the leak [20]. Embolization has a much higher success rate: if the thoracic duct can be intubated successfully, the procedure is successful in well over 90% of cases [18, 20, 21]. Percutaneous embolization can even lead to healing in patients who have been unsuccessfully treated with surgery.

In conclusion, the grade of evidence for optimum management of chyle leakage post esophageal resections is poor to date. There is, moreover, no universal management algorithm due to unique clinical factors impacting therapy such as age, functional status, local expertise, and rates of chyle accumulation. There is a paucity of high-quality prospective studies directly comparing treatment modalities; therefore, approaches are based upon clinical experience and low-quality reports. The improved nomenclature, and the advent of IR approaches, presents an opportunity to advance our understanding and management of this occasionally complex problem across the spectrum of its clinical presentation.

Key Points

- The most frequent causes of chylothorax today are surgery mainly esophagectomy and tumors.
- Clinically, chylothorax manifests non-specifically as a pleural effusion, typically with a triglyceride content of over 110 mg/dL.
- The diagnosis is confirmed by demonstrating the presence of chylomicrons in the aspirate.
- Untreated Chylothorax can lead to severe nutritional consequences and eventually high morbidity and mortality.
- As a rule, conservative treatment is tried first. The aim is to bring about spontaneous closure of a lymph leak by reducing the flow of lymph.

- The cornerstones of conservative and supportive treatment are adequate fluid and electrolyte replacement along with appropriate nutrition
- If conservative treatment fails, the next option to consider is surgery. This may be in the form of thoracic duct ligation, pleurodesis, or placement of a pleuroperitoneal shunt.
- Surgical treatment is successful in most of the cases, although some patients have to undergo several procedures
- Other alternatives available today are interventional radiological procedures such as percutaneous thoracic duct embolization.
- Individual case management is determined by the clinical situation and local availability of the various treatment options, since no prospective studies are available as a basis for guidance.

References

1. Lagarde SM, Omloo JM, de Jong K, Busch OR, Obertop H, van Lanschot JJ. Incidence and management of chyle leakage after esophagectomy. Ann Thorac Surg. 2005;80:449–54.
2. Shah RD, Luketich JD, Schuchert MJ, et al. Post esophagectomy chylothorax: incidence, risk factors, and outcomes. Ann Thorac Surg. 2012;93:897–903.
3. Pillay TG, Singh B. A review of traumatic chylothorax. Injury. 2016;47:545–50.
4. Soto-Martinez M, Massie J. Chylothorax: diagnosis and management in children. Paediatr Respir Rev. 2009;6:8.
5. Skouras V, Kalomenidis I. Chylothorax: diagnostic approach. Curr Opin Pulm Med. 2010;16:387–93.
6. Breaux J, Marks C. Chylothorax causing reversible T-cell depletion. J Trauma. 1988;28:705–7.
7. McGrath EE, Blades Z, Anderson PB. Chylothorax: aetiology, diagnosis and therapeutic options. Respir Med. 2010;105:1–8.
8. Shackcloth MJ, Poullis M, Lu J, Page RD. Preventing of chylothorax after oesophagectomy by routine pre-operative administration of oral cream. Eur J Cardiotharac Surg. 2001;20:1035–6.
9. Lai FC, Chen L, Tu YR, Lin M, Li X. Prevention of chylothorax complicating extensive esophageal resection by mass ligation of thoracic duct: a random control study. Ann Thorac Surg. 2011;91:1770–4.
10. You X, Fu J-H, Wang X, Zhang L-J, Liu Q-W, Luo K-J, et al. Prophylactic thoracic duct ligation has unfavorable impact on overall survival in patients with resectable oesophageal cancer. Eur J Surg Oncol. 2014;40:1756–62.
11. Crucittia P, Mangiamelia G, Petittib T, Condolucia A, Roccoa R, Francesca Gallo I, Longoa F, Rocco G. Does prophylactic ligation of the thoracic duct reduce chylothorax rates in patients undergoing oesophagectomy? A systematic review and meta-analysis. Eur J Cardiothorac Surg. 2016;50:1019–24.
12. Nair SK, Petko M, Hayward MP. Aetiology and management of chylothorax in adults. Eur J Cardiothorac Surg. 2007;32:362–9.
13. DePew ZS, Iqbal S, Nichols FC, Mullon JJ, Maldonado F. The role for tunneled indwelling pleural catheters in patients with persistent benign chylothorax. Am J Med Sci. 2013:1–4.
14. Ilczyszyn A, Ridha H, Durrani AJ. Management of chyle leak post neck dissection: a case report and literature review. J Plast Reconstr Aesthet Surg. 2011;64:e223–30.
15. Pui MH, Yueh TC. Lymphszintigraphy in chyluria, chyloperitoneum and chylothorax. J Nucl Med. 1998;39:1292–6.

16. Yu-XX MXX, Wang Q, Zhang Y, Li C-F. Morphological changes of the thoracic duct and accessory lymphatic channels in patients with chylothorax: detection with unenhanced magnetic resonance imaging. Eur Radiol. 2013;23:702–11.
17. Maldonado F, Cartin-Ceba R, Hawkins FJ, Ryu JH. Medical and surgical management of chylothorax and associated outcomes. Am J Med Sci. 2010;339:314–8.
18. Itkin M, Krishnamurthy G, Naim MY, Bird GL, Keller MS. Percutaneous thoracic duct embolization as a treatment for intrathoracic chyle leaks in infants. Pediatrics. 2011;128:e237.
19. Orringer MB, Bluett M, Deeb GM. Aggressive management of chylothorax complicating transhiatal esophagectomy without thoracotomy. Surgery. 1988;104:720–6.
20. Cope C, Kaiser L. Management of unremitting chylothorax by percutaneous embolization and blockage of retroperitoneal lymphatic vessels in 42 patients. J Vasc Interv Radiol. 2002;13:1139–48.
21. Boffa DJ, Sands MJ, Rice TW, et al. A critical evaluation of a percutaneous diagnostic and treatment strategy for chylothorax after thoracic surgery. Eur J Cardiothorac Surg. 2008;33:435–9.
22. Cerfolio RJ, Allen MS, Deschamps C, Trastek VF, Pairolero PC. Postoperative chylothorax. J Thorac Cariovasc Surg. 1996;112:1361–5.
23. Zabeck H, Muley T, Dienemann H, Hoffmann H. Management of chylothorax in adults: when is surgery indicated. Thorac Cardiovasc Surg. 2011;59:243–6.
24. Sahn SA. Management of malignant pleural effusions. Monaldi Arch Chest Dis. 2001;56:394–9.
25. Gupta D, Ross K, Piacentino V, et al. Use of LeVeen pleuroperitoneal shunt for refractory high-volume chylothorax. Ann Thorac Surg. 2004;78:e9–12.
26. Alejandre-Lafont E, Krompiec C, Rau WS, Krombach GA. Effectiveness of therapeutic lymphography on lymphatic leakage. Acta Radiol. 2011;52:305–11.
27. Nadolski GJ, Itkin M. Thoracic duct embolization for nontraumatic chylous effusion: experience in 34 Patients. Chest. 2013;143:158–63.
28. Itkin M, Kucharczuk JC, Kwak A, Trerotola SO, Kaiser LR. Non-operative thoracic duct embolization for traumatic thoracic duct leak: experience in 109 patients. J Thorac Cardiovasc Surg. 2010;139:584–9.

Post Thoracotomy Neuralgia in Post Esophagectomy Patients

31

Himanshu Shukla, Ashwani Sharma, and Surender Dabas

31.1 Introduction

Wide exposure thoracotomy requires a muscle cutting incision, involving several muscle layers, rib resection or rib split, and continuous motion due to respiration. Management of acute post-thoracotomy pain is essentially very important to minimize post op pulmonary complications. Proper pain control enables patients to be ambulatory and to breathe at normal pace as well as deep inspiration. Contrary to acute pain. The effect of chronic post-thoracotomy pain is rather less detrimental to work of respiration but can be very incapacitating for patients making life miserable.

International Association for the Study of Pain (IASP) has defined Post-thoracotomy pain syndrome or post- thoracotomy neuralgia as 'pain that recurs or persists along a thoracotomy incision at least 2 months following the surgical procedure'. Usually the nature of pain is burning and stabbing with or without dysesthesia typical of neuropathic pain [1]. This nature of pain is increasingly reported by Pain Specialists and Thoracic surgeons [2].

31.2 Prevalence of Post-thoracotomy Pain

Post-thoracotomy neuralgic pain was commonly seen by treating physicians in Second World War victims with surgery for chest trauma. Majority of patients usually do not see treating doctor for their pain as they think it as usual side effects of surgery, but they mention it only when specifically asked. Contrary to common

H. Shukla (✉) · A. Sharma · S. Dabas
Department of Surgical Oncology and Robotic Surgery, BLK MAX Superspeciality Hospital, New Delhi, India

K. Sood Sharma et al. (eds.), *Complications of Cancer Therapy: Best Practices in Prevention and Management*, https://doi.org/10.1007/978-981-99-0984-1_31

belief post-thoracotomy pain is neither transient, nor it decreases significantly over time. According to ....et al. incidence of long-term post-thoracotomy pain has been reported to be 80% at 3 months, 75% at 6 months, and 61% at 1 year after surgery; incidence of severe pain is 3–5%, and pain that interferes with normal life is reported by about 50% of patients [3]. Roughly 50–66% of the patients with this kind of pain received treatment for post thoracotomy pain [4]. In another study, more than 70% of the cases with post thoracotomy pain received more than three treatment modalities and regimens. Out of these patients, none have become free of symptoms with treatment, and a significant patients claimed that therapy was rather more disabling than pain while some reported worsening of pain [5].

Post thoracotomy neuralgia patients usually report intense pain with a gentle stimulation with significant disturbance in routine daily activities. Type of procedure usually does not make a difference for the long term persistent pain at 3–18 months [6, 7]. Some authors concluded that the use of video-assisted thoracic surgery for thoracic surgery may decrease the incidence of chronic persistent pain when compared with open thoracotomy [8, 9].

Data suggest wide variation and difference in incidence probably due to non standardised definition of pain but post-thoracotomy pain is seen as most common complication of thoracotomy procedure [10].

31.3 Pathophysiology

Various mechanisms for post thoracotomy pain have been proposed but no definitive consensus regarding exact pathophysiology exists till date.

1. Surgical trauma to Intercostal nerve—Surgical handling in form of traction, crushing or severing of nerve has been proposed as a cause for this neuralgia as the nerve is superficial on the caudal end of the rib. Sometimes it is included in the suture while closure of thoracotomy included in a suture when closing the incision. Other possible causes of nerve damage may be compression with retractor, damage due to rib fracture, entrapment of nerve in callus during healing thus causing pain symptoms. The spectrum of this neuralgia ranges from allodynia to hyperalgesia and usually in the distribution of nerve is usually characteristic feature of post thoracotomy neuralgia [11]. Some studies reported total conduction block during Neurophysiological assessment of the intercostal nerve denoting nerve injury during rib retraction [12, 13]. Higher the impairment of the nerve greater the incidence of post thoracotomy neuralgia. This was shown in a study of 24 patients after a month post thoracotomy [14].
2. Tumor recurrence—this may be the earliest sign of tumour recurrence especially in malignant cases. This observation is supported by many studies [15, 16].
3. Type of incision—data is conflicting regarding this mechanism. Some author suggest improvement in incidence of pain with muscle sparing incision while others show no significant advantage over classical posterolateral incisions [17].

In conclusion with available data the various incisions and surgical modifications failed to show reduced incidence of post surgical pain [18].

4. Personality Traits: Studies suggest that type of personality also has strong predictive factors in the overall incidence of post-thoracotomy pain. One study showed that Preoperative anxiety and fear appeared to play a major role [19].
5. Excessive traction during the procedure may cause dysjunction of costochondral and costovertebral joints which may be the cause of persistent pain.
6. Muscle injury: During thoracotomy division of posterior and lateral chest wall muscles especially serratus anterior muscles and latissimus dorsi cause ipsilateral shoulder disability ultimately leading to frozen shoulder which may results in persistent pain.
7. Suprasensitization: Studies has shown that management of acute pain with effective afferent pathway blockade may reduce the incidence of chronic postoperative pain. A study conducted by Katz et al. [20] showed that aggressive and effective management of early postoperative pain causes decrease incidence of neuralgia by preventing suprasensitization of CNS. Various regiments and combinations of analgesia has been reported to have better outcome.
8. Others—Preoperative anxiety appears to play a major role [19]. The costochondral and costovertebral junctions may be disarticulated due to extensive rib retraction, and ipsilateral shoulder disability is also common as a result of division of serratus anterior muscles and latissimus dorsi. Injuries to the muscles responsible for moving the shoulder as well as insufficiently treated pain lead to inadequate rehabilitation and may produce frozen shoulder.

31.3.1 Management of Post-thoracotomy Pain

(a) Pharmacological management: Post thoracotomy pain is usually managed using same principle of neuropathic pain.

Antidepressants: The role of this class of drug was recognised in early 1982. Tricyclic antidepressant were particularly very effective in treating diabetic and post herpetic neuralgia. The analgesic action was similar in in all patients irrespective of depression status. The involved mechanism is inhibition of serotonin reuptake in descending inhibitory fibres of pain pathway.

Newer class of drug selectively inhibiting monoamine reuptake like duloxetine and velnafexine have good efficacy in management of neuropathic pain and have better side effect profile.

Anticonvulsants: First drug of this group used for this kind of pain is carbamazepine which is drug of choice for trigeminal neuralgia. The other drug gabapentin and pregabalin controls this pain by blocking voltage dependent calcium channels.

Topical local Anesthetics: Lidocaine patches and gels has been used with limited success. They have several advantages like lack of systemic side effects, ease of application without dose titration. Hence, they may be useful in localized neuropathic pain. Cochrane review has supported the use [21].

Topical Capsaicin: This is active content of chilli peppers. This causes localised desensitisation after a period of initial irritation by depleting substance P and other chemical transmitters [22].

Opiods—this has controversial role because of side effect profile, long term efficacy, drug abuse and addiction. Newer groups of drug such as tramadol and tapentadol have better side effect profile and low potential for drug abuse has been used to treat such pain. Tapentadol is relatively newer and is similar to tramadol in its dual mechanism of action but only has weak effects on the reuptake of serotonin [23]. Tapentadol is not a pro-drug and its pharmacokinetics is more predictable with less potential for drug interactions [24]. The studies to date have been of inconclusive clinical significance in efficacy outcomes [25].

Botulinum toxin A: This drug inhibit the release of local nociceptive neuropeptides, which may play a role in suppressing peripheral sensitisation [26].

The Neuropathic Pain Special Interest Group (NeuPSIG) published updated recommendations in 2015 based on a systematic review, which incorporated large, unpublished data and recent high quality clinical trials [27].

TCAs, SNRI antidepressants duloxetine and venlafaxine, and gabapentinoids are used as first-line therapy. Tramadol, lidocaine patches and high concentration capsaicin patches are proposed as second-line therapy. Strong opioids and botulinum toxin A have been reserved as third-line therapy.

Regional Nerve blockade: Epidural analgesia has been gold standard for post thoracotomy pain with substantial risk of hypotension, spinal cord injury and significant failure rates. Hence, newer techniques of paravertebral and intercostal nerve block has emerged. Pharmacological agents used in regional nerve blockade are often a combination of local anaesthetic drugs and opioids. Levo-bupivacaine and ropivacaine are commonly used. These are weak bases, which temporarily block sodium channels along neurons and disrupting electrical transmission along the nociceptive pathway. The addition of opioids appears to enhance its analgesic effect. A double-blind, randomised controlled trial demonstrated that 0.15% ropivacaine with 5 mcg/ml fentanyl was significantly better than plain 0.2% ropivacaine [28].

Pharmacological prevention stategies: Pre-emptive thoracic epidural analgesia should theoretically target the process of central sensitisation and reduce the inflammatory mediators in the nociceptive pathway. However, studies have not clearly demonstrated a reduction in PTPS [29]. Given the complex mechanism of the development of PTPS, a multimodal pharmacological strategy perioperatively is recommended in pre-empting chronic pain.

The various drugs used as analgesic adjuncts are Magnesium, Clonidine/dexmedetomidine, β2-agonist, Anti-depressants—TCA, SNRI, Topical lidocaine.

Topical capsaicin, NSAIDS, Gabapentine and ketamine. Although evidences for the use of all these drugs is weak.

Large prospective observational trials are need of the hour to determine the natural history of postthoracotomy pain as well as the extent of the problem. The neuropathic features and objective evidence from studies suggest that intercostal nerve damage is a major factor in the cause of this pain. Once precise mechanism of intercostal nerve injury is known then only strategies will be directed towards treating postthoracotomy pain. Detailed studies of surgical technique should be performed. This will finally cause modification of operative techniques to reduce the incidence of chronic postthoracotomy pain.

31.4 Conclusion

Post-thoracotomy pain is a serious and highly underrated condition. Incidences ranges up to 50% of patients with thoracotomy and disabling in 5–10%. Exact mechanism is unknown and it rarely diminishes over time. Intercostal nerve damage at thoracotomy is most likely a cause for postthoracotomy pain. All the patients need to be consented for the possibility of chronic postthoracotomy pain irrespective of the type of surgery or incision.

References

1. Koehler RP, Keenan RJ. Management of postthoracotomy pain: acute and chronic. Thorac Surg Clin. 2006;16(3):287–97.
2. Gottschalk A, Cohen SP, Yang S, Ochroch EA. Preventing and treating pain after thoracic surgery. Anesthesiology. 2006;104(3):594–600.
3. Perttunen K, Tasmuth T, Kalso E. Chronic pain after thoracic surgery: a follow-up study. Acta Anaesthesiol Scand. 1999;43(5):563–7.
4. Kalso E, Perttunen K, Kaasinen S. Pain after thoracic surgery. Acta Anaesthesiol Scand. 1992;36(1):96–100.
5. Conacher ID. Therapists and therapies for post-thoracotomy neuralgia. Pain. 1992;48(3):409–12.
6. Furrer M, Rechsteiner R, Eigenmann V, Signer C, Althaus U, Ris HB. Thoracotomy and thoracoscopy: postoperative pulmonary function, pain and chest wall complaints. Eur J Cardiothorac Surg. 1997;12(1):82–7.
7. Maguire MF, Ravenscroft A, Beggs D, Duffy JP. A questionnaire study investigating the prevalence of the neuropathic component of chronic pain after thoracic surgery. Eur J Cardiothorac Surg. 2006;29(5):800–5.
8. Forster R, Storck M, Schafer JR, Honig E, Lang G, Liewald F. Thoracoscopy versus thoracotomy: a prospective comparison of trauma and quality of life. Langenbeck's Arch Surg. 2002;387(1):32–6.
9. Landreneau RJ, Mack MJ, Hazelrigg SR, Naunheim K, Dowling RD, Ritter P, Magee MJ, Nunchuck S, Keenan RJ, Ferson PF. Prevalence of chronic pain after pulmonary resection by thoracotomy or video-assisted thoracic surgery. J Thorac Cardiovasc Surg. 1994;107(4):1079–85.
10. Karmakar MK, Ho AM. Postthoracotomy pain syndrome. Thorac Surg Clin. 2004;14(3):345–52.
11. Gotoda Y, Kambara N, Sakai T, Kishi Y, Kodama K, Koyama T. The morbidity, time course and predictive factors for persistent post-thoracotomy pain. Eur J Pain. 2001;5(1):89–96.
12. Rogers ML, Henderson L, Mahajan RP, Duffy JP. Preliminary findings in the neurophysiological assessment of intercostal nerve injury during thoracotomy. Eur J Cardiothorac Surg. 2002;21(2):298–301.
13. Maguire MF, Latter JA, Mahajan R, Beggs FD, Duffy JP. A study exploring the role of intercostal nerve damage in chronic pain after thoracic surgery. Eur J Cardiothorac Surg. 2006;29(6):873–9.
14. Benedetti F, Vighetti S, Ricco C, Amanzio M, Bergamasco L, Casadio C, Cianci R, Giobbe R, Oliaro A, Bergamasco B, Maggi G. Neurophysiologic assessment of nerve impairment in posterolateral and muscle-sparing thoracotomy. J Thorac Cardiovasc Surg. 1998;115(4):841–7.

15. Keller SM, Carp NZ, Levy MN, Rosen SM. Chronic post thoracotomy pain. J Cardiovasc Surg. 1994;35(6 Suppl. 1):161–4.
16. Kanner R. Diagnosis and management of neuropathic pain in patients with cancer. Cancer Investig. 2001;19(3):324–33.
17. Ochroch EA, Gottschalk A, Augoustides JG, Aukburg SJ, Kaiser LR, Shrager JB. Pain and physical function are similar following axillary, muscle-sparing vs posterolateral thoracotomy. Chest. 2005;128(4):2664–70.
18. Khan IH, McManus KG, McCraith A, McGuigan JA. Muscle sparing thoracotomy: a biomechanical analysis confirms preservation of muscle strength but no improvement in wound discomfort. Eur J Cardiothorac Surg. 2000;18(6):656–61.
19. Bachiocco V, Morselli-Labate AM, Rusticali AG, Bragaglia R, Mastrorilli M, Carli G. Intensity, latency and duration of post-thoracotomy pain: relationship to personality traits. Funct Neurol. 1990;5(4):321–32.
20. Katz J, Jackson M, Kavanagh BP, Sandler AN. Acute pain after thoracotomy predicts long-term post-thoracotomy pain. Clin J Pain. 1996;12:50–5.
21. Derry S, Wiffen PJ, Moore RA, Quinlan J. Topical lidocaine for neuropathic pain in adults. Cochrane Database Syst Rev. 2014;(7):CD010958.
22. Moore RA, et al. Topical analgesics for acute and chronic pain in adults. Cochrane Database Syst Rev. 2010;(7).
23. Singh DR, Nag K, Shetti AN, Krishnaveni N. Tapentadol hydrochloride: a novel analgesic. Saudi J Anaesth. 2013;7(3):322–6.
24. Raffa RB, Buschmann H, Christoph T, et al. Mechanistic and functional differentiation of tapentadol and tramadol. Expert Opin Pharmacother. 2012;13(10):1437–49.
25. Santos J, Alarcão J, Fareleira F, et al. Tapentadol for chronic musculoskeletal pain in adults. Cochrane Database Syst Rev. 2015;(5).
26. Aoki KR. Future aspects of botulinum neurotoxins. J Neural Transm (Vienna). 2008;115(4):567–73.
27. Finnerup NB, Attal N, Haroutounian S, et al. Pharmacotherapy for neuropathic pain in adults: a systematic review and meta-analysis. Lancet Neurol. 2015;14(2):162–73.
28. Macias A, Monedero P, Adame M, Torre W, Fidalgo I, Hidalgo F. A randomized, double-blinded comparison of thoracic epidural ropivacaine, ropivacaine/fentanyl, or bupivacaine/fentanyl for postthoracotomy analgesia. Anesth Analg. 2002;95(5):1344–50.
29. Gerner P. Postthoracotomy pain management problems. Anesthesiol Clin. 2008;26(2):355–67.

TACE and TARE Associated Complications in Liver Tumours

32

Kausar Makki, Saurabh Kumar, and Suhail Farooq

32.1 Introduction

Hepatocellular cancer (HCC) is the fifth most common cancer and the third most common cause of cancer related deaths in the world. Ideally surgical resection or liver transplant in case of coexisting liver disease form the mainstay of treatment of HCC. However, due to late detection, most patients are unable to undergo curative therapy. Also, patients who do undergo surgical resection, end up with a recurrence (true recurrence or de-novo tumours) within 5 years [1].

Liver transplant is an option available only to a few due to limited donor pool. Conversely, all patients may not be able to undergo surgical resection due to presence of cirrhosis. For such patients TACE (Trans Arterial Chemo Embolization) and TARE (Trans Arterial Radio Embolization) forms the mainstay of treatment for HCC. TACE entails selective and super-selective access to arteries feeding tumours and then embolization of such a vessel followed by instillation of a chemotherapeutic agent. The most commonly used chemotherapeutic drugs are Doxorubicin, Mitomycin C, Epirubicin, Cisplatin and Mitoxantrone.

TARE entails using radionuclides like Yttrium-90 microspheres, Iodine-131 labelled Iodized oil (Lipiodol), Rhenium- 188, Phosphorus-32 and Holmium-166 microspheres for delivering a radiation dose to a localized area of the liver

K. Makki (✉)
Department of Liver Transplant, Fortis Hospital, Noida, India

S. Kumar
Department of Interventional Radiology, FMRI, Gurugram, Haryana, India

S. Farooq
Department of Liver Transplant, FEHI, Okhla, Delhi, India

K. Sood Sharma et al. (eds.), *Complications of Cancer Therapy: Best Practices in Prevention and Management*, https://doi.org/10.1007/978-981-99-0984-1_32

containing the tumour. Occlusion of a feeding tumour vessel of HCC by TACE or TARE can be used as a bridge to liver transplants in patients on the waiting list for organ donation.

32.2 TACE Associated Complications

TACE is the most commonly used therapy for patients with HCC and has been shown to provide a survival benefit in those with unresectable disease. A detailed description of the procedure is beyond the scope of this chapter. The complications and management of TACE and TARE are discussed below

32.2.1 Post Embolization Syndrome (PES)

PES is seen in 60% -80 % of patients undergoing TACE. A clinical syndrome manifesting as fever, nausea, vomiting and right upper quadrant pain. It is mediated by an inflammatory response to the chemotherapeutic drug or embolization itself. Possible causes include tumor necrosis, ischemia of liver parenchyma, gall bladder ischemia, higher doses of chemoembolic agent or pulmonary embolism of iodised oil. More commonly seen with conventional TACE (iodised oil) as compared to DC bead (DEB) TACE [2–6].

PES as per literature occurs in 1/3rd to 2/3rd of patients undergoing TACE within 72 h of procedure [2, 4, 7]. Though mostly self-limited, PES does add to increased hospital stay and patient discomfort. Pain is caused by acute ischemia of liver parenchyma and distension of liver capsule. Gall bladder ischemia may also cause pain secondary to inadvertent embolization of cystic artery. Symptoms are usually managed with antipyretics, steroids, analgesics and anti-emetics. PES is a common complication in patients with advanced, unresectable HCC. In the setting of other well-established prognostic factors,

PES is an early predictor of worse overall survival for this population of patients. The biological basis of this association may be related to the inflammatory nature of PES. DEB-TACE is associated with a decreased risk of PES and should be preferred whenever possible. For patients at an increased risk of PES, more aggressive strategies such as Trans-arterial radio embolization should be considered [8].

32.2.2 Acute Liver Failure

Acute liver failure with HCC undergoing TACE, is defined as increased Child-Pugh score $\geq$2, increase in serum bilirubin $\geq$2 mg/dL, or new ascites/encephalopathy within 2 weeks of the procedure

This is one of the most serious complications that can occur following TACE. It occurs in 12 to 15% of patients undergoing TACE with some studies quoting rates as high as 48% [9–12]. Acute liver failure generally presents within 2 weeks of

TACE [12]. It is more common in patients with Child C cirrhotic chronic liver disease, biliary obstruction and patients with portal vein thrombosis (PVT). Especially in patients with PVT, TACE needs to be super selective only for the tumour feeding arteries, and with reduced amount of chemo embolic agents.

In cases of PVT with Child C disease, it is advisable to avoid TACE keeping in mind high risk of liver failure. Patients who develop acute liver failure after TACE present with raised bilirubin and high INR. Some patients with post-TACE liver failure may develop acute ascites and encephalopathy. Higher dose of chemo embolic agents may also predispose to development of liver failure. A study by Min, et al concluded that presence of PVT, high AST, low albumin, low sodium, high serum bilirubin and low AFP levels were predictors for development of post TACE acute liver failure [13]. In most cases, liver failure after TACE is reversible.

32.2.3 Liver Infarction

TACE can cause infarction of non-tumorous portions of the liver. Generally, these areas are small. Risk of infarction of normal liver parenchyma increases with non-selective TACE, use of both iodised oil and gelatin sponge and in patients with portal vein thrombosis and biliary obstruction.

Infarction of liver can further predispose to formation of liver abscess or bilomas, sepsis and acute hepatic failure.

32.2.4 Liver Abscess (Fig. 32.1)

Incidence of liver abscess is 0.5–2% after TACE [7]. It is a potentially fatal complication of TACE. Patient generally presents with high grade fever, raised white cell count and abdominal pain.

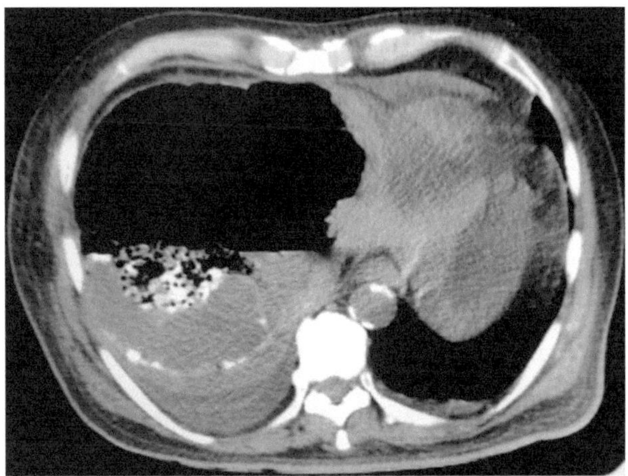

Fig. 32.1 Liver abscess post TACE

When suspecting liver abscess, radiological investigations like ultrasonography or Computed tomography along with percutaneous needle aspiration can be helpful in establishing a diagnosis. Antibiotics and percutaneous drainage are helpful in management of such patients. Timely management is of essence as liver abscesses can even lead to life threatening sepsis.

Portal vein thrombosis (PVT), biliary obstruction, presence of bilio-enteric anastomosis, sphincter of Oddi dysfunction and metastatic tumours are all related to increased risk of development of liver abscess. Infection can occur during TACE procedure itself or can be due to secondary bacterial infection of the necrosed tissue following TACE [14]. In patients with risk factors for development of liver abscess, prophylactic antibiotics can help. Bowel preparation can reduce the risk of liver abscess in patients with bilio-enteric anastomosis.

32.2.5 Sepsis

Sepsis following TACE is a rare phenomenon. It is more commonly seen in patients who develop liver abscess following TACE. Consequently, risk factors for sepsis include portal vein thrombosis, biliary anomalies including obstruction or presence of bilio-enteric anastomosis. Patients generally present with fever. Blood cultures may be positive. It is important to rule out liver abscess or bilomas in these patients. Appropriate antibiotics and treatment of any underlying abscess or biloma forms the mainstay of treatment.

32.2.6 Bile Duct Injury

As bile duct is mainly supplied by the hepatic artery, TACE can lead to ischemia of the peri-biliary plexus of the bile duct. It is more common with selective distal arterial embolization. It can occur in up to 12% patients and presents as focal/multiple biliary strictures, biloma or dilatation of the intra hepatic bile radicles (IHBR) [15]. It is more common in patients with metastatic liver tumours. Most patients are asymptomatic. However, if symptoms occur, management with antibiotics and drainage are recommended.

32.2.7 Acute Pancreatitis

It can occur due to reflux of embolic material into pancreaticoduodenal artery which causes ischemia of the pancreas. This can manifest clinically as acute pancreatitis or patient may remain asymptomatic depending on the extent of pancreas involved. The use of a micro catheter for super selective embolization can help prevent this complication [1].

32.2.8 Extra-hepatic Non-Target Embolization

Non-target embolization is infrequent if a diagnostic angiogram is carefully performed. However, even with utmost precautions non-target embolization may occur wherein a vessel other than the vessel feeding the tumour is accidentally embolised.

(a) **Gall bladder injury**: Gall bladder is the most common non-target organ which gets embolised. This can occur due to cystic artery embolization during TACE. This presents with pain in right upper quadrant. Usually it runs a self-limited course. Sometimes patients can develop gall bladder perforation, gangrene of the gall bladder or emphysematous cholecystitis [1]. Treatment in such a setting is usually surgical i.e. cholecystectomy or percutaneous drainage of the gall bladder (cholecystostomy). Hence it is necessary to ensure identification of the cystic artery and ensuring chemo embolic infusion distal to the cystic artery.
(b) **Supra-umbilical skin rash**: It occurs when lipiodol is accidentally injected into a patent falciform artery. Prevention entails coil embolization of a falciform artery if seen on DSA [1].
(c) **Non-target embolization of internal mammary artery and Intercostal arteries:** Collaterals may connect internal mammary artery and intercostal artery to the vessels feeding the tumours. In such a situation, non-target embolization of these vessels may occur. It manifests usually as painful induration and discoloration of the overlying skin. Rarely trans-mural necrosis may occur [1]. Such a situation may require grafting even.
(d) **Gastroduodenal ulcers:** They may occur by inadvertent embolization of accessory left gastric artery, left hepatic artery or right gastric artery. It is managed by coil embolization of bleeding vessel. If embolization fails, patient may need surgery for controlling the bleeding.
(e) **Pulmonary embolism**: It generally presents between 2nd day to 5th day after TACE. This occurs due to presence of arteriovenous hepatic shunts which cause embolization of iodized oil into pulmonary vascular network. Patient presents with cough, difficulty in breathing and haemoptysis. ABG shows hypoxemia. There can be accumulation of lipiodol in the lung fields, which may lead to consolidation and pleural effusion [1].

    Symptoms depend on the amount of lipiodol embolised. Larger amounts of lipiodol to the lung can produce a chemical pneumonitis and may be fatal. Lipiodol volume exceeding 20 mL has been identified as a risk factor for pulmonary embolization.

    Usually symptoms start resolving in a couple of weeks. This can be easily prevented by recognition and embolization of intra hepatic arterio-venous shunts prior to chemo-embolization. Proper identification of hepatic artery and selective TACE of hepatic artery also helps reduce the chances of pulmonary embolism [16, 17].

(f) **Inadvertent intra-cardiac embolization**: This may occur if there is a right to left sided shunt via a patent foramen ovale or intrapulmonary shunts. It may lead to potentially lethal cerebral lipoidal embolism once it reaches the systemic circulation.

32.2.9 Acute Renal Failure

Iodinated contrast used in TACE can lead to increased risk of renal failure especially in patients with liver cirrhosis who may already have a degree of acute kidney injury owing to peripheral vasodilatation leading to reduced renal perfusion, ascites, and prolonged diuretic use. TACE itself may induce renal vasoconstriction and cause pre-renal acute renal failure [18, 19]. Usually reversible with fluid hydration and conservative line of management.

32.2.10 Iatrogenic Hepatic Artery Injury

Use of guide wire, lipiodol and chemotherapeutic agents during TACE may lead to hepatic artery spasm or occlusion. This is usually reversible and heals spontaneously in most patients. However, hepatic artery stenosis can occur in certain cases along with irreversible occlusion of the hepatic artery [20, 21].

This can especially be a problem for patients who undergo TACE as a bridging procedure prior to liver transplant owing to the difficulty in obtaining arterial inflow. It can also be a problem for patients who need to undergo repeated TACE. Dissection of visceral arteries may occur with TACE. This may manifest post TACE as pseudo aneurysm. Common sites for iatrogenic injury are the celiac axis and the Hepatic artery proper.

32.3 TARE Associated Complications

TARE entails using radionuclides like Yttrium-90 microspheres, Iodine-131 labelled Iodized oil (Lipiodol), Rhenium-188, Phosphorus-32 and Holmium-166 microspheres for delivering a radiation dose to a localized area of the liver containing the tumour. TARE is the preferred modality in cases of advanced liver disease, portal vein thrombosis, neuroendocrine tumors and multifocal cancers. It provides a better quality of life and has a better toxicity profile with improved survival benefit as compared to TACE. After TARE, most complications are related to non-target radiation injury. These are easily preventable by comprehensive angiographic evaluation [22].

32.3.1 Post Embolization Syndrome (PES):

As compared to TACE, the incidence of post embolization syndrome is less [23]. PES after TARE is seen in 20–55%. Post TARE, PES is much milder leading to ease of patient management and outpatient treatment possibility with TARE [24, 25]. It mainly presents with fatigue, abdominal discomfort and nausea. Usually it is not severe enough to warrant hospitalization.

32.3.2 Radiation Cholecystitis

It occurs in less than 1% cases [26]. It is more frequent when cystic artery originates from segmental hepatic artery. In post radiation cholecystitis, imaging findings include gall bladder oedema, enhancement of gall bladder wall and mural disruption. Treatment of this condition entails a cholecystectomy.

32.3.3 Biliary Complications

Incidence of biliary complications after TARE is <10% [26]. These can occur either due to radiation induced biliary injury or due micro-embolization of small blood vessels of the biliary system. These manifest as bilomas, abscesses and radiation induced cholangitis. These may require drainage along with antibiotics. Imaging can help in early diagnosis once biliary complications are suspected. More common in patients with surgeries/procedures violating the integrity of the ampulla of Vater or in patients on polychemotherapy. Biliary complication incidence is also higher in patients who have had polychemotherapy.

32.3.4 Gastroduodenal Ulcer

The incidence is less than 5% in cases after TARE [26]. Radiation injury can occur due to non-target administration of microspheres into the accessory left gastric artery, the right gastric artery and the gastro duodenal artery. This can lead to gastric ulcers which are generally refractory to medical management as these generally form on the serosal surface as opposed to normal mucosal ulcers. Patients often present with severe epigastric pain. Surgical resection remains the treatment option in such cases.

32.3.5 Radiation Pneumonitis

It is quite uncommon. Incidence after TARE is less than 1% [26]. This low incidence after TARE is due to mandatory quantification of pre- treatment lung shunting and dosimetry. Technetium-99 Macroaggregated Albumin Scan (Tc-99 MAA scan) is used to assess splanchnic and pulmonary shunting. Lung shunt fraction (LSF) is used to calculate the dose to be delivered to the lungs and adjustment minimizes the risk of radiation pneumonitis after radio embolization. In patients with, lung shunting fraction of >13% or when the right inferior phrenic artery (most common extra hepatic collateral artery) supplies the tumour, special caution is needed to prevent radiation pneumonitis in such a case. This is because the right inferior phrenic artery commonly accompanies pulmonary shunting. Radiation pneumonitis presents as restrictive ventilatory dysfunction. CT chest shows a typical bat wing appearance. It is advised to keep lung doses less than 30 Gy per treatment and cumulative dose less than 50 Gy.

32.3.6 Radiation-Induced Liver Disease (RILD)

RILD can be seen in up to 4% of patients [27]. Patients present with jaundice, ascites, increased alkaline phosphatase levels, and thrombocytopenia. It occurs 1–2 months after TARE [28]. Liver biopsy shows extensive sinusoidal congestion affecting peri-venular areas with focal hepatic atrophy, areas of necrosis around central veins with fresh thrombosis, and some cholestasis in peri-portal areas. The exact tolerable dose to the liver by TARE is not known. The ratio of true absorbed dose to the normal liver tissue is extremely difficult to assess. Thus, the easiest and most definitive way to prevent radiation-induced liver disease is to avoid whole liver irradiation in single treatment or sequential treatment. Prior exposure of the liver to external beam radiation therapy (EBRT) may lead to increased liver toxicity after radioembolization. This depends on fractional liver exposure and dose level. Radioembolization appears to be safe for the treatment of hepatic malignancies only in patients who have had limited hepatic exposure to prior EBRT.

32.3.7 Portal Hypertension

TARE leads to fibrosis which may manifest as portal hypertension. It is usually seen with bilobar treatment and in patients with chemotherapy associated steatohepatitis (CASH). Pre-existing cirrhosis may aggravate portal hypertension.

32.3.8 Vascular Injury

There is low incidence of vascular injury and arterial dissection after TARE.

32.3.9 Lymphopenia

It can be mild to moderate. As the most radiosensitive cells of the hematopoietic system, lymphocytes residing within or circulating through a radiation portal are frequently depleted by radiation therapy. This is usually reversible after recovery of bone marrow.

32.4 Conclusion

Treatment of HCC is challenging in the most ideal of circumstances. TACE and TARE are a relatively modern addition to the armamentarium of clinicians in treating HCC. Complications following these Trans arterial interventions are not infrequent. Fatal, life threatening complications after TACE and TARE are rare. Complications like Post Embolization syndrome are relatively very frequent. Overall, complications after TACE are more common than after TARE.

References

1. Jarnagin WR, Blumgart LH. Blumgart's surgery of the liver, biliary tract and pancreas. 6th ed. Philadelphia, PA: Elsevier; 2017.
2. Dhand S, Gupta R. Hepatic transcatheter arterial chemoembolization complicated by postembolization syndrome. Semin Intervent Radiol. 2011;28(2):207–11.
3. Okuda K, Ohtsuki T, Obata H, Tomimatsu M, Okazaki N, Hasegawa H, et al. Natural history of hepatocellular carcinoma and prognosis in relation to treatment. Study of 850 patients. Cancer. 1985;56(4):918–28.
4. Paye F, Farges O, Dahmane M, Vilgrain V, Flejou JF, Belghiti J. Cytolysis following chemoembolization for hepatocellular carcinoma. Br J Surg. 1999;86(2):176–80.
5. Shin SW. The current practice of transarterial chemoembolization for the treatment of hepatocellular carcinoma. Korean J Radiol. 2009;10(5):425–34.
6. Clark TW. Complications of hepatic chemoembolization. Semin Intervent Radiol. 2006;23(2):119–25.
7. Chung JW, Park JH, Han JK, Choi BI, Han MC, Lee HS, et al. Hepatic tumors: predisposing factors for complications of transcatheter oily chemoembolization. Radiology. 1996;198(1):33–40.
8. Mason MC, Massarweh NN, Salami A, Sultenfuss MA, Anaya DA. Post-embolization syndrome as an early predictor of overall survival after transarterial chemoembolization for hepatocellular carcinoma. HPB (Oxford). 2015;17(12):1137–44.
9. Chan AO, Yuen MF, Hui CK, Tso WK, Lai CL. A prospective study regarding the complications of transcatheter intraarterial lipiodol chemoembolization in patients with hepatocellular carcinoma. Cancer. 2002;94(6):1747–52.
10. Katsushima S, Inokuma T, Oi H, Okamura J, Higashi T, Takeuchi R, et al. Acute hepatic failure following transcatheter arterial embolization for the treatment of hepatocellular carcinoma. Digestion. 1997;58(2):189–95.
11. Marelli L, Stigliano R, Triantos C, Senzolo M, Cholongitas E, Davies N, et al. Transarterial therapy for hepatocellular carcinoma: which technique is more effective? A systematic review of cohort and randomized studies. Cardiovasc Intervent Radiol. 2007;30(1):6–25.
12. Huang YS, Chiang JH, Wu JC, Chang FY, Lee SD. Risk of hepatic failure after transcatheter arterial chemoembolization for hepatocellular carcinoma: predictive value of the monoethylglycinexylidide test. Am J Gastroenterol. 2002;97(5):1223–7.
13. Min YW, Kim J, Kim S, Sung YK, Lee JH, Gwak GY, et al. Risk factors and a predictive model for acute hepatic failure after transcatheter arterial chemoembolization in patients with hepatocellular carcinoma. Liver Int. 2013;33(2):197–202.
14. Xia J, Ren Z, Ye S, Sharma D, Lin Z, Gan Y, et al. Study of severe and rare complications of transarterial chemoembolization (TACE) for liver cancer. Eur J Radiol. 2006;59(3):407–12.
15. Kobayashi S, Nakanuma Y, Terada T, Matsui O. Postmortem survey of bile duct necrosis and biloma in hepatocellular carcinoma after transcatheter arterial chemoembolization therapy:

relevance to microvascular damages of peribiliary capillary plexus. Am J Gastroenterol. 1993;88(9):1410–5.
16. Chung JW, Park JH, Im JG, Han JK, Han MC. Pulmonary oil embolism after transcatheter oily chemoembolization of hepatocellular carcinoma. Radiology. 1993;187(3):689–93.
17. Lee DH, Hwang JC, Lim SM, Yoon HK, Sung KB, Song HY. Pleural and pulmonary staining at inferior phrenic arteriography mimicking a tumor staining of hepatocellular carcinoma. Cardiovasc Intervent Radiol. 2000;23(2):109–13.
18. Burney IA. Acute tumor lysis syndrome after transcatheter chemoembolization of hepatocellular carcinoma. South Med J. 1998;91(5):467–70.
19. Huo TI, Lee SD. Management of inoperable hepatocellular carcinoma. J Gastroenterol Hepatol. 2004;19:272–8.
20. Belli L, Magistretti G, Puricelli GP, Damiani G, Colombo E, Cornalba GP. Arteritis following intra-arterial chemotherapy for liver tumors. Eur Radiol. 1997;7(3):323–6.
21. Kwok PC, Lam TW, Chan SC, Chung CP, Wong WK, Chan MK, et al. A randomized clinical trial comparing autologous blood clot and gelfoam in transarterial chemoembolization for inoperable hepatocellular carcinoma. J Hepatol. 2000;32(6):955–64.
22. Mosconi C, Calandri M, Javle M, Odisio BC. Interventional radiology approaches for intrahepatic cholangiocarcinoma. Chin Clin Oncol. 2020;9(1):8.
23. Salem R, Lewandowski RJ, Mulcahy MF, Riaz A, Ryu RK, Ibrahim S, et al. Radioembolization for hepatocellular carcinoma using Yttrium-90 microspheres: a comprehensive report of long-term outcomes. Gastroenterology. 2010;138(1):52–64.
24. Salem R, Gilbertsen M, Butt Z, Memon K, Vouche M, Hickey R, et al. Increased quality of life among hepatocellular carcinoma patients treated with radioembolization, compared with chemoembolization. Clin Gastroenterol Hepatol. 2013;11(10):1358–65.
25. Steel J, Baum A, Carr B. Quality of life in patients diagnosed with primary hepatocellular carcinoma: hepatic arterial infusion of Cisplatin versus 90-Yttrium microspheres (Therasphere). Psychooncology. 2004;13(2):73–9.
26. Riaz A, Lewandowski RJ, Kulik LM, Mulcahy MF, Sato KT, Ryu RK, et al. Complications following radioembolization with yttrium-90 microspheres: a comprehensive literature review. J Vasc Interv Radiol. 2009;20(9):1121–30.
27. Kennedy AS, McNeillie P, Dezarn WA, Nutting C, Sangro B, Wertman D, et al. Treatment parameters and outcome in 680 treatments of internal radiation with resin 90Y-microspheres for unresectable hepatic tumors. Int J Radiat Oncol Biol Phys. 2009;74(5):1494–500.
28. Sangro B, Gil-Alzugaray B, Rodriguez J, Sola I, Martinez-Cuesta A, Viudez A, et al. Liver disease induced by radioembolization of liver tumors: description and possible risk factors. Cancer. 2008;112(7):1538–46.

33 Prevention and Management of Early Bleed After Pancreatic Resections

Ashish George, Vaibhaw Kumar, and Ajitabh Srivastava

33.1 Introduction

Pancreatic resectional surgeries have come a long way with a significant decrease in the mortality associated with the surgery [1, 2] over the last few decades. Despite the same, a morbidity in the range of 30–60% is very high compared to other abdominal surgeries [3]. After postoperative pancreatic fistula, bleeding is one of the most devastating complications for the patient as well as the surgeon. Development of post pancreatectomy haemorrhage(PPH) in the post operative period is associated with a significant increase in morbidity and mortality for these patients [4, 5]. The discussion in this chapter would be restricted primarily to early PPH.

33.2 Definition

The incidence of PPH varies between 6% and 10% [5]. In 2007, International Study Group of Pancreatic Surgery (ISGPS) introduced a definition and classification of PPH which has helped to bring uniformity in reporting and has helped to formulate algorithms to treat the same. PPH is defined on three criteria, including time of onset (less than or greater than 24h), location (intraluminal or extraluminal)

A. George (✉) · A. Srivastava
Department of GI Surgery and Liver Transplantation, Aakash Healthcare Super Specialty Hospital, Delhi, India

V. Kumar
Department of Liver Transplant and GI Surgery, Metro Group of Hospitals, Faridabad, Noida, India

K. Sood Sharma et al. (eds.), *Complications of Cancer Therapy: Best Practices in Prevention and Management*, https://doi.org/10.1007/978-981-99-0984-1_33

Table 33.1 ISGPS definition and classification for Post-pancreatectomy haemorrhage [6]

Time of onset	Early	Less than 24 h from the time of surgery
	Late	More than 24 h from the time of surgery
Location	Intraluminal	Within the lumen of the bowel
	Extraluminal	In the abdominal cavity, evident through the drain
Severity	Mild	Less than 3 g drop in haemoglobin
		Mild clinical impairment
		Up to 2–3 units blood transfusions within 24 h from surgery *or* 1–3 units requirement more than 24 h from surgery
		No major therapeutic implications
	Severe	≥3 g/dL drop in Haemoglobin
		Need for invasive therapy including surgery/ radiological or endoscopic procedures
		Evidence of hemodynamic instability or oliguria, requirement of >3 units blood
Grade A	Early (intra or extraluminal) **and** Mild	No clinical implications, may need ICU care
Grade B	Early **and** Severe	Very rarely life threatening
	Late **and** Mild	Need for therapeutic endoscopy, radiological procedures or re-exploration
Grade C	Late **and** Severe	Significant impairment, life threatening
		Any interventional procedure for management

and severity of the bleed (mild or severe). PPH is classified into three grades(A, B and C) based on the different permutations of the above mentioned criteria (Table 33.1) [6].

33.3 Etiopathogenesis, Diagnosis and Treatment

In their analysis of more than 1600 consecutive patients, Yekebas et al found three primary reasons for the development of early PPH (ePPH). Technical failures resulting from improper haemostasis, slipped ligatures in the surgical field, invariably led to extraluminal bleeds. In the presence of bleed from the suture line of the gastroenteric anastomosis or the other entero-enteric anastomoses, the bleed was intraluminal. Bleeding from the resection cavity i.e. DPPHR (duodenum preserving pancreatic head resection) or transection surface (pancreaticoduodenectomy or distal pancreatic resections) would lead to bleed into the lumen in only half the cases as in the other half the bleeding was identified fallaciously as extraluminal [7]. Wente et al also ascribe technical failure and peri-operative coagulopathy as the major causes for early post-operative bleeding. The bleeding can be from arterial, venous sources or from the suture line of the various anastomoses like the pancreatico-jejunostomy/ gastrostomy, hepaticojejunostomy, gastrojejunostomy or the jejunojejunostomy. The other sites include the areas of resection i.e. the pancreatic stump or the retroperitoneum [6]. Bleeds from eroded/ruptured pseudoaneurysms or anastomotic ulcers are usually not associated with ePPH.

Of all the pancreatic resection surgeries, the incidence of bleeding is probably higher in DPPHR [8, 9]. This may be due to the presence of the rich anastomotic pancreaticoduodenal plexus, which is usually preserved but direct injury to it or its branches or their exposure may precipitate a significant number of bleeding episodes. Gao et al retrospectively evaluated 423 patients undergoing pancreaticoduodenectomy and found three factors associated with ePPH. These include vascular reconstruction, history of previous upper abdominal surgery and pre-operative albumin level [10].

According to the ISGPS classification, ePPH is classified only as Grade A or B. Patients with grade A PPH have similar outcomes to patients without PPH. Early and severe PPH has been classified along with late and mild PPH, in the same grade i.e., grade B PPH. Comparing these two subclasses, there is a significant increase in the need for ICU care in the ePPH group (22.1 vs. 6.7%, $p = 0.05$) but no difference in 90-day mortality, readmission rate or the length of hospital stay. Surgery was performed in management of 81.2% of ePPH compared to only 10.1% in the late and mild group, which was most commonly managed with observation [11]. Intuitively it may come across, that patients with early and severe PPH have minimal morbidity and mortality and may portend a false sense of safety to the reader. However, complications from the inadequate/incomplete or occasionally the sequelae of the bleed, may lead to major morbidity and sometimes mortality. Thus, all bleeds must be identified, evaluated and treated with utmost urgency and expertise, to minimise/arrest the unwanted manifestations of the complication.

Once an ePPH is identified, the diagnostic and treatment algorithm should be initiated. The CT scan finding as well as the haemodynamic stability of the patient guides further diagnostic and therapeutic interventions.

If despite adequate resuscitation, the patient continues to be hemodynamically unstable, then surgical re-exploration becomes the most appropriate intervention. The aim of the surgery would be to identify the site of bleed and control the same while minimising injury to the multiple reconstructions. Management of bleeding from the arterial and venous stumps as well as the retroperitoneal dissection planes may be easier to manage in the early post-operative period as they may be easily approachable, Also, early bleed by definition occurs within the first 24h and thus it is rarely associated with major inflammation which may prevent proper suture ligation of the bleeding. After satisfactory control of these bleeds, one may use absorbable hemostatic materials to decrease the risk of a rebleeding episode. These hemostats can be used to provide mild tamponade especially in the region of the meso-uncinate where it may be sandwiched between the pancreatic body anteriorly and the retroperitoneum posteriorly.

On the other hand, bleeding from the pancreatico-enteric anastomosis may be more difficult to tackle without dismantling the anastomosis. One way to avoid taking down the anastomosis is to create an enterotomy slightly distal to the pancreatico-enteric anastomosis and evert the anastomosis through the enterotomy after evacuation of the clots for better visibility and control. This may bring the pancreatic cut surface in view for performing a proper hemostasis. This may not always be possible and sometimes it may be necessary to open the anterior layer of the pancreatico-enteric anastomosis or occasionally dismantle the complete anastomosis to control the bleed.

The jejuno-jejunal anastomosis may be one of the less commonly suspected sites of bleeds. The bleeding may be from the cut edge or sometimes from the mesenteric vessels near the cut edge bleeding either intraluminally or extraluminally. In our experience, these bleeds may be more commonly associated with an end to side anastomosis compared with a side-to-side anastomosis.

In a hemodynamically stable patient with danger signs, usually a multiphasic CT scan may best delineate the site of bleed. In a persistent intraluminal bleed, management with endoscopy may be tried and is usually successful. However, there is data implying that endoscopy may mislead and delay appropriate treatment. It may frequently be needed to be supplanted with other therapeutic measures [3, 12, 13]. However, proper use of endoscopy as a diagnostic and therapeutic option is still important. A bleed from the gastrojejunostomy, pancreaticogastrostomy, jejuno-jejunal anastomosis are relatively easy to evaluate and manage using endoscopy. However, it requires an experienced endoscopist to reach the bilio-enteric and the pancreatico-jejunal anastomoses, for which, endoscopic procedure may fail more often. Also, the use of endoscopy comes with its own set of problems across the freshly assembled anastomoses. These include the need to distend the bowel with air for adequate visualisation and control of bleeding, as well as the need for movement of the scope across multiple anastomoses to reach the more distal of the bleed sites. It may thus be advisable for an experienced endoscopist to use minimal insufflation and gentle handling of the scope across the anastomoses to avoid causing injury to bowel or disruption of the sutures.

Radiological interventions may be the first line of management in patients in whom the bleeding site is localised during the CT scan. Interestingly, according to Gaudon et al, in up to 55% of cases, an MDCT was not able to localise the exact site of bleed. Despite the same, a MDCT is irreplaceable in the evaluation of PPH as it helps to provide a roadmap, identify vascular anatomical variations and other factors which may make the procedure difficult or alter the route to be taken to reach the bleeding vessel radiologically [14]. It is easier to manage bleeding occurring from arterial and major venous branches, however if the bleed is from a distal small vessel, access radiologically may not be possible for want of smaller catheters. Similarly, bleeds evident only in the delayed phase of the CT scan may not always be amenable to radiological interventions. The overwhelming evidence for radiological management of PPH is in the late PPH subset. However, in the patient with right indication, it may help to manage ePPH and thus avoid a re-exploration. Any failure of minimally invasive procedures requires the patient to be subjected to a surgical exploration. The treatment algorithm to be followed after an ePPH is identified, is shown in Fig. 33.1.

Apart from the management of ePPH once it is evident, various intra-operative manoeuvres may help to decrease the incidence of this problem.

The use of hemostatic stay sutures along the pancreatico-duodenal groove, before the DPPHR decreases the bleeding during surgery and also in the

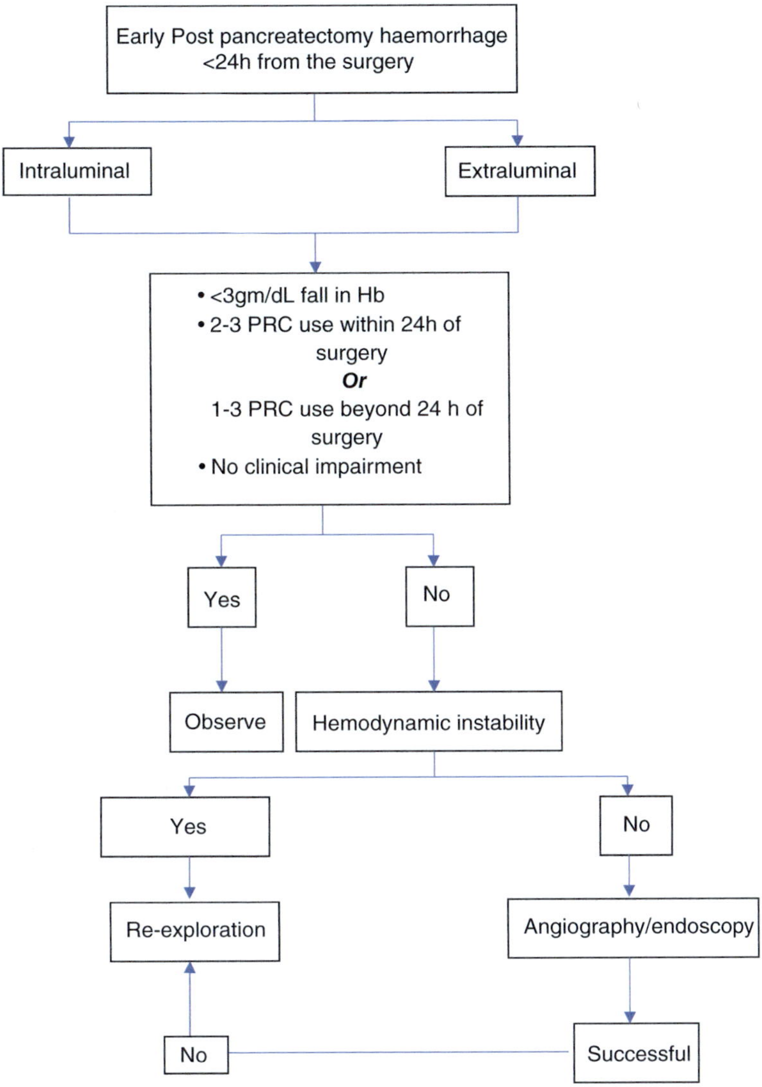

Early Post pancreatectomy haemorrhage <24h from the surgery

Intraluminal

Extraluminal

- <3gm/dL fall in Hb
- 2-3 PRC use within 24h of surgery **Or** 1-3 PRC use beyond 24 h of surgery
- No clinical impairment

Yes

No

Observe

Hemodynamic instability

Yes

No

Re-exploration

Angiography/endoscopy

No

Successful

Fig. 33.1 Algorithm for management of Early post-pancreatectomy haemorrhage

post-operative period by controlling the vessels in the pancreaticoduodenal arcade. The use of energy sources like harmonic scalpel are expected to seal the vessels at the resection margin, but this may not always be the case. Their use may lead to the possibility of post-operative bleed(early or late). The use of bipolar forceps to control bleeding points at the pancreatic resection/excision margin is helpful. At the end of the resection, a gauze piece to rub the cut edge gently to open up cut vessels and individually suture ligating them may help to decrease the incidence of bleeding in the post-operative period [15].

For intraluminal bleeds, the presence of oedema at the time of anastomosis may contribute, as the sutures might become loose once the oedema starts to settle. The role of the anaesthetist to manage the fluid balance during the surgery to avoid bowel oedema cannot be over emphasized. Hence, the use of restrictive fluid therapy or goal directed therapy may be beneficial in avoiding bowel oedema towards the end of the resection phase and decrease the incidence of anastomotic bleed. The use of haemostatic interlocking sutures to avoid loosening of the sutures may be tried. This may lead to the theoretical decrease in the vascularity at the site of the anastomosis. Division of major blood vessels especially the gastroduodenal artery needs special mention. It is preferable to doubly ligate the stump of the GDA for safety. Also, the division of the GDA should be performed after leaving a short stump of the proximal artery and flush division at its origin should be avoided. Bleeds occurring from the stump of the GDA divided flush at its origin are extremely difficult to control. Suturing the bleeding vessel flush at its origin may compromise the hepatic blood flow secondary to narrowing. Also, during radiological management of a bleeding GDA stump, plug embolization cannot be performed if there is no stump. The only option that remains in such situation, is to place a covered stent either intra-operatively or at a later opportune moment. Another potential site of major postoperative arterial bleed includes the inferior pancreaticoduodenal artery (IPDA). All efforts should be made for a direct ligation of the IPDA, as mass ligation of the tissue to the right of the superior mesenteric artery (SMA) may lead to slippage of the ligature and thus an early torrential bleed from the IPDA. The jejunal branches of the SMA should also be carefully handled during the surgery [16]. During the performance of the pancreatico-enteric anastomosis, one should avoid leaving a gap of more than 3–4 mm between two successive sutures or perform the gastrojejunostomy (which usually may be performed by the surgical resident or by a tired surgeon towards the end of the surgery) in a hurried fashion [17].

33.4 Conclusion

Grade B ePPH is a potentially life-threatening complication of major pancreatic resections. With increasing expertise in surgery and improving diagnostic modalities, its incidence, diagnosis and management are improving. Surgery remains the mainstay of management of such bleeds which fail conservative trial. Endoscopy and interventional radiological techniques have limited but certain role in the properly selected patient.

References

1. Lewis R, Drebin JA, Callery MP, Fraker D, Kent TS, Gates J, et al. A contemporary analysis of survival for resected pancreatic ductal adenocarcinoma. HPB. 2013;15(1):49–60.
2. van Rijssen LB, Koerkamp BG, Zwart MJ, Bonsing BA, Bosscha K, van Dam RM, et al. Nationwide prospective audit of pancreatic surgery: design, accuracy, and outcomes of the Dutch Pancreatic Cancer Audit. HPB. 2017;19(10):919–26.

3. Mañas-Gómez MJ, Rodríguez-Revuelto R, Balsells-Valls J, Olsina-Kissler JJ, Caralt-Barba M, Pérez-Lafuente M, et al. Post-pancreaticoduodenectomy hemorrhage. Incidence, Diagnosis, and Treatment. World J Surg. 2011;35(11):2543–8.
4. Miura F, Asano T, Amano H, Yoshida M, Toyota N, Wada K, et al. Management of postoperative arterial hemorrhage after pancreato-biliary surgery according to the site of bleeding: re-laparotomy or interventional radiology. J Hepatobiliary Pancreat Surg. 2009;16(1):56–63.
5. Wolk S, Grützmann R, Rahbari NN, Hoffmann RT, Plodeck V, Weitz J, et al. Management of clinically relevant postpancreatectomy hemorrhage (PPH) over two decades—a comparative study of 1450 consecutive patients undergoing pancreatic resection. Pancreatology. 2017;17(6):943–50.
6. Wente MN, Veit JA, Bassi C, Dervenis C, Fingerhut A, Gouma DJ, et al. Postpancreatectomy hemorrhage (PPH)–An International Study Group of Pancreatic Surgery (ISGPS) definition. Surgery. 2007;142(1):20–5.
7. Yekebas EF, Wolfram L, Cataldegirmen G, Habermann CR, Bogoevski D, Koenig AM, et al. Postpancreatectomy hemorrhage: diagnosis and treatment: an analysis in 1669 consecutive pancreatic resections. Ann Surg. 2007;246(2):269–80.
8. Schäfer M, Müllhaupt B, Clavien PA. Evidence-based pancreatic head resection for pancreatic cancer and chronic pancreatitis. Ann Surg. 2002;236(2):137.
9. Ho C, Kleeff J, Friess H, Büchler MW. Complications of pancreatic surgery. HPB. 2005;7(2):99–108.
10. Gao F, Li J, Quan S, Li F, Ma D, Yao L, et al. Risk factors and treatment for hemorrhage after pancreaticoduodenectomy: a case series of 423 patients. Biomed Res Int. 2016;2016:1–9.
11. Duarte Garcés AA, Andrianello S, Marchegiani G, Piccolo R, Secchettin E, Paiella S, et al. Reappraisal of post-pancreatectomy hemorrhage (PPH) classifications: do we need to redefine grades A and B? HPB. 2018;20(8):702–7.
12. Rajarathinam G, Kannan DG, Vimalraj V, Amudhan A, Rajendran S, Jyotibasu D, et al. Post pancreaticoduodenectomy haemorrhage: outcome prediction based on new ISGPS Clinical severity grading. HPB. 2008;10(5):363–70.
13. Ansari D, Tingstedt B, Lindell G, Keussen I, Ansari D, Andersson R. Hemorrhage after major pancreatic resection: incidence, risk factors, management, and outcome. Scand J Surg. 2017;106(1):47–53.
14. Gaudon C, Soussan J, Louis G, Moutardier V, Gregoire E, Vidal V. Late postpancreatectomy hemorrhage: predictive factors of morbidity and mortality after percutaneous endovascular treatment. Diagn Interv Imaging. 2016;97(11):1071–7.
15. Lakshmanan A, Ravichandran P, Jeswanth S, Sukumar R. Bleeding complication after pancreatic surgery: role of harmonic scalpel. Indian J Surg. 2013;75(S1):436–8.
16. Das S, Ray S, Mangla V, Mehrotra S, Lalwani S, Mehta N, et al. Post pancreaticoduodenectomy hemorrhage: a retrospective analysis of incidence, risk factors and outcome. Saudi J Gastroenterol. 2020;26(6):337.
17. Wente MN, Shrikhande SV, Kleeff J, Müller MW, Gutt CN, Büchler MW, Friess H. Management of early hemorrhage from pancreatic anastomoses after pancreaticoduodenectomy. Dig Surg. 2006;23:203–8.

Post-operative Liver Failure in Hepatic Resections

34

Niteen Kumar and Abhideep Chaudhary

34.1 Introduction

34.1.1 Concept of Liver Failure

Liver failure per se is temporary or permanent cessation of its function which maintains body homeostasis. Liver performs myriad of functions which are loosely categorized as excretory, synthetic and detoxifying function. The cessation of its function would lead to accumulation of may toxic products in the body. The bilirubin is the surrogate marker of accumulated toxic products, and thus finds first place in the definition of liver failure along with coagulopathy [1]. Historically, in the context of acute liver failure, this rise in bilirubin and coagulopathy will be accompanied prominently with mental changes. Not only this onset of mental change defines liver failure it would also portend poor prognosis [2]. Although, brain dysfunction, is the most prominent, liver failure leads to other end-organ damage which has bearing on the prognosis like lung injury, kidney dysfunction and circulatory dysfunction and so on. Whereas brain dysfunction is the most prominent and defining symptom of adult acute liver failure, it is conspicuous by its absence in the definition of neonatal acute liver failure for want of near impossible assessment of mental status changes in neonates. Here, liver failure means hyperbilrubinemia and coagulopathy!! [3]. In the context of post hepatectomy liver failure, rise in bilirubin and accompanying coagulopathy naturally defines this condition. However, development of brain dysfunction (hepatic encephalopathy) is considered as important complication and marker of worsening prognosis. The post hepatectomy liver failure is frequently complicated by sepsis and patient might be having what is called

N. Kumar (✉) · A. Chaudhary
Department of HPB and Liver Transplant, BLK Max Hospital, Delhi, India

K. Sood Sharma et al. (eds.), *Complications of Cancer Therapy: Best Practices in Prevention and Management*, https://doi.org/10.1007/978-981-99-0984-1_34

septic encephalopathy. In this case it will not be prudent to wait for the development of the hepatic encephalopathy, to define liver failure. Interventions prior to this, like search for operative complications, septic foci would change the course of disease and help recover the patient.

34.1.2 Defining Postoperative Liver Failure

Against this background it not difficult to understand that definition of PHLF essentially has varying combination of serum bilirubin level, prothrombin time, ascites and end organ damage. This simplistic approach however, was marred for a long time by the arbitrarily chosen cut offs [4]. This confused the entire literature of PHLF, created problem of heterogeneity and difficulties in analysing various study results. No wonder incidence of PHLF and its mortality varies widely in literature (see below: epidemiology). In this interesting journey of defining PHLF, curtain came down with emergence of 50–50 criteria [5] which based its definition's cut off on meticulous scientific evaluation. Few more studies followed on to validate the 50–50 criteria and then to defining PHLF with new cut offs. However, this criterion was largely not applicable to those with raised preoperative bilirubin levels and those with chronic liver disease undergoing resection (Table 34.1) [5–7], Also, not many patients fell into the category of PHLF according to this definition when applied prospectively. Hence idea of having any cut off was done away with and International Study Group of Liver Surgery (ISGLS) (Table 34.2) came up with a definition which was applicable to even those with chronic liver disease and preoperatively raised bilirubin level. An important aspect of influence of end organ damage with prognostic implications was also added, recognising that not all fulfilling criteria of liver failure will have similar outcome [4]. Many of them would not be requiring any intervention or deviation from usual management and therefore recover completely without any sequel. It is for this reason that grades of severity of liver failure have been introduced to help clinician in making early decisions and determining intensity of management change.

A broader understanding of the normal recovery pattern of liver function test is important to recognize the ensuing liver failure. What is equally important to

Table 34.1 Commonly used definitions for PHLF

Definition	Description
"50–50 criteria" [5]	Prothrombin time < 50% of normal (INR > 1.7) and serum bilirubin >50 mmol/L (>2.9 mg/dL) on postoperative day 5
"Edinburgh criteria" [7]	The definition is based on serum concentrations of total bilirubin and lactate, prothrombin time, and signs of encephalopathy, categorized into 3 levels each, and points were given for each level, and summarized to provide a score which indicated four grades of PHLF (none/mild/moderate/severe)
Peak bilirubin criterion >120 mmol/mL [6]	Postoperative peak serum bilirubin >120 mmol/mL (>7 mg/dL)

Table 34.2 The current International Study Group of Liver Surgery (ISGLS) definition of post-hepatectomy liver failure (PHLF) [4]. A postoperatively acquired deterioration in the ability of the liver to maintain its synthetic, excretory, and detoxifying functions characterized, on postoperative day 5

If pre-operative LFTs Normal:	If pre-operative LFTs abnormal:
– Increasing INR (or need of clotting factors to maintain INR) – Hyperbilirubinemia	– Increasing INR or prothrombin time (compared to the day before) – Increasing bilirubin (compared to the day before)

Grade A	**Grade B**	**Grade C**
Abnormal laboratory parameters but requiring no change in the clinical management of the patient	Deviation from the regular clinical Management but manageable without invasive treatment	Deviation from the regular clinical management and requiring invasive treatment

LFTs liver function tests, *INR* international normalized ratio

understand the setting in which the recovery pattern is being analysed. For a quite good period of time, studies pertaining to recovery of LFT failed to show consistent results [8, 9]. Probably earlier researchers failed to recognize the importance and influence of set of other variables. For example, recovery pattern of PT post-operatively cannot be studied, if patients were transfused large amount of fresh frozen plasma (FFP). FFPs would affect the values of PT. Likewise, Serum bilirubin may rise itself owing to severe postoperative complications or other extrahepatic factors. Therefore, later studies trying to recognize the recovery pattern of LFTs and PT considered a subgroup of population which had a normal preoperative liver function test, no postoperative complications and were not transfused FFPs [10]. Nonetheless, this limited its wider applicability. It is important to note that an early decrease in postoperative PT occurs irrespective of the extent of resection, irrespective of the normal liver or patients with chronic liver disease. From here, however, things change in what happens in normal liver vis a vis in chronic liver disease. For initial dip in PT, short half-life of factor VII, plasma volume and patient temperature may be responsible [11–13]. These factors become very important in the initial postoperative period. Thereafter, PT recovers rapidly in 'normal' liver, and normalizes mostly by day 5, which may not happen if liver fails to regenarate owing to underlying disease or other reasons (see below). It is quite conceivable that PT might not get influenced by the extent of liver resection per se. The situation is very different in the case of serum bilirubin. It has a longer half-life, and peaks between POD 3 and 5 after major resection per se. And it is impacted by the extent of resection and remnant liver and probably the more sensitive indicator of liver dysfunction especially in living donors (as they have invariably preoperative normal liver).

34.1.3 Pathophysiology of Post-hepatectomy Liver Failure

It would be difficult if not impossible to understand process of liver failure without going into the nitty gritty of liver regeneration. Premises of partial hepatectomy is based on the regenerative capacity of the liver i.e the ability of the 'remaining' hepatocyte to increase in number and size (a similar regenerative capacity is shown by other hepatic cells, like cholangiocytes, liver sinusoidal endothelial cells (LSEC), hepatic stellate cells (HSC) etc., a phenomenon called phenotypic fidelity). Generally, after a two third hepatectomy, liver regenerate to maintain 100% liver body size ratio. Liver regeneration is an intricately orchestrated process with a number of redundant pathways which ensures liver regeneration proceeds smoothly and surely [14]. It is equally remarkable to note that not all hepatocyte enter regeneration at once and 'wave' of regeneration seen starting from periportal area to the pericentral area. This ensures that while liver is regenerating, certain population of hepatocytes is reserved for discharging essential liver function [15]. Liver failure is simply the manifestation of failed regeneration. Whether it is acute liver failure, acute on chronic liver failure, chronic liver disease or post-hepatectomy liver failure, inability of liver, due to any reason (see risk factors below) to regenerate is in the root of all evils!! Although it is out of the scope of this chapter to discuss in detail the process of 'partly known' liver regeneration, certain points pertaining to explain PHLF will be explained here. One question that comes to mind is that, why liver regeneration fails at all. As widely accepted, that excessive portal blood flow to the remnant liver inflicts sinusoidal endothelial damage, initiating a cascade of events, that shuts down regeneration. It is interesting to know however that, it is essentially, this increased portal flow which initiates regeneration. 'At least in animals,' after two third hepatectomy there is mathematically threefold increase in portal flow per unit of liver tissue. This increased portal flow (and pressure) also brings in increased amount of hepatotropic factors to the remnant liver, providing perhaps with essential ingredients of regeneration. Although, the connect between increased portal flow and extracellular matrix modulation (ECM modulation, an important initial molecular event in the regeneration of liver) remains elusive to this date, undoubtedly, it is the, most important event. It is not difficult to understand that, there lies a fine balance between what is increased versus excessive portal flow. Whatever, may be the underlying molecular mechanism, this balance will be disturbed whenever, critical mass (in numbers or functional) of liver remnant is not maintained. Hence, in general more than two third hepatectomy in any animal fails to initiate liver regeneration, thus leading to post hepatectomy liver failure [16].

34.1.4 Epidemiology

Liver failure following liver resection is a dreaded and preventable complication. There are multiple factors that play role in postoperative liver failure. There has been tremendous improvement in the preoperative evaluation of liver function, hepatic reserve, surgical and anaesthetic techniques and postoperative care. As a result, the survival has improved considerably over the years. Mortality after hepatic resection now ranges from 0% in highly selected patients to 5% in large clinical series. However, the incidence for PHLF still remains around 5–9%. Depending on severity and the used definition of PHLF, the perioperative mortality still ranges between 40% and 60% [17]. In a large study, PHLF criteria were satisfied in 70% of patients who died following a liver resection for all indications, with PHLF being the direct cause of death in over half of those [18]. Thus, PHLF still represents the single most important reason for death after major and extended hepatectomy. There is still significant and ongoing efforts have been to reduce it further. One of the important focuses of research had been to identify the reliable early markers of liver failure which could help in instituting early effecting therapies, identifying high risk patients to improve further outcomes by avoiding deaths.

34.1.5 Risk Factors of Post-hepatectomy Liver Failure

The risk factor for PHLF is controversial. Age more than 65 is widely considered as an independent risk factor for PHLF owing to impaired regeneration [19]. However, recent data reveal that with advancing age regeneration is only delayed and liver is ultimately restored to 100% of body weight [14]. Likewise, diabetes and high BMI also considered important patient related risk factors. Insulin although not directly mitogenic to the hepatocyte, it is indispensable for regeneration and hepatocyte function [16]. Advancing age brings in many other risk factors, like comorbidity of diabetes, impaired immune function, thus predisposing more for infection, which can impair regeneration. Hence, patient related risk factors should not be seen in isolation, for eventual outcome may be the result of complex interplay amongst various other factors (see Table 34.3). it is noteworthy that liver resection is an

Table 34.3 Biological marker and clinical risk factor for PHLF. Reproduced with permission (Shen et al. 2018)

Biological markers	Patient-related factors	Liver quality-related factors	Surgery-related factors
AST	Male sex	Hepatitis	Extent of resection
ALT	Age ≥ 65 years	Cirrhosis	Intraoperative blood loss > 1000 mL
GGT	Diabetes	Steatosis	Intraoperative hypotension
TB	BMI ≥ 30 kg/m^2	Cholestasis	Vascular reconstruction
LDH	Malnutrition	Portal hypertension	Prolonged in-flow occlusion
ALP	ASA score ≥ 3	Neo-adjuvant chemotherapy	Postoperative hemorrhage
ALB	Sepsis		
CRE			
PT			
PLT			
INR			

injury to the liver and predictably there is striking similarities between wound healing and liver regeneration, with some differences [16]. It might therefore be possible that factors affecting wound healing would affect liver regeneration as well. As discussed earlier, it is ultimately, inadequate critical remnant mass (in number or function) which is responsible for impaired liver regeneration and thus for PHLF. Hence quality of remnant liver is immensely important. Although the limits of safe hepatic resection [20] in each category of the compromised liver quality can be challenged, there is no denying of fact that depreciating function has to be replaced with increasing mass of liver (Fig. 34.1). One of the biggest challenge clinicians face today is not in determining the remnant liver volume limits but in finding optimal tools which could accurately assess quality of liver preoperatively.

34.1.6 Assessment of Liver Function

Table 34.4 enumerates the various liver function tests. Qualitative tests only measure activity or concentration of substance in the blood and is influenced by factors other than liver itself. For example, serum bilirubin can be affected by extrahepatic factors, Prothrombin time can get affected by administration of fresh frozen plasma, albumin level with generalized hypoproteinaemia. Similarly, quantitative test analyses certain aspect of liver functioning. Amongst the quantitative tests indocyanine green test is perhaps the most studies and in authors opinion most useful. Earlier studies based on ICG retention rate at 15 min of distribution phase and calculated as ratio of the ICG plasma concentration at 15 min to its initial concentration and expressed as a percentage (%). It is worth mentioning here that ICGR at 15 min was developed for determining extent of resection in patient with HCC [21]. Perioperative factors like blood loss, postoperative complications, ischemia reperfusion injury play important role in the development of PHLF. Extent of resection thereby impacting FLRV is important. However, precisely what level of % FLRV is required in normal liver to prevent PHLF remains controversial. The general consensus is 20–30% according to the different authors [20]. In contrast, precise safe limit

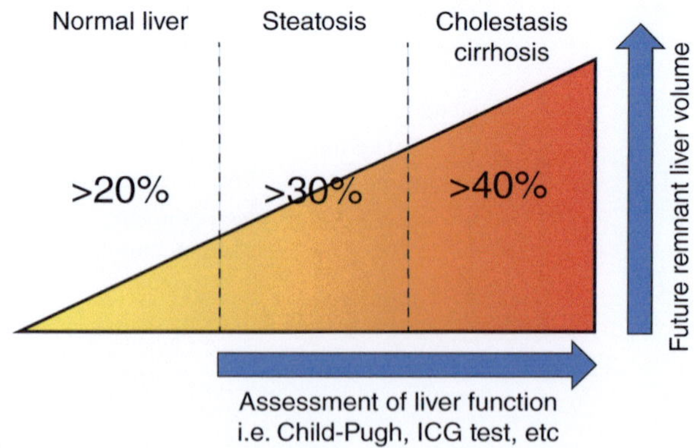

Fig. 34.1 Limits of safe resection. (Reproduced with permission (Guglielmi et al. 2012))

Table 34.4 Liver function tests

Qualitative or conventional tests	Quantitative tests
Serum bilirubin	Aminopyrine breath test
Serum bile acids	Antipyrine clearance
Alkaline phosphatase	Caffeine clearance
Gamma-glutamyl transpeptidase transaminases	Lidocaine clearance (MEGX)
Coagulation factors, prothrombin time	Methacetin breath test
Albumin	Galactose elimination capacity (GEC)
	Low-dose galactose clearance
	Sorbitol clearance
	Indocyanine green disappearance
	99mTc-GSA

MEGX monoethylglycinexylidide, *99mTc-GSA* technetium-99 m galactosyl human serum albumin

remains unqualified in patients with chronic liver disease. However, decision tree based on ICGR15, Child Peugh score is useful.

34.1.7 Prediction Models

Various combination of assessing tools have been used in developing prediction model and nomograms. These prediction model frequently combine serum bilirubin level, coagulopathy, ascites, platelet count, serum albumin level, parameters of portal hypertension, parameters of future liver remnant volume etc. It cannot be overemphasized that these prediction models have been developed and applied to a specific population of patients, lack external validation and thus devoid of general applicability. Limiting patient population though decreases generalization it increases the accuracy and vice versa. It has been observed that vast majority of studies have FLRV and parameters of portal hypertension in their prediction models of PHLF consistent with specific patient population of HCC. Addition of intraoperative factor in prediction model does not further improve its accuracy suggesting that preoperative factors may be more important in predicting PHLF. Despite these limitations, prediction models when used in their specific population of patients, can accurately predict PHLF and in such situation exercising preventing strategy as well as those models which include postoperative factors, can help in early recognition of PHLF and institution of treatment thereby improving outcome. Perioperative platelet may be considered relevant and important prognostic factor for PHLF; however, most studies are retrospective and majority of patients had minor hepatectomy [22].

34.1.8 Preventive Measures

Given the stormy postoperative course of patient developing PHLF it is extremely important that by utilizing available tools, a reasonable prediction of PHLF is made and preventive strategies accordingly applied to improve outcomes. With increasing

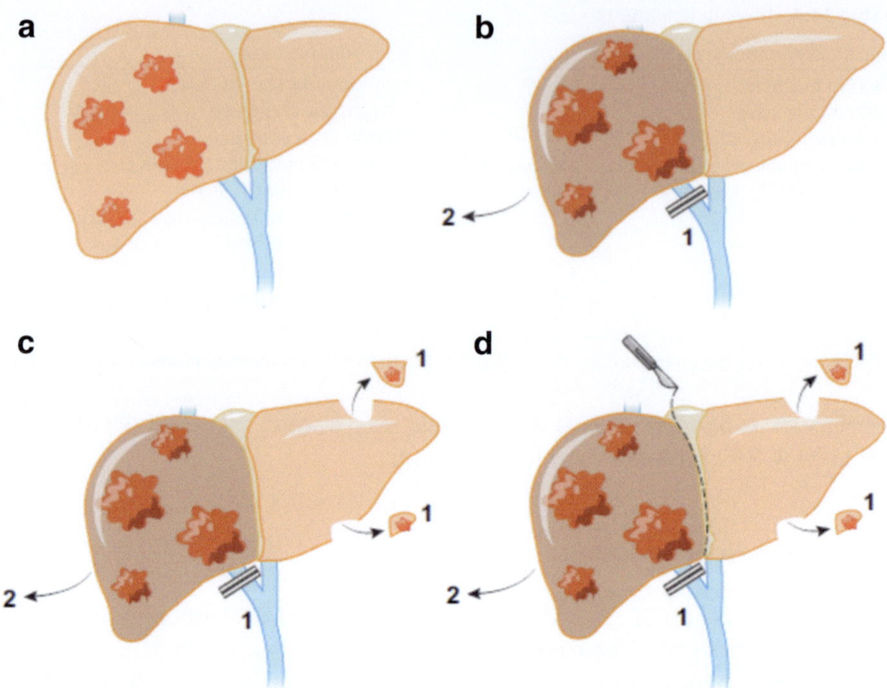

Fig. 34.2 Visualization of pre- or perioperative interventions and their effect on liver remnant volume. (**a**) Malignant liver disease (**b**) Embolization/ligation of the right portal branch (1) results in atrophy of the right hemi-liver and compensatory growth of the left hemi-liver, which can be removed when appropriate hypertrophy has been achieved (2). (**c**) Removal of tumours from the left hemi-liver and occlusion of the right portal branch (1). After 4–6 weeks, the volume of the left hemi-liver is increased and the right hemi-liver can be removed (2). (**d**) Removal of tumours from the left hemi-liver, in situ splitting of the hemi-livers, and simultaneous ligation of the right portal vein branch (1). After 1-week, augmented hypertrophy of the left hemi-liver permits removal of the right hemi-liver (2). (With permission: van Mierlo et al. (2016))

refinements in techniques of surgery, more and more patient will undergo major liver resection. More and more patient will have comorbid condition, compromised liver function and a smaller remnant. Hence, one of the principals of prevention is to enlarge remnant liver [23]. Figure 34.2 enumerates the various preoperative and intraoperative strategies of enlarging FLRV. Another important principal is preoperative optimisation of liver function like liver steatosis can be reduced by a preoperative very-low calorie diet, as has been shown in potential liver transplant donors [24], preoperative biliary drainage in patients with obstructive jaundice [25], chemotherapy free interval to reduce the impact of chemotherapy associated liver injury (CALI) and possibly platelet infusion in chronic liver disease patients [26]. Limiting hepatic hemodynamic imbalance (see pathophysiology) is another important principal. Both surgical (Splenic artery ligation, splenectomy) and pharmacological (terlipressin, octreotide) modulation of portal flow can help prevent portal hyper perfusion there by limiting sinusoidal endothelial injury [27, 28]. The importance of meticulous surgery in limiting blood loss, less manipulation of liver, minimum duration of pringle manoeuvre or ischemic preconditioning cannot be overemphasized [29–31]. Much of the improvement in patient outcome following major liver resection as of today can be ascribed to refinements in patient selection and surgical technique.

34.2 Management of PHLF

By now, we are well aware that occurrence and resolution of PHLF is intricately intertwined with liver regeneration and hence all therapeutic measures essentially aim to promote it. Since liver regeneration underlies the development of liver failure, management principals also remain same across all liver failure categories. That is why, general principles of management of acute liver failure (ALF) and organ dysfunction apply in PHLF also [32]. These have remained the same over the years and incorporate principles of management of ALF from any cause, goal-directed therapy for organ dysfunction, and identifying and treating reversible factors in the postoperative period. In general, in the early postoperative period surgical complications should be actively looked for. Post operative hyperbilirubinemia if develops, obstructive cause should be ruled out and corrected either surgically or radiologically. Torsion of remnant liver is a real possibility and should be looked for, which can result in congestive hepatopathy and may further jeopardise regenerative process. Vascular thromboses should be actively identified with the help of ultrasound doppler studies. Postoperative collection of fluids is the source of sepsis and aggressively looked for and drained. Although postoperative prophylactic antibiotics are not routinely indicated, experience from ALF suggest that prophylactic antibiotics can modify outcome.

34.2.1 Management of Circulatory Dysfunction

Fluid resuscitation should be goal-directed to maintain adequate tissue perfusion. It should be realized that in PHLF due to hemoglobinemia, there is capillary leakage and excessive fluid administration can lead to extravasation and tissue oedema. At the same time a high vasoconstrictor use can cause ischemia in the already struggling remnant liver.

34.2.2 Management of Kidney Dysfunction and Dyselectrolytemia

Acute kidney injury is quite common in PHLF patients. An excessive fluid administration can lead to pulmonary oedema. As total body water increases, it causes hypervolemic hyponatremia. Liver regeneration induces hypokalaemia (along with hyperaldosteronism) and hypophosphatemia. Importance of expeditious replacement and correction of dyselectrolytemia cannot be overemphasized. If need patient might require renal replacement therapy. In comparison to ALF, PHLF patient have a postoperative status, along with imaging studies causing further renal dysfunction. It is recommended to institute early renal replacement therapy if there is evidence of fluid overload. Continuous RRT is better than intermittent, however, evidence for optimal rate is lacking.

34.2.3 Management of Pulmonary Complication

Acute lung injury or acute respiratory distress syndrome gravely impact PHLF patient. Early institution of mechanical ventilation with lung preserving setting is recommended. However, clinician should be mindful of the impact of the prolonged positive pressure ventilation on the hepatic hemodynamic.

34.2.4 Management of Neurological Complication

Development of cerebral oedema in ALF is an ominous sign and portends a extremely poor prognosis if corrective measures not instituted. Specific management of hepatic encephalopathy in ALF have been extensively studied and meat analyses recommend use of Rifaximin. Serum ammonia level correlate with the cerebral oedema and predict mortality in ALF. Continuous venovenous hemofiltration (CVVHF) is also useful in ammonia clearance and increasing rate of hemofiltration increases ammonia clearances. Although specific management of HE in relation to PHLF has not been studied, general management is as that of ALF with expectant management of early grades (Grade 1 or 2) of HE and early intubation with mechanical ventilation for higher grades of HE (Grade 3 or 4). Hypothermia and administration of hypertonic saline is recommended. Routine use of hyperventilation and steroids is not beneficial.

34.2.5 Management of Coagulopathy

Patients with PHLF invariably present with coagulopathy. As in ALF it is an important prognostic marker and rarely is the cause of bleeding. Hence correction of coagulopathy is not routinely advised except when an invasive procedure is planned. It is important to note that coagulopathy with worsening grades of PHLF can lead to gastrointestinal bleeding and high index of suspicion and expeditious management including correction of coagulopathy is advised.

Amongst the drug, although many centres routinely use N-Acetyl cysteine (NAC) postoperatively in patents deemed to be at high risk of developing PHLF, data is scarce on its benefits or otherwise [33].

34.2.6 Liver Specific Management

Artificial liver support—extra-corporal liver support devices (ELSD): Although extension of studies of ESLD in ALF can be applied to the PHLF patient, this is not universally accepted. Molecular Adsorbent Recirculating System (MARS) treatment is safe and feasible in patients with PHLF however cannot be recommended as standard of care as yet [34]. Theoretically, the only definitive and potentially curative management of irreversible PHLF would be a salvage liver transplantation. However, experience is very limited [35] and deals with the issue of scarce organ availability in case of deceased donor liver transplant and ethical issue of possible donor coercion in living donor liver transplant.

References

1. Sen S, Jalan R, Williams R. Extracorporeal albumin dialysis in acute-on-chronic liver failure: will it stand the test of time? Hepatology. 2002;36(4):1014–6.
2. Sherlock S. Emergencies in general practice BRrrisH 1383 medical journal emergencies in general practice acute hepatic failure.
3. Taylor SA, Whitington PF. Neonatal acute liver failure. Liver Transpl. 2016;22(5):677–85.
4. Rahbari NN, Garden OJ, Padbury R, Brooke-Smith M, Crawford M, Adam R, et al. Posthepatectomy liver failure: a definition and grading by the International Study Group of Liver Surgery (ISGLS). Surgery. 2011;149(5):713–24.
5. Balzan S, Belghiti J, Farges O, Ogata S, Sauvanet A, Delefosse D, et al. The "50-50 criteria" on postoperative day 5: an accurate predictor of liver failure and death after hepatectomy. Ann Surg. 2005;242(6):824–9.
6. Mullen JT, Ribero D, Reddy SK, Donadon M, Zorzi D, Gautam S, et al. Hepatic insufficiency and mortality in 1,059 noncirrhotic patients undergoing major hepatectomy. J Am Coll Surg. 2007;204(5):854–62.
7. Schindl MJ, Redhead DN, Fearon KCH, Garden OJ, Wigmore SJ. The value of residual liver volume as a predictor of hepatic dysfunction and infection after major liver resection. Gut. 2005;54(2):289–96.
8. Kubota K. Measurement of liver volume and hepatic functional reserve as a guide to decision-making in resectional surgery for hepatic tumors. Hepatology. 1997;26(5):1176–81.
9. Parikh AA, Gentner B, Wu TT, Curley SA, Ellis LM, Vauthey JN. Perioperative complications in patients undergoing major liver resection with or without neoadjuvant chemotherapy. J Gastrointest Surg. 2003;7:1082–8.
10. Yigitler C, Farges O, Kianmanesh R, Regimbeau JM, Abdalla EK, Belghiti J. The small remnant liver after major liver resection: How common and how relevant? Liver Transpl. 2003;9(9):S18–25.
11. Johnston TD, Chen Y, Reed RL. Functional equivalence of hypothermia to specific clotting factor deficiencies. J Trauma. 1994;37(3):413–7.
12. van Os EC, Kamath PS, Gostout CJ, Heit JA. Gastroenterological procedures among patients with disorders of hemostasis: evaluation and management recommendations. Gastrointest Endosc. 1999;50(4):536–43.
13. Ruttmann TG, James MF, Aronson I. In vivo investigation into the effects of haemodilution with hydroxyethyl starch (200/0.5) and normal saline on coagulation. Br J Anaesth. 1998;80(5):612–6.

14. Michalopoulos GK, Bhushan B. Liver regeneration: biological and pathological mechanisms and implications. Nat Rev Gastroenterol Hepatol. 2021;18:40–55.
15. Michalopoulos GK. Principles of liver regeneration and growth homeostasis. Compr Physiol. 2013;3(1):485–513.
16. Michalopoulos GK. Liver regeneration. J Cell Physiol. 2007;213(2):286–300.
17. Gilg S, Sandström P, Rizell M, Lindell G, Ardnor B, Strömberg C, et al. The impact of post-hepatectomy liver failure on mortality: a population-based study. Scand J Gastroenterol. 2018;53(10–11):1335–9.
18. Jara M, Reese T, Malinowski M, Valle E, Seehofer D, Puhl G, et al. Reductions in post-hepatectomy liver failure and related mortality after implementation of the LiMAx algorithm in preoperative work-up: a single-centre analysis of 1170 hepatectomies of one or more segments. HPB. 2015;17(7):651–8.
19. Xing Y, Liu ZR, Yu W, Zhang HY, Song MM. Risk factors for post-hepatectomy liver failure in 80 patients. World J Clin Cases. 2021;9(8):1793–802.
20. Guglielmi A, Ruzzenente A, Conci S, Valdegamberi A, Iacono C. How much remnant is enough in liver resection? Dig Surg. 2012;29(1):6–17.
21. Imamura H, Sano K, Sugawara Y, Kokudo N, Makuuchi M. Assessment of hepatic reserve for indication of hepatic resection: decision tree incorporating indocyanine green test. J Hepato-Biliary-Pancreat Surg. 2005;12(1):16–22.
22. Yoshino K, Yoh T, Taura K, Seo S, Ciria R, Briceño-Delgado J. A systematic review of prediction models for post-hepatectomy liver failure in patients undergoing liver surgery. HPB. 2021;23:1311–20.
23. van Mierlo KMC, Schaap FG, Dejong CHC, Olde Damink SWM. Liver resection for cancer: new developments in prediction, prevention and management of postresectional liver failure. J Hepatol. 2016;65:1217–31.
24. Doyle A, Adeyi O, Khalili K, Fischer S, Dib M, Goldaracena N, et al. Treatment with optifast reduces hepatic steatosis and increases candidacy rates for living donor liver transplantation. Liver Transpl. 2016;22(9):1295–300.
25. Farges O, Regimbeau JM, Fuks D, le Treut YP, Cherqui D, Bachellier P, et al. Multicentre European study of preoperative biliary drainage for hilar cholangiocarcinoma. Br J Surg. 2012;100(2):274–83.
26. Matsuo R, Nakano Y, Ohkohchi N. Platelet administration via the portal vein promotes liver regeneration in rats after 70% hepatectomy. Ann Surg. 2011;253(4):759–63.
27. Ren YS, Qian NS, Tang Y, Liao YH, Liu WH, Raut V, et al. Benefcial effects of splenectomy on liver regeneration in a rat model of massive hepatectomy. Hepatobiliary Pancreat Dis Int. 2012;11(1):60–5.
28. Fahrner R, Patsenker E, de Gottardi A, Stickel F, Montani M, Stroka D, et al. Elevated liver regeneration in response to pharmacological reduction of elevated portal venous pressure by Terlipressin after partial hepatectomy. Transplantation. 2014;97(9):892–900.
29. van den Broek MAJ, Shiri-Sverdlov R, Schreurs JJW, Bloemen JG, Bieghs V, Rensen SS, et al. Liver manipulation during liver surgery in humans is associated with hepatocellular damage and hepatic inflammation. Liver Int. 2013;33(4):633–41.
30. Simillis C, Robertson FP, Afxentiou T, Davidson BR, Gurusamy KS. A network meta-analysis comparing perioperative outcomes of interventions aiming to decrease ischemia reperfusion injury during elective liver resection. Surgery. 2016;159(4):1157–69.
31. Miki C, Hiro J, Ojima E, Inoue Y, Mohri Y, Kusunoki M. Perioperative allogeneic blood transfusion, the related cytokine response and long-term survival after potentially curative resection of colorectal cancer. Clin Oncol. 2006;18(1):60–6.
32. Søreide JA, Deshpande R. Post hepatectomy liver failure (PHLF)—recent advances in prevention and clinical management. Eur J Surg Oncol. 2021;47(2):216–24.
33. Kemp R, Mole J, Gomez D. Current evidence for the use of N-acetylcysteine following liver resection. ANZ J Surg. 2018;88(6):E486–90.

34. Sparrelid E, Gilg S, van Gulik TM. Systematic review of MARS treatment in post-hepatectomy liver failure. HPB. 2020;22(7):950–60.
35. Chan SC, Sharr WW, Chan ACY, Chok KSH, Lo CM. Rescue living-donor liver transplantation for liver failure following hepatectomy for hepatocellular carcinoma. Liver Cancer. 2013;2(3–4):332–7.

Prevention and Treatment of Pancreatic Fistulae and Leaks in Carcinoma Pancreas

35

Imtiakum Jamir, Niteen Kumar, Gaurav Sood, and Abhideep Chaudhary

35.1 Introduction

Post operative Pancreatic fistula (POPF) is the most dreaded complication after a pancreatic resection and the major determinant of morbidity and mortality [1]. The recent study estimates the incidence of clinically relevant POPF in 19% following pancreatoduodenectomy and 15.1% following distal pancreatectomy [2, 3]. The leak associated with distal pancreatectomy is less burdensome. The consequences of POPF are many: prolonged hospital stay, economic burden, delays in initiation of adjuvant therapy, and negatively impact on overall survival [4]. The recent universal definition of POPF has helped to examine the various risk factors, prediction models and mitigation strategies. Despite plethora of studies and trials describing novel strategies to ameliorate the risk of POPF formation, the rates of POPF have remained plateaued [5]. In recent years the understanding of post-operative acute pancreatitis (POAP) and acinar density as important risk factors has helped understand the underlying mechanism of POPF which may not always necessarily be due to the mechanical failure of pancreatico-enteric anastomosis [6, 7].

The current aim of the chapter will be to review the evidence for prevention of the occurrence of postoperative pancreatic fistula (POPF), mitigation strategies and the treatment of clinically relevant fistula.

I. Jamir (✉) · N. Kumar · A. Chaudhary
Department of HPB Surgery and Liver Transplantation, BLK MAX Super Speciality Hospital, Delhi, India

G. Sood
Department of Liver and GI Surgery, BLK Super Speciality Hospital, New Delhi, India

K. Sood Sharma et al. (eds.), *Complications of Cancer Therapy: Best Practices in Prevention and Management*, https://doi.org/10.1007/978-981-99-0984-1_35

35.2 Definition of Pancreatic Fistula (Fig. 35.1)

The definition and management of pancreatic fistulas has become more standardized, and data driven over the years. In 2005 the International Study Group of Pancreatic Fistula (ISGPF) defined POPF as "an abnormal communication between the pancreatic ductal epithelium and another epithelial surface containing pancreas-derived, enzyme rich fluid" [8]. This pancreatic juice leakage occurs on the site of the surgical resection following pancreatojejunostomy in case of pancreaticoduodenectomy or pancreatic surface as in distal pancreatectomy/enucleation by the impaired sealing of the pancreatic parenchyma. In 2017, a new definition and grading system was proposed by ISFPF which is now universally accepted. The former "grade A postoperative pancreatic fistula" is now redefined and called a "biochemical leak," because it has no clinical importance and is no longer referred to a true pancreatic fistula [1]. Currently postoperative pancreatic fistula is now said to be clinically relevant only if the drain output of any measurable volume of fluid with an amylase level >3 times the upper limit of institutional normal serum amylase activity is associated with a clinically relevant development/condition related directly to the postoperative pancreatic fistula. In the updated version Grade B was defined as when drains were either left in place for >3 weeks or repositioned through endoscopic/percutaneous procedures. Grade C postoperative pancreatic fistula

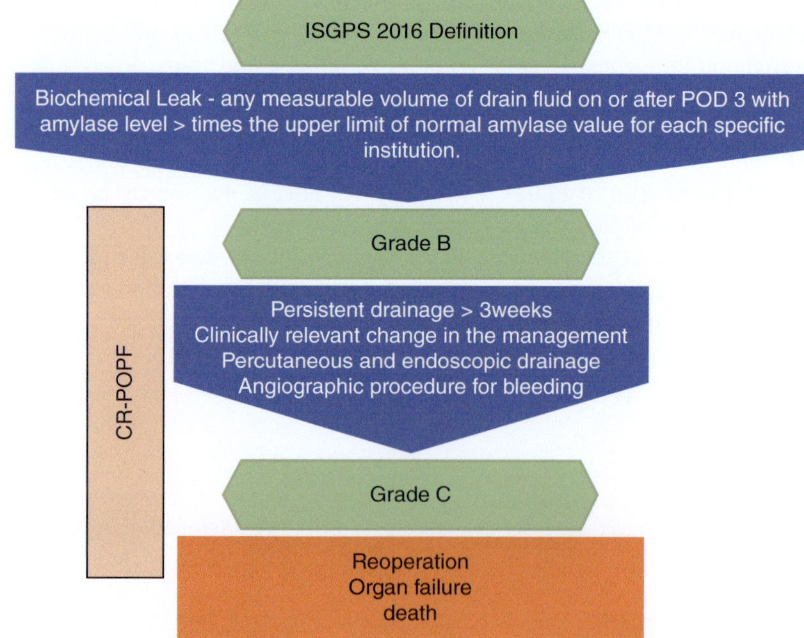

Fig. 35.1 ISGPS definition of postoperative pancreatic fistula. *CR-POPF* clinically relevant postoperative pancreatic fistula, *ISGPS* the International Study Group for Pancreatic Surgery [1]

refers to those postoperative pancreatic fistulae that require reoperation or lead to single or multiple organ failure and/or mortality. The standardization of definition has permitted a more rigorous search and awareness of risk factors, predictors, prevention strategies and ways to mitigate the modifiable factors to minimize this dreaded complication. Unfortunately, the final POPF grade can only be assessed posteriori after the complete resolution of the clinical condition or death.

35.3 Current Risk Stratification Systems

Various studies over the past few decades have developed numerous prediction nomograms based on combination of various preoperative, operative and postoperative factors like male sex, body mass index, pre-operative serum albumin, bilirubin, pancreas related factors-texture, duct size, pathology, relationship of tumour to portal vein, blood loss, intra-abdominal fat thickness and POD drain amylase [9]. The attempt of these risk scores was aimed to stratify and predict patients who might develop serious pancreatic fistula. Prediction scores are used for counselling patients pre-operatively, application of mitigation strategies during surgery, proactive identification of POPF as well as consideration for early removal of drains leading to potential minimization of adverse events in patients who are at risk.

The most widely accepted and validated score is the Callery model (also known as the Fistula Risk Score) consisting of pancreatic gland texture, duct size diameter, pathology and perioperative blood loss based on surgeon's assessment (Table 35.1) [10]. However, it failed to consider other factors such as patients undergoing

Table 35.1 FRS for the prediction of POPF after pancreaticoduodenectomy [10]

Risk factors	Parameters	Points
Gland texture	Firm	0
	Soft	2
Pathology	Pancreatic adenocarcinoma or pancreatitis	0
	Ampullary, duodenal, cystic, islet cells, etc.	1
Intraoperative blood loss	≥5 mm	0
	4 mm	1
	3 mm	2
	2 mm	3
	≤1 mm	4
	≤400 mL	0
	401–700 mL	1
	701–1000 mL	2
	≥1000 mL	3
Total points	0–10 points	

Reproduce from Callery et al. [10]

pancreaticoduodenectomy (PD) following neoadjuvant radiation therapy which has a protective effect on POPF. Mungroop et al. developed and proposed an alternate Fistula Risk Score which included three factors: pancreatic texture, duct size and BMI initially for minimally invasive pancreatectomy and later validated open pancreaticoduodenectomy [11]. Furthermore, an updated alternate FRS score included male sex as an added risk factor [12].

A recent first systematic review and meta-analysis of risk factors associated with POPF following PD, 52,774 patients from 122 studies were included (13 studies adopted the 2016 ISGPF definition of CR-POPF). Out of 176 variables, the study identified 24 and 17 factors that were associated with an overall POPF rate of 27% and CR-POPF in 19% [13]. The study demonstrated that several risk factors associated with CR-POPF were not used within current available risk prediction models hence a better prediction model was required which would incorporate all the factors responsible for CR-POPF. The Samsung medical centre attempted to develop an artificial intelligence Risk prediction platform (AUC 0.74) for POPF incorporating multiple (sixteen) identified risk factors for POPF [14]. This web based POPF prediction platform is available at https:/popfrisk.smchbp.org. and can be helpful in determining perioperative management pathways to mitigate the risk of POPF.

Histological study at the resection margins has demonstrated that acinar cell density ≥60% and not fat was associated with POPF. Also, the presence of fibrosis confers a protective effect on POPF. Acinar cell density is a now accepted as a key factor in the POPF and postoperative acute pancreatitis POAP [7, 15]. POAP with or without elevation of C-reactive protein was associated with increased CR-POPF [16].

The use of this risk score promotes a better preparedness and suggests the best pathway to prevent and mitigate POPF specially in High-risk pancreatic anastomosis.

35.4 The Impact of Centralization and Centre Volume

Currently the trend in the west is toward a referral based high volume centric pancreatic surgery practice as it has shown to significantly decrease hospital mortality [17–20]. More so these high-volume centres have vast surgical experience in the management of pancreatic complications, provide better resources and have a multidisciplinary team of experts comprising of radiologists, interventional radiologists and endoscopists. However, this practice of centralization did not demonstrate a decrease in POPF rates, length of stay and costs in Sweden, suggesting factors other than centralization which need to be explored [21].

35.5 Intraoperative Technical Considerations

The pancreatic surgeon should properly plan the surgery and assess the risk for potential POPF. Meticulous dissection and minimal blood loss is critical. A careful approximation especially for a duct-to-mucosa anastomosis using operating loupes or even microscopes reduce the incidence of PF by allowing precise reconstruction of the pancreatic anastomosis. Avoiding technical errors by ensuring adequate bites of pancreatic duct and jejunal mucosa, correct knot placement, avoidance of crossing of the sutures and air knots is crucial [22]. Proper needle size and suture material as per pancreatic diameter is essential. The pancreatic neck is an area of vascular watershed and avoidance of long remnant neck by performing a full neck resection (transection ≥7 mm at the left side of the portal vein) was shown to provide a protective effect for CR-POPF after PD [23]. Best technique for transection of the neck (surgical scalpel, diathermy or harmonic scalpel) is not known. Since the advent of minimally access pancreatic surgery the use of harmonic has become more common [22, 24]. The fear of using energy is thermal injury of pancreatic stump thereby increasing the risk of POAP and resultant POPF.

35.6 Use of Surgical Drains to Mitigate POPF

The routine use of prophylactic drains in pancreatic surgery is an ongoing controversy. Cochrane database of systematic reviews have shown that no drain insertion/early drain removal to be associated with earlier discharge from hospital [25, 26]. Despite weak data to support routine use of prophylactic drains most surgeons continue to use intraperitoneal drains. However, the non-use of surgical drains may be harmful. In a recent publication of risk-adjusted analysis of drain use in pancreaticoduodenectomy, the use of single or multiple drains in intermediate or high-risk cases was found to mitigate the course of anticipated pancreatic leaks and omission of drains was associated with significant increase in complications and mortality [27]. The placement of drains gives sentinel information which potentially prevents the patient from worsening beyond salvage. Hence the use of FRS score as a harbinger for POPF thereby warranting prophylactic drain placement is beneficial. The best policy as per current evidence is to selectively use drains in high-risk patients (soft pancreas, small duct and high BMI) and to consider for an early drain removal on POD3 if the drain amylase on POD1 is <666 U/L and POD3 drain amylase is <252 U/L [28, 29]. A recent international survey on drain use among pancreatic surgeons worldwide concluded that drain management was very diverse in terms of the type of drains used, enzyme testing and removal schedules. Interesting to note was that only 5% of the total respondents completely omitted a prophylactic drain [30].

35.7 Surgical Anastomosis Techniques and Development of POPF

The quest for the best surgical anastomotic technique is still ongoing for the pancreatic surgeons. The type of anastomotic reconstruction is broadly classified into two categories pancreaticogastrostomy (PG) and pancreatojejunostomy (PJ). In order to answer which is the best technique, the latest Cochrane metanalysis reviewed 7 out of 10 RCTs and concluded that there was little or no difference between PJ and PG in development of postoperative pancreatic fistula (PJ 24.3%; PG 21.4%; RR 1.19, 95% CI 0.88–1.62), clinically significant pancreatic fistula and risk of postoperative mortality (3.9 vs. 4.8%) [31]. The jury is still debating as to which is the best technique. Different methods of anastomosis of the pancreatic stump with the jejunum include end-to-side duct-to-mucosa anastomosis, end-to-side or end-to-end invagination techniques (dunking). The most frequently used technique for pancreatojejunostomy is the end-to-side duct-to-mucosa anastomosis. Peng's binding pancreatojejunostomy after PD was initially demonstrated to significantly reduce the risk of pancreatic leak. Ensuing western studies did not demonstrate any reduction in the postoperative pancreatic fistula rate [32, 33]. Despite numerous efforts on technical modification, it should be noted that currently no single reconstructive technique for pancreatic anastomosis is superior to the others, the preference of technique is purely centre based and the individual surgeon's discretion.

Currently the impact of Ante vs. Retro GJ also did not have any influence on leak rate [34]. An isolated Roux loop to compartmentalize the biliary and pancreatic limbs does not decrease the risk of POPF however it prevents the activation of pancreatic secretions thereby ameliorating the course of POPF [35, 36].

35.8 Techniques of PJ

In 2020, a systematic review and meta-analysis of two most common PJ techniques in a total of 2412 patients, almost equal number of cases underwent Blumgart anastomosis (BA) which involved both duct-to-mucosa and a full-thickness pancreatic "U" stitch (mattress stitch) and another half underwent non-Blumgart anastomosis. BA was associated with significantly lower rates of grade B/C POPF (OR 0.38, 0.22–0.65; $P = 0.004$) as compared to the non-Blumgart anastomosis (Cattell-Warren anastomosis (CWA) and Kakita anastomosis (KA). Subgroup analysis of soft pancreatic texture showed that though the incidence of POPF (grade B/C) was lower in the BA group vs. the conventional PJ group (27.3 vs. 41.2%), it was not statistically significant (OR 0.46, 0.14–1.53; $P = 0.21$). Therefore, it is possible that a soft pancreas led to higher incidence of pancreatic fistula, regardless of which way the PJ anastomosis was done. A subsequent multi-center randomized controlled trial (RCT) comparing Blumgart vs. Cattell Warren techniques of PJ following pancreato-duodenectomy, of the 236 patients there was no demonstrable overall reduction in CR-POPF with the Blumgart technique (BA 13 (5.5%), CWA 14 (5.9%), $p = 0.857$) [37]. A most recent Cochrane review on duct-to-mucosa versus other types of pancreaticojejunostomy (e.g., invagination pancreaticojejunostomy, binding pancreaticojejunostomy) for the prevention of postoperative pancreatic fistula following pancreaticoduodenectomy could not demonstrate superiority of one over the other [38].

According to current evidence, no technique seems to mitigate POPF, and the choice of technique is dependent on the surgeon's experience in a particular centre.

35.9 Use of Stents; Internal or External Stents and Type of Material Used

Use of pancreatic duct anastomosis stents is another possible way to reduce fistula formation. The rationale for trans-anastomotic stent (TAS) placement includes diversion of pancreatic enzymes, decompression of the pancreatic remnant and assistance in suturing of the pancreatic-enteric anastomosis. However, the use of internal trans-anastomotic stents (ITS) has not shown any benefit in alleviating development of POPF consistently in various clinical trials [39–41]. On the contrary, selective use of external trans-anastomotic stents (ETS) unlike most trials in pancreatic surgery has shown to decrease POPF and hence is now accepted as a standard method for reduction of POPF in patients mainly in high-risk patients [42–44]. Phase 3 RCT comparing use of ETS in pancreaticojejunostomy vs. ETS in pancreaticogastrostomy for patients with high-risk pancreatic anastomosis the CR-POPF was similar, however the pancreaticogastrostomy group had an increased incidence of Clavien-Dindo grade 3 or above complications. The trial recommended the use of PJ with the use of externalized stent and octreotide omissions for patients with high risk for pancreatic fistula, as a mitigation strategy [45].

Lately, pancreatic surgeons have tried TAS with different materials. The use of simple infant feeding tube for ETS led to stent dislodgement. In a pilot study, ITS with coronary artery stents (CAS) was compared with external stents and the use of CAS as ITS was found to be a safe and secure mitigating strategy for high-risk PJ anastomosis with not a single stent displacement compared to one fourth in the ETS group. Further trials are the need of the hour to demonstrate whether change in material of stent produces a better result for ITS [46].

35.10 Use of Pancreatic Sealants and Glues

Since 1978 various sealants have been used in pancreatic surgery to prevent pancreatic fistula after resection of the pancreatic head and tail. The use of glue around the PJ has been tried with the intent to prevent leak of pancreatic juice by reinforcing the pancreatic anastomoses. However, across various RCTS, multicentric studies and Cochrane review, a significant decrease in the incidence of POPF could not be demonstrated [47, 48]. Since they seemed to be inert and caused no untoward ill effects, they could be used in high-risk pancreatic anastomosis.

The occlusion of the main pancreatic duct after PD is an easy-to-perform procedure and can be considered in cases where a complication can be life threatening specially in elderly with comorbidities, soft and small pancreatic ducts [49, 50]. The use of occlusive glues particularly with a permanent occlusive sealant such as neoprene can triple the risk of diabetes at 1 and 3 years and should be used with caution [51].

35.11 Pharmacological Strategies to Prevent POPF

35.11.1 Somatostatin Analogs

The physiological effect of somatostatin and its analogs has an inhibitory effect on pancreatic exocrine secretion volume. Hence it was presumed to potentially alleviate the natural course of POPF and facilitate closure of PF. However, studies have yielded mixed results and most trials have demonstrated the ineffectiveness of POPF closure [52–55]. In fact, large clinical series after risk-adjustment by the FRS revealed that octreotide may be harmful as their use escalated the risk for CR-POPF and recommended the omission of octreotide in high-risk patients [56].

In 2014, a single-centre RCT by Allen and colleagues demonstrated the ability of pasireotide, a somatostatin analogue that has a longer half-life than octreotide to significantly reduce the CR-POPF rate (absolute risk reduction of 12% from 21% in the placebo group to 9% in pasireotide group) and proposed that pasireotide may provide some clinical advantage in patients undergoing either PD or DP [57]. Similarly, a recent real-world data on the use of pasireotide during routine pancreatic surgery from Kunstman et al. showed a clinically significant reduction in pancreatic leak rate (13.3%) comparable to Allen et al. [57, 58]. There can be a more widespread use of pasireotide in pancreatic surgeries if it's limiting factors such as increased cost and availability issues are eliminated [59]. A recent meta-analysis confirmed that routine administration of pasireotide was also associated with decreased POPF rates for PD and lesser readmission rates [60].

35.11.2 Perioperative Use of Steroids

Two small RCTs have shown that perioperative hydrocortisone compared to placebo was effective in reducing major complications after PD and the rate of POPF after DP. The mechanism of these actions is believed to be the anti-inflammatory effects at the site of pancreatic transection thereby providing a niche for healing. In a non-inferiority single centre trial comparing hydrocortisone with the more expensive pasireotide, both were found to be equivalent. Hence the use of steroid before transection should be considered in most cases. Prophylactic administration of these corticosteroid agents can reduce the severity of pancreatitis as indicated by various histopathologic markers, serum amylase and IL-6 levels and thereby may reduce the POPF rate [61].

35.12 Clinical Presentation

POPF is associated with different clinical presentations. It might be asymptomatic or, when not adequately drained there is deviation from normal post operative course with nonspecific complaints associated with abdominal discomfort, nausea, tachycardia and fever. Laboratory parameters may report an increase in counts and C-reactive protein. POPF may contribute to the development of further complications such as intra-abdominal abscess, bleeding, wound infection, pneumonia, sepsis and postoperative mortality. An algorithm based early recognition and minimal invasive management using a smart phone app was shown to decrease the overall 90 days mortality by almost 50%. There was also reduction of relaparotomy from 15% to 8% with this proactive algorithm. The algorithm guided the treating team when to do abdominal CT, radiological drainage, start antibiotic treatment, and remove abdominal drains [62].

35.13 Treatment of CR-POPF (Fig. 35.2)

Patients who are clinically stable should be managed by a Step-up approach [63]. This intervention aims to convert undrained collections into controlled external fistula, prevention and detection of sequelae such as bleed and sepsis and wait for the spontaneous closure of fistula. There is no requirement for this specific intervention and most POPF can be management in a non-ICU setting. The uncomplicated low output fistula (<200 mL per day) can be managed conservatively with timely imaging and drainage of intraabdominal collection with the support of IR and most of them will close with non-operative management. High output fistulae are more problematic and associated with excessive fluid and electrolytes. The care of these drains is paramount, which need to be secured in order to prevent dislodgement as peri drain leakages can result in severe excoriations. Initially on detection of CR-POPF, empirical wide spectrum antibiotics were administered in all patients and final antibiotic treatment was decided based on the results of blood and drain fluid culture sensitivity reports. The monitoring of drain fluid bacterial culture and assessment for the presence of candida needs to be done as it is associated with severe infectious complications [64, 65]. With this conservative measure fistula closure will usually occur within 4 weeks in almost more than 90%.

Skin care around the percutaneous drains needs to be meticulously taken care of to prevent skin breakage from digestive fluid, as these drains would be present for a considerable period. The intrastromal therapist should be involved in difficult cases.

The use of somatostatin and its analogues is debateable with no clear-cut guideline. The intuitive thinking of decreased secretion thereby decreasing the output and facilitating fistula closure is not conclusively agreed by the pancreatic surgeons.

Careful monitoring for signs of fever, counts and inflammatory markers and/or sentinel bleed need to be kept in mind. Patients may require bed side USG or urgent CT with or without contrast based on clinical judgement. Patients with POPF related sepsis and or bleed would require appropriate supportive care. These patients may require ICU admission, inotropic infusion, high end antibiotics and antifungals, ventilatory support, coagulopathy correction, renal support and blood transfusions.

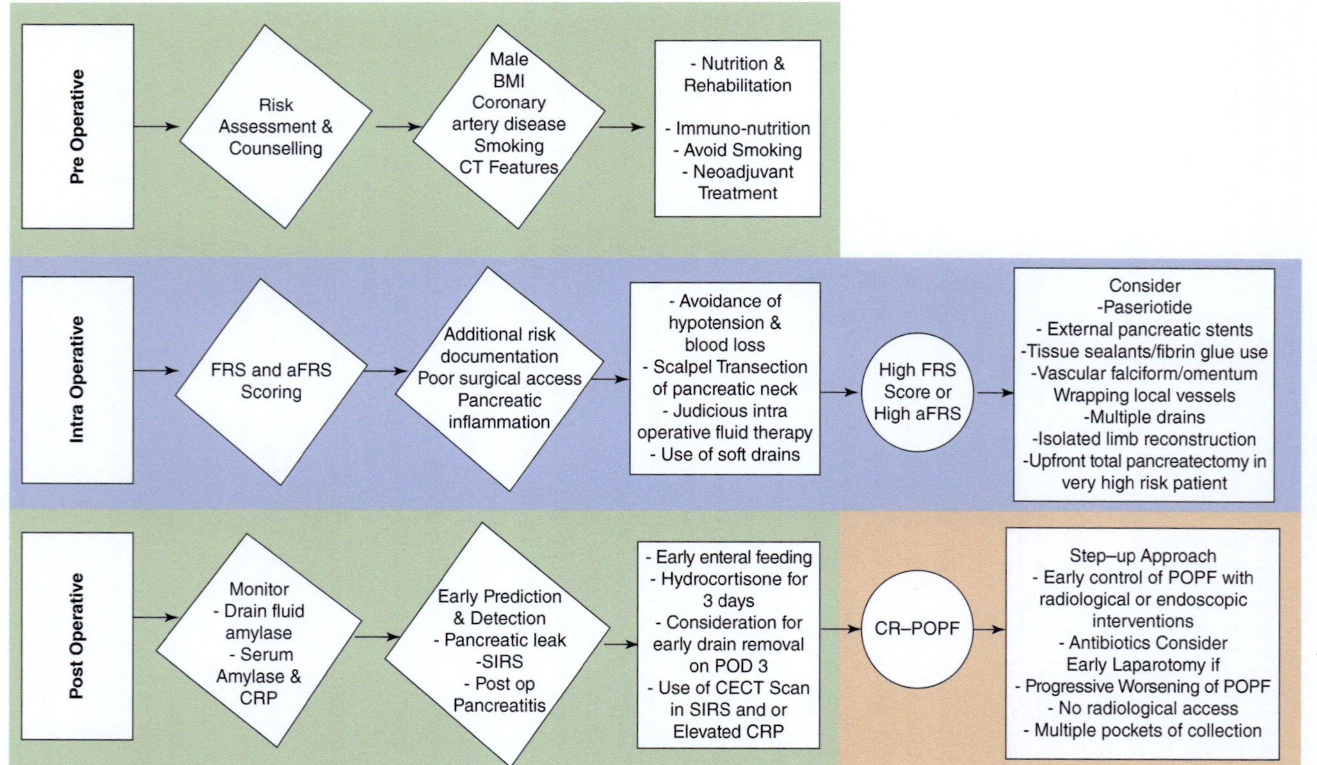

Fig. 35.2 An overview of the preventive, mitigation strategies using FRS score and an early recognition and algorithm-based management adopted form Dutch Pancreatic Cancer Group [62]. *POPF* postoperative pancreatic fistula, *CECT* contrast enhanced tomography, *FRS* fistula risk score, *aFRS* alternate fistula risk score, *CRP* C-reactive protein

35.14 Nutrition: Parental and Enteral Nutrition

Earlier, keeping nil per mouth was vital in the management of POPF, which prevented food induced stimulation of pancreatic exocrine secretion. However, it led to impaired wound healing and nutritional, fluid and electrolyte depletion specially in high-output POPF (>200 mL of daily drain output). The use of enteral jejunal feed through a feeding jejunostomy or nasojejunal tube allows resting of exocrine pancreatic secretion and prevention of atrophy of intestinal mucosa thereby inhibiting bacterial translocation. Parenteral nutrition should be used for supplementation till caloric requirement is met enterally since long term PN is associated with septicaemia, wound infections and metabolic complications (hyperglycaemia). An open label randomized controlled clinical trial demonstrated the faster rate of fistula closure with EN compared to PN [66]. Routine prophylactic tube placement should be considered in patients with poor nutritional status and in pancreaticoduonectomy with high risk to develop POPF. Use of immunonutrition supplements during peri-operative phase of PD was shown to be beneficial in prevention of POPF [67].

35.15 Minimally Invasive Radiological Techniques and Angiographic Interventions

In recent years the advancement in minimally invasive IR intervention has achieved high technical success in management of peripancreatic collections reducing the need for unplanned laparotomies following pancreatic resections which carried very high morbidity and mortality [68].

The development of peripancreatic fluid collection in PD is likely to get infected with enteric bacteria as it involves the opening of intestine unlike DP. The presentation may be asymptomatic or may have vague abdominal pain and fever. In most cases image guided drainage prevents a relaparotomy, thereby avoiding general anaesthesia and surgical stress. This drainage may be USG or CT guided depending on access and local expertise. The fluid is sent for microbiological cultures. The catheter may require upsizing depending on the consistency of the fluid. The patient may require repositioning and/or additional multiple catheters if the collections are not adequately drained. Fluid in the lesser sac should be drained by an expert endoscopist via a trans gastric route using an Endoscopic Ultrasound [69].

In case of suspicion of bleed, urgent CT angiography should be done for identification of site of pseudoaneurysm which may require embolization or stent placement bridging the bleed site.

35.16 Surgical Management

Surgical management is a last-ditch salvage effort when primary percutaneous catheter drainage approach fails. However, it should be considered early in patients showing no improvement after radiological interventions before the onset of multiorgan dysfunction and when drainage of fluid collections is not technically feasible, in peritonitis and/or perforations.

In a recent retrospective multicentre cohort study published by the Dutch pancreatic study group, 3% required relaparotomy, and majority underwent pancreas-preserving procedures and the rest one fifth underwent a completion pancreatectomy. The surgical management of grade C POPF is challenging involving a high risk of mortality for completion pancreatectomy 56 vs. 32% for pancreas-preserving [70].

Relaparotomy is difficult in view of adhesions, friable tissues with risk of inadvertent injury to the surrounding viscera. Moreover, there are no guidelines for decision making and relies wholly on intraoperative findings, surgical experience and discretion. The surgical intervention will depend on the stability of the patients, remnant pancreatic duct size and remnant pancreas viability. Broadly the surgeon has two options: parenchyma preserving or rescue completion pancreatectomy.

Various modifications for parenchyma preservation have been described by different authors with the intent to preserve the pancreatic stump, namely simple drainage and lavage, external wirsungostomy, salvage pancreaticogastrostomy, pancreatic duct occlusion with suture closure with or without subtotal resection. Simple drainage involves debridement, lavage of peripancreatic regions and placement of multiple drains when anastomosis is relatively intact and when local peripancreatic condition may not permit an aggressive approach. In external wirsunostomy, PJ is dismantled and jejunal opening is closed and a small calibre catheter is inserted into the main pancreatic duct and exteriorized in the epigastric region [71, 72]. The rationale is to prevent mixing of bili-enteric secretion with pancreatic secretion and to convert an active PF into a pure PF. These patients frequently require relaparotomy, and secondary abdominal wall closure [73]. Patients who survive wirsungostomy can be planned for repeat pancreatic jejunal anastomosis months later to preserve pancreatic function [74].

The temptation to revise a PJ anastomosis during the acute phase should not be considered as it is inevitably bound to fail. In selective cases a telescoped 2-layer salvage PG can be attempted. The procedure involves taking down PJ, sharp debridement of 2–3 cm of the necrotic pancreatic stump, sufficient mobilization of the pancreatic stump and finally telescoping into the gastric lumen [75].

35.17 Completion Pancreatectomy

The desperate attempt in salvaging a severe pancreatic leak is completion pancreatectomy consisting of resection of the remaining body and tail of the pancreas [70]. The aim of this most aggressive strategy is to completely remove the focus of intra-abdominal leakage and associated inflammation in cases of POPF complicated by haemorrhage or associated with uncontrollable leakage of the pancreatoenteric anastomosis and post pancreatectomy acute necrotizing pancreatitis [76]. In a recent multicentre cohort study and meta-analysis by Groen et al., there was a significantly high mortality after completion pancreatectomy (56 vs. 32%) compared to pancreas preserving procedures [70]. Over the years high volume pancreatic centres have achieved satisfactory perioperative outcomes with CP. The option of performing total pancreatectomy to avoid morbidity related to high risk pancreatico-jejunostomy anastomosis is being evaluated by an ongoing RCT [77, 78].

35.18 Distal Pancreatectomy

The incidence of POPF remains high (around 30%) regardless of centre volume or surgical expertise [2]. The best practice of stump closure in distal pancreatectomy for avoiding POPF remains an unresolved issue. Different techniques proposed to ameliorate the occurrence of POPF are sharp transection with handsewn closure (using mattress or fish-mouth sutures), use of mechanical stapler for transection, transection with energy-based devices (diathermy, ultrasonic devices, with or without ligation of the main pancreatic duct), the use of additional supportive sealant at site or even anastomosis of the pancreatic stump to a Roux-en-Y jejunal limb or as a pancreaticogastrostomy [79–82]. None of these techniques have demonstrated a clear superiority over the others in randomized controlled trials. The use of drains after DP is currently the norm since DP has high POPF [83]. The progression of POPF after DP less frequently leads to severe complications but contributes to prolonged drain related problems and longer hospital stay.

Key Points

- Despite its current limitations, use of risk scores should be used to counsel and stratify patients in order to plan clinical management.
- Studies have not demonstrated superiority of one surgical technique over the other in preventing CR-POPF and mitigating pancreatic leaks, leaving it to the surgeon to adopt the best technique based on their experience.
- Externalized stents should be considered in high-risk pancreatojejunostomy anastomosis.
- Use of prophylactic drain placement in pancreaticoduodenectomy remains controversial except in high-risk patients.
- Efficacy of perioperative somatostatin analogues to reduce POPF requires further evaluation.
- Perioperative hydrocortisones prevent POAP by their anti-inflammatory mechanisms and thereby reduce POPF.
- CR-POPF should be conservatively managed by step-up approach, however few patients may require surgical intervention.
- Completion pancreatectomy may be required as a salvage procedure in severe leaks.
- Algorithm based early recognition and management has shown to remarkably reduce the overall morbidity and mortality of pancreatic surgery.

35.19 Conclusions

POPF remains the most significant challenge faced by pancreatic surgeons. Prevention, mitigation and management are an integral part of the proactive strategy for the amelioration of POPF. The need of the hour is bench to bed side research and collaborative clinical trials for identifying newer treatment strategies. A risk-based algorithm for early recognition and management will help in homogenizing treatment pathways for decreasing the incidence of POPF.

References

1. Bassi C, Marchegiani G, Dervenis C, Sarr M, Abu Hilal M, Adham M, et al. The 2016 update of the international study group (ISGPS) definition and grading of postoperative pancreatic fistula: 11 years after. Surgery. 2017;161(3):584–91.
2. Ecker BL, McMillan MT, Allegrini V, Bassi C, Beane JD, Beckman RM, et al. Risk factors and mitigation strategies for pancreatic fistula after distal pancreatectomy: analysis of 2026 resections from the international, multi-institutional distal pancreatectomy study group. Ann Surg. 2019;269(1):143–9.
3. Zhou L, Xiao WM, Li CP, Gao YW, Gong WJ, Lu GT. Impact of fatty pancreas on postoperative pancreatic fistulae: a meta-analysis. Front Oncol. 2021;11:5054.
4. Maggino L, Malleo G, Bassi C, Allegrini V, McMillan MT, Borin A, et al. Decoding grade B pancreatic fistula: a clinical and economical analysis and subclassification proposal. Ann Surg. 2019;269(6):1146–53.
5. Pedrazzoli S. Pancreatoduodenectomy (PD) and postoperative pancreatic fistula (POPF): a systematic review and analysis of the POPF-related mortality rate in 60,739 patients retrieved from the English literature published between 1990 and 2015. Medicine. 2017;96(19):e6858.
6. Ikenaga N, Ohtsuka T, Nakata K, Watanabe Y, Mori Y, Nakamura M. Clinical significance of postoperative acute pancreatitis after pancreatoduodenectomy and distal pancreatectomy. Surgery. 2021;169(4):732–7.
7. Nahm CB, Brown KM, Townend PJ, Colvin E, Howell VM, Gill AJ, et al. Acinar cell density at the pancreatic resection margin is associated with post-pancreatectomy pancreatitis and the development of postoperative pancreatic fistula. HPB. 2018;20(5):432–40.
8. Bassi C, Dervenis C, Butturini G, Fingerhut A, Yeo C, Izbicki J, et al. Postoperative pancreatic fistula: an international study group (ISGPF) definition. Surgery. 2005;138(1):8–13.
9. Eskander MF, Cloyd JM. Predicting post-operative pancreatic fistula: one size may not fit all. Hepatobiliary Surg Nutr. 2021;10(1):11315–115.
10. Callery MP, Pratt WB, Kent TS, Chaikof EL, Vollmer CM Jr. A prospectively validated clinical risk score accurately predicts pancreatic fistula after pancreatoduodenectomy. J Am Coll Surg. 2013;216(1):1–14.
11. Mungroop TH, Klompmaker S, Wellner UF, Steyerberg EW, Coratti A, D'Hondt M, et al. Updated alternative fistula risk score (ua-FRS) to include minimally invasive pancreatoduodenectomy: pan-European validation. Ann Surg. 2021;273(2):334–40.
12. Mungroop TH, van Rijssen LB, van Klaveren D, Smits FJ, van Woerden V, Linnemann RJ, et al. Alternative fistula risk score for pancreatoduodenectomy (a-FRS): design and international external validation. Ann Surg. 2019;269(5):937–43.
13. Kamarajah SK, Bundred JR, Lin A, Halle-Smith J, Pande R, Sutcliffe R, et al. Systematic review and meta-analysis of factors associated with post-operative pancreatic fistula following pancreatoduodenectomy. ANZ J Surg. 2021;91(5):810–21.

14. Han IW, Cho K, Ryu Y, Shin SH, Heo JS, Choi DW, et al. Risk prediction platform for pancreatic fistula after pancreatoduodenectomy using artificial intelligence. World J Gastroenterol. 2020;26(30):4453–64.
15. Laaninen M, Bläuer M, Vasama K, Jin H, Räty S, Sand J, et al. The risk for immediate postoperative complications after pancreaticoduodenectomy is increased by high frequency of acinar cells and decreased by prevalent fibrosis of the cut edge of pancreas. Pancreas. 2012;41(6):957–61.
16. Bonsdorff A, Helanterä I, Tarvainen T, Sirén J, Kokkola A, Sallinen V. Prediction and consequences of postoperative pancreatitis after pancreaticoduodenectomy. BJS Open. 2022;6(2):zrac012.
17. Meguid RA, Ahuja N, Chang DC. What constitutes a "high-volume" hospital for pancreatic resection? J Am Coll Surg. 2008;206(4):622.e1–9.
18. Hunger R, Seliger B, Ogino S, Mantke R. Mortality factors in pancreatic surgery: a systematic review. How important is the hospital volume? Int J Surg. 2022;101:106640.
19. Polonski A, Izbicki JR, Uzunoglu FG. Centralization of pancreatic surgery in Europe. J Gastrointest Surg. 2019;23(10):2081–92.
20. Alsfasser G, Leicht H, Günster C, Rau BM, Schillinger G, Klar E. Volume-outcome relationship in pancreatic surgery. Br J Surg. 2016;103(1):136–43.
21. Williamsson C, Ansari D, Andersson R, Tingstedt B. Postoperative pancreatic fistula-impact on outcome, hospital cost and effects of centralization. HPB (Oxford). 2017;19(5):436–42.
22. Wada K, Traverso LW. Pancreatic anastomotic leak after the Whipple procedure is reduced using the surgical microscope. Surgery. 2006;139(6):735–42.
23. Bardol T, Delicque J, Hermida M, Herrero A, Guiu B, Fabre JM, et al. Neck transection level and postoperative pancreatic fistula after pancreaticoduodenectomy: a retrospective cohort study of 195 patients. Int J Surg. 2020;82:43–50.
24. Wu CH, Chen CH, Ho TW, Shih MC, Wu JM, Kuo TC, et al. Pancreatic neck transection using a harmonic scalpel increases risk of biochemical leak but not postoperative pancreatic fistula after pancreaticoduodenectomy. HPB (Oxford). 2021;23(2):301–8.
25. Zhang W, He S, Cheng Y, Xia J, Lai M, Cheng N, et al. Prophylactic abdominal drainage for pancreatic surgery. Cochrane Database Syst Rev. 2018;6(6):CD010583.
26. Cheng Y, Xia J, Lai M, Cheng N, He S. Prophylactic abdominal drainage for pancreatic surgery. Cochrane Database Syst Rev. 2016;10(10):CD010583.
27. Brubaker LS, Casciani F, Fisher WE, Wood AL, Cagigas MN, Trudeau MT, et al. A risk-adjusted analysis of drain use in pancreaticoduodenectomy: some is good, but more may not be better. Surgery. 2022;171(4):1058–66.
28. Seykora TF, Maggino L, Malleo G, Lee MK, Roses R, Salvia R, et al. Evolving the paradigm of early drain removal following pancreatoduodenectomy. J Gastrointest Surg. 2019;23(1):135–44.
29. Caputo D, Angeletti S, Ciccozzi M, Cartillone M, Cascone C, la Vaccara V, et al. Role of drain amylase levels assay and routinary postoperative day 3 abdominal CT scan in prevention of complications and management of surgical drains after pancreaticoduodenectomy. Updat Surg. 2020;72(3):727–41.
30. Pergolini I, Schorn S, Goess R, Novotny AR, Ceyhan GO, Friess H, et al. Drain use in pancreatic surgery: results from an international survey among experts in the field. Surgery. 2022;172(1):265–72.
31. Cheng Y, Briarava M, Lai M, Wang X, Tu B, Cheng N, et al. Pancreaticojejunostomy versus pancreaticogastrostomy reconstruction for the prevention of postoperative pancreatic fistula following pancreaticoduodenectomy. Cochrane Database Syst Rev. 2017;2017(9):CD012257.
32. Casadei R, Ricci C, Silvestri S, Campra D, Ercolani G, D'Ambra M, et al. Peng's binding pancreaticojejunostomy after pancreaticoduodenectomy. An Italian, prospective, dual-institution study. Pancreatology. 2013;13(3):305–9.
33. Wang W, Zhang Z, Gu C, Liu Q, Liang Z, He W, et al. The optimal choice for pancreatic anastomosis after pancreaticoduodenectomy: a network meta-analysis of randomized control trials. Int J Surg. 2018;57:111–6.

34. Hüttner FJ, Klotz R, Ulrich A, Büchler MW, Probst P, Diener MK. Antecolic versus retrocolic reconstruction after partial pancreaticoduodenectomy. Cochrane Database Syst Rev. 2022;1(1):CD011862.
35. el Nakeeb A, Hamdy E, Sultan AM, Salah T, Askr W, Ezzat H, et al. Isolated Roux loop pancreaticojejunostomy versus pancreaticogastrostomy after pancreaticoduodenectomy: a prospective randomized study. HPB. 2014;16(8):713–22.
36. Ozdemir E, Gokler C, Gunes O, Kaplan K, Aydin MC, Sumer F, et al. Isolated roux loop versus conventional pancreaticojejunostomy following pancreaticoduodenectomy. Ann Ital Chir. 2022;93:248–53.
37. Halloran C, Neoptolemos JP, Platt K, Jackson R, Reddy S, Oreilly D, et al. PANasta Trial: Cattell Warren versus Blumgart techniques of pancreatico-jejunostomy following pancreatoduodenectomy—A double-blinded multi-centered trial, trial results. J Clin Oncol. 2020;38(15 suppl):4619. https://doi.org/10.1200/JCO20203815_suppl4619.
38. Hai H, Li Z, Zhang Z, Cheng Y, Liu Z, Gong J, et al. Duct-to-mucosa versus other types of pancreaticojejunostomy for the prevention of postoperative pancreatic fistula following pancreaticoduodenectomy. Cochrane Database Syst Rev. 2022;2022(3):CD013462.
39. Winter JM, Cameron JL, Campbell KA, Chang DC, Riall TS, Schulick RD, et al. Does pancreatic duct stenting decrease the rate of pancreatic fistula following pancreaticoduodenectomy? Results of a prospective randomized trial. J Gastrointest Surg. 2006;10(9):1280–90.
40. Smyrniotis V, Arkadopoulos N, Kyriazi MA, Derpapas M, Theodosopoulos T, Gennatas C, et al. Does internal stenting of the pancreaticojejunostomy improve outcomes after pancreatoduodenectomy? A prospective study. Langenbecks Arch Surg. 2010;395(3):195–200.
41. Zhou Y, Zhou Q, Li Z, Chen R. Internal pancreatic duct stent does not decrease pancreatic fistula rate after pancreatic resection: a meta-analysis. Am J Surg. 2013;205:718–25.
42. McMillan MT, Ecker BL, Behrman SW, Callery MP, Christein JD, Drebin JA, et al. Externalized stents for pancreatoduodenectomy provide value only in high-risk scenarios. J Gastrointest Surg. 2016;20(12):2052–62.
43. Jiang Y, Chen Q, Wang Z, Shao Y, Hu C, Ding Y, et al. The prognostic value of external vs internal pancreatic duct stents in CR-POPF after Pancreaticoduodenectomy: a systematic review and meta-analysis. J Investig Surg. 2021;34(7):738–46.
44. Guo C, Xie B, Guo D. Does pancreatic duct stent placement lead to decreased postoperative pancreatic fistula rates after pancreaticoduodenectomy? A meta-analysis. Int J Surg. 2022;103:106707.
45. Andrianello S, Marchegiani G, Malleo G, Masini G, Balduzzi A, Paiella S, et al. Pancreaticojejunostomy with externalized stent vs pancreaticogastrostomy with externalized stent for patients with high-risk pancreatic anastomosis: a single-center, phase 3, randomized clinical trial. JAMA Surg. 2020;155(4):313–21.
46. Huscher C, Perri G, Lazzarin G, Marchegiani G, Malleo G, Salvia R, et al. Coronary artery stent for securing high-risk pancreatico-jejunal anastomosis after pancreatoduodenectomy: a pilot series. Ann Surg. 2022;275(4):E665–8.
47. Deng Y, He S, Cheng Y, Cheng N, Gong J, Gong J, et al. Fibrin sealants for the prevention of postoperative pancreatic fistula following pancreatic surgery. Cochrane Database Syst Rev. 2020;3(3):CD009621.
48. Serra F, Bonaduce I, Rossi EG, de Ruvo N, Cautero N, Gelmini R. The using of sealants in pancreatic surgery: a systematic review. Ann Med Surg (Lond). 2021;64:102244.
49. Giuliani A, Avella P, Segreto AL, Izzo ML, Buondonno A, Coluzzi M, et al. Postoperative outcomes analysis after pancreatic duct occlusion: a safe option to treat the pancreatic stump after Pancreaticoduodenectomy in low-volume centers. Front Surg. 2021;8:804675.
50. Suc B, Msika S, Fingerhut A, Fourtanier G, Hay JM, Holmières F, et al. Temporary fibrin glue occlusion of the main pancreatic duct in the prevention of intra-abdominal complications after pancreatic resection: prospective randomized trial. Ann Surg. 2003;237(1):57–65.
51. Mazzaferro V, Virdis M, Sposito C, Cotsoglou C, Droz Dit Busset M, Bongini M, et al. Permanent pancreatic duct occlusion with neoprene-based glue injection after pancre-

atoduodenectomy at high risk of pancreatic fistula: a prospective clinical study. Ann Surg. 2019;270(5):791–8.

52. Yeo CJ, Cameron JL, Lillemoe KD, Sauter PK, Coleman JA, Sohn TA, et al. Does prophylactic octreotide decrease the rates of pancreatic fistula and other complications after pancreaticoduodenectomy? Results of a prospective randomized placebo-controlled trial. Ann Surg. 2000;232(3):419–29.
53. Yoon SJ, Lee O, Jung JH, Shin SH, Heo JS, Han IW. Prophylactic octreotide for postoperative pancreatic fistula in patients with pancreatoduodenectomy: risk-stratified analysis. Medicine. 2022;101(22):e29303.
54. Jin K, Zhou H, Zhang J, Wang W, Sun Y, Ruan C, et al. Systematic review and meta-analysis of somatostatin analogues in the prevention of postoperative complication after pancreaticoduodenectomy. Dig Surg. 2015;32(3):196–207.
55. You DD, Paik KY, Park IY, Yoo YK. Randomized controlled study of the effect of octreotide on pancreatic exocrine secretion and pancreatic fistula after pancreatoduodenectomy. Asian J Surg. 2019;42(2):458–63.
56. McMillan MT, Christein JD, Callery MP, Behrman SW, Drebin JA, Kent TS, et al. Prophylactic octreotide for pancreatoduodenectomy: more harm than good? HPB. 2014;16(10):954–62.
57. Allen PJ, Gönen M, Brennan MF, Bucknor AA, Robinson LM, Pappas MM, et al. Pasireotide for postoperative pancreatic fistula. N Engl J Med. 2014;370(21):2014–22.
58. Kunstman JW, Goldman DA, Gönen M, Balachandran VP, D'Angelica MI, Kingham TP, et al. Outcomes after pancreatectomy with routine pasireotide use. J Am Coll Surg. 2019;228(2):161–170.e2.
59. Goyert N, Eeson G, Kagedan DJ, Behman R, Lemke M, Hallet J, et al. Pasireotide for the prevention of pancreatic fistula following pancreaticoduodenectomy: a cost-effectiveness analysis. Ann Surg. 2017;265(1):2–10.
60. Dalton EC, Johns MS, Rhodes L, Iii WTM, Petrelli NJ, Tiesi GG. Meta-analysis on the effect of pasireotide for prevention of postoperative pancreatic fistula. Am Sur. 2020;86(5):429–36.
61. Cecire J, Adams K, Pham H, Pang T, Burnett D. Pharmacological prevention of post-operative pancreatitis: systematic review and meta-analysis of randomized controlled trials on animal studies. ANZ J Surg. 2022;92(6):1338–46.
62. Smits FJ, Henry AC, Besselink MG, Busch OR, van Eijck CH, Arntz M, et al. Algorithm-based care versus usual care for the early recognition and management of complications after pancreatic resection in The Netherlands: an open-label, nationwide, stepped-wedge cluster-randomised trial. Lancet. 2022;399(10338):1867–75.
63. Rangelov E, Valente R, del Chiaro M. "Step-up approach" for the treatment of postoperative severe pancreatic fistula: is it really possible and useful? JAMA Surg. 2017;152(6):548–9.
64. Abe K, Kitago M, Shinoda M, Yagi H, Abe Y, Oshima G, et al. High-risk pathogens and risk factors for postoperative pancreatic fistula after pancreatectomy; a retrospective case-controlled study. Int J Surg. 2020;82:136–42.
65. Demir E, Abdelhai K, Demir IE, Jäger C, Scheufele F, Schorn S, et al. Association of bacteria in pancreatic fistula fluid with complications after pancreatic surgery. BJS Open. 2020;4(3):432–7.
66. Klek S, Sierzega M, Turczynowski L, Szybinski P, Szczepanek K, Kulig J. Enteral and parenteral nutrition in the conservative treatment of pancreatic fistula: a randomized clinical trial. Gastroenterology. 2011;141(1):157–63.
67. Wang SY, Hung YL, Hsu CC, Hu CH, Huang RY, Sung CM, et al. Optimal perioperative nutrition therapy for patients undergoing pancreaticoduodenectomy: a systematic review with a component network meta-analysis. Nutrients. 2021;13(11):4049.
68. Smits FJ, van Santvoort HC, Besselink MG, Batenburg MCT, Slooff RAE, Boerma D, et al. Management of severe pancreatic fistula after pancreatoduodenectomy. JAMA Surg. 2017;152(6):540–8.
69. Ang TL, Teoh AYB. Endoscopic ultrasonography-guided drainage of pancreatic fluid collections. Dig Endosc. 2017;29(4):463–71.

70. Groen JV, Smits FJ, Koole D, Besselink MG, Busch OR, den Dulk M, et al. Completion pancreatectomy or a pancreas-preserving procedure during relaparotomy for pancreatic fistula after pancreatoduodenectomy: a multicentre cohort study and meta-analysis. Br J Surg. 2021;108(11):1371–9.
71. Ma T, Bai X, Chen W, Li G, Lao M, Liang T. Pancreas-preserving management of grade-C pancreatic fistula and a novel bridging technique for repeat pancreaticojejunostomy: an observational study. Int J Surg. 2018;52:243–7.
72. Denost Q, Pontallier A, Rault A, Ewald JA, Collet D, Masson B, et al. Wirsungostomy as a salvage procedure after pancreaticoduodenectomy. HPB. 2012;14(2):82–6.
73. Standop J, Glowka T, Schmitz V, Schäfer N, Overhaus M, Hirner A, et al. Operative re-intervention following pancreatic head resection: indications and outcome. J Gastrointest Surg. 2009;13(8):1503–9.
74. Paye F, Lupinacci RM, Kraemer A, Lescot T, Chafaï N, Tiret E, et al. Surgical treatment of severe pancreatic fistula after pancreaticoduodenectomy by wirsungostomy and repeat pancreatico-jejunal anastomosis. Am J Surg. 2013;206(2):194–201.
75. Bachellier P, Oussoultzoglou E, Rosso E, Scurtu R, Lucescu I, Oshita A, et al. Pancreatogastrostomy as a salvage procedure to treat severe postoperative pancreatic fistula after pancreatoduodenectomy. Arch Surg. 2008;143(10):966–70.
76. Hoffmann K, Kulu Y, Feisst M, Hinz U, Lang M, Goeppert B, Albrecht T, Strobel O, Büchler MW, Hackert T. Completion pancreatectomy after pancreatoduodenectomy: who needs it? Ann Surg. 2023;278(1):e87–93. https://doi.org/10.1097/SLA.0000000000005494.
77. Salvia R, Lionetto G, Perri G, Malleo G, Marchegiani G. Total pancreatectomy and pancreatic fistula: friend or foe? Updat Surg. 2021;73(4):1231–6.
78. Total pancrEaTectomy vs High-Risk Pancreatic anastomosiS—Full Text View—ClinicalTrials.gov. https://clinicaltrials.gov/ct2/show/NCT05212350
79. Hassenpflug M, Bruckner T, Knebel P, Diener MK, Büchler MW, Werner J. DISCOVER trial-distal resection of the pancreas with or without coverage of the pancreatic remnant: study protocol of a randomised controlled trial. Trials. 2013;14(1):1–7.
80. Hüttner FJ, Mihaljevic AL, Hackert T, Ulrich A, Büchler MW, Diener MK. Effectiveness of Tachosil® in the prevention of postoperative pancreatic fistula after distal pancreatectomy: a systematic review and meta-analysis. Langenbeck's Arch Surg. 2016;401(2):151–9.
81. Andrianello S, Marchegiani G, Bannone E, Vacca P, Esposito A, Casetti L, et al. Predictors of pancreatic fistula healing time after distal pancreatectomy. J Hepatobiliary Pancreat Sci. 2021;28(12):1076–88.
82. Diener MK, Seiler CM, Rossion I, Kleeff J, Glanemann M, Butturini G, et al. Efficacy of stapler versus hand-sewn closure after distal pancreatectomy (DISPACT): a randomised, controlled multicentre trial. Lancet. 2011;377(9776):1514–22.
83. Machado MCC, Machado MAC. Drainage after distal pancreatectomy: still an unsolved problem. Surg Oncol. 2019;30:76–80.

36 Complications of Surgery for Urinary Bladder Cancer

Sumit Bansal, Abhinav Jain, Abhiyutthan Singh Jadaon, and Vikas Jain

36.1 Transurethral Resection of Bladder Tumour (TURBT)

36.1.1 Introduction

Transurethral resection of bladder tumour (TURBT) is certainly the first and most common surgical procedure carried out for a urinary bladder tumour. It is therapeutic in non muscle invasive tumours and serves as a diagnostic tool for muscle invasive or advanced tumours. TURBT is generally a safe endourological procedure with most complications being minor and without future disability or morbidity.

The important complications of TURBT are:

1. Urinary Tract Infection (UTI): UTI is one of the commonest complications of urogenital tract interventions including TURBT. The spectrum includes post operative fever, epidedymo-orchitis or prostatitis in males and rarely septicemia. The incidence of UTI varies between 16–24% in various studies [1, 2]. Risk factors for a postoperative UTI are preoperative positive urine culture, long term indwelling foley's catheter, inadequate sterilization of surgical equipments, increased operative time and excessive bleeding. Preoperative urine culture and adequate antibiotic therapy is the one most important factor in prevention of

S. Bansal (✉)
Department of Urology and Kidney Transplant, Narayana Superspeciality Hospital, Gurgaon, Haryana, India

A. Jain · A. S. Jadaon
Dharamshila Narayana Superspeciality Hospital, Delhi, India

V. Jain
Fortis Hospital Shalimar Bagh and Fortis Hospital Vasant Kunj, Delhi, India

K. Sood Sharma et al. (eds.), *Complications of Cancer Therapy: Best Practices in Prevention and Management*, https://doi.org/10.1007/978-981-99-0984-1_36

UTI. Most of the available guidelines recommend a sterile urine culture before the procedure.

2. Bleeding: Minor intraoperative and postoperative bleeding is very common in TURBT with bleeding requiring transfusion seen in 2–3% cases [3, 4]. Main risk factors for excessive and avoidable bleeding are large tumour, sessile base, history of antiplatelets intake and coughing or bucking of the patient during extubation from a general anesthesia. Good intraoperative fulguration of the tumour base is very important and avoids majority of postoperative bleeding The use of a wide bore (20–24 fr) three way foleys catheter postoperatively with normal saline irrigation takes care of most post operative bleedings and re-exploration is hardly required. The surgeon should examine the resection site carefully with partially full bladder with special focus over bladder neck and dome as these sites are notaries to harbour bleeders. Also, the final examination should be done after the tumour chips are evacuated because the bladder wash itself might increase oozing. Proper history of antiplatelet intake is imperative and should be discussed with the cardiologist regarding stopping it before surgery. We prefer to stop all kinds of antiplatelets and anticoagulants before the procedure if it doesn't increase cardiac risk.
3. Urinary retention: Like any endourological procedure, per urethral instrumentation, anesthesia and narcotic use increase the chances of urinary retention, specially in males. Elderly male patients should be started on alfa blocker therapy immediately post operatively and removal of foley's catheter can be delayed to third or fourth day. Small bladder clots may block the catheter and are generally cleared by bedside wash with Toomy's syringe. Larger bladder clots may require re-exploration and clot evacuation.
4. Bladder perforation: Urinary bladder perforation is the most significant complication of TURBT. The incidence varies from 1.3% to 3.5% in different studies [3, 4].

   The main risk factors for bladder wall perforation and tips for prevention are:

   (a) Large and broad based tumours requiring complex resection: Because of the extensive resection required, large tumours carry an increased risk of bladder wall perforation. Surgeon experience is very important in such cases. The fullness of urinary bladder should be checked continuously during the procedure to prevent resecting full thickness if bladder is deflated in between.
   (b) Tumours located inside diverticulae: Urinary bladder diverticulae lack muscularis propria layer and are therefore very likely to perforate during resection within them. This risk is increased if it has a narrow neck. Excluding very small diverticular tumours in which careful resection can be done, majority diverticular tumours are better dealt with by cystectomy-partial or radical [5]
   (c) Lateral bladder wall tumours: Resection over lateral bladder walls may stimulate the obturator nerve resulting in strong adduction of the thigh. The resectoscope may perforate the bladder wall during this jerk. A general anesthesia or an obturator nerve block is recommended with regional anesthesia to prevent this jerk. We prefer a general anesthesia during lateral wall resec-

tion. Other tips and tricks to avoid the obturator jerk are avoidance of bladder overfilling, reduced cutting current, use of short and intermittent burst current, use of bipolar cautery [6]

Most of the perforations are extraperitoneal and placement of a drain with long term foley's catheter heals the rent. Small intraperitoneal perforations can also be managed similarly with large ones requiring exploration and repair. Resection should be immediately stopped after necessary hemostasis, once a perforation is identified. Reduced outflow fluid with abdominal distention clinches the diagnosis. Immediate postoperative intravesical instillation of chemotherapy (e.g. mitomycin c), if planned, should not be given in case of perforation. There is a theoretical risk of tumour after bladder perforation and some studies suggest systemic chemotherapy. However, there is no framed consensus or guideline to start a systemic chemotherapy in such cases

5. Transurethral resection syndrome: Transurethral resection (TUR) syndrome occurs due to systemic absorption of irrigation fluid causing hypervolemia and hyponatremia which may progress to hypotension, oliguria, acidosis, renal failure and mental status changes. This syndrome is more typically associated with transurethral resection of prostate and rarely with TURBT. The chances are increased with unidentified bladder wall perforation and irrigation fluid getting absorbed through peritoneum. With the advent of bipolar current during resection allowing normal saline as irrigation fluid has decreased the incidence of TUR syndrome to virtually nil.
6. Injury to ureteric orifices leading to stricture: Resection of tumours located in proximity to the ureteric orifices may lead to damage and ureteric stricture. Coagulation current should be minimized near to ureteric orifices [5] and a double J stent can be placed if such injury occurs.
7. Obturator jerk: Electrocautery use over lateral wall of bladder may stimulate the obturator nerve resulting in sudden adduction of hip. This sudden jerk may lead to perforation from the resectoscope. With a lateral wall tumour it is wise to resect with an obturator block or general anesthesia with muscle paralysis.
8. Rare complications like pulmonary embolism, Arrythmias, Multiorgan failure (due to urosepsis) and death. With a less than 1% incidence, these grave complications are possible with any major surgical procedure including TURBT.

36.2 Complications of Radical Cystectomy with Urinary Diversion

Radical cystectomy is the surgery of curative intent for muscle invasive bladder tumours, recurrent high grade non muscle invasive bladder tumours and selective cases of locally advanced bladder tumours. This surgery involves removal of the urinary bladder along with prostate in males and uterus, fallopian tubes, ovaries, anterior vaginal wall and urethra in females. Urine is diverted outside most commonly by creating an ileal conduit (ileostomy with ureters anastomosed to the ileal pouch and urine continuously draining into ileostomy bag) followed by formation of a neobladder using ileum. Less common procedures are continent cutaneous urinary diversion and ureterosigmoidostomy. Despite the advances in minimally invasive modalities including robotics, radical cystectomy with urinary diversion remains a morbid surgery with complication rates as high as 28–64% [7–9].

The complications can broadly be divided in perioperative (which includes intraoperative and early complications) and late complications.

36.2.1 Perioperative and Early Complications

1. Bleeding requiring blood transfusion: Various series report an average transfusion rate of 2–3 units per patient. High blood loss is also associated with higher chances of other complications.

   Tips to prevent and management:

   - Bleeding from deep venous complex(DVC) in males: Opening endopelvic liberally on both sides of prostate and careful suture ligation of the DVC before cutting. Barbed sutures are sometimes very helpful.
   - Bleeding from vascular pedicles: Suture or clip ligation of the vascular pedicles. Selective use of energy sources like Harmonic and Ligasure.
   - Bleeding from urethral margin and vaginal wall: Relook and hemostasis after specimen is out.
2. Urine leak: Early urine leak is more common with neobladder than ileal conduit.

   Tips to prevent and management:

   - Ureteroileal anastomotic stenosis: Use of ureteral stent across the ureteroileal anastomosis reduces the chances of urine leak [10]. We commonly perform ileal conduit and use feeding tubes as ureteral stent which are fixed to the ileal loop with an absorbable suture and the outer end kept in ileostomy bag.
   - Mucus plugs blocking the outflow of urine: This may cause give way of the anastomosis. Gentle wash of the ileum pouch or the neobladder with normal saline reduces mucus accumulation. We use an indwelling foley's catheter in the ilial conduit pouch for continuous drainage of mucous for a couple of days. Catheter is kept for longer in neobladder.
   - Unrecognized early leaks: Placement of passive abdominal drain close to the ileal conduit pouch or the neobladder helps in early recognition of the leak thus preventing peritonitis and septicemia.
3. Bowel related complications: Namely paralytic ileus, intestinal obstruction, anastomotic leak and enteric fistula.

   Tips to prevent and management:

   - Poor nutritional status: Bowel related complications are higher with poor preoperative nutritional status of the patient. Use of long term steroids, chemotherapy and diabetes mellitus are also associated with higher bowel complications. Post operative infusion of amino acids and albumin is helpful in selected cases. Strict blood sugar control is very important in diabetic patients.

- Electrolyte imbalance: Hypokalemia is associated with paralytic ileus so adequate postoperative replenishment is important.
- Post operative ambulation/physical mobilization: Early mobilization prevents bowel related complications.
- Nasogastric decompression for a few days post op helps prevent vomiting and reduces bowel related complications.

4. Infections: Infection is a common complication of this major surgery and can present as pyelonephritis, wound infection, chest infection etc.

   Tips to prevent and management:

   - Fecal soiling of surrounding tissues: Care should be taken while handling bowel to minimize fecal soiling of the skin and surrounding tissues. We separate abdominal cavity with proper draping while bowel anastomosis.
   - Improper cleansing of ileal pouch: Ileal pouch should be washed adequately till a clear efflux is obtained.
   - Adequate broad spectrum antibiotic coverage in the perioperative period is very helpful.
   - Chest infection due to stasis: Adequate analgesia, early mobilization, spirometry and chest physiotherapy reduces chest infections.

5. Pelvic lymphocele: Radical cystectomy involves bilateral pelvic lymphadenectomy which may sometimes cause lymphorrhea and lymphocele formation.

   Tips to prevent and management:

   - Ligation of lymphatics during lymph node dissection usually prevents excessive lymph drainage.
   - Passive abdominal drain placement- prevents lymphocele formation and related complications.
   - It usually subsides on its own and abdominal drain is kept until the output decreases below 50–100 mL/day.

6. Nerve injury: Obturator nerve is present in obturator fossa beneath the external iliac vein. It is skeletonized during pelvic lymph node dissection and can be accidently injured. Deficit presents as difficulty in hip adduction and a small area of sensory loss over inner thigh. The genitofemoral nerve is a relatively thin and filmsy nerve which traverses over psos bed. It forms the lateral limit of pelvic node dissection. Inadvertent injury results in sensory loss over femoral triangle, scrotum in males and labia in females. Femoral nerve runs lateral to psoa muscle and then coursing beneath the inguinal ligament. It is not exposed during radical cystectomy and may be occasionally injured by compression under retractor blades or prolonged lithotomy position. It is motor nerve of the quadriceps and sensory to anterior thigh.

   Tips to prevent and management:

   - Minimizing use of cautry during dissection in obturator fossa and near genitofemoral nerve.
   - Use of sharp dissection rather than finger or forceful blunt dissection near the nerves.
   - Careful positioning of self retaining retractors and avoidance of exaggerated lithotomy positioning.

- Nerve transections identified intraop can be sutured with fine sutures with or without graft. Physiotherapy, limb exercises, and early mobilization are helpful in the post operative period and most deficits recover.

7. Deep venous thrombosis(DVT): Radical cystectomy carries a significant risk of DVT, as is the case with any major pelvic surgery. Thromboprophylaxis, DVT pump and early ambulation are recommended for its prevention.

36.2.2 Late Complications

1. Ureteroenteric anastomotic stricture: Except cutaneous ureterostomy, all methods of urine diversion involve uretero bowel anastomosis. Various anastomotic techniques are used which can broadly be refluxing or non refluxing. The incidence varies between 1.3–10% and mostly seen during first 2 years [11, 12]. Usually the cause is some sort of ureteral ischemia or fibrosis due to urine leak and infection. Rarely the cause can be recurrence of malignancy at anastomotic site. It is the most common cause of deteriorating renal function in the long run.

   Tips to prevent and management:
   - Preserving the blood supply of ureter during surgery by not skeletonizing it and minimizing use of cautry.
   - Use of a stent across the anastomosis.
   - Judicious use of broad spectrum antibiotics.
   - Addressing and treating any urine leak.
   - Management involves antigrade or retrograde stenting, placement of nephrostomy, balloon dilatation, endoureterotomy and sometimes revising the anastomosis.
2. Urinary tract infection: Due to some reflux of intestinal secreations into the ureter UTI episodes are common, more so in Neobladders. Majority of patients are however asymptomatic and treatment is advocated if symptoms develop or there is declining renal function due to recurrent infection.

   Tips to prevent and management:
   - Regular emptying of the neobladder by clean intermittent catheterization.
   - Creation of non refluxing anastomosis.
   - Judicious treatment with antibiotics where indicated.
3. Renal failure: As discussed earlier, the prime reasons for renal failure are anastomotic stenosis, reflux of urine and recurrent infections. These factors slowly damage the nephrons and may gradually warrant renal replacement therapy. The tips for prevention have already been discussed.
4. Stone formation in Neobladder: Improper emptying leading to urine stasis and recurrent infection is primarily responsible for stone formation in the neobladder. Absorption for urine leading to metabolic abnormalities also play a role.

   Tips to prevent and management:
   - Use of urine alkalizers containing citrate.
   - Avoidance and early management of UTI, specially proteus species.
   - Regular emptying of neobladder.

- Management is similar to other urinary calculi using endoscopic or laparoscopic routes.

5. Urinary retention: Milder retention in neobladder can be due to urethral stricture presenting with difficulty voiding, decreased urine output, abdominal distention and UTI. Inadequate emptying also causes retention. Chronically untreated and neglected cases may present with perforation of neobladder advancing to peritonitis, septicemia and death.

   Tips to prevent and management:
   - Regular clean intermittent catheterization.
   - Self emptying is facilitated by applying suprapubic pressure and bending forwards while voiding.
   - Endoscopic treatment of urethral stricture.

6. Recurrence: Recurrence is a risk with any treated cancer and bladder cancer is no different. 5 years recurrence risk for high grade muscle invasive bladder cancer is as high as 45% [13]. Recurrence can be either local or distant and carries a poor prognosis. Preoperative predictive factors are high grade disease, Lymphovascular invasion, obesity, smoking, positive lymph nodes, and the presence of micropapillary or neuroendocrine features on histopathology.

   Tips to prevent and management:
   - Achieving complete resection with negative margins.
   - Lymph node dissection with a minimum yield of 8–12.
   - Post operative chemotherapy if positive margins or lymph nodes.
   - Role of neoadjuvant chemotherapy is debatable.
   - Management depends upon the site and extent of recurrence and generally requires systemic therapy.

7. Parastomal hernia: Parastomal hernia is the protrusion of intestinal contents through stoma site and forming adhesions to stoma wall. Majority are small and asymptomatic which can be left as such. These are more common with obesity and smoking.

   Tips to prevent and management:
   - Creating adequate sized stoma.
   - Creating the stoma through rectus sheath and fixing serosa with the sheath.
   - Larger hernias require repair with or without mesh and sometimes relocation of the stoma.

8. Metabolic complications: These are an important set of complications associated with the use of bowel in urinary diversion and are discussed in detail elsewhere in the text.

36.3 Conclusion

Complications arising after urinary bladder tumour surgeries are not uncommon owing to complexity of and variedness of the surgical procedures involved. There is no substitute to clinical experience in preventing these complications and managing them successfully if they occur.

Key Points

- TURBT involves resecting the bladder tumour endoscopically and forms the mainstay of diagnosis as well as treatment of superficial bladder tumours
- Important complications associated with TURBT are perforation of bladder, injury to ureteric orifices, obturator jerk, uncontrolled bleeding with bladder clot retention and UTI.
- Resecting with partially filled bladder, obturator block or general anesthesia, use of bipolar electrocautry, careful resection with hemostasis and use of normal saline bladder irrigation post op are very useful in preventing the complications
- Muscle invasive bladder tumours require radical removal of the bladder (Radical cystectomy) with bilateral pelvic lymph node dissection with urinary diversion which is a major surgery.
- Radical cystectomy can be complicated with excessive bleeding, nerve injuries(obturator, genitofemoral, femoral), residual disease, and injury to surrounding viscera.
- Pelvic lymph node dissection may lead to pelvic lymphocele
- Urinary diversion is mainly done by forming and ileal conduit with ureteroileal anastomosis or creating a neobladder with ileum.
- Important complications associated with urinary diversion are urine leak, anastomotic stricture, renal failure, recurrent UTI, stone formation in neobladder, and metabolic complications.
- Long term follow up is required after these surgeries to detect these complications or recurrences early and manage them adequately.

References

1. Dick A, Barnes R, Hadley H, Bergman RT, Ninan CA. Complications of transurethral resection of bladder tumors: prevention, recognition and treatment. J Urol. 1980;124:810–1.
2. Pycha A, Lodde M, Lusuardi L, Palermo S, Signorello D, Galantini A, et al. Teaching transurethral resection of the bladder: still a challenge? Urology. 2003;62:46–8.
3. Nieder AM, Meinbach DS, Kim SS, Soloway MS. Transurethral bladder tumor resection: intraoperative and postoperative complications in a residency setting. J Urol. 2005;174:2307–9.
4. Collado A, Chéchile GE, Salvador J, Vicente J. Early complications of endoscopic treatment for superficial bladder tumors. J Urol. 2000;164:1529–32.
5. Burger M, Oosterlinck W, Konety B, et al. ICUD-EAU international consultation on bladder cancer 2012: non-muscle-invasive urothelial carcinoma of the bladder. Eur Urol. 2013;63:36–44. https://doi.org/10.1016/j.eururo.2012.08.061.
6. Panagoda PI, Vasdev N, Gowrie-Mohan S. Avoiding the obturator jerk during TURBT. Curr Urol. 2018;12:1–5. https://doi.org/10.1159/00044722.
7. Stein JP, Lieskovsky G, Cote R, et al. Radical cystectomy in the treatment of invasive bladder cancer: long-term results in 1,054 patients. J Clin Oncol. 2001;19(3):666–75.
8. Shabsigh A, Korets R, Vora KC, et al. Defining early morbidity of radical cystectomy for patients with bladder cancer using a standardized reporting methodology. Eur Urol. 2009;55(1):164–76.
9. Hautmann RE, de Petriconi RC, Volkmer BG. Lessons learned from 1,000 neobladders: the 90-day complication rate. J Urol. 2010;184(3):990–4.

10. Mattei A, Birkhaeuser FD, Baermann C, Warncke SH, Studer UE. To stent or not to stent perioperatively the ureteroileal anastomosis of ileal orthotopic bladder substitutes and ileal conduits? Results of a prospective randomized trial. J Urol. 2008;179(2):582–6. https://doi.org/10.1016/j.juro.2007.09.066.
11. Nazmy M, Yuh B, Kawachi M, et al. Early and late complications of robot-assisted radical cystectomy: a standardized analysis by urinary diversion type. J Urol. 2014;191:681–7.
12. Lobo N, Dupré S, Sahai A, Thurairaja R, Khan MS. Getting out of a tight spot: an overview of ureteroenteric anastomotic strictures. Nat Rev Urol. 2016;13:447–55.
13. Alfred Witjes J, Lebret T, Comperat EM, et al. Updated 2016 EAU guidelines on muscle-invasive and metastatic bladder cancer. Eur Urol. 2017;71(3):462–75.

Complications of Carcinoma Prostate Surgery

37

Abhiyutthan Singh Jadaon, Vikas Jain, and Abhinav Jain

37.1 Introduction

Surgical treatment for prostate cancer can be divided into either curative (radical prostatectomy), or for the purpose of androgen deprivation (bilateral orchidectomy), or for the lower urinary tracts symptoms in cancer prostate patients (channel Transurethral resection of prostate).

37.2 Complications of Radical Prostatectomy

Radical prostatectomy (RP) is one of the first-line treatments for clinically organ-confined prostatic cancer [1, 2]. However, there are several complications and adverse events related to the surgical procedure.

With regard to intraoperative complications, nerve injury due to patient positioning, blood loss during RP, intestinal injuries mostly in form of rectal injuries, ureteral injury.

Early complications related to surgical procedures were surgical site infection (SSI), anastomotic leaks (intraperitoneal urinary leak), persistent lymph drainage, lymphocele, deep vein thrombosis, obturator nerve injury.

Late complications such as anastomotic stricture (bladder neck stricture), erectile dysfunction and stress urinary incontinence have been the common ones [3].

A. S. Jadaon (✉) · V. Jain · A. Jain
ILBS, Hospital, Delhi, India

K. Sood Sharma et al. (eds.), *Complications of Cancer Therapy: Best Practices in Prevention and Management*, https://doi.org/10.1007/978-981-99-0984-1_37

37.3 Common Complications

- Blood loss/hemorrhage
  Incidence: <1% patient require blood transfusion.
  Ways to prevent it: Good exposure, suture or clip ligation, packing, proper control of dorsal vein complex.
  In troublesome bleeding from DVC, surgeon should completely divide the DVC over urethra and oversew the end [4].
- Thromboembolic event
  DVT with pulmonary embolism is one the major cause of morbidity after RP.
  Measures to prevent it: Careful patient position during surgery, intermittent compression devices, early ambulation, low molecular weight heparin.
  Treatment: LMWH (s.c.) twice a day, intravenous unfractionated heparin [5].
- Bladder neck contracture
  Incidence: 0.5%.
  Cause: Inadequate coaptation of mucosal surfaces during surgery, prevention of urinary extravasation or distraction of bladder neck due to hematoma.
  Clue towards diagnosis: Poor urinary stream post operatively or prolonged unexplained urinary incontinence.
  Treatment: Endoscopic dilatation, cold knife incision at 3,6,and 9 o'clock. Injection of triamcinolone acetate with cold incisions [6].
- Urinary incontinence
  Incidence: <6%.
  Prevention: Preserve striated sphincter during apical dissection, mucosa-to-mucosa anastomosis of UB neck to urethra without tension.
  Treatment: Avoid alcohol, caffeinated drinks, medicine like alpha agonist and imipramine are helpful [7].
- Erectile dysfunction
  Incidence: <4%.
  Cause: Neurovascular bundle injury.
  Techniques to prevent it: High anterior release of neurovascular bundle [8].
  Treatment: PDE5 inhibitors.
- Surgical complication of Bilateral orchidectomy
  Its one of the most cost effective and quick way to decrease the testosterone level to less then 50 ng/dL.
  Bleeding, hematoma, surgical site infection and pain are few of the surgical complications of this surgery [9].
  To prevent bleeding or hematoma the pedicles of testis is doubly ligated and closure of wound is done after proper check of hemostasis.
- Surgical complication of Channel TURP
  Channel TURP is a procedure in which resection of visually obstructing tissue without extension to the prostatic capsule in a patient with metastatic or locally advanced disease to improve voiding symptoms [10].
  Its complications can be hemorrhage leading to transfusion, infections, urethral strictures, failure to void, urinary incontinence, and TUR syndrome [11].

- Urinary incontinence
  Incidence: <1%.
  Its mostly temporary, usually settles within 3 months, but if sphincter is either involved by the disease or got traumatised during resection (TURP) it can be permanent.
  Treatment: Perineal muscle strengthening exercises, artificial sphincters, continuous or intermittent catheterization [10].

Key Points

- Radical prostatectomy(RP) is one of the first line treatment for clinically organ-confined prostate carcinoma.
- Intra operative complications of RP can be nerve injury due to positioning during the surgery, blood loss, thromboembolic events which can be life threatening.
- Few of the most troubling post operative complications of Radical prostatectomy are, urinary incontinence and erectile dysfunction.
- Bilateral orchidectomy is one of the most cost effective and quick way to decrease *S. testosterone*. i.e. androgen deprivation therapy for Locally advanced and/or Metastatic carcinoma prostate.
- Bleeding, surgical site infection are few of the minor complications of pretty much straight forward surgery.
- Complications due to testosterone deficiency can manifest after few days to months.eg loss of libido to bone density loss.
- Channel TURP is a procedure for Lower urinary tract symptoms in Carcinoma prostate patients.
- Intra-operative complications of Channel TURP can be, hemorrhage leading to transfusions, TUR syndrome.
- Post operative complications of Channel TURP can be urinary tract infections, Failure to void, urethral stricture and dreaded complication of urinary incontinence.
- Most of carcinoma prostate surgical complications are manageable and should not prevent a patient from receiving ideal treatment for Ca prostate.

References

1. Hisasue S-i, et al. Early and late complications of radical retropubic prostatectomy: experience in a single institution. Jpn J Clin Oncol. 2004;34(5):274–9.
2. Maffezzini M, Seveso M, et al. Evaluation of complications and results in a contemporary series of 300 consecutive radical retropubic prostatectomies with the anatomic approach at a single institution. Urology. 2003;61(5):982–6.
3. Shekarriz B, Upadhyay J, Wood DP, Shekarriz B, et al. Intraoperative, perioperative, and long-term complications of radical prostatectomy. Urol Clin North Am. 2001;28(3):639–53.
4. Reiner WG, Walsh PC. An anatomical approach to the surgical management of the dorsal vein and Santorini's plexus during radical retropubic surgery. J Urol. 1979;121(2):198–200.

5. Büller HR, Davidson BL, Decousus H, et al. Subcutaneous fondaparinux versus intravenous unfractionated heparin in the initial treatment of pulmonary embolism. N Engl J Med. 2003;349(18):1695–702.
6. Breyer BN, McAninch JW. Management of recalcitrant bladder neck contracture after radical prostatectomy for prostate cancer. Endoscopic and open surgery. J Urol. 2011;185(2):390–1.
7. Kim PH, Pinheiro LC, Atoria CL, et al. Trends in the use of incontinence procedures after radical prostatectomy: a population based analysis. J Urol. 2013;189(2):602–8.
8. Nielsen ME, Schaeffer EM, Marschke P, et al. High anterior release of the levator fascia improves sexual function following open radical retropubic prostatectomy. J Urol. 2008;180(6):2557–64.
9. Anheuser P, Kranz J, Will J, Dieckmann KP. Complications associated with inguinal orchiectomy and scrotal orchiectomy. Urologe A. 2014;53(5):676–82.
10. Mazur AW, Thompson IM. Efficacy and morbidity of 'channel' TURP. Urology. 1991;38(6):526–8.
11. Sheng XJ, Zhu YJ, Ye M, Chen JH, Zhang L, Kong L. Experience in treating advanced prostate cancer with bladder outlet obstruction. Ai Zheng. 2005;24(10):1284–6.

Metabolic Complications of Urological Surgeries

38

Abhinav Jain, Abhiyutthan Singh Jadaon, and Vikas Jain

38.1 Introduction

With the urological problems especially benign prostatic enlargement and carcinoma urinary bladder on a rise and so the surgeries for them, it is imperative to know about the various metabolic complications that can arise during the operations for them. This text will highlight them with a special focus on prevention and treatment.

38.2 TUR Syndrome

Prostatic resections are one of the commonest procedures that an elderly male undergoes next only to cataract surgery. Use of irrigating fluids during resections is an imperative part and enables to keep the vision clear for better surgical outcomes. The incidence of this dreadful entity is decreasing nowadays but still this is not unheard of and may still be encountered. This occurs due to absorption of irrigation fluid in the systemic veins [1]. This entity is defined as a constellation of signs and symptoms involving mainly neurological and cardiovascular systems. Pressures more than 10 mm Hg have a propensity to cause TUR syndrome as beyond these pressures, fluid can get into systemic circulation.

A. Jain (✉) · A. S. Jadaon · V. Jain
Fortis Hospital Shalimar Bagh and Fortis Hospital Vasant Kunj, Delhi, India

K. Sood Sharma et al. (eds.), *Complications of Cancer Therapy: Best Practices in Prevention and Management*, https://doi.org/10.1007/978-981-99-0984-1_38

38.2.1 Incidence and Risk Factors

Several risk factors have been implicated that include prostate size exceeding 45 g [2], resection for more than 90 min, placing irrigant at height more than 60 cm, pre-existing hyponatremia and dehydrated patient. Although the incidence is on a decline, it has been described in up to 0.8–2% of all patients undergoing transurethral resections [3]. Most common causes are dilutional hyponatremia that may result from intravascular overload, loss of sodium in periprostatic space and inappropriate high release of atrial natriuretic peptide by glycine leading to natriuresis. Others implicated are rise in serum ammonia levels when glycine (by its inhibitory properties cause damage to heart and retina) is being used as resection fluid. The following are the various pathophysiological causes:

1. **Circulatory overload:** The fluid absorption may be directly into intravascular compartment (prostate size determines this) or in the interstitial periprostatic space (directly related to break in prostatic capsule). The desired fluid absorption in 1 h should be kept below 1 L keeping in mind that on an average 20 mL fluid [4, 5] gets into systemic circulation a minute. Cerebral and pulmonary oedema will thus ensue from reduced serum osmolarity thus causing the neurological and respiratory manifestations.
2. **Water intoxication:** May result when the serum sodium levels falls drastically beyond 20 mEq of the baseline value.
3. **Hypotension:** Caused by blood loss and release of substances from resection bed.
4. **Visual disturbances:** Transient blindness, fogginess and seeing halos around objects returning to normal within 48 h are typical. Loss of pupillary responses and preservation of blink reflexes is the rule.

38.2.2 Early Warning Signs and Diagnostic Work up

Signs and symptoms depend whether the operation is being done in regional or general anesthesia. Neurological manifestations in regional anesthesia may be yawning, restlessness, confusional state, nausea, altered sensorium, visual changes, lethargic state, headache, dizziness, unconsciousness, seizures and comatose state. Cardiovascular responses may be refractory bradycardia, tightness in chest, hypertension that may be fatal and progress to hypotension and circulatory collapse. Diagnosis of the syndrome may be difficult in general anesthesia and may include several ECG changes.

38.2.3 Management

Prompt recognition of the error and timely abandonment of the procedure holds the key. Frusemide may help. Deterioration in respiratory system to be managed as per individual need. Correct hyponatremia with hypertonic saline not exceeding 1 mEq/h.

38.2.4 Tips and Tricks to Prevent Complications

Preoperatively, hyponatremia to be treated and corrected before taking the patient for TURP. Good antibiotic coverage needed especially in positive urine cultures. Restrict height of irrigant and minimize the operating time. Ideal height at which irrigation fluid is to be kept has been found to be 60 cm in various studies that maintains between a balance between clear view during surgery and minimises fluid absorption in the system [6]. A positive correlation has been found between the height of irrigant and amount of fluid being absorbed systemically with the risk doubling with 10 cm increase in height. Replenish blood in case of significant losses. Avoid opening capsule and venous sinuses. Adequate fluid supplementation in the pre-operative period is prudent. Bipolar resection can certainly be helpful as it uses saline and would prevent absorption of hypoosmolar fluid. Serum electrolytes can be done after the surgery or intraoperatively if the suspicion is high (when the prostatic venous sinuses have been opened, large prostate and high resection time). Care should be taken in large resections of the possibility of subtrigonal passage being created that will hinder the further excursions of the resectoscope.

38.2.5 Conclusion

TUR syndrome is a rarity nowadays but still needs to be kept in mind in view of the increasing elderly population that requires surgeries on prostate as a routine. One has to be cautious starting right from the preoperative period. Prompt recognition is the key. Role and coordination of anesthetist cannot be undermined. This condition has varied pathophysiological mechanisms and manifestations may be different under regional and general anesthesia. Adequate intraoperative precautions need to be followed and even if the syndrome occurs, can be managed in expert hands.

38.3 Post Obstructive Diuresis (POD)

38.3.1 Introduction

Bilateral hydronephrosis/obstructive uropathy is very common scenario in urological clinics. This may either be a result of chronic urinary retention secondary to bladder outlet obstruction or underactive detrusor, bilateral obstructive calculi, ureteric calculus in solitary kidney or bilateral hydronephrosis/hydronephrosis in solitary functioning kidney secondary to pelvic malignancies (urinary bladder, uterus, cervix, prostate or rectum) or compression by malignant lymph nodes. Post obstructive diuresis (POD) may result when obstruction in such kidneys is relieved by means of urinary catheterization/DJ stenting or PCN (per cutaneous nephrostomy/ies) and is characterized by high urinary output. This condition becomes important to recognize as it can cause its own morbidities and turn out to be fatal. This assumes significance as our center is high burden oncology institute such patients are commonly seen here. No clear cut definition exists however, but we take it to be an hourly urine output of more than 300 mL for two consecutive hours at our place.

38.3.2 Risk Factors

The patients who have already been initiated on dialysis before renal decompression have practically not found to have POD as renal replacement therapy renders them euvolemic. Higher the serum creatinine and fluid overload, the higher are the chances of POD. The duration since which the kidneys are obstructed is inversely proportional to the occurrence and degree of POD. Use of medicines (especially anticholinergics) or precipitated urinary retention may be villainous.

38.3.3 Mechanism

1. **Osmotic diuresis**: Increased urea in renal tubules exerts high osmotic pressure thus driving water in the tubular lumen.
2. **Natriuresis** [7]**:** Increased Atrial and Brain Natriuretic peptides (ANP/BNP) drive water out of the renal tubules along with sodium.
3. **Loss of concentrating ability:** Kidneys lose their concentrating ability secondary to ischemic insult following obstruction.
4. **Tubular dysfunction** [8]
5. **Fluid overload:** The patients with bilateral obstructive uropathy/obstruction in single functioning kidney often present in emergency with fluid overload due to inability of diseased renal units to remove extra intra and extra vascular fluid out from the body. POD results when the obstruction is reversed.
6. **Unresponsiveness to ADH:** The diseased kidneys are often not properly responsive to the water retaining action of antidiuretic hormone (ADH) thus causing post obstructive diuresis.

38.3.4 Management

Two types are existent: Physiological post obstructive diuresis (electrolyte and volume loss are maximum during the first day) and Pathological post obstructive diuresis. Tubules are the first to recover their lost function followed by recovery of glomerulus after that. These recoveries make sure that maximum patients who have a diuresis have it on a transient (physiological) basis with a return to baseline renal functions in a fortnight. Hence it is clear by the above discussions that physiological POD are self-limited and do not require any specific management apart from fluid considerations. Due to paucity of guidelines entailing the management, we have developed our own protocol.

1. **Monitoring:** Urine output is monitored hourly. Vitals are checked every 3 hourly. Serum electrolytes are checked every 12 h followed by decreasing their frequency as they are replete. Special emphasis is placed on replacement of calcium.
2. **Fluid management:** We do 100% replacement if hourly urine output is less than 300 mL. However if the same is more than or equal to 300 mL per hour, we do 80% replacement. Replacement with isotonic or hypertonic saline depends on the serum electrolytes. Replacement can be done orally or intravenously in case the patient is not able to take enough oral fluids or in cases having hemodynamic instability. The down side of 100% replacement is that the vicious cycle continues and the urine output will continue to get chased instead of the diuresis resolving.
3. **Pathological diuresis:** May need to estimate urine and serum osmolarity and may require replacement with hypertonic saline in cases of salt losing nephropathies. Nephrotoxic antibiotics and antihypertensives may need to be withdrawn. Imaging in the form of ultrasonography or CT scan for determination of resolution of hydronephrosis may be prudent. Do not forget to monitor acid and base status of the patient and their timely and appropriate correction goes a long way in the management of such patients.

38.3.5 Tips and Tricks to Prevent Complications

There is no effective means to prevent post obstructive diuresis. However, prompt identification of the possible patient who may land into the same is extremely important to prevent the associated morbidities and a possible mortality in worst of cases. An idea could be obtained based on the retention volume drained after urinary bladder catheterization or DJ stent/percutaneous nephrostomy. The degree of hydronephrosis may be an indirect predictor of the ominous entity. The thickness of renal parenchyma and cortical echogenicity can predict the occurrence of POD with decreased parenchyma or higher echogenicity effectively if not completely ruling it out.

38.3.6 Conclusion

Post obstructive diuresis which is usually seen in obstructive uropathy is an easily manageable entity if promptly detected. A high index of suspicion should be maintained and patients should be properly counselled.

38.4 Metabolic Complications of Urinary Intestinal Diversion

38.4.1 Introduction

Candidates for this sort of surgery are the patients who are undergoing cystectomy for curative/palliative carcinoma of urinary bladder. These patients needs some segment from the gastrointestinal tract for subsequent reconstruction. This assumes significance as the incidence of urinary bladder carcinoma is gradually on a rise and such mixed reconstructive and extirpative surgeries are being increasingly performed especially at high volume oncology centres of which our centre is a prime example. A uro oncologist needs to be fully aware of the metabolic complications after these sort of procedures as these are not uncommon and understanding of the pathophysiology and management is extremely crucial for such already compromised patients.

38.4.2 Risk Factors

Several risk factors dictate the occurrence and severity of metabolic complications after intestinal urinary diversion. Type of segment of gastrointestinal tract used is probably the most important determinant with the unique set of complications associated with each described later on. The length of the segment and the duration of time for which the mucosa remains in contact with urine is also crucial. Since the job of the surgeon is not only to operate upon a patient but to treat him as a whole, associated renal, hepatic illness, age and other comorbidities should not be forgotten as all these can have independent bearing on the outcome. The chances of complications will escalate significantly in neobladders as compared to conduits which is directly linked to the amount of intestine utilized for the reconstruction. Operating dehydrated patients is a big no and should be avoided in cases where stomach is to be used as an interposition tissue.

38.4.3 Mechanism

The defects and aberrations stem out from two basic principals: the remaining bowel has decreased absorptive area and the segment used for reconstruction continues to both secrete and absorb at the same time and thus behaves like the parent tissue till the compensatory mechanisms of the body overpower them or the mucosa atrophies due to non-contact with feces for a long period of time.

38.4.4 Pathophysiology

1. **Deteriorating renal functions:** It would be hard to believe that renal function follows a decline after these sorts of surgeries even in the patients with normal

GFR preoperatively. Such decline in GFR has been estimated variously in different studies to the tune of up to 20% on an average for a follow up of around 10 years. Ureteroileal anastomotic stricture (s), recurrent urinary tract infections and urinary calculi can be the proposed villains here.

2. **Acid Base Abnormalities:** Metabolic acidosis with compensation by respiratory mode is the most frequent abnormality in these patients. In majority of the cases though it is mild, it can be refractory and persistent in up to 15% of them [9]. This is linked with presence of leaky junctions which are least in number in colon hence, making it the most stable segment as far as occurrence of acid base derangements are concerned. Most of the times in ileal/colonic diversions, sodium and bicarbonate are secreted in exchange for hydrogen and chloride resulting in hyperchloremic acidosis which if persists can lead to fatigue, anorexia and weakness with ammonia and chloride directly getting absorbed from urine also being responsible. Probably the most dangerous of all is hypochloremic hyperkaemic hyponatremic acidosis with the use of jejunum which can lead to a concomitant dehydration. Acidosis can be corrected using oral sodium bicarbonate, sodium citrate, nicotinic acid or chlorpromazine.
3. **Chemotherapeutics:** Many drugs after being secreted in urine are let into the blood stream again after getting reabsorbed in the gut specially drugs used in chemotherapy. Caution should be exercised in their administration as the altered dynamics can increase their levels in the systemic circulation
4. **Calculi in urinary tract** [10]**:** Not an uncommon and surprising complication, calcium stones can get formed because of acidosis and increased excretion of calcium in urine. Free oxalates in gut lumen due to calcium chelating effect of bile salts can precipitate oxalate stones in the urinary tract with dehydration exaggerating the risk. Understandably, more the length of the gut segment, higher the stone forming propensity.
5. **Altered bowel function:** Diarrhea is the most often reported symptom due to loss of surface of gut and can also happen after colonic loss due to it being unable to handle excessive small intestinal alkaline secretions. Chronic diarrhea, steatorrhoea, bacterial overgrowth, Vitamin B 12 deficiency, deficiency of fat soluble vitamins and altered fat digestion can happen when the terminal ileum is divided which in today's world is not the preferred segment for these obvious reasons.
6. **Electrolyte abnormalities:** Secondary to intestinal losses and renal wasting by both transcellular and paracellular routes, deficiencies of potassium, magnesium and calcium can become clinically significant in a few patients. Exuberant correction of potassium can worsen the already existent acidosis
7. **Hepatic toxicity:** Hepatic impairment in the form of altered sensorium, encephalopathy and coma is a rarity after conduit but not so uncommon after neobladder. Urinary tract obstruction and infection with the feared urease producing bacteria can increase the ammonia load to liver thus exacerbating the liver damage.
8. **Bone metabolism:** Various theories for bony demineralization include compensation of acidosis by bone minerals, inadequate renal handling of calcium, Vitamin D not getting converted into active form by kidneys, less surface area of

gut meaning less absorption of calcium and bony resorption by the secondary activation of osteoclasts. Demineralization so severe as to cause osteomalacia and rickets is very rare with the aberration being commoner in children.

38.4.5 Tips and Tricks to Prevent Complications

Needless to say, proper patient selection, type and length of the gut segment to be deployed form the most important points to be pondered over before operating.

38.4.6 Conclusion

Due to the complexity of these procedures and the associated risk of significant metabolic abnormalities that can be problematic for the patients, the surgeons need to be fully aware of how to avoid and minimize these complications.

38.5 Summary

1. Metabolic complications after urological surgeries are not very uncommon.
2. It is very essential for the urosurgeons to be aware of the renal physiology.
3. The correct patient choice is of utmost significance.
4. Before taking the patient for TURP, it is essential to correct dehydration, hyponatremia and urinary tract infections.
5. Careful surgery avoiding breaching prostatic capsule, venous sinuses, taking the height of irrigant under consideration and staging a long procedure may be wise.
6. It is imperative to know and judge which patient can have pathological post obstructive diuresis.
7. Correction of diuresis and electrolyte abnormalities is a must with special emphasis on the fact that the urine output should not be chased.
8. Precise knowledge of metabolic abnormalities after cystectomy and intestinal urinary diversion is must.
9. Hyperchloremic metabolic acidosis being the commonest aberration after urinary diversion which can be persistent in a few patients.
10. Lifelong follow up after intestinal diversion after cystectomy is a must as gradual renal function deterioration is the rule rather than exception even if the preoperative renal parameters are normal.

References

1. Hagstorm RS. Studies on fluid absorption during transurethral resection of prostate. J Urol. 1955;73(5):852–9.
2. Mebust WK, Holtgrewe HL, Cockett AT. Transurethral prostatectomy: immediate and post-operative complications. A cooperative study of 13 participating institutions evaluating 3,885 patients. J Urol. 1989;141(2):243–7.
3. Ahyai SA, Gilling P, Kaplan SA. Meta-analysis of functional outcomes and complications following transurethral procedures for lower urinary tract symptoms resulting from benign prostatic enlargement. Eur Urol. 2010;58(3):384–97.
4. Olsson J, Nilsson A, Hahn RG. Symptoms of the transurethral resection syndrome using glycine as the irrigant. J Urol. 1995;154:123–8.
5. Hahn RG, Ekengren JC. Patterns of irrigating fluid absorption during transurethral resection of the prostate as indicated by ethanol. J Urol. 1993;149:502–6.
6. Madsen PO, Naber KG. The importance of the pressure in the prostatic fossa and absorption of irrigating fluid during transurethral resection of the prostate. J Urol. 1973;109(3):446–52.
7. Widmaier EP, Raff H, Strang T. Vander's human physiology. McGraw-Hill Higher Education; 2007.
8. Kumar P, Clark M. Clinical medicine. Saunders Elsevier; 2009.
9. Mc Dougal WS. Bladder reconstruction following cystectomy by uretero-ileo-colourethrostomy. J Urol. 1986;135:698–701.
10. Terai A, et al. Urinary calculi as a late complication of the Indiana continent urinary diversion: comparison with the Kock pouch procedure. J Urol. 1996;155:66–8.

Complications of Nephrectomy 39

Vikas Jain, Abhinav Jain, and Sumit Bansal

39.1 Introduction

The first nephrectomy was performed for benign pathology that is the treatment of ureterovaginal fistula. Since then we have come a long way forward in the management of other renal conditions be it benign or malignant causes. Initially open nephrectomies were the answer to these sorts of kidney problems. As our understanding of the renal anatomy and the complications stemming from some of the surgeries has evolved, we have moved forwards and progressed. Now are the days of minimally invasive renal surgeries. As we move forwards, we can encounter the surgical complications, though not so common nowadays due to the enhancement in vision, instruments and surgical prowess. Therefore, for flawless decision making and a smooth perioperative course of the patient, a thorough knowledge of the surgical anatomy is needed. The same is beyond the scope of this chapter. Since the advent of donor nephrectomies, one more indication of nephrectomy has been added to the existent long list. Ours is a high volume center for renal transplant besides being a high burden hospital for malignancies. We ought to discuss the various surgical complications that may arise during nephrectomy and the appropriate steps to prevent and treat the same.

Appropriate patient selection and proper counseling of the family is essential for any treatment to be effective and successful. For this not only disease centric but an approach is needed that focusses on the patient as a whole. A thorough history and assessment of the all the risk factors that can influence the surgical outcome are essential. A patient with normally functioning both kidneys is the least likely to experience complications in the form of drop in GFR post operatively. Baseline

V. Jain (✉) · A. Jain · S. Bansal
Manipal Hospital Dwarka, Delhi, India

K. Sood Sharma et al. (eds.), *Complications of Cancer Therapy: Best Practices in Prevention and Management*, https://doi.org/10.1007/978-981-99-0984-1_39

serum creatinine, functioning of the opposite kidney, age of the patient, cardiopulmonary reserves of the patient, and any underlying comorbidities including hepatic dysfunction should be made note of as presence of any one of these may have a bearing on the incidence of complications and the final outcome of the patient [1].

39.2 Pre Operative Renal Arterial Embolization

Appears to be a tempting approach especially in large renal tumours that appear to be difficult to be managed during surgery. It is claimed to facilitate dissection by causing edema in the planes, can decrease intra operative blood loss and facilitate clamping of renal vein first [2]. However it is notorious to cause infraction syndrome consisting of nausea, vomiting, fever and pain. In some series, it is even thought to increase perioperative blood loss possibly due to increased tissue edema. In our experience, we like to usually subject the patient to pre op embolization in case of huge renal masses with exaggerated blood supply form dilated tortuous collaterals.

39.3 DVT Prophylaxis

Although American Urological Association is in favour of mechanical prophylaxis in all patients who are being subject to open nephrectomy, we in our clinical practice make use of DVT pump in the operation theatre and till the time the patient is made to ambulate. After the patient is mobile, we do not recommend the use of mechanical prophylaxis. We believe in enhanced recovery after surgery (ERAS) protocol, and thus ambulate the patient on the very first day after surgery, negating the need of any sort of prophylaxis after that. Pharmacological prophylaxis may be initiated in high risk patients if deemed absolutely necessary and the same is started when the risk of bleeding is considered to be minimal.

39.4 Incision and Exposure Related Problems

We have in our personal experience been able to complete all the nephrectomies to date (including donor nephrectomies) in a minimally invasive fashion and can boost of a zero conversion to open. This does not however mean that the surgeon should not have the surgical skill to complete a nephrectomy in open fashion. A clinical should be abreast thoroughly with the complications and problems that can arise in all of the possible treatment options and be ready to successfully cope with each of them. Injury to subcostal nerve can be one of these complications encountered after open nephrectomies. This preventable entity results in injury to the aforementioned nerve that supplies sensations to anterior abdominal wall and also gives a motor supply to anterior abdominal wall musculature. This can be avoided by curving the incision gently downwards at the mid axillary line when are incising from the lateral border of sacrospinalis and moving anteriorly. A transcostal approach to the kidney requires cutting of a rib which can be painful in the post-operative period. A supracostal [3] approach may be necessitated for a partial nephrectomy where control of the renal hilum is essential or removal of a upper polar renal mass where a subcostal approach fails. This approach can be notorious for inadvertent injuries to the neurovascular bundle running in the inferior aspect of the rib. A prudent approach to avoid the neurovascular bundle would be to stay as close as possible to the superior rib aspect. Injury and inadvertent entry into the pleura is a possibility in supracostal exposure while trying to reflect the pleura medially. Dorsal lumbotomy approach is favored in this adults and in pediatric patients. However the prone position required in this position required in this exposure may be poorly tolerated by the patient having poor cardiopulmonary reserves, in individuals with thoracic outlet syndrome and in patients following chest wall trauma. Mediastinal pressures may rise leading to venous engorgement. Reduced cerebral blood flow for a prolonged period of time and increased work of respiration may have its own consequences. Lung injuries may be encountered in thoracoabdominal approach to the kidney. This exposure is deemed necessary for large upper polar/suprarenal masses and tumours with venous thrombus.

39.5 Chest Complications

Can be expected (basal atelectasis) in patients with bad respiratory reserve especially those who are chronically addict to tobacco. Abstinence from smoking for a minimum period of 4 weeks is an ideal approach in case the pathology does not require an emergent surgical management. Post-operative incentive spirometry and deep breathing exercises are a must and facilitate early and smooth recovery. A robust support of good physiotherapy team is one of the integral pillars in management of such patients which is not difficult to find in a high volume oncology set up as ours.

39.6 Surgical Site Infections

Largely unheard of in this era where special emphasis is laid on surgical prophylaxis and antisepsis. The patients vulnerable are the ones with co-existing morbidities, immunocompromised state or especially those who have uncontrolled diabetes. Strict control of blood sugars before taking the patient to the OT is a prudent approach. We prefer to give antibiotic prophylaxis just before induction with a cephalosporin. We prefer a third generation one. We in our clinical practice do not start the patient with antibiotics pre operatively unless specifically indicated. We do not prefer mechanical bowel preparation in clear cut cases unless intra-abdominal adhesions are suspected due to previous abdominal surgeries.

39.7 Complications Due to Patient Positioning

Trendelenburg position is usually employed after the retrieval of kidney is done to facilitate closure of abdominal wall and preventing bowel from falling on the pfannenstiel retrieval incision. The same can increase cardiac output which can be helpful. However it can be counterproductive also and can cause raise intracranial and intraocular pressures. Facial edema and cyanosis can also result in this position. Right lateral position which is employed for facilitating laparoscopic left nephrectomies may cause decreased cardiac output by putting compression on the inferior vena cava. We employ the position for nephrectomy as detailed. The dependent leg is flexed at the hip and knee with the other leg being kept straight. Care is taken to insulate the pressure points at all times which in this case are the knees, axilla and heel of the patients. Complications can emanate from failure to adequately support these points and can be seen in the post-operative period as pain at these points or axillar neuropathy. Since the top arm is hyperextended and goes to the other side, shoulder pain can also be seen after the surgery during the hospital stay but is usually a rarity in the hands of expert technicians who manage the operating room and the patient positioning.

39.8 Complications Due to Pneumoperitoneum

1. **Respiratory and acid base problems:** Due to increased intraabdominal pressure and the excursion of the diaphragm upwards, there is reduced total lung volume and compliance and increase of respiratory resistance [4, 5]. A ventilator perfusion mismatch can lead to hypoxemia albeit rare in health persons undergoing laparoscopic surgeries. Acid base anomalies seen after insufflation include hypercapnoea and acidosis due the carbon dioxide being rapidly absorbed in the systemic circulation. This all may result in increased intraarterial carbon dioxide levels and elevated ET CO_2 levels. The increase in the blood carbon dioxide levels can be prolonged and achieving normal levels can take several hours even after desufflation of the abdomen. Surgeon and anesthetist should beware of pulmonary edema, carbon dioxide embolism, atelectasis, pneumothorax/mediastinum/pericardium and subcutaneous emphysema.
2. **Cardiovasular effects:** Moderate to severe hypercarbia can have direct myocardial depressant effect. Depression in stroke volume, and cardiac output and elevation of mean arterial blood pressure is usually seen as a response to pneumoperitoneum. Tachycardia may result [6, 7]. Hypertension is usually seen at the starting of the surgery due to drop in splanchnic pressure and increase in cardiac pre load. Keep a strict eye on hypotension which can be a life threatening complication and has been seen to occur in 10–15% of the laparoscopic operations [8]. Vagal stimulation due to the stretching of peritoneum can be seen in some surgeries resulting in bradycardia.

3. **Renal changes:** Oliguria is the rule owing to decreased renal blood flow and cortical vasoconstriction due to activation of RAAS pathway. Transient rise in serum creatinine has been observed during laparoscopy during many studies. The rise of serum creatinine can be attributed to production of free radicals and acute tubular toxicity.
4. **Splanchnic circulation:** 10–15 mmHg of elevation of intraabdominal pressures can decrease blood flow up to around 50% in stomach, average 30% in jejunum, 40–50% in colon, 30–40% in liver, and 50–70% in peritoneum [9].

39.9 Injury to Surrounding Structures

Liver injuries may occur in right sided nephrectomies and can range from minor lacerations to significant trauma. Minor trauma can be repaired just as renoraphy is done after partial nephrectomy. Similarly minor splenic injuries in the form of sub capsular tears and minor laceration can be managed with electro cautery and topical hemostatic agents. Duodenal trauma can occasionally go unnoticed and the patient may present in the post-operative period with acute abdomen. These sorts of injuries can occur with the current from electro cautery being transmitted from a nearby working area or the non-insulated limb of harmonic scalpel touching the bowel inadvertently. This is a serious and potentially life threatening event and has to managed emergently. Presence of gastro surgeon is desired in such settings. Surrounding large gut may be injured especially in cases of non-functioning small shrunken kidneys harboring pus. These kidneys usually pose a surgical challenge and are a nightmare for us. Pre-operative planning has to be immaculate in such cases and a low threshold should be maintained for open conversion in these difficult nephrectomies. Sub capsular nephrectomy is one valid and viable option in such cases and this means to remove as much tissue of the kidney that can be excised without causing harm to the surrounding structures. A rim of renal capsule can be left behind that is usually densely adherent. One more challenging scenario is when the hilum of the kidney is stuck due to enlarged lymph nodes or previous disease processes causing dense inflammation and scarring. Renal hilum can be clamped and divided en bloc in such cases with the occurrence of arterio venous fistula being practically nonexistent although a few cases having been reported in literature. Pancreatic injury can occur as the tail of the pancreas comes in relation to the spleen. A practical approach that we always follow during laparoscopic nephrectomy is to dissect as close as possible to the kidney and to divide the structures only in the immediate vicinity of the kidney. These sorts of mishaps can be detected by the increasing abdominal drain output and high level of amylase and lipase in the drain fluid. Management depends on the amount and severity of such injuries. Occasionally diaphragm can get opened in cases of large upper polar renal or adrenal masses that are densely stuck. Intracorporeal repair of the defect with placement of intercostal drainage tube appears to be the most practical approach. Injury to lumbar veins is a dreaded thing to happen as the cut ends of the veins usually retract inside psoas muscle and become out of sight rendering it impossible to clip or control and can cause torrential retroperitoneal bleeding and circulatory collapse.

39.10 Chylous Ascites

This complication has been seen especially following donor nephrectomies and characterized by chylous drainage in the abdominal drain or abdominal distension if the patient does not have a drainage tube in situ. Postulated to be caused by dissection of lymphatics during donor nephrectomy. A practical approach to the prevention is to carefully ligate all the lymphatics encountered during dissection. Can be managed by a low fat diet. Severe recalcitrant cases may need exploration and ligation of the responsible lymph channels.

39.11 Complications During Regional Lymphadenectomy

Sometimes there is a need for dissection and removal of lymph nodes located at a level above left renal hilum. This dissection which is to be done in interaortocaval groove should be done with caution as many vital structures are there in this area which are prone to injury including duodenum, pancreas, celiac trunk, superior mesenteric artery and cisterna chyli and injury to any of the above can have devastating and long lasting impact on the patient. Damage to the intestinal vasculature can again be a catastrophic event. The inferior mesenteric artery and vein can be safely ligated if the marginal artery of Drummond is intact. Superior mesenteric vessels should be preserved at any cost failing which bowel edema and venous engorgement can result leading to systemic/splanchnic hypertension.

39.12 Port Site Recurrence

Since the practice of open nephrectomy for renal masses slowly going in disrepute, and with the advancements in laparoscopy, most centers are now increasingly opting for minimally invasive nephrectomies. While the concern for port side recurrence is a genuine one, most of the studies show that this seeding is not statistically significant. The causes are multitude and can be attributed to cancer aggressiveness and the immunity of the person undergoing the surgery. Most common attributable factor being tumour spillage. The incidence is less than 0.2% in majority of the series [10], retrieval should be careful. Although as per animal studies, the chances of port site seeding increase significantly by the contact of malignant cells with the port site, there has not been enough human studies to defend the common practice of using a specimen bag during retrieval of the specimen.

39.13 Local Recurrence

Defined as isolated recurrence in the renal bed, regional lymph nodes or adrenal gland without distant spread. This entity is a rarity. With limited reports and papers available addressing this issue, the maximum reported incidence has been 1.8%. Targeted therapy or open surgical excision in selected cases may provide benefit.

39.14 Complications of Partial Nephrectomy

With nephron sparing surgery becoming increasingly common to preserve maximum number of nephrons especially in CKD patients, individuals with diabetes and hypertension, syndromic bilateral renal masses or kidney masses in the solitary functioning kidney, a background information and knowledge about the procedure is must in todays world of advancements.

1. **Urinomas:** Urinomas and urinary leakage occur when the pelvicalyceal system is opened during resection of the masses. The same can be confirmed by instillation of methylene blue retrogradely via ureteric catheter after the tumour has been excised. The PCS need to be meticulously repaired using non absorbable suture and the adequacy of the sealing of repair need to be confirned. It is our normal practice to repair the PCS over a double J stent and to put an abdominal drain and wide bore urinary catheter during the procedure. The usual sequence of removal of the above mentioned tubes followed by us is removal of the urinary catheter usually on the fourth or fifth post operative day. The abdominal drain may be removed subsequently if it continues to drain minimally. Many studies are in favor of keeping the abdominal drain in situ for a week to 10 days as the maximal chances of urinary leakage are around that time only. Urinary collections with double J stent, abdominal drain and urinary catheter usually resolve spontaneously.
2. **Hematoma:** This can occur when the renoraphy of the renal cortex has not been achieved meticulously.
3. **Delayed bleeding:** Bed rest, serial monitoring of hematocrit and vital charting should be done. Usually occurs due to secondary infections and here lies the role of selective renal angioembolizations. Most of times, bleeding can be successfully managed like this.
4. **Hyperfiltration injury:** Increased glomerular capillary perfusion pressures is a common occurrence when a large amount of kidney cortex has been sacrificed and the blood is received by the remaining lesser number of nephrons. Single nephron filtration increases leading to what is called hyperfiltration. This can manifest as proteinuria or glomerulosclerosis as a mark of injury to the remaining nephrons. It may take decades to manifest and is a common phenomenon when total nephron mass is lessened by around 80% or more.

39.15 Conclusion

1. There is a long list of possible complications during nephrectomy.
2. A careful selection of the patient is the key with a special focus on age, baseline renal and hepatic function, and comorbidities.
3. Suitability for laparoscopic resections should be assessed thoroughly before moving ahead with the operation.
4. A low threshold should exist for open conversion in case of pyonephrotic adhered kidney or where difficulties are anticipated.
5. Patient should be properly positioned to avoid position related complications.
6. Importance of sound anesthetist and critical care team cannot be ignored.
7. Long term follow up is essential.

References

1. Fleisher LA, et al. ACC/AHA 2007 guidelines on perioperative cardiovascular evaluation and care for noncardiac surgery: a report of the American College of Cardiology/American Heart Association Task Force on Practice Guidelines (Writing Committee to Revise the 2002 Guidelines on Perioperative Cardiovascular Evaluation for Noncardiac Surgery): developed in collaboration with the American Society of Echocardiography, American Society of Nuclear Cardiology, Heart Rhythm Society, Society of Cardiovascular Anesthesiologists, Society for Cardiovascular Angiography and Interventions, Society for Vascular Medicine and Biology, and Society for Vascular Surgery. Circulation. 2007;116(17):418–99.
2. Wszolek MF, et al. Surgical management of large renal tumours. Nat Clin Pract Urol. 2008;5(1):35–46.
3. Turner Warwick RT, et al. The supracostal approach to the renal area. Br J Urol. 1965;37(6):671–2.
4. Makinen MT, Yli-Hankala A. The effect of laparoscopic cholecystectomy on respiratory compliance as determined by continuous spirometry. J Clin Anesth. 1996;8:119–22.
5. Pelosi P, et al. Effects of carbon dioxide insufflation for laparoscopic cholecystectomy on the respiratory system. Anaesthesia. 1996;51:744–9.
6. Shuto K, et al. Hemodynamic and arterial blood gas changes during carbon dioxide and helium pneumoperitoneum in pigs. Surg Endosc. 1995;9:1173–8.
7. Nguyen NT, Cronan M, Braley S. Duplex ultrasound assessment of femoral venous flow during laparoscopic and open gastric bypass. Surg Endosc. 2003;17:285–90.
8. Lopez-Herranz GP. Complicaciones transoperatorias asociadas al capnoperitoneo en cirugia laparoscopica. Rev Med Hosp General Mexico. 2002;65:149–58.
9. Schilling MK, et al. Splanchnic microcirculatory changes during CO2 laparoscopy. J Am Coll Surg. 1997;184:378–82.
10. Shimokihara K, et al. Port site recurrence after laparoscopic radical nephrectomy. J Med. 2017;11:151.

Prevention and Management of Intraoperative Urological Injuries

40

Hemlata Garg, Megha Nandwani, and Satinder Kaur

40.1 Introduction

The female pelvis is complicated area where urinary and genital tract are in a close proximity to each other and intertwined. Intraoperative injuries encountered during gynaecological surgeries occur because of the complexity of the involved anatomy and intimate relationship of these various structure. Most of the pelvic tumours have the ability to invade and compromise the surrounding tissues and distort the anatomy and making it difficult to recognize. The incidence of Operative injuries to the urinary tract system while performing major gynaecological surgeries is estimated to be 1–2% and 75% of these injuries occur during hysterectomy (Daniel l, Clarke pearson). These injuries can occur anywhere in the urinary tract from ureter, bladder or urethra. When route of surgery is compared the incidence of bladder injury is 1% for abdominal route, 2.1% for laparoscopic route and 1.2% for vaginal route [1]. Blackwell et al. reported a 0.78% rate of ureteral injury during gynaecological surgeries which is grossly underestimated, with nearly 62% of those being unrecognized during surgery.

The detailed knowledge of anatomy is the mainstay of prevention of GU tract injuries. The ureter are retroperitoneal, 25–30 cm long structure that run from the renal pelvis to the bladder and can be injured during pelvic surgery at any point along their distal course. Most common sites of injuries are at the pelvic brim during clamping of infundibulo-pelvic ligament, at the bifurcation of common iliac artery during internal iliac artery ligation, lateral pelvic wall above the uterosacral

H. Garg (✉) · S. Kaur
Dharamshila Narayana Superspeciality Hospital, Delhi, India

M. Nandwani
Chittaranjan National Cancer Institute Kolkata, Kolkata, West Bengal, India

K. Sood Sharma et al. (eds.), *Complications of Cancer Therapy: Best Practices in Prevention and Management*, https://doi.org/10.1007/978-981-99-0984-1_40

ligament, base of broad ligament where ureter passes under the uterine artery, at ureteric canal during Wertheim's hysterectomy, at Intramural portion near the insertion into the trigone when base of bladder is injured or repaired and upper vagina during clamping of vaginal angle. Bladder injuries are more common during gynaecologic procedures. The bladder is at risk for injury during a hysterectomy during the creation of a bladder flap when the bladder dome is dissected from the lower uterine segment or from veress needle while creating the pneumo peritoneum. Urethral injuries are uncommon and rarely life threatening in isolation, however they are quite devastating injuries due to long term sequel including strictures, incontinence.

Gynaecological oncologist perform a wide array of surgical procedure from staging laparotomy, radical hysterectomy, retroperitoneal lymphadenectomy, debulking surgery for cancer ovary, radical vulvectomy, exenteration surgeries and surgeries post radiation and chemotherapy. Even in most of the expert hands due to anatomical considerations iatrogenic injuries cannot be avoided.

40.2 Bladder Injuries

Intraoperative recognition is the key. The bladder injury is suggested by the presence of gas filling up the Foleys bag or visibly bloody urine in the Foleys or fluid pooling in the abdominal or pelvic cavity. If a bladder injury is suspected, the bladder should be filled with methylene blue colored saline. The flow of blue colored fluid indicated the bladder injury and repair can be performed in two layers with absorbable sutures. A urethral catheter should be left for 7–10 days to ensure adequate healing and decrease the risk for subsequent vesicovaginal fistulas.

Postoperative presentation can mimic ureteral injuries with abdominal distension, ileus, fever, chills, leukocytosis, and increased drainage from pelvic drains. Diagnosis is established with a computed tomography cystogram. Intraperitoneal leaks are managed with robotic or open repair in two layers with absorbable sutures. On occasion, when a small, contained extraperitoneal leak is evident, management can be conservative with urethral catheter drainage. Often after hysterectomy, definitive repair of extensive bladder injury is the best option as the patient would be at risk for vesicovaginal fistula formation.

40.3 Ureteric Injuries

Mechanisms of ureteral injury are very diverse ranging from pinpoint thermal injury that can be asymptomatic in the vast majority, to complete ligation and transluminal or partial transection. Partial or complete transections are the most commonly identified problems and are managed intraoperatively. Ligation and thermal injury have a more delayed presentation. Devascularization of the ureter can lead to delayed stricture formation or necrosis.

The best way to avoid ureteral injuries is to identify the ureter as early as possible, certainly before ligation of critical pedicles [2]. It is crucial to keep in mind important landmarks for the ureter during an ongoing surgery. The ureter can be injured proximally as it is in close proximity to the gonadal vessels. Later along its course, other common areas of injury are as it courses over the iliac vessels at the level of the pelvic brim. In the deep pelvis, the ureter can be damaged as it courses below the uterine vessels in the female patient.

A high index of suspicion is necessary to detect ureteral injuries. Depending on the operation performed, the surgeon must be cognizant of the locations at which ureteral injuries can happen. Certain anatomic landmarks can be used to help identify the ureter. In the upper abdomen, the ureter is in close proximity to the gonadal vessels and the lower pole of the kidney. In the lower abdomen, the pelvic brim is an excellent landmark. The ureter crosses over the common iliac artery, and one can dissect and isolate it and trace it from this location. If a ureter is injured with a needle that pierced transmurally, the suture must be removed and a ureteral stent placed endoscopically at the end of the procedure. The same principles can be applied for limited inadvertent thermal injuries to the ureter with monopolar devices and bipolar sealing devices. Transection of the ureter requires more expertise, especially when one is willing to repair it laparoscopically. Partial tears with very reduced tissue loss and deterioration and no need for debridement can be closed primarily with 4.0 or 5.0 absorbable sutures after placing a stent through the ureterostomy. The stent will be left 4–8 weeks to allow enough time for healing. When complete transection of the ureter occurs, the location of the injury mandates the repair strategy. For proximal transections in the upper two-thirds of the ureter, ultimately above the pelvic inlet, an open, laparoscopic, or robotic ureteroureterostomy can be performed after trimming both edges and performing adequate spatulated anastomosis. A stent should be left for optimal drainage. Delayed recognition can lead to development of urinoma, ileus, sepsis, and shock with the need for nephrostomy tube diversion [3]. Early recognition can have a great impact on morbidity, and the need for nephrostomy in early versus delayed recognition of ureteral injury was 2.3% and 23.4%, respectively.

Role of Universal Cystoscopy

- The idea of using cystoscopy as a routine screening tool in major gynaecologic procedures continues to intrigue surgeons. However, it remains unclear whether its universal use should be advocated. Overall ureteric injury rate in Benign Gynaecological surgeries is 0.3% but only 18% of ureteric injuries can be detected without a cystoscopy based on intra operative findings, with cystoscopy the detection rate increases to 95%.

Non fistulous urological complications like voiding dysfunction, incontinence, hydronephrosis are usually seen following radical pelvic surgery done for carcinoma cervix. Despite being common problem it shows significant improvement within 12 months of surgery. However urodynamic studies should be a mandatory investigation in patients complaining.

Voiding Dysfunction

1. Early Post op Voiding Dysfunction seen in 70–85% patients.
2. Decreased Urinary sensation and Voiding by abdominal Straining.
3. Treatment: Bladder training and clean Intermittent Self Catheterization.
4. Spontaneous recovery expected within 6–12 months after surgery.
5. Persistent late changes mostly irritative.
6. Long term Voiding dysfunction seen in 30% cases.

Incontinence

1. ≥15% of women report regular urinary incontinence prior to surgery.
2. The incidence of involuntary urinary leakage 6 weeks after surgery is 48–53%, dropping to 30% at 3 months and remaining relatively constant thereafter.
3. Around 15% of women seek further medical treatment for their urinary incontinence 12 months after treatment.
4. The first choice of treatment for genuine stress incontinence is a mid-urethral tension-free sling.
5. Less-invasive treatment alternatives such as bulking-agent urethral-injection-therapy could be valid options for Urgency, increased frequency of voiding and incontinence.

Low Compliance Bladder

1. Urgency, increased frequency of voiding and incontinence
2. Cause is Detrusor overactivity due to Non nerve sparing RH, post op radiation and voiding with abdominal pressure at 3 months after surgery
3. Treatment:
   (a) Oral anti-cholinergic drugs
   (b) Intra-vesical instillation of the chondroitin sulphate solution, or the sodium hyaluronate solution
   (c) Intravesical injections of botulinum toxin, or neuromodulation

Hydronephrosis

1. Incidence:
   (a) Intravenous urography 2 weeks after surgery has shown hydronephrosis in 21% of women causes of hydronephrosis
2. Causes:
   (a) Reduction of peristaltic movements due to surgical denervation of the ureter
   (b) Iatrogenic lesions, scar-tissue formation or local oedema of the distal ureters by surgical trauma
3. In 74–100% of patients, hydronephrosis resolved spontaneously within 6 months of surgery
4. Less than 1% require intervention

40.4 Conclusion

Although the surgical urological complications are not so common but they cause significant morbidity to the patient. Precise anatomical knowledge is the corner stone in prevention of these injuries. Early diagnosis and intervention is necessary to prevent lifelong complications.

Key Points

- Due to close proximity of urogenital system to female reproductive tract, urological injuries are not so uncommon.
- Precise anatomical knowledge is the keystone for prevention.
- Bladder injuries are more common than ureteric injuries.
- Gentle dissection of the tissues is the first rule for avoiding injuries.
- In case of dense adhesions ureter should be identified anterior to the bifurcation of iliac vessels and then dissected distally to the area of concern.
- Always keep high degree of suspicion in case of suspected injury.
- Intraoperative repairs have better prognosis than late repairs.
- Identify risk factors associated with urological injuries.
- There is no evidence that pre operative ureteric stenting can prevent ureteric injuries.
- Even in most of the expert hands sometimes due to anatomical consideration injuries cannot be prevented.

References

1. Johnson N, Barlow D, Lethaby A, Tavender E, Curr E, Garry R. Surgical approach to hysterectomy for benign gynaecological disease. Cochrane Database Syst Rev. 2006;(2):CD003677. https://doi.org/10.1002/14651858.CD003677.pub3. Update in: Cochrane Database Syst Rev. 2009;(3):CD003677
2. Permpongkosol S, Link RE, Su LM, Romero FR, Bagga HS, Pavlovich CP, Jarrett TW, Kavoussi LR. Complications of 2,775 urological laparoscopic procedures: 1993 to 2005. J Urol. 2007;177(2):580–5.
3. Blackwell RH, Kirshenbaum EJ, Shah AS, Kuo PC, Gupta GN, Turk TMT. Complications of recognized and unrecognized iatrogenic ureteral injury at time of hysterectomy: a population based analysis. J Urol. 2018;199(6):1540–5.

Gastrointestinal Injuries in Gynaecological Surgeries

41

Hemlata Garg, Megha Nandwani, and Satinder Kaur

41.1 Introduction

Gastrointestinal injury remains one of the most serious complication if happens during surgery. Bowel injuries are difficult to diagnose intra operatively unless suspected, and can result in serious morbidity and mortality with delayed diagnosed postoperatively. The incidence of gastrointestinal tract injuries after hysterectomy can range from 0.1% to 1%, with an average of 0.3% for open and 0.2% for laparoscopic surgeries [1].

Types of gastrointestinal injuries: There are three types of bowel injuries that can occur during surgery: Thermal injury, direct mechanical damage, and indirect injury due vascular injury to mesentery.

1. **Mechanism of thermal injury**
    (a) Direct application when a surgeon inadvertently touches the monopolar cautery while the instrument is inside the patient.
    (b) Direct coupling when a monopolar device is activated while in contact with metal graspers retracting tissue.
    (c) Induced current when a monopolar device is activated when in contact with a metal suction cannula, which in turn is in contact with tissue.
    (d) Electrosurgical device touches the bowel during activation, where there is a microscopic insulation defect.
2. **Direct mechanical Injury**
    (a) During adhesiolysis by blunt or sharp instrument.

H. Garg (✉) · S. Kaur
Dharamshila Narayana Superspeciality Hospital, Delhi, India

M. Nandwani
Chittaranjan National Cancer Institute Kolkata, Kolkata, West Bengal, India

K. Sood Sharma et al. (eds.), *Complications of Cancer Therapy: Best Practices in Prevention and Management*, https://doi.org/10.1007/978-981-99-0984-1_41

(b) Laparoscopic instrument i.e. veress needle or trocar placement.

3. **Vascular injuries** are a result of interruption of the blood supply through the mesentery to the bowel.

41.2 Threat Factors for Bowel Injury

Presence of intra abdominal adhesions accounts for 11% of bowel injuries, and 38.2% of bowel injuries occur during adhesiolysis. Adhesions may be due to previous caesarean section or abdominal surgeries particularly laparotomy via vertical incision, endometriosis, history of pelvic abscess, perforation of bowel, pelvic and abdominal radiation therapy in the past [2].

Identification of Injury—thermal injuries to the bowel are the ones that can go unrecognized at the time of surgery. However, high degree of suspicious is required and inspection may reveal pale spots on the serosal surface of the bowel. If left undiagnosed, a thermal injury often has a delayed course. The common signs and symptoms of bowel injury are fever, nausea, vomiting, abdominal distension, and leukocytosis. Acute abdomen usually does not develop for several days to weeks postoperatively.

Direct injury to the bowel is more often recognized at the time of surgery, either as a breach in the serosal surface or as a full-thickness trauma to the bowel. However, even with careful inspection of the bowel, smaller defects may go unnoticed. Serosal tears may develop into perforations later. The classic signs and symptoms of a bowel perforation include fever leukocytosis, nausea, vomiting, and an acute abdomen. The diagnosis is usually confirmed by an X-ray abdomen and erect suggestive of free air under diaphragm and abdominal and pelvic CT with oral contrast.

Vascular injury to the bowel usually has a progressive course, being diagnosed later in the postoperative period. The classic signs and symptoms of bowel injury may not be apparent. When injury to the recto-sigmoid colon is suspected, a "bubble test" may be useful intra operatively. A proctoscope is inserted transanally, and saline is put in the pelvis to cover the area of colon in question. Proximally, the colon is occluded by hand compression. The recto-sigmoid is then insufflated with air through the proctoscope. If bubbles appear in the saline, a defect in the colon must then be located and repaired.

Prevention of bowel injuries: Prevention of bowel injuries should be started while planning for the surgery. Surgical history of the patient should be thoroughly taken; the entire previous scar marks should be well depicted in the diagram. Surgery on obese or lean patients, previous abdominal and pelvic surgery (in particular having midline scar), severe endometriosis, and complicated pelvic pathology i.e. previous radiation given for malignancy or frozen pelvis must increase the surgeon's awareness of potential complications during surgical procedures. Pre-operative bowel preparation for complicated surgery may not show any benefits in reducing the bowel injuries but has been used by many gynaecologists. This has potential benefits in reducing infection and anastomotic leakage if resection is done intra operatively [3].

During laparoscopic surgery veress needle is used to create a pneumo-peritoneum. Therefore, various safety tests have been done to determine its correct position like palmer saline test and double click test. Traditionally, Veress needles are inserted at the base of the umbilicus because this area is very thin. In patients having low midline scars, or previous abdominal surgeries palmer point entry for the Veress needle is recommended. Palmer's point is 2–3 cm below the left sub-costal margin. However, previous splenectomy and splenomegaly might be a contraindication for Palmer point entry. In addition, before inserting veress needle, stomach should be deflated by placing nasogastric tube to avoid stomach injury.

During primary trocar insertion Trendelenburg position should be avoided because it can make the angle of insertion more perpendicular. In an average patient, the distance between the anterior abdominal wall and major retroperitoneal blood vessels is normally 3–4 cm which can be increased to 5.6 cm (range 4–8 cm) by creating a pneumo-peritoneum pressure of 20–25 mmHg. The Royal College of Obstetricians and Gynaecologists recommend achieving a pressure of 20–25 mmHg before inserting the trocar. This increases splinting and allows the trocar to be more easily inserted through the abdominal wall. Careful inspection for omental and bowel adhesions prior to insertion of other trocars is important. Trocar screwing motion rather than direct pushing gives better control. The secondary trocars should be placed under direct vision to avoid vascular and internal organ injuries. Using optical trocars did not reduce bowel injury.

41.3 Management of Bowel Injuries

Early involvement of gastrointestinal surgeon is recommended whenever an intestinal injury is suspected during gynaecological surgery. Injury caused by the Veress needle can be managed conservatively since its small diameter leaves no defect and the muscular layer will close the defect. Trocar injuries may require a laparotomy for repair. When trocar injury occurs, leaving the trocar in place may be useful to identify the site of injury. The extent of bowel injury caused by bipolar electro surgery can be easily identified. Nevertheless, it is difficult to evaluate and identify those resulting from monopolar electro surgery. Therefore, excision of the damaged area and up to 5 cm around the margin of injury is recommended to prevent subsequent perforation. Primary closure in two layers using 3/0 Vicryl or PDS sutures is usually sufficient for majority of small bowel injuries. In case of a large bowel injury, the treatment options include primary repair, segmental resection, or colostomy. Segmental resection is more common in thermal injuries. There is strong evidence supporting primary repair of the colon and avoiding a colostomy especially in hemodynamically stable patients [4].

41.4 Conclusion

Intra operative bowel injuries can increase morbidity and mortality of the patient. Careful planning before surgery, meticulous surgical dissection, high degree of suspicion and intra operative identification of trauma and appropriate surgical management can avert the disaster.

Key Points

- Overall incidence of bowel injury is low in gynaecologic minimally invasive techniques, including conventional laparoscopy, robot-assisted laparoscopy, and laparoendoscopic single site surgery.
- Risk of bowel injury is highest in patients with prior abdominal surgery, adhesive disease, or endometriosis but can occur in women with no risk factors.
- The best prevention strategy for bowel injury is careful patient selection and meticulous surgical technique.
- When bowel injury occurs, outcomes are optimized with early diagnosis and intraoperative repair, which can be performed by an experienced gynecologist or other surgical consultant. Minimally invasive gynecologic procedure.

References

1. Llarena NC, Shah AB, Milad MP. Bowel injury in gynecologic laparoscopy: a systematic review. Obstet Gynecol. 2015;125(6):1407–17.
2. Elbiss HM, Abu-Zidan FM. Bowel injury following gynecological laparoscopic surgery. Afr Health Sci. 2017;17(4):1237–45.
3. Eisner IS, Wadhwa RK, Downing KT, Singhal PK. Prevention and management of bowel injury during gynecologic laparoscopy: an update. Curr Opin Obstet Gynecol. 2019;31(4):245–50.
4. Clarke-Pearson DL, Geller EJ. Complications of hysterectomy. Obstet Gynecol. 2013;121(3):654–73. https://doi.org/10.1097/AOG.0b013e3182841594.

42 Pedal Lymphedema After Lymphadenectomy for Pelvic Cancers

Megha Nandwani, Hemlata Garg, and Satinder Kaur

42.1 Introduction

When extreme amount of fluid gets collected in the interstitial spaces resulting in tissue swelling, this condition is commonly defined as lymphedema. Lymphedema is of two types:

1. Primary: that results due to congenital vascular deformities.
2. Secondary: that results after surgery, radiotherapy, infections or due to systemic disorders. It is acquired [1].

Pedal lymphedema which occurs commonly after lymphadenectomy for pelvic cancers is secondary lymphedema. Lymphadenectomy in pelvic cancers involves pelvic lymph node dissection and para-aortic lymph node dissection. For vulvar cancers, inguinal lymphadenectomy is done that also leads to pedal lymphedema in majority of the patients.

The incidence of pedal lymphedema reported in various studies is 2.4–41% after pelvic lymph node dissection done for gynecologic malignancies [2]. For patients who undergo inguinofemoral lymph node dissection for vulvar cancers, the incidence calculated from previous literature is around 28.8%. There is a five times increased risk of lymphedema in patients who are subjected to complete inguinal lymphadenectomy as compared to sentinel lymph node biopsy. Radiotherapy

M. Nandwani (✉)
Chittaranjan National Cancer Institute, Kolkata, India

H. Garg
Dharamshila Narayana Superspeciality Hospital, Delhi, New Delhi, India

S. Kaur
Gyn Oncology, Dharamshila Narayana Superspeciality Hospital, Delhi, New Delhi, India

K. Sood Sharma et al. (eds.), *Complications of Cancer Therapy: Best Practices in Prevention and Management*, https://doi.org/10.1007/978-981-99-0984-1_42

post-surgery is an important risk factor for developing pedal lymphedema in these women [3].

As lymphedema leads to increased morbidity in patients, its timely management is crucial. Patient education is a vital part of the management and the gold standard for treatment of pedal lymphedema is decongestive therapy [2].

42.2 Pathophysiology

The main role of lymphatic channels in our body is interstitial microcirculation [1]. The removal of large particulate matter from extravascular space is carried out by lymphatics. During lymphadenectomy, these lymphatics and lymph nodes are removed. This results in the accumulation of macromolecules in the interstitial spaces, leading to modification in the osmotic and hydrostatic pressures in the tissue spaces. The T lymphocytes and Langerhans cells are also carried out of the tissue spaces by an exit pathway via these lymphatics. And hence, the immunological function also gets impaired after the lymph node dissection procedure. So, due to thee patho-physiological changes that occur after lymphadenectomy, swelling of the tissue spaces occur leading to lymphedema. As the immunological process is also affected, the chances of secondary infection are also increased [4, 5].

42.3 Presentation and Diagnosis

Pedal lymphedema post lymphadenectomy presents as bilateral lower limb swelling. This presentation can be within 6 weeks, 3 months or even after 24 months post-surgery. The incidence of lymphedema by 24 months of surgical procedure is reported as 45%, when presented by patients themselves and 37% when measured by health care professionals [6]. Persistent lymphedema is reported in 60% of these cases [6].

When patients present with bilateral lower limb swelling, the first thing that has to be ruled out is deep vein thrombosis. Other conditions that mimic pedal lymphedema should be considered especially renal and cardiac conditions before starting any kind of management. Morbid obesity, Chronic venous insufficiency, cardiac/renal failure, hypoalbuminemia, infection, obstructive sleep apnea, lipedema are few disease states that mimic lower limb lymphedema [7].

The key for diagnosing lymphedema is history and physical examination. The European society of lymphology has described three stages of development of lymphedema [7].

Stage 0 (or Ia): Latent or sub-clinical condition where swelling is not evident despite impaired lymph transport.

Stage I: Early accumulation of fluid relatively high in protein content which subsides with limb elevation. Pitting may occur. An increase in proliferating cells may also be seen.

Stage II: In this stage limb elevation alone rarely reduces tissue swelling and pitting is manifest. Late in Stage II, the limb may or may not pit as tissue fibrosis supervenes.
Stage III: Lymphostatic elephantiasis where pitting is absent and trophic skin changes such as acanthosis, fat deposits, and warty overgrowths develop.

The international society of lymphology has also graded lymphedema into mild (less than 20% increase in volume), moderate (20–40% increase in volume) and severe (more than 40% increase in volume) [8].

Another grading system recommended by CTCAE or the National Cancer institute's common terminology for adverse events for lymphedema is as follows [9]:

Grade 1 involves trace thickening or faint skin discoloration.
Grade 2 is when patient's daily activities are limited. It is characterized by marked skin discoloration, lethargy texture, papillary formation.
Grade 3 involves severe symptoms limiting self-care and activities of daily living.

Pedal lymphedema is commonly assessed by the above-mentioned grades and by measuring limb volume. A water volumeter is used for measurement of the same. This method is not complaint to patients most of the times and especially with lower limbs lymphedema, even though it is an easy procedure to learn and perform [10–12]. The difference in limb circumference when measured using a non-elastic tape is also another tool used for diagnosing lymphedema. A 2 cm difference between the normal and affected limb is considered to be of diagnostic value [13, 14]. The drawback of this method is that in cases of bilateral lower limb lymphedema, it cannot be used. The Frustum formula is also used for measuring lymphoedema. It uses the principle of limb being conical in shape and hence calculating the volume of the cone for diagnosis [15]. Another instrument used for measuring lymphedema is the perometer that uses light emitting diodes for measurement purposes. Its high cost restricts its usage [14]. Other instruments like tissue tonometer have also been in used in the recent past [16]. A reliable diagnostic tool in measuring lymphedema in patients of gynecologic malignancies is the bioimpedance spectroscopy that uses the concept of low tissue resistance seen in tissues with high water content [17].

Imaging modalities like lymphography, commuted tomography with use of radionuclide dye is also a useful method for detecting pedal lymphedema [18]. Many questionnaires have also been used to assess lymphedema in patients post surgery [13].

42.4 Pedal Lymphedema and Gynecologic Cancers

The largest prospective trial conducted for assessment of lymphedema in gynecologic cancer or the LEG study (GOG 244) was published in the year 2020 [19]. This study evaluated 1054 women with endometrial, cervical and vulvar malignancies. All patients were diagnosed with lymphedema based on leg volume. This was measured by taking the limb diameter at 10 cm intervals from heel to inguinal crease. The starting point of measurement was 10 cm above the bottom line of the heel. The results of the study showed that maximum number of cases of lymphedema occurred after 4–6 weeks of surgery. It was seen that women who were more than 65 years of age showed decreased limb volume change. Also, for endometrial cancer patients when a greater number of lymph nodes were removed during surgery increased incidence of limb volume change was noted.

42.5 Prevention and Management

The old saying of prevention is better than cure is very apt here as it aims to decrease patient morbidity and improve their quality of life. Though there are limited studies on lower limb lymphedema prevention, recent data shows the benefit of sentinel lymph node in early stages of gynecologic cancers (cervix, endometrium and vulva) to be of some benefit. Thus, where appropriate, the use of sentinel lymph node biopsy should be considered as compared to complete lymph node dissection [20].

For the management of pedal lymphedema at early stages (stages 0 and 1), compression bandaging reduces limb volume significantly. The application of manual lymphatic drainage along with use of multilayered bandaging has shown to reduce the limb volume by 31% at 24 weeks as compared to individual use of these techniques [21]. Care of the skin and physiotherapy exercises form an important aspect of treatment of lymphedema. Use of intermittent pneumatic compression also reduces lymphedema with time. It is a safe procedure that can be used for prolonged periods with daily therapy. It reduces lymphedema especially over mid-calf and above the ankle while improving elasticity of the lymphatics [22].

Complete decongestive therapy is a cost-effective method for management of pedal lymphedema. It involves manual massage and use of compression bandaging. Once educated about the technique, it can be used by the patient themselves. It has shown to improve quality of life score significantly in patients with lower limb lymphedema [23, 24].

For patients who present with higher stages of lymphedema, compression bandaging may not always be effective. Surgical interventions involving anastomosis of lymphatics can be useful for these cases. The anastomosis can be done between lymphatic channels that is lympho-lymphatic or between lymphatics and venous channels that is lympho-venous or between lymphatics and subcuticular lymphatics that is lymphaticovenular [25]. These procedures help in restoring the physiology of the affected limb and relieving lymphedema.

Other surgical interventions that are not commonly used include ablative procedures. These involve removal of layers of fat and affected tissues up to superficial and deep fascia. One of these procedures is the Charles procedure that is the most radical one. It includes removal of the skin along with all layers of tissue till the muscle layer and then using grafts for closure [26]. The Sistrunk procedure is less extensive that removes tissue layer up to the deep fascia followed by primary closure [27]. A modification of the Charles procedure is the Honnan surgery that involves preservation of the subdermal plexus [28, 29].

Another promising technique for management of lymphedema is liposuction. The use of compression bandaging after liposuction has shown improved quality of life in lymphedema patients for a long time [30].

The transfer of a lymph node with its blood supply to the affected side has also shown to improve the symptoms of lymphedema. This vascularized lymph node transfer has shown to act like a pump for lymphatic drainage [31]. The use of lymph node flap is also being used for the same. All these procedures have shown promising results in patients with higher stage (Stages 2 and 3) lymphedema [32, 33].

Thus, the management of early stages of lymphedema mostly involves compression bandaging and physiotherapy while for advanced stages, surgery should be considered. Medical management can be considered for shorter periods. It includes use of diuretic and antibiotics for treatment of cellulitis. Coumarin has limited role in reducing lymphedema [34–36].

Vulvar cancer patients undergoing inguinofemoral lymphadenectomy are at a high risk of developing postoperative lymphedema. Omental free flaps containing gastroepiploic vessels has also shown efficacy to treat lymphedema in these patients [37].

Newer treatment modalities are being explored for the management of lymphedema. Genetic basis for development of secondary lymphedema in cases of breast cancer surgery have been studied [38] but the role of genetic markers for predicting risk of pedal lymphedema post gynecologic cancer surgeries still needs to be reviewed. Role of vascular endothelial growth factor-C for management of lymphedema is also being evaluated as it helps in regeneration of lymphatics and its deficiency or genetic disorder is often responsible for primary lymphedema [39].

42.6 Conclusion

Lymphedema is a major complication in patients of gynecologic malignancies post-surgery. High body mass index (BMI), adjuvant radiation therapy contributes in increasing the risk of occurrence of pedal lymphedema. Education of patient and applying preventive strategies seem to be crucial for lymphedema management. Timely treatment of this condition helps in improving quality of life for patients with pelvic malignancies. Further research is advocated in this field for designing guidelines and treatment protocols.

References

1. Grada AA, Phillips TJ. Lymphedema: pathophysiology and clinical manifestations. J Am Acad Dermatol. 2017;77(6):1009–20.
2. Bakar Y, Tuğral A. Lower extremity lymphedema management after gynecologic cancer surgery: a review of current management strategies. Ann Vasc Surg. 2017;44:442–50.

3. Huang J, Yu N, Wang X, Long X. Incidence of lower limb lymphedema after vulvar cancer. Medicine. 2017;96(46):e8722.
4. Mallon EC, Ryan TJ. Lymphedema and wound healing. Clin Dermatol. 1994;12:89–93.
5. Farrell R, Gebski V, Hacker NF. Quality of life after complete lymphadenectomy for vulvar cancer: do women prefer sentinel lymph node biopsy? Int J Gynecol Cancer. 2014;24:813–9.
6. Hayes SC, Janda M, Ward LC, Reul-Hirche H, Steele ML, Carter J, Quinn M, Cornish B, Obermair A. Lymphedema following gynecological cancer: results from a prospective, longitudinal cohort study on prevalence, incidence and risk factors. Gynecol Oncol. 2017;146(3):623–9.
7. Greene AK, Goss JA. Diagnosis and staging of lymphedema. Semin Plast Surg. 2018;32(1):12–6.
8. Cheng MH, Chang DW, Patel KM, editors. Principles and practice of lymphedema surgery. Oxford: Elsevier Inc.; 2015. ISBN: 978-0-323-29897-1.
9. National Institutes of Health (NIH). The National Cancer Institute common terminology criteria for adverse events. 2019.
10. Executive C. The diagnosis and treatment of peripheral lymphedema: 2016 consensus document of the International Society of Lymphology. Lymphology. 2016;49:170–84.
11. Shaitelman SF, Cromwell KD, Rasmussen JC, Stout NL, Armer JM, Lasinski BB, et al. Recent progress in the treatment and prevention of cancer-related lymphedema. CA Cancer J Clin. 2015;65:55–81.
12. Mihara M, Hara H, Araki J, Kikuchi K, Narushima M, Yamamoto T, et al. Indocyanine green (ICG) lymphography is superior to lymphoscintigraphy for diagnostic imaging of early lymphedema of the upper limbs. PLoS One. 2012;7:e38182.
13. Carter J, Raviv L, Appollo K, Baser RE, Iasonos A, Barakat RR. A pilot study using the gynecologic cancer lymphedema questionnaire (GCLQ) as a clinical care tool to identify lower extremity lymphedema in gynecologic cancer survivors. Gynecol Oncol. 2010;117:317–23.
14. Sharkey AR, King SW, Kuo RY, Bickerton SB, Ramsden AJ, Furniss D. Measuring limb volume: accuracy and reliability of tape measurement versus perometer measurement. Lymphat Res Biol. 2018;16:182–6.
15. Karges JR, Mark BE, Strikeleather SJ, Worrell TW. Concurrent validity of upper-extremity volume estimates: comparison of calculated volume derived from girth measurements and water displacement volume. Phys Ther. 2003;83:134–45.
16. Thorne CH, Gurtner GC, Chung KC, Gosain A, Mehrara B, Rubin P, Spear SL, editors. Grabb and Smith's plastic surgery. 7th ed. Philadelphia: Wolters Kluwer/Lippincott Williams & Wilkins; 2014.
17. Warren AG, Janz BA, Slavin SA, Borud LJ. The use of bioimpedance analysis to evaluate lymphedema. Ann Plast Surg. 2007;58:541–3.
18. O'Donnell TF Jr, Rasmussen JC, Sevick-Muraca EM. New diagnostic modalities in the evaluation of lymphedema. J Vasc Surg Venous Lymphat Disord. 2017;5:261–73.
19. Carlson JW, Kauderer J, Hutson A, Carter J, Armer J, Lockwood S, Nolte S, Stewart BR, Wenzel L, Walker J, Fleury A, Bonebrake A, Soper J, Mathews C, Zivanovic O, Richards WE, Tan A, Alberts DS, Barakat RR. GOG 244-the lymphedema and gynecologic cancer (LEG) study: incidence and risk factors in newly diagnosed patients. Gynecol Oncol. 2020;156(2):467–74.
20. Chow S, Karam A. Role of sentinel lymph node biopsy for gynecologic cancers. Curr Opin Obstet Gynecol. 2022;34(1):15–9.
21. Badger CM, Peacock JL, Mortimer PS. A randomized, controlled, parallel-group clinical trial comparing multilayer bandaging followed by hosiery versus hosiery alone in the treatment of patients with lymphedema of the limb. Cancer. 2000;88:2832–7.
22. Zaleska M, Olszewski WL, Durlik M. The effectiveness of intermittent pneumatic compression in long-term therapy of lymphedema of lower limbs. Lymphat Res Biol. 2014;12:103–9.
23. Lasinski BB, McKillip Thrift K, Squire D, Austin MK, Smith KM, Wanchai A, et al. A systematic review of the evidence for complete decongestive therapy in the treatment of lymphedema from 2004 to 2011. PM R. 2012;4:580–601.

24. Kim SJ, Park YD. Effects of complex decongestive physiotherapy on the oedema and the quality of life of lower unilateral lymphoedema following treatment for gynecological cancer. Eur J Cancer Care (Engl). 2008;17:463–8.
25. Campisi C, Bellini C, Campisi C, Accogli S, Bonioli E, Boccardo F. Microsurgery for lymphedema: clinical research and long-term results. Microsurgery. 2010;30:256–60.
26. Charles RH. Elephantiasis scroti. London: Churchill; 1912.
27. Sistrunk WE. Contribution to plastic surgery: removal of scars by stages; an open operation for extensive laceration of the anal sphincter; the Kondoleon operation for elephantiasis. Ann Surg. 1927;85:185–93.
28. Homans J. The treatment of elephantiasis of the legs. A preliminary report. N Engl J Med. 1936;215:1099–104.
29. Miller TA, Wyatt LE, Rudkin GH. Staged skin and subcutaneous excision for lymphedema: a favorable report of long-term results. Plast Reconstr Surg. 1998;102:1486–98.
30. Brorson H. Liposuction in lymphedema treatment. J Reconstr Microsurg. 2016;32(01):56–65.
31. Chen HC, O'Brien BM, Rogers IW, Pribaz JJ, Eaton CJ. Lymph node transfer for the treatment of obstructive lymphoedema in the canine model. Br J Plast Surg. 1990;43(5):578–86.
32. Raju A, Chang DW. Vascularized lymph node transfer for treatment of lymphedema: a comprehensive literature review. Ann Surg. 2015;261(5):1013–23.
33. Cheng MH, Chen SC, Henry SL, Tan BK, Lin MC, Huang JJ. Vascularized groin lymph node flap transfer for postmastectomy upper limb lymphedema: flap anatomy, recipient sites, and outcomes. Plast Reconstr Surg. 2013;131(6):1286–98.
34. Moseley AL, Carati CJ, Piller NB. A systematic review of common conservative therapies for arm lymphoedema secondary to breast cancer treatment. Ann Oncol. 2007;18(4):639–46.
35. Szuba A, Rockson SG. Lymphedema: classification, diagnosis and therapy. Vasc Med. 1998;3(2):145–56.
36. Kligman L, Wong RK, Johnston M, Laetsch NS. The treatment of lymphedema related to breast cancer: a systematic review and evidence summary. Support Care Cancer. 2004;12(6):421–31.
37. Kenworthy EO, Nelson JA, Verma R, Mbabuike J, Mehrara BJ, Dayan JH. Double vascularized omentum lymphatic transplant (VOLT) for the treatment of lymphedema. J Surg Oncol. 2018;117:1413–9.
38. Finegold DN, Baty CJ, Knickelbein KZ, Perschke S, Noon SE, Campbell D, Karlsson JM, Huang D, Kimak MA, Lawrence EC, Feingold E, Meriney SD, Brufsky AM, Ferrell RE. Connexin 47 mutations increase risk for secondary lymphedema following breast cancer treatment. Clin Cancer Res. 2012;18(8):2382–90.
39. Schindewolffs L, Breves G, Buettner M, Hadamitzky C, Pabst R. VEGF-C improves regeneration and lymphatic reconnection of transplanted autologous lymph node fragments: an animal model for secondary lymphedema treatment. Immun Inflamm Dis. 2014;2(3):152–61.

43 Venous Thromboembolism After Gynecologic Malignancies

Megha Nandwani, Hemlata Garg, and Satinder Kaur

43.1 Introduction

Venous thromboembolism (VTE) comprises of deep vein thrombosis (DVT) and pulmonary embolism (PE) and is a major complication of patients with gynecologic malignancies leading to significant morbidity and mortality. Cancer patients are more prone to develop venous thromboembolism. The incidence for the same has been reported to be around 20% [1]. Women suffering from gynecologic cancers have an incidence of VTE ranging from 0% to 41.5% as seen from different studies in the literature [2–7].

Patients of gynecologic cancers often have risk factors like advanced age, increased body mass index (BMI), undergo prolonged surgery, hormonal and chemotherapy, remain immobile for longer periods of time and suffer from comorbidities like diabetes and hypertension. All these factors are contributory in development of venous thromboembolism [8].

The first presentation of malignancy can also be symptoms of venous thromboembolism. Patients present with bilateral or recurrent deep vein thrombosis. VTE of unknown cause has a 2–5 times increased incidence of occult cancer. This increase is often seen in malignancies of internal organs like brain, pancreas and ovary [9].

An American study conducted on 104,368 patients undergoing gynecological surgeries for cancer was conducted to evaluate the rate of occurrence of this vital complication. They reported the incidence of VTE of 1.8%. For individual cancers,

M. Nandwani (✉)
Chittaranjan National Cancer Institute, Kolkata, India

H. Garg
Dharamshila Narayana Superspeciality Hospital, Delhi, New Delhi, India

S. Kaur
Gyn Oncology, Dharamshila Narayana Superspeciality Hospital, Delhi, New Delhi, India

K. Sood Sharma et al. (eds.), *Complications of Cancer Therapy: Best Practices in Prevention and Management*, https://doi.org/10.1007/978-981-99-0984-1_43

it was observed that VTE occurred 1.5 times more in patients with carcinoma ovary as compared to endometrial, cervical and vulval cancers. They also noted a 64% decreased risk of venous thromboembolism in patients undergoing minimally invasive surgeries as compared to open surgery [10].

43.2 Pathophysiology of VTE

The pathophysiology of VTE can be explained by understanding the Virchow's triad that involves changes in blood flow or stasis of the blood, changes in vessel wall that is represented by vessel wall injury and changes in the properties of blood that is seen as hypercoagulability of blood. All these factors are increased in gynecologic malignancy patients that leads to activation of the clotting factor pathways [11]. The factors that contribute in activation of the components of Virchow's triad include perioperative immobility in patients, huge pelvic masses and iatrogenic lymphocysts and hematomas leading to venous stasis, vessel wall injury occurring during surgery and decreased fibrinolytic activity associated with the procedure. Also, cancer cells themselves can lead to activation of procoagulants and hence lead to a state of hypercoagulability [12].

43.3 Clinical Presentation and Diagnosis

Patients with deep vein thrombosis present with leg swelling, pain, cramps or soreness of calf and skin discoloration. Patients can also be affected with DVT without any noticeable symptoms. On examination, there is calf tenderness, pitting edema, increased skin temperature, superficial venous dilatation, swelling below the knee in cases of distal deep vein thrombosis and up to the groin in proximal deep vein thrombosis. In cases with severe obstruction, cyanosis can also occur [13].

The possibility of DVT can be assessed by measuring the leg diameter. This measurement is done 10 cm below the tibial tuberosity. A 3 cm or more difference between the affected and the asymptomatic leg increases the chances of DVT [14]. Homan's sign was a test to diagnose DVT in ancient times with low sensitivity [15]. Studies have shown that Homan's sign was elicited in almost 21% patients without thrombus and in patients having acute thrombosis, only one-third patients could be diagnosed [16]. Thus, these tests are no longer used these days.

Wells criteria is often used to assess the probability of occurrence of DVT [17]. The old version of the criteria involved nine factors to divide patients into low, intermediate and high risk [18]. The revised addition of the Wells criteria also includes history of previous DVT and the post-operative duration as 4–12 weeks. On the basis of this criteria the chances of developing DVT ranges from 6% to 28% that is unlikeliness and likeliness to develop DVT [19]. According to the NICE guidelines, the sensitivity of Wells criteria was around 77–98% and the specificity was 38–58% [20].

D dimer assay has also been used for diagnosing DVT with a sensitivity of 75–100% and a specificity of 26–83% [20]. This is often combined with Wells score to determine the probability of DVT.

Imaging modalities play a key role in diagnosing deep vein thrombosis. Ultrasound is the most safe and accessible tool to diagnose DVT [21, 22]. When ultrasound modality is used with duplex and color flow doppler, the sensitivity of the same increases. The diagnosis of proximal DVT with use of ultrasound is more accurate as compared to distal DVT. It was reported that the pooled sensitivity to diagnose proximal DVT was 94.2% as compared to 63.5% for distal DVT [23].

Contrast venography, CT venography and MR venography are the other imaging modalities used in the diagnosis of DVT. Using venography is considered to be gold standard. In contrast venography, dye is injected into the vascular system and filling defect on imaging confirms DVT [22, 24]. Ct venography is also based on the same principle with the advantages of being non-invasive, easily available with high sensitivity and specificity [25]. It is also of diagnostic importance in patients having suspected pulmonary embolism. MR venography is similar to CT venography with lesser exposure to radiation but has higher cost [26].

The patients with pulmonary embolism present with breathlessness, chest pain, cough, hemoptysis, syncope, palpitations, chest tightness and cardiopulmonary arrest. It is a medical emergency and if not treated immediately leads to 100% mortality. The signs of PE include tachypnea, tachycardia, hypertension, rales on chest auscultation, phlebitis, cardiac murmur, cyanosis, increased temperature and diaphoresis [27]. The diagnosis of PE is similar to that of DVT. Wells criteria, D-dimer assay and imaging modalities help in its diagnosis. The gold standard investigation for PE diagnosis is computed tomography pulmonary angiography [27]. It has high diagnostic accuracy. The only disadvantage of the test is that a silent PE of unknown significance will also be picked up. Ventilation perfusion scans or VQ scans are also an alternate choice of investigation with lesser radiation exposure. Intermediate probability VQ scans will need further investigations whereas a low probability scan will rule out and a high probability will confirm PE [28].

43.4 Risk Stratification and Scoring

Many scoring systems were developed to assess the risk of VTE in peri-operative patients. The efficacy of any of these scores in not of any clear benefit. One such score or predictive model for diagnosis of venous thromboembolism in surgical patients is the Joseph Caprini risk assessment score. This score gives points 1, 2 or 3 based on risk factors of thromboembolism like age, presence or absence of comorbidities, past history of VTE, sepsis, duration of surgery, etc. If the total score is more than or equal to 9 then patient is given thromboprophylaxis for 30 days, if the score is between 5 and 8 then thromboprophylaxis is to be given for 10 days and if it is 0–4 then no thromboprophylaxis is needed [29].

43.5 Prevention and Management

If oncological patients are not given preventive treatment for VTE then the risk of development of postoperative thromboembolism is estimated to be around 38%. Pulmonary embolism which is a component of VTE is the chief cause of death in women undergoing surgery for gynecologic cancers attributing to 3% of these deaths [30]. Thus, it is crucial to give thromboprophylaxis to patients of gynecologic malignancies before taking them up for surgical procedures although its role is not very clear for minimally invasive surgery.

Prevention of VTE involves screening the patients and risk stratification (as described above) and application of preventive measures. Early ambulation post-surgery and implementing the ERAS (early recovery after surgery) protocol are one of the measures adopted for VTE prevention in patients with gynecologic malignancies [31]. Mechanical methods like use of DVT stockings pre and post operatively, use of intermittent pneumatic compression devices during surgery are used especially in patients with high risk for development of DVT [32]. Minimally invasive surgeries for early-stage gynecologic cancers significantly decrease the risk of development of thromboembolism [33].

Pharmacologic measures for VTE prevention include the use of anti-coagulants like low molecular weight heparin and oral anticoagulants (factor Xa inhibitors). They decrease the risk of embolism by almost 50–70% [34].

Once the diagnosis of VTE is established, its management includes use of anticoagulant drugs that is unfractionated heparin and low molecular weight heparin (LMWH). Due to better safety profile, LMWH is the preferred drug. Swift management is needed for these cases. The acute phase of VTE lasts for 5–10 days. The patient should be hospitalized and heparin started parenterally. After the acute phase has passed, patient can be started on oral anticoagulants [35–37].

Vitamin K antagonists like warfarin are not in popular use due to drug interactions, delayed onset of anticoagulation and frequent monitoring needs. Direct oral anticoagulants like dabigatran, rivoraxaban, apixaban and edoxaban are now being considered for treatment of VTE due to lesser monitoring requirements and better patient compatibility. They have shown to be efficacious in the management of VTE [35, 37, 38].

43.6 Conclusion

To conclude venous thromboembolism is a deadly complication of patients with gynecologic cancers. At risk patients should be identified earlier and timely thromboprophylaxis started. Use of adequate measures to prevent DVT and further PE can help reduce the rate of venous thromboembolism to a great extent and hence prevent patient morbidity and mortality. Further research is needed to define protocols for prevention and management of this salient complication.

References

1. Heit JA, et al. Relative impact of risk factors for deep vein thrombosis and pulmonary embolism: a population-based study. Arch Intern Med. 2002;162:1245–8.
2. Dusenbery KE, Carson LF, Potish RA. Perioperative morbidity and mortality of gynecologic brachytherapy. Cancer. 1991;67:2786–90.
3. Sivanesaratnam V, Sen DK, Jayalakshmi P, Ong G. Radical hysterectomy and pelvic lymphadenectomy for early invasive cancer of the cervix: 14-year experience. Int J Gynecol Cancer. 1993;3:231–8.
4. Rodriguez AO, et al. Venous thromboembolism in ovarian cancer. Gynecol Oncol. 2007;105:784–90.
5. Timp JF, Braekkan SK, Versteeg HH, Cannegieter SC. Epidemiology of cancer-associated venous thrombosis. Blood. 2013;122:1712–23.
6. Trugilho IA, Renni MJP, Medeiros GC, Thuler LCS, Bergmann A. Incidence and factors associated with venous thromboembolism in women with gynecologic cancer. Thromb Res. 2020;185:49–54.
7. Walker AJ, Card TR, West J, Crooks C, Grainge MJ. Incidence of venous thromboembolism in patients with cancer: a cohort study using linked United Kingdom databases. Eur J Cancer. 2013;49:1404–13.
8. Cohen A, Lim CS, Davies AH. Venous thromboembolism in gynecological malignancy. Int J Gynecol Cancer. 2017;27:1970–8.
9. Klein A, Shepshelovich D, Spectre G, Goldvaser H, Raanani P, Gafter-Gvili A. Screening for occult cancer in idiopathic venous thromboembolism—systemic review and meta-analysis. Eur J Intern Med. 2017;42:74–80.
10. Graul A, Latif N, Zhang X, et al. Incidence of venous thromboembolism by type of gynecologic malignancy and surgical modality in the National Surgical Quality Improvement Program. Int J Gynecol Cancer. 2017;27:581–7.
11. Nielsen HK. Pathophysiology of venous thromboembolism. Semin Thromb Hemost. 1991;17(Suppl 3):250–3.
12. Wang X, Fu S, Freedman RS, Kavanagh JJ. Venous thromboembolism syndrome in gynecological cancer. Int J Gynecol Cancer. 2006;16(Suppl 1):458–71.
13. Kruger PC, Eikelboom JW, Douketis JD, Hankey GJ. Deep vein thrombosis: update on diagnosis and management. Med J Aust. 2019;210(11):516–24.
14. Ng AH, Gupta E, Bianty J, Williams JL, Bruera E. Calf measurements screening for deep vein thrombosis in acute inpatient cancer rehabilitation. Int J Ther Rehabil. 2019;26(1):1–5.
15. Ambesh P, Obiagwu C, Shetty V. Homan's sign for deep vein thrombosis: a grain of salt? Indian Heart J. 2017;69(3):418–9.
16. Haeger K. Problems of acute deep venous thrombosis: the interpretation of signs and symptoms. Angiology. 1969;20:219–23.
17. Wells PS, Anderson DR, Bormanis J, et al. Value of assessment of pretest probability of deep-vein thrombosis in clinical management. Lancet. 1997;350:1795–8. https://doi.org/10.1016/S0140-6736(97)08140-3.
18. Wells PS, Owen C, Doucette S, et al. Does this patient have deep vein thrombosis? JAMA. 2006;295:199–207. https://doi.org/10.1001/jama.295.2.199.
19. Wells PS, Anderson DR, Rodger M, et al. Evaluation of D-dimer in the diagnosis of suspected deep-vein thrombosis. N Engl J Med. 2003;349:1227–35. https://doi.org/10.1056/NEJMoa023153.
20. Langford N, Stansby G, Avital L. The management of venous thromboembolic diseases and the role of thrombophilia testing: summary of NICE guideline CG144. Acute Med. 2012;11:138–42.
21. Kearon C, Julian JA, Newman TE, et al. Noninvasive diagnosis of deep venous thrombosis. McMaster diagnostic imaging practice guidelines initiative. Ann Intern Med. 1998;128:663–77.

22. Min SK, Kim YH, Joh JH, et al. Diagnosis and treatment of lower extremity deep vein thrombosis: Korean practice guidelines. Vasc Specialist Int. 2016;32:77–104.
23. Goodacre S, Sampson F, Thomas S, et al. Systematic review and meta-analysis of the diagnostic accuracy of ultrasonography for deep vein thrombosis. BMC Med Imaging. 2005;5:6. https://doi.org/10.1186/1471-2342-5-6.
24. Guyatt GH, Norris SL, Schulman S, et al. Methodology for the development of antithrombotic therapy and prevention of thrombosis guidelines: Antithrombotic Therapy and Prevention of Thrombosis, 9th ed: American College of Chest Physicians Evidence-Based Clinical Practice Guidelines. Chest. 2012;141:53S–70S.
25. Thomas SM, Goodacre SW, Sampson FC, et al. Diagnostic value of CT for deep vein thrombosis: results of a systematic review and meta-analysis. Clin Radiol. 2008;63:299–304.
26. Sampson FC, Goodacre SW, Thomas SM, et al. The accuracy of MRI in diagnosis of suspected deep vein thrombosis: systematic review and meta-analysis. Eur Radiol. 2007;17:175–81.
27. Toplis E, Mortimore G. The diagnosis and management of pulmonary embolism. Br J Nurs. 2020;29(1):22–6.
28. Kruger PC, Eikelboom JW, Douketis JD, Hankey GJ. Pulmonary embolism: update on diagnosis and management. Med J Aust. 2019;211(2):82–7.
29. Grant PJ, Greene MT, Chopra V, Bernstein SJ, Hofer TP, Flanders SA. Assessing the Caprini score for risk assessment of venous thromboembolism in hospitalized medical patients. Am J Med. 2016;129(5):528–35.
30. Liakou C, Thomakos N. Postoperative thromboembolism in gynecologic oncology patients. Still a lethal but preventable complication. Br J Res. 2017; https://doi.org/10.21767/2394-3718.100031.
31. Bogani G, Sarpietro G, Ferrandina G, Gallotta V, Di Donato V, Ditto A, Pinelli C, Casarin J, Ghezzi F, Scambia G, Raspagliesi F. Enhanced recovery after surgery (ERAS) in gynecology oncology. Eur J Surg Oncol. 2021;47(5):952–9.
32. Anderson DR, Dunbar M, Murnaghan J, Kahn SR, Gross P, Forsythe M, Pelet S, Fisher W, Belzile E, Dolan S, et al. Aspirin or rivaroxaban for VTE prophylaxis after hip or knee arthroplasty. N Engl J Med. 2018;378:699–707.
33. Jorgensen EM, Li A, Modest AM, Leung K, Moore Simas TA, Hur H-C. Incidence of venous thromboembolism after different modes of gynecologic surgery. Obstet Gynecol. 2018;132:1275–84.
34. Samama MM, Cohen AT, Darmon JY, Desjardins L, Eldor A, Janbon C, Leizorovicz A, Nguyen H, Olsson CG, Turpie AG, et al. A comparison of enoxaparin with placebo for the prevention of venous thromboembolism in acutely ill medical patients. N Engl J Med. 1999;341:793–800.
35. Streiff MB, Agnelli G, Connors JM, et al. Guidance for the treatment of deep vein thrombosis and pulmonary embolism. J Thromb Thrombolysis. 2016;41:32–67.
36. Garcia DA, Baglin TP, Weitz JI, et al. Parenteral anticoagulants: Antithrombotic Therapy and Prevention of Thrombosis, 9th ed: American College of Chest Physicians Evidence-Based Clinical Practice Guidelines. Chest. 2012;141:e24S–43S.
37. Konstantinides S, Torbicki A. Management of venous thrombo-embolism: an update. Eur Heart J. 2014;35:2855–63.
38. Holbrook A, Schulman S, Witt DM, et al. Evidence-based management of anticoagulant therapy: Antithrombotic Therapy and Prevention of Thrombosis, 9th ed: American College of Chest Physicians Evidence-Based Clinical Practice Guidelines. Chest. 2012;141:e152S–84S.

Surgical Complications in Management of Musculoskeletal Oncology Cases

44

Lokesh Garg

44.1 Introduction

Through limb salvage surgery (LSS), musculoskeletal oncology patient gain a chance at an active, disease-free life, and goal is to preserve function, prevent tumor recurrence, and enable the rapid administration of chemo- or radiation therapy [1]. In recent years the number of limbs sparing surgeries for bone tumors has increased due to advances in imaging techniques, chemotherapy, radiation therapy, and operations that increase patient survival. Bone tumor excision often develops a large defect in the bone, prompting physicians to look for an appropriative function-preserving alternative after massive resection of the bone tumor and affected soft tissue. There are several methods for preserving limb length and filling bone defects after excision of the tumor include: megaprosthesis (custom made, modular replacement, endoprosthesis), allograft-prosthetic composite, and allograft alone.

The limb salvage operation usually needs to do an extensive dissection in a host in poor medical status. Therefore, the occurrence of complications is related to multiple factors, like: (1) age (physis open or closed), (2) site involved (central or axial), (3) method of reconstruction chosen (biological or prosthesis), (4) biology of tumor, (5) tumor extension and structure involved, (6) timing of adjuvant treatment, (7) plastic reconstruction (needed or not). Since some problems are still encountered, we offer a systematic understanding for complications in the management of musculoskeletal tumors that we have encountered so far.

The complications which may be originated from the resection could be divided into two main groups as age-independent and age-dependent. Age-independent complications can further be grouped as biological and endoprosthetic etiology; the

L. Garg (✉)
Musculoskeletal/Orthopaedic Oncology, Dharamshila Narayana Superspeciality Hospital, Delhi, New Delhi, India

K. Sood Sharma et al. (eds.), *Complications of Cancer Therapy: Best Practices in Prevention and Management*, https://doi.org/10.1007/978-981-99-0984-1_44

former including infection and non-union, and the latter laxity, shortness, implant failure and restricted range of motion. Age-dependent complications can be categorized as three subgroups: physis loss, definite physis injury, and radiotherapy-induced injury. Physeal loss presents with shortness, partial loss of physis with deformity, and sequel of radiotherapy with deformity and pelvis asymmetry.

In 2014, Hendersons published a modified classification of failure after limb salvage surgery [2]. Types of failure after endoprosthetic reconstruction. *Type 1 failures: soft-tissue failure*. Soft-tissue failures are classified as failure of function (type 1A) and failure of cover (type 1B). Functional failures resulting in dysfunction as a result of instability, such as dislocation or symptomatic subluxation of a joint, excessive soft-tissue resection, tendon rupture, and poor soft-tissue ingrowth into the prosthesis. Failures of cover involve aseptic wound dehiscence. A failure of cover may lead to deep infection, but if an infection occurs secondary to inadequate soft-tissue cover. *Type 2 failures: aseptic loosening*. In order to accommodate these temporal and aetiological differences, failures causing aseptic loosening have been subclassified as early (<2 years, type 2A) and late (>2 years, type 2B). *Type 3 failures: structural failure*. Structural failures have been subclassified according to the site of dysfunction. Implant wear or breakages requiring revision are considered type 3A and peri-prosthetic fractures are considered type 3B. *Type 4 failures: infection*. Further classified into early infection (<2 years, type 4A), and late (>2 years, type 4B). *Type 5 failures: recurrence of disease*. Failure of limb salvage due to a recurrent tumour as a consequence of contamination at the time of the endoprosthetic reconstruction has been subclassified to differentiate between recurrence within the soft tissues (type 5A) and recurrence within bone (type 5B). *Type 6 failures: failure of limb salvage in paediatric patients*. The lengthening mechanism of expandable implants may fail and this is considered to be a structural failure, or type 3A. However, types of failures include Physeal arrest (type 6A) and joint dysplasia (type 6B).

Types of failure after biological reconstruction. *Type 1 failure: soft-tissue failure*. Type 1A is functional loss due to insufficient musculo-ligamentous attachment. Type 1B is due to aseptic wound dehiscence. *Type 2 failures: non-union at the graft–host junction*. Subclassified to reflect the local biological healing capacity of the host, hypertrophic (type 2A) and atrophic non-union (type 2B), thereby indicating whether an improvement in stability is likely to result in union at the allograft–host junction. *Type 3 failures: structural failure*. These failures have been subclassified as failure of fixation (type 3A) and fracture of the allograft (type 3B). *Type 4 failures: infection*. Allograft infections are subclassified as early (A) and late (B), defined as within or beyond 6 months of implantation. *Type 5 failures: recurrent disease*. Similar to endoprostheses, failures due to recurrent tumour are subclassified according to the site of recurrence owing to differences in the treatment required for each location. Soft-tissue recurrences abutting an allograft (type 5A), or Bony recurrence (type 5B). *Type 6 failures: salvage after failure in paediatric patients*. Subclassified as premature Physeal arrest (type 6A) and joint dysplasia (type 6B).

Incidence and factors affecting complications:

1. *Infection*: The extensive excision of tumor and the surrounding soft tissue without a good soft tissue reconstruction is usually complicated by wound necrosis and subsequent infection. In addition, prolonged exposure during the operation makes bacteria seeding followed by wound infection a potential problem. It may postpone the planned adjuvant chemotherapy and, at times, the limb may end up with an amputation. Incidence of infection ranges from 6% to 30% in different studies [3].
2. *Flap necrosis*: Major factors is site, size and feasibility of large incision for tumor dissection. Chances of flap necrosis increases with large dissection, long surgical time, previous wrong biopsy that led to unusual incision. Incidence were increased with adjuvant radiation to the surgical site.
3. *Neuro-vascular injury*: The malignant bone tumors usually abut and, at times, encase the major neurovascular bundles. Thus, the dissection of tumor usually has a possibility to cause a neurovascular injury. Vascular injury may occur as a venous thrombosis, arterial or venous intimal damage, direct laceration of vessels, or pulmonary embolism in the early postoperative period. Neurapraxia is an early complication of limb salvage, and may take at least a year to resolve. Tumour encasement of a nerve may require the sacrifice of a nerve during resection. Etiologies include direct traction and dissection during surgery and neurotoxicity of chemotherapeutic agents. In the lower extremity, common peroneal neurapraxia is seen in approximately 14% of cases [4]. The condition is most common after upper extremity reconstructions, where the radial and ulnar nerves are usually affected in approximately 34% of cases [5].
4. *Joint contracture (stiffness)*: A comprehensive rehabilitation program is essential for the restoration of the limb function, such as range of motion, muscle strength, joint stability, etc. Unfortunately, the loss of extensive myofascial tissue after wide resection of malignant tumor and the general weakness of the patients may hinder a vigorous rehabilitation program of the involved joint. The lengthening replacement with a longer segment, on the other hand, will induce a contracture. The proximal tibial reconstructions are immobilized for 3–6 more weeks to provide healing of reconstructed extensor mechanism. Thus, a temporary stiffness may occur in the early postoperative period.
5. *Non-union*: This complication is relatively higher in limb salvage group than trauma fracture fixation, due to higher operating time, large and extensive dissection and periosteal striping, leading to devascularisation if bone. Nonunion of the allograft–host bone junction is reported to occur in 4–50% of cases, making it the most common cause of failure [6]. Nonunion is affected by radiation therapy and chemotherapy. After the course of chemotherapy is complete, healing should occur. However, radiation has longer-term effects and may reduce healing at the allograft–host junction permanently.
6. *Endoprosthesis failure*: Hardware fracture is another late complication, which is seen more frequently in limb salvage and revision arthroplasty when compared with conventional joint replacement surgery. This is because limb salvage is performed in a younger, more active patient population. There is less soft tissue support in the surgical resection site and larger, more constrained

implants. The larger implants create strong bending forces through a long lever arm [7]. Immediate clinical outcomes of the endoprosthetic reconstruction of extremity is promising, however, the long-term survival of the prosthesis deteriorated year by year. Prosthesis survival is determined by many parameters, such as prosthesis design, site, fabrication techniques, extent of resection of soft tissue and its reconstruction, wound healing, etc. The prosthetic survival was 89% for proximal femur, and for distal femur, 59%, for proximal tibia. The overall general endoprosthetic survival rate was 85–91% at 3 years, 79–87% at 5 years, 65–80% at 10 years, 56% at 15 years, and 53% achieved 20 years survival [8]. Telemetric studies by Taylor et al. have demonstrated that offset of the tip of prosthesis from weight bearing axis is important for future survival of endoprosthesis. An increment in offset will increase the bending moment around the prosthesis and cause loosening [9]. The overall complication rate was 20–41%, including mechanical failure rate: 5–16%, dislocation or instability rate: 5–8%, prosthetic failure 5%, loosening rate: 2–7%, polyethylene wear, 2%, local recurrence 4–11%, wound complication 6%, infection 5–15%, neuropraxia 5%. The expandable prosthesis has the highest complication rate, may be up the 70%. The early detection and early correction of minor complications, such as worn polyethylene bushing, resulted in a significant reduction of implant failure, thus it may prevent the occurrence of major complications, such as an accelerated process of bone resorption, aseptic loosening, secondary osteoarthritis, fatigue, etc.

7. *Allograft failure or fracture*: Structural failures of allograft occur in 6–42% of cases and are usually fractures of the graft. Allografts usually incorporate themselves at approximately 8 months but may take as long as 18 months. Nonunion rates are as high as 6–33%. Causative factors of nonunion include the effects of chemotherapy and radiation therapy, inadequate soft tissue coverage, infection, and poor nutritional status of the patient as well as immunologic factors. Non irradiated graft have less fracture and more union rate.
8. *Limb length discrepancy*: The potential of limb growth impaired after the involved major growth plate was removed during resection of tumor tissue. The resultant leg length discrepancy is common and may compromise the function in the Pediatric patients.
9. *Physeal damage*: Incidence could be ranged from 10% to 30% depending on extent of tumor and distance between tumor and physis.
10. *Aseptic loosening of implant*: Conventional aseptic loosening due to resorption of bone, usually due to microscopic polyethylene debris. Technical issues may also play a role as, like, under sizing of uncemented implants or poor cementing technique for cemented implants. Patients undergoing adjuvant treatments may present with an early form of aseptic loosening resulting from poor bone ingrowth and the formation of a fibrous bone–implant junction. Extramedullary callus formation and bone ingrowth at the bone–prosthesis interface should be seen on follow-up radiography within the first 3–6 months. The early signs of aseptic loosening include focal osteopenia and cortical thinning followed by

frank osteolysis. Aseptic loosening is very unusual in the upper extremity but is seen in association with 2–20% of lower-extremity endoprostheses [10].

11. *Local recurrence*: Local recurrence after limb salvage means a complete failure in the tumor management effort. The common possible factors are related to the aggressiveness of the tumor with wide extension resulting in causing poor response to chemotherapy, difficult to achieve a wide safe margin, and poor local circumstance for other adjuvant therapy, such as radiation, etc. The local recurrence rate in patients treated with primary amputation is 2.4%, the 4–11% local recurrence rate after endoprosthetic reconstruction is acceptable [11].
12. *Dislocation or subluxation of endoprosthesis*: Most dislocation/subluxation of the joint are related to the inadequate soft tissue repair and improper use of the patients. The common contributory factors to a dislocation of endoprosthesis include mechanical failure of the joint mechanism, poor muscles and fascia constraints, improper orientation of the prosthesis, accidental trauma or falls, etc. Dislocation or subluxation of the knee endoprosthesis is uncommon, as compared to the femoral or humerus head component in the hip or shoulder hemiarthroplasty. Dislocation or subluxation of an endoprosthesis is most frequent with upper-extremity replacements, occurring in 5–11% of cases [12].
13. *Periprosthetic fracture*: The periprosthetic fracture may occur after an accident. The contributory factors include local periprosthetic osteopenia, loosening of stem, stress shielding effect, etc. Local osteolysis usually makes a thin cortex around the stem in the long run. Thus a minor force may cause the periprosthetic fracture.

Treatment of complication depends on the complication extent, type of resection and reconstruction done previously.

1. *Infection*: It can be deal with antibiotic or incision and drainage, if only superficial infection happens. If deep infection happened, incision and drainage with antibiotic coverage. Treatment of allograft or endoprosthetic infections generally requires removal of the graft or implant and a two-stage revision procedure using another allograft, a prosthesis, a vascularised autograft or a combination of these implants.
2. *Vascular or nerve injury*: Careful dissection reduces the incidence of nerve palsy. This complication can be deal with repair of defect with the help of plastic or vascular surgeon.
3. *Flap necrosis*: Treatment usually depend on extent of necrosis, can be treated with debridement, revision flap, skin grafting, vacuum dressing.
4. *Positive margins*: Chances of positive margins increases in cases of previously done wrong biopsy, scar and drain exit. Revision surgery may be required, plan depending on site of margin, planning and histology of tumor. In case of STS or Ewings Sarcoma and planned closed margin, adj. RT can help. In case of osteosarcoma, Chondrosarcoma, revision is must, in some cases amputation may be required.

5. *Joint contracture (stiffness)*: The joint stiffness may be associated an increased local torsional stress and bending force, resulting in prosthetic failure or loosening. Therefore, an early closed or open manipulation is usually needed if the range of motion cannot recover in the first 2 months. The manipulation should be careful because of the local osteopenia in the cortex after endoprosthetic reconstruction.
6. *Implant failure*: Revision surgery will be required and sometime amputation or Rotationplasty needs to be done, depending of remaining bone stock and functional need of patient.
7. *Dislocation or subluxation of endoprosthesis*: Careful repair of surrounding soft tissue to form a balanced soft tissue cuff and stable fibrous sleeve, proper assemble of the joint component, correct prosthetic orientation, postoperative bracing and casting, tendon transfers and/or myotenodesis, as well as appropriate protection in the initial postoperative period may all decrease the incidence of dislocation or subluxation of component. The use of Merseline tape or Dacron vascular graft material around the reconstructed joint can help prevent this complication [12].
8. *Non-union*: Osteoarticular fractures are usually remediated by conventional total joint replacement. To prevent fracture, dual reconstruction plates or intramedullary nails should span the length of the graft. Bone-allograft junction non-union can be treated with help of revision rigid fixation and bone grafting. While doing Allograft prosthesis composite, care must take to ensure that no cement was caught on the graft–host interface.
9. *Allograft fracture or failure*: Failures of fixation typically occur early in the post-operative period, prior to union at the allograft–host junction, and may be treated by revision of the fixation. Allograft fractures occur both early and late. Typically early fractures occur at the allograft–host junction; periarticular fractures, resulting from subchondral resorption of bone causing inadequate support of the articular surface. Late allograft fractures occur secondary to creeping substitution and revascularisation of the graft, typically near or around screw holes. The graft is strongest at implantation and weakest as incorporation occurs [13]. Not all allograft fractures require replacement of the allograft, as some may heal with revision of the fixation and autograft placement.
10. *Local recurrence*: Some patients have a chance of re-excision of the recurrent tumor, however, some patients may end up with amputation. Strict selection of surgical indication and adjuvant therapy, adequate wide resection, postoperative local therapy for possibly contaminated margin, help reduce the local recurrence through the local tumoricidal effect. Regular follow-up protocol for the early detection and treatment of the local recurrence is very important.
11. *Limb length discrepancy (LLD)*: Minor LLD can be due to human error of measurement while resection, need close follow-up or can be treated with shoe raise. Multiple operations are usually needed to address the leg length discrepancy. Major LLD can be treated with osteotomy and illizarov. In Pediatric cases with open physis, LLD can be prevented with epiphysiodesis of contralateral epiphysis. Deformity correction might be needed for major deformity.

Therefore, some surgeons argue primary amputation for the Pediatric patients. The development of the expandable prosthesis provides a temporary solution at the expense of higher rate of complications, and these patients almost require major revision before or at skeletal maturity [14]. These expandable endoprostheses may be lengthened invasively through multiple operations with a higher risk of infection. New generation growing endoprosthesis can be lengthened by the external magnetic field.

12. *Aseptic loosening*: This can be prevented with proper implant sizing and cementing. Careful watch over the progression and timely intervention is important to prevent periprosthetic fracture.
13. *Restricted range of motion*: Treated with physical therapy, or soft tissue release.
14. *Periprosthetic fracture*: Such a situation is difficult to treat because of the poor bone quality. A plate-wire system may provide a good solution to this difficult situation.

Some complications are specific to the procedure with sterilization of bone graft with liquid nitrogen. We kept this in separate section due its technically demanding and difference from other procedure. In contrast to the hyperthermic methods, liquid nitrogen sterilization of primary malignant bone tumors retains the osteoinductive potential of the recycled bone [15].

1. *Skin necrosis*: Usually happened in pedicle freezing when soft tissue not protected sufficiently. Care must be taken to keep pedicle away from margin of container. Can be managed with regular dressing for superficial necrosis, may need flap coverage for deep and extensive necrosis.
2. *Fracture of graft*: This can happen because of water volume expansion during freezing. Chances are increases if lesion is sclerotic and dense. This can be prevented by making one or two cortical holes drilled (with a 2.5-mm drill bit) into the medullary canal, preferably in the same direction in which the cortical screws of the plate to fix the graft would be passed.
3. *Resorption of autograft*: This is the unique late complication with Liquid nitrogen treated autograft. Most of the patient does not need any intervention, careful observation and protected weightbearing with a brace was recommended to prevent a pathologic fracture. Usually with time, new bone formation happens, may need revision with endoprosthesis or revised reconstruction with allograft. This can be decreased with the use of vascularised fibula grafting with autograft.

Complication due to amputation: Ablative surgery may be the final strategy to achieve cure, but it will still permit the patient to ambulate on a prosthetic limb. A stump neuroma may develop after nerve transection, and this may be quite painful. A neuroma is the body's attempt at nerve regeneration characterized by disorganized, elongating axons. Flap necrosis at stump, prosthetic fitting is complication after amputation.

44.2 Conclusion

A limb sparing surgical approach to achieve success depends on the recognition of the anatomy of tumoral tissues by appropriate radiological methods, complete resection of tumor, biological destruction of tumor, conservation of surrounding healthy tissues, and reparation and restoration of the tissue remained after resection. The selection of limb salvage modality needs to consider carefully the radiological staging, pathological staging and clinical status. The custom-made metallic endoprosthesis can permit an immediate rehabilitation program and provide a durable and functional limb after operation, while biological reconstruction is more tedious and complicated but once succeed gives excellent long-term results. More understanding of the biology of sarcoma, introduction of new effective chemotherapeutic agents, development of new techniques concerning the surgical resection, advances in diagnostic methods, and improvements in reconstructive surgery all make a major contribution to limb salvage surgery. In addition to a well-planned operation and comprehensive postoperative rehabilitation, the proper prosthesis design, good soft tissue coverage/healing, and adequate stability of reconstruction all contribute the final outcomes. The common complications include wound problem, infection, aseptic loosening, fatigue fracture, dislocation/subluxation, mechanical failure, polyethylene failure, etc., and may occur early or late. Careful attention to preoperative planning and intraoperative technique help minimize their incidence. Furthermore, continued early detection and correction of the minor complications may reduce the occurrence of major complication, prolong the survival of the reconstruction, and improve the functional outcomes of limbs for the oncologic patients.

Key Points

- Surgeon should be well versed with the procedure and should know how to deal with complications.
- Patient and relatives should be well informed about procedures and different options available, their benefit, possible functional outcome and chances of complications.
- Biopsy should always be done by Orthopaedic Onco Surgeon for Musculoskeletal Onco cases, to prevent extra-compartmental contamination of tumor.
- Before planning biopsy, surgeon should have provisional diagnosis, and possible surgical options in his mind.
- Pre-operative planning includes (a) MRI discussion with onco-radio, (b) use of modern technique where needed, e.g., 3D printing, Computer navigation, keeping bone model in operating room.
- All cases should be passed through multi-disciplinary tumor board discussion, for planning the treatment of complications and its implication on adjuvant treatment options.
- Meticulous planning and calculation of bone resection and its resection is very important for preventing limb length discrepancy.
- High volume centres have low chances of complications, as musculoskeletal oncology surgery have long learning curve.

- Orthopaedic Onco Surgeon, Plastic Surgeon and Vascular Surgeon should work as team to execute the big resection and reconstruction.
- Execution of planning intra-operatively, immediate acceptance and identification of any mistake done, and strict & immediate action to improve it. Nothing should be left in doubt.

References

1. Simon MA, Springfield D. Surgery for bone and soft tissue tumors. Philadelphia: Lippincott–Raven Publishers; 1998. p. 227–31.
2. Henderson ER, O'Connor MI, Ruggieri P, Windhager R, Funovics PT, Gibbons CL, Guo W, Hornicek FJ, Temple HT, Letson GD. Classification of failure of limb salvage after reconstructive surgery for bone tumours: a modified system including biological and expandable reconstructions. Bone Joint J. 2014;96-B(11):1436–40. https://doi.org/10.1302/0301-620X.96B11.34747.
3. Jeys LM. Periprosthetic infection in patients treated for an orthopaedic oncological condition. J Bone Joint Surg Am. 2005;87-A:842–9.
4. Safran MR, Kody MH, Namba RS, et al. Endoprosthetic reconstruction for patients with primary tumors involving bone. Contemp Orthop. 1994;29:15–25.
5. Wittig JC, Bickels J, Kellar-Graney KL, et al. Osteosarcoma of the proximal humerus: long term results with limb sparing surgery. Clin Orthop. 2002;397:156–76.
6. Mankin HJ, Gebhardt MC, Jennings LC, Springfield DS, Tomford WW. Longterm results of allograft replacement in the management of bone tumors. Clin Orthop Relat Res. 1996;324:86–97.
7. Peabody TD, Eckhardt JJ. Complications of prosthetic reconstructions. In: Simon MA, Springfield D, editors. Surgery for bone and soft tissue tumors. Philadelphia: Lippincott–Raven Publishers; 1998. p. 467–79.
8. Mittermayer F, Windhager F, Dominkus M, et al. Revision of the Kotz type of tumour endoprosthesis for the lower limb. J Bone Joint Surg. 2002;84B:401–6.
9. Taylor S, Perry J, Adler J, et al. The telemetry of forces in vivo developed in massive orthopaedic implants: the first 18 months, results from walking. In: Tan SK, editor. Limb salvage: current trends. Singapore: ISOLS; 1993. p. 560.
10. Eckhardt JJ, Eilber FR, Rosen G, et al. Endoprosthetic replacement for stage IIB osteosarcoma. Clin Orthop. 1991;270:202–13.
11. Picci P, Sangiorgi L, Bahamonde L, Aluigi P, Bibiloni J, Zavatta M, Mercuri M, Briccoli A, Campanacci M. Risk factors for local recurrences after limb-salvage surgery for high-grade osteosarcoma of the extremities. Ann Oncol. 1997;8(9):899–903.
12. Asavamongkolkul A, Eckhardt JJ, Eilber FR, et al. Endoprosthetic reconstruction for malignant upper extremity tumors. Clin Orthop. 1999;360:207–20.
13. Wilkins RM. Complications of allograft reconstructions. In: Simon MA, Springfield D, editors. Surgery for bone and soft tissue tumors. Philadelphia: Lippincott–Raven Publishers; 1998. p. 487–97.
14. Eckardt JJ, Kabo JM, Kelley CM, et al. Expandable endoprosthesis reconstruction in skeletally immature patients with tumors. Clin Orthop. 2000;373:51–61.
15. Tsuchiya H, Wan SL, Sakayama K, Yamamoto N, Nishida H, Tomita K. Reconstruction using an autograft containing tumour treated by liquid nitrogen. J Bone Joint Surg Br. 2005;87:218–25.

Part III

Miscellaneous Complications

45 Prevention and Treatment of Infective Complications During Cancer Therapy

Gitali Bhagawati and Sania Paul

45.1 Introduction

Although there is advancement in the treatment and overall management of cancer leading to significant improvement in prolonged survival of cancer patients, infections still remain a significant cause of morbidity and mortality in this group of patients with neoplastic diseases. Neutropenia and subsequent infectious complications are among the most serious treatment-related toxicities of cancer treatment and result in preventable morbidity and mortality [1, 2]. However, with the increasing antimicrobial resistance (AMR), both in pre and post-Covid-19 era, it has become a challenging task for the clinicians to treat infections among these patients who are prone to such infections because of a complicated matrix of host's immunodeficiency, local tumor effect, treatment-induced immunosuppression and environmental effect. AMR-related infections claim at least 50,000 lives each year across Europe and the US alone, with many hundreds of thousands more dying in other areas of the world but the reliable estimates of the true burden are scarce [3].

Prolonged hospital stay of host in health care organization (HCO) for cancer care is again a double-edged sword which can lead to health care-associated infections (HAI) with the multi-drug resistant organism (MDRO), extensively drug resistant (XDR) or pan-drug resistant (PDR) organisms.

In high-income countries, approximately 30% of patients in intensive care units (ICU) are affected by at least one HAI which is two to threefold higher in low- and

G. Bhagawati (✉)
Department of Microbiology and Infection Control, Dharamshila Narayana Superspeciality Hospital, Delhi, New Delhi, India

S. Paul
Department of Microbiology, Dharamshila Narayana Superspeciality Hospital, Delhi, New Delhi, India

K. Sood Sharma et al. (eds.), *Complications of Cancer Therapy: Best Practices in Prevention and Management*, https://doi.org/10.1007/978-981-99-0984-1_45

middle-income countries (LMIC) [4]. In India, the overall prevalence of HAIs was found to be 7%, and surgical site infections (SSI) were the most common (33%) [5]. HAI risk is found to be more amongst cancer patients with MDRO leading to increased therapeutic failure and high mortality rates [6–9]. Neutropenic patients or patients with hematological malignancies (HM) are more vulnerable to infections as compared to patients with solid tumors [9].

Covid-19 pandemic was a major challenge for the oncologists to deliver continuous quality care with minimum patients' risk of exposure to Covid-19 infection. The negative impact was more evident in LMICs; contributing factors include poor laboratory infrastructure for prompt diagnosis, population burden, shortage of human resource in HCO, Covid-19 infected health care workers, shortage of personal protective equipment (PPE), poor access to technology, etc. leading to lack of ability to provide and deliver critical care, cessation of cancer screening and delayed hospital visits [10–13].

A good multidisciplinary hospital infection prevention and control (ICP) program plays a keen role in prevention of both is community-acquired infections and HAIs. These measures should be stringently implemented and monitored among immunocompromised group of patients to break the chain of transmission of infections. Another multidisciplinary approach that plays a great role in this era of MDR, XDR and PDR organisms is Antimicrobial stewardship program (AMSP) which is the utmost need of the hour for optimum utilization of prevailing antimicrobial with standard dose and duration while minimizing negative consequences such as development of bacterial resistance.

Here, we shall mainly focus on infections and its preventive measures and treatment for the infective complications in the cancer care setting.

45.2 Infectious Complications of Cancer and Cancer Treatment

45.2.1 Epidemiological Triad

A classic epidemiological triad model of infectious disease shows that an infectious disease results from a combination of agent, host, and environmental factors (Fig. 45.1). Infectious agent can be any pathogen including bacteria, virus, fungus, parasite, etc. Agent and host interactions occur in a cascade of stages that include infection, disease, and recovery or death [14].

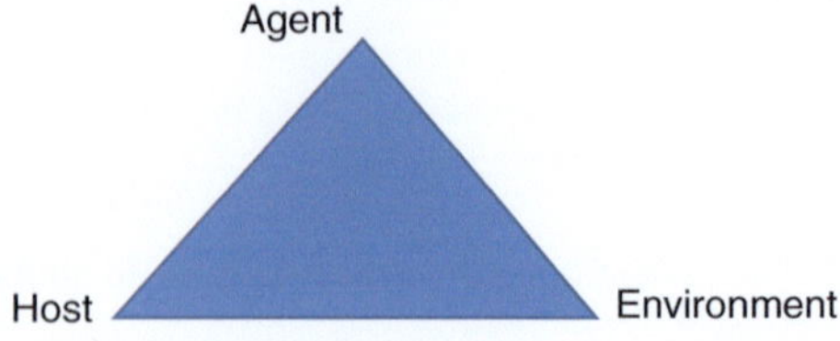

Fig. 45.1 Classical epidemiological triad

Cancer patients are those immunocompromised 'Host' who has defects in their body's normal defence mechanisms that predispose the person to infections that can be often life threatening which would not be otherwise occur in inmmunocompetent one. Infections are common during the course of disease and its treatment; 80% patients with acute leukemia, 40–60% with lung cancer and 50% with lymphoma, develop infection at some point in the course of the illness [15].

Clinical manifestation of disease may also be different in this group of patients, which include [16]:

- Rapid progression of disease
- Abnormal radiological/laboratory findings
- Less pain perception while on sedation, etc.

Literature has shown various infection rates in both solid tumour and haematological malignancies [HM]. Blood stream infection rates are similar in both the cases; 32.53% [17], 17% [18] in solid tumour; 33.33% [17], 11.8–40% [19] in HM. Respiratory tract infections are found to be more in solid tumour; 34.93% [17], 10% [20] as compared to HM 19.2% [17], 3.3% [21] (Table 45.1).

Cancer chemotherapy and organ transplantation are just two examples of medical treatments that leave the patient highly vulnerable to bacterial infections (Table 45.1).

Table 45.1 List of host factors in cancer patients leading to infectious complications [15, 16]

Serial no.	Defect at the level of	Example
1	Skin	• Cancer itself example, basal cell carcinoma • Surgical incisions • Indwelling intravenous lines • Trauma or damage to skin induced by irradiation/chemotherapy
2	Mucous membrane	• Poor oral hygiene (especially in head and neck cancers) • Mucositis induced by irradiation/chemotherapy • Endotracheal tube/nasogastric tube insertion • Foley catheterisation
3	Obstruction of natural body passage	• Seen in many cancers like carcinoma oesophagus, carcinoma lung, carcinoma ovary, etc.
4	Abnormal granulocyte number and function	• Acute leukemia, hairy cell leukemia • Bone marrow transplant recipients • Chemotherapy induced
5	Impairment of cell-mediated immunity (CMI)	• Bone marrow transplant recipients • Chemotherapeutic agents: purine analogues, particularly fludarabine, cladribine, etc.
6	Abnormal humoral immunity	• Bone marrow transplant recipients • Chronic lymphocytic leukaemia • Multiple myeloma, etc.

45.2.2 Major Nosocomial Infection Causing Organisms

ESKAPE pathogens are responsible for majority of nosocomial bacterial infections both in pre and post Covid era. It includes:

- *Enterococcus faecium* [MDRO—Vancomycin resistant Enterococcus (VRE)]
- *Staphylococcus aureus* [MDRO—Methicillin Resistant *Staphylococcus aureus* (MRSA)]
- *Klebsiella pneumonia* [MDRO—Carbapenem resistant Enterobacterales (CRE)]
- *Acinetobacter baumanii* [MDRO—Carbapenem resistant *Acinetobacter baumanii* (CRAB)]
- *Pseudomonas aeruginosa* [MDRO—Carbapenem resistant *Pseudomonas aeruginosa* (CRPA)]
- *Enterobacter* spp. [MDRO—Carbapenem resistant Enterobacterales (CRE)]

45.2.3 Other Opportunistic Organisms Causing Disease in Cancer Patients

45.2.3.1 Bacteria

- Coagulase negative Staphylococcus (CONS)
- *Streptococcus* spp. (Viridans Streptococci, *Streptococcus pneumoniae*, *Streptococcus pyogenes*)
- *Enterococcus* spp.
- *Escherichia coli*
- *Listeria monocytogenes*
- *Legionella* spp.
- *Bacteroides* spp.
- *Clostridium* spp.

45.2.3.2 Fungi

- *Candida albicans*
- Non-albicans Candida (NAC) (includes *C. tropicalis*, *C. glabrata*, *C. krusei*, *C. auris*, etc.)
- *Trichosporon* spp.
- *Aspergillus* spp.
- Zygomycetes (Mucor, Rhizopus, etc.)
- Other molds (Fusarium, *Pseudoallescheria boydii*, *Scedosporium* spp., etc.)

45.2.3.3 Viruses

- Herpes virus group
- Measles virus
- Adenovirus
- Enterovirus
- Respiratory syncytial virus (RSV)

- Influenza virus

45.2.3.4 Protozoa

- *Plasmodium* spp.
- *Strongyloides stercoralis*, etc.

45.2.4 Antimicrobial Resistance (AMR) and Cancer

Among Gram negative bacterial isolates, CRE, CRPA and CRAB are growing cause of HAIs. According to the latest report from Indian Council of Medical Research (ICMR)—AMR surveillance network, resistance to imipenem was found in 28%, 55% and 80% in *E. coli*, *K. pneumoniae* and *A. baumannii* respectively. Hypervirulent carbapenem-resistant (CR) *K. pneumoniae* strains present an additional threat in Indian hospitals with a potential for global dissemination [22].

CRE is increasingly observed to cause bacteremia among HM patients due to increased colonization. One Indian study showed *E. coli* as the most common (83.2%) CRE, followed by *Klebsiella* spp. (9.6%). ^{bla}NDM-1 was the most common gene (57.3%), followed by ^{bla}OXA-48 (37.8%); 26.8% isolates found to carry both ^{bla}NDM-1 and ^{bla}OXA-48 genes [23].

The magnitude of the AMR has been accepted worldwide; it is estimated that by 2050, 10 million lives a year are at risk due to the rise of infections by MDROs if we do not find proactive solutions. Even today, 700,000 people die of resistant infections every year. AMR can be a cause of failure of treatment despite modern treatment modalities used for cancer patients [24].

Resistance to antimicrobials is a natural phenomenon that has been observed since the first antibiotics were discovered. However, AMR has increasingly become a problem in recent times because of overuse and misuse of antimicrobials and we lack new drugs to challenge these new superbugs [24].

Most invasive 'dirty' surgeries (involving gut) among cancer patients are usually 'de-risked' by effective antimicrobial prophylaxis used prior to surgery with re-dosing as per half-life of the drug. However, this could be challenging if the antibiotic stops its function. Intubated cancer patients in ICU experience very high rates of MDR, XDR and PDR-infections and the mortality risk associated with this rises with depletion of treatment options for such infections [24].

45.2.5 Covid-19 Infection, AMR and Cancer [25]

A comparative analysis on bacterial isolates and antimicrobial susceptibility pattern (ASP) was done from admitted patients with respiratory tract infection (RTI) from both Covid-19 positive group (CPG) and Covid-19 Negative group (CNG). Out of 36 CPG, only 12 had cancer-comorbidity (33.33%) while in 102-CNG, 79 patients (77.45%) had cancer. No statistically significant difference was observed in bacterial isolates as well in their ASP (Fig. 45.2).

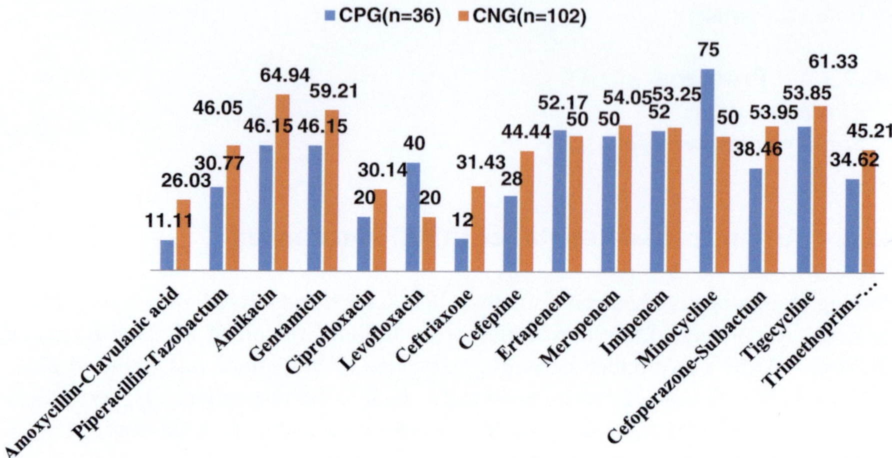

Fig. 45.2 Comparative analysis of antimicrobial susceptibility pattern of Enterobacterales in both CPG and CNG

Table 45.2 Components of standard precautions

1. Hand hygiene
2. Use of personal protective equipment (e.g., gloves, masks, eyewear)
3. Biomedical waste management (BMWM)
4. Sharps safety (engineering and work practice controls)
5. Safe injection practices
6. Sterilization and disinfection
7. Environmental cleaning
8. Respiratory hygiene/cough etiquette

45.3 Strategies to Prevent HAIs and AMR [26, 27]

45.3.1 Standard Precautions (SP)

Standard precautions, previously called universal precautions, are a set of infection control practices that apply to all patient care, regardless of suspected or confirmed infection status of the patient, in any setting where health care is delivered.

For cancer care, although each component of SP plays an important role, overall hygiene contributes the major part in infection prevention (Table 45.2).

45.3.2 Hygiene

45.3.2.1 Hand Hygiene

Poor hand hygiene (HH) among healthcare workers (HCWs) is identified as one of the major causes of HAIs, which is much higher among immuocompromised group. Microorganisms are capable of surviving on HCWs' hands for at least several minutes following contamination, and if HH practices are suboptimal, microbial colonization is more easily established and help in transmission of HAIs through direct or indirect contact [28]. After being scientifically proven, HCWs are reversing back to the basics of infection preventions by simple measures such as HH which alone can significantly reduce HAI rate up to 40% [29].

Among HH practices (Tables 45.3 and 45.4), hand washing is mandatory during patient care in following conditions:

- Visibly soiled hands
- While dealing patients with diarrhoea

Note: Alcohol-based handrubs may not be effective against *C. difficile.* PPE and handwashing with a non-antimicrobial or antimicrobial soap and water following glove removal are highly recommended for *C. difficile* associated diarrhoea

Covid-19 pandemic has spread adequate awareness regarding HH over the globe but to implement the awareness in attitude and practice, continuous motivation of HCWs is necessary. Celebration of World Hand Hygiene Day on May fifth every year should be a part of the motivational programs.

45.3.2.2 Chlorhexidine Bathing

Daily chlorhexidine bathing can decrease acquisition of MRSA by 32% and VRE by 50% thereby reducing colonization leading to reduction in blood stream infections in ICU patients. Another multicenter study involving 9 ICUs and BMT units in six hospitals demonstrated a 23% reduction in MDRO acquisition and a 28% reduction in hospital-associated blood-stream infections with daily chlorhexidine bathing [32]. World Health Organisation (WHO) suggests moderate evidence to bath or shower prior to surgery either with plain soap or an anti-microbial soap to reduce the rate of surgical site infection (SSI) [33, 34].

45.3.2.3 Oral Hygiene

Oral pathogenic organisms can be the potential source of both oral and systemic infection and the reason of failure of successful cancer surgeries with flap reconstruction which can again lead to mortality in neutropenic cancer patients. Oral and

Table 45.3 Types of hand hygiene methods [30]

Types of hand hygiene	Definition	Duration
Hand wash	Washing hands with plain or antimicrobial soap and water (antiseptic agent 4% chlorhexidine)	40–60 s
Hand rub (antiseptic handrub)	Applying an antiseptic handrub to reduce or inhibit the growth of microorganisms; no water or towel is required (antiseptic agent—70–80% ethyl alcohol with or without 0.5–4% chlorhexidine)	20–30 s
Surgical hand scrub	Surgical hand preparation with antimicrobial soap and water (antiseptic agent 4% chlorhexidine)	3–5 min

Table 45.4 'My 5-moments of hand hygiene' includes [31]

5-Moments of hand hygiene	Example
Before touching a patient	Shaking hands, taking pulse, blood pressure, chest auscultation, abdominal palpation, etc.
Before clean/aseptic procedures	Secretion aspiration, skin lesion care, wound dressing, subcutaneous injection; catheter insertion, etc.
After body fluid exposure risk	Secretion aspiration, skin lesion care, wound dressing, subcutaneous injection, drawing and manipulation any fluid sample, opening draining system, endotracheal tube insertion and removal, etc.
After touching a patient	Shaking hands, taking pulse, blood pressure, chest auscultation, abdominal palpation, etc.
After touching patient's surroundings	Changing bed linen, perfusion speed adjustment, holding a bed rail, clearing the bedside table, etc.

periodontal examination is necessary for all patients of head and neck cancer undergoing irradiation/surgery [35].

45.3.2.4 Cleaning, Disinfection and Sterilization

Healthcare facilities must have adequate water and sanitation infrastructure to perform environmental cleaning according to best practices (Table 45.5).

Cleaning is removal of visible dirt, soil, organic matter and other debris which should be performed either manually or mechanically. Before disinfecting, use a cleaning product to remove all organic material and soil.

The patient care items/equipment/instruments used in healthcare have been classified (by Spaulding) according to the degree of risk of infection involved in use of these items [36].

45.3.2.5 Use of Personnel Protective Equipment (PPE)

The PPE provides a physical barrier between micro-organisms and the wearer and prevents transmission of germs from the wearer to other patients and staff. It includes gloves, gowns, masks and respirators, goggles and face shield.

Use of Gloves

- Most patient care activities require the use of a single pair of non-sterile gloves made of either latex, nitrile, or vinyl.
- Sterile surgical gloves (1/2 pairs) are worn by surgeons and other healthcare personnel who perform invasive patient procedures.
- Re-usable heavy-duty gloves made of latex or nitrile are worn by environmental services personnel for cleaning environmental surfaces and to handle biomedical waste. It can reduce the incidence of needle stick injuries.

Do's of Glove Use

- Work from clean to dirty area.
- Limit touch contamination—protect yourself, others, and the environment.

Table 45.5 Spaulding criteria and method of sterilization and disinfection

Device classification	Type of contact	Minimum inactivation level	Example	Method
Critical	Sterile areas of the body including blood contact	Sterilization—free from all viable microorganisms	Surgical instruments, cardiac and urinary catheters, implants, and ultrasound probes	Single use device (SUD)/ autoclave/ ethylene oxide (ETO)/plasma sterilization
Semi-critical	Mucous membranes or non-intact skin	High level disinfection—effective against all microbial pathogens, with the exception of large number of bacterial spores	Aanesthesia equipment, some endoscopes, laryngoscope blades, esophageal manometer probes, cystoscopes, etc.	Glutaraldehyde (>2.0%) Hydrogen peroxide—HP (7.5%) Peracetic acid—PA (0.2%) HP (1.0%) and PA (0.08%) HP (7.5%) and PA (0.23%) Glut (1.12%) and phenol (1.93%) Ortho-phthalaldehyde (OPA) 0.55%
Non-critical items	Intact skin	Physical removal—by cleaning • Low level disinfection—effective against certain bacteria, viruses and fungi • Intermediate level disinfection—effective against bacteria, myco-bacteria, most viruses and fungi, but not spores	Bedpans, BP cuffs, computers	Quaternary ammonium compounds Ethyl or isopropyl alcohol (70–90%) Sodium hypochlorite

(continued)

Table 45.5 (continued)

Device classification	Type of contact	Minimum inactivation level	Example	Method
Non-critical environmental surface	Noncritical environmental surfaces frequently touched by hand	Low level disinfection	Bed rails, utensils, bedside tables, patients' furniture and floors	Quaternary ammonium compounds

Table 45.6 Air-borne transmission related organisms

Evidence for airborne transmission	Fungi	Bacteria	Viruses
Numerous reports in health-care facilities	*Aspergillus* spp. *Mucorales* (*Rhizopus* spp.)	*Mycobacterium tuberculosis*	*Measles (rubeola) virus*, *Varicella-zoster virus*
Occasional reports in health-care facilities	*Acremonium* spp. *Fusarium* spp. *Pseudoallescheria boydii*	*Acinetobacter* spp. *Bacillus* spp. *Brucella* spp. *Staphylococcus aureus* Group A *streptococcus*	*Smallpox virus* (*variola*) Influenza viruses Respiratory syncytial virus Adenoviruses Norwalk-like virus

- Do hand hygiene before and after removal of gloves.
- Discard as per biomedical waste management (BMWM) policy.
- Change if torn or heavily soiled.

Don't of Glove Use

- Don't touch face or adjust PPE with contaminated gloves.
- Don't touch environmental surfaces with contaminated gloves.

Other PPE

Type of PPE should be worn depending on mode of transmission of diseases and risk of exposure.

Perform hand hygiene before and after removing PPE.

PPE should be removed before exiting the patient environment.

PPE should be discarded as per BMWM policy.

45.3.2.6 Transmission Based Precaution Policy

Based on the mode of transmission in hospital environment, precautions can be of three types:

1. Air borne precautions
2. Droplet precautions
3. Contact precautions

1. *Airborne precaution*: Airborne precautions are for containment of airborne transmission that occurs by dissemination of airborne nuclei (<5 μm). Cancer patients are more prone to infections by organism (Table 45.6) spread by airborne droplets.

   Recommendation includes:

   (a) Single room with a separate exhaust to outside (pressure differential should be >−2.5 Pa)
   (b) Clean-to-dirty airflow in room should be towards the patient
   (c) Alerting all care providers of additional precautions needed (i.e., "air borne precautions" sign on resident's door, chart)
   (d) PPE for direct resident care includes:
      - Double face mask/N 95 mask or care of residents within factious pulmonary tuberculosis
      - Removal of PPE on leaving the room
      - Hand hygiene after removing PPE

2. *Droplet precautions*: Droplet precautions are for containment of droplet transmission that occurs by dissemination of respiratory droplets (>5 μm in size) that are generated by coughing, sneezing, talking, suctioning, endotracheal intubation, cardiopulmonary resuscitation, etc. Area of defined risk is about 3 ft around the patient.

   Example: *B. pertussis*, *Influenza virus*, *adenovirus*, *rhinovirus*, *M. pneumoniae*, SARS-associated coronavirus (SARS-CoV), Covid-19, Group A *Streptococcus* and *N. meningitides.*

   Recommendation includes:

   (a) Single room
   (b) Encourage resident for hand hygiene
   (c) Surgical mask/N95 respirator
   (d) Encourage respiratory etiquette practices
   (e) Encourage use of appropriate PPE when providing care
   (f) Removal of PPE on leaving the room
   (g) Hand hygiene after removing PPE

3. *Contact precautions*:

   Diseases requiring contact isolation mainly concerned with cancer patients include all MDR, XRD, PDR organisms; mostly spread via the hands of healthcare workers (Table 45.7).

   Recommendations include proper HH (Tables 45.3 and 45.4) and single room/cohorting.

Table 45.7 Mode of contact transmission

Direct contact	Indirect contact
• Via percutaneous injury (needle stick injury) • Mites from a scabies-infested	• **Hands of healthcare personnel** • Patient-care devices (glucose monitoring) • Shared toys (HM patients) • Improperly decontaminated instruments

45.3.2.7 Adequate Microbiological Infrastructure

For Antimicrobial Stewardship Program (AMSP)

Adequate microbiological infrastructure is necessary for proper functioning of AMSP system.

Identification and antimicrobial susceptibility pattern (ASP) of isolates: Samples of cancer patients should be collected appropriately and processed following standard operating procedure (SOP) for proper identification and ASP.

Antibiogram should be made based on cumulative data at an interval of 4–6 months and that has to be communicated with the oncologists. Both Medical and Surgical Antibiotic policy should be formulated based on antibiogram of the HCO for judicious use of prophylactic and empiric antibiotics.

Culture should be sent prior to the initiation of antibiotic therapy. Escalation and de-escalation of antibiotics should be followed as per ASP.

AMSP can be monitored by front end strategy a (restriction of formulary) or by back end strategy (antibiotic prescription audit, audit of restricted antibiotic usage, etc.)

For Outbreak Prevention

Species level identification and AMS following proper sample collection can act as a primer for prevention of outbreaks in cancer care set ups which is very common by MDROs. With prompt species level identification, stringent infection control measures and continuous monitoring, we could be able to control MDR *C. auris* spread in our hospital [37].

For Surveillance of CRE in Rectal Swab Samples

Gut colonization with CRE has been postulated to be a risk factor for CRE bacteremia, which is associated with high mortality among cancer patients. In a study from Italy, 86% of patients with CRE bacteremia in HM patients were found to be colonized [38]. In our study on HM patients, the incidence of CRE bacteremia in CRE colonized patients was 18% (17/94), and mortality in those with CRE bacteremia was 100% [39].

For surveillance purpose, rectal swab screening for microbiological evaluation of CRE can be done or for the rapid diagnosis, polymerase chain reaction (PCR) or real-time qualitative PCR tests are available for the identification of carbapenemase expressing genes (KPC, IMP, VIM, NDM and OXA-48 like variants) [22]. These surveillance screening can be helpful in taking appropriate IPC measures among the cancer patients.

For Surveillance of Environmental Samples

There are various studies suggesting association between environmental contamination and HAIs with MDROs [40, 41]. Literature suggests relation of damp environmental reservoirs (sink drains, traps and the horizontal drainage system) with MDR coliforms [41]. There are many articles in favour of MDR *K. pneumoniae* persistently harboring in sink and related pipes leading to outbreaks in ICUs [41–43].

Stringent implementation of water surveillance program along with immediate corrective action against the root cause of contamination should be mandatory in each HCO.

45.4 Conclusion

Infection and infectious complications are countless in cancer patients, especially in neutropenic category if adequate IPC measures are not taken seriously. In the era of MDR, XDR and PDR organisms along with the effect of novel virus Covid-19, IPC has become a social responsibility which should be dedicatedly followed when it comes for cancer care. Oncologists should maintain a high index of clinical suspicion for infective complications so that proper sample should be sent for proper diagnostic purpose to for proper management of the patient. Since newer antibiotics are almost nil in the pipeline, irrational or overuse of antibiotic has to be stopped. All surveillance activities and preventive care should get priority in cancer care institute. Microbiological evaluation with AST of the isolates following AMSP should be mandatory to preserve those few left over antibiotics for the future. Otherwise, cancer care without antibiotic for infective complication will remain questionable for its overall success.

References

1. Herbst C, Naumann F, Kruse EB, Monsef I, Bohlius J, Schulz H, Engert A. Prophylactic antibiotics or G-CSF for the prevention of infections and improvement of survival in cancer patients undergoing chemotherapy. Cochrane Database Syst Rev. 2009;1:CD007107.
2. Lyman GH, Michels SL, Reynolds MW, Barron R, Tomic KS, Yu J. Risk of mortality in patients with cancer who experience febrile neutropenia. Cancer. 2010;116:5555–63.
3. An antimicrobial resistance: tackling a crisis for the health and wealth of nations. The Review on Antimicrobial Resistance, Chaired by Jim O'Neill, Dec 2014.
4. https://www.cdc.gov/hai/data/portal. Accessed 2/1/22.
5. Kumar A, Biswal M, Dhaliwal N, Mahesh R, Appannanavar SB, Gautam V, et al. Point prevalence surveys of healthcare-associated infections and use of indwelling devices and antimicrobials over three years in a tertiary care hospital in India. J Hosp Infect. 2014;86:272–4.
6. Montassier E, Batard E, Gastinne T, Potel G, de la Cochetière MF. Recent changes in bacteremia in patients with cancer: a systematic review of epidemiology and antibiotic resistance. Eur J Clin Microbiol Infect Dis. 2013;32:841–50.
7. Neidell NJ, Cohen B, Furuya Y, Hill J, Jeon CY, Glied S, et al. Costs of healthcare- and community-associated infections with antimicrobial-resistant versus antimicrobial-susceptible organisms. Clin Infect Dis. 2012;55:807–15.
8. Kollef MH, Fraser VJ. Antibiotic resistance in the intensive care unit. Ann Intern Med. 2011;134:298–314.
9. Cornejo-Juárez P, Vilar-Compte D, García-Horton A, López-Velázquez M, Ñamendys-Silva S, Volkow-Fernández P. Hospital-acquired infections at an oncological intensive care cancer unit: differences between solid and hematological cancer patients. BMC Infect Dis. 2016;16:274.
10. Bong CL, Brasher C, Chikumba E, et al. The COVID-19 pandemic: effects on low- and middle-income countries. Anesth Analg. 2020;131:86–92.

11. Osseni IA. COVID-19 pandemic in sub-Saharan Africa: preparedness, response, and hidden potentials. Trop Med Health. 2020;48:48.
12. McMahon DE, Peters GA, Ivers LC, et al. Global resource shortages during COVID-19: bad news for low-income countries. PLoS Negl Trop Dis. 2020;14:e0008412.
13. Ranganathan P, Sengar M, Cinnaswamy G, Agrawal G, Arumugham R, Bhatt R. Impact of COVID-19 on cancer care in India: a cohort study. Lancet Oncol. 2021;22(7):970–6.
14. Snieszko SF. The effects of environmental stress on outbreaks of infectious diseases of fishes. In: Environmental Protection Agency workshop: pathologic effects of chemicals on aquatic organisms, Pensacola, Florida, 8 May 1973.
15. Safdar N, Crnich CJ, Maki DG. Chapter 76: Infectious complications of cancer therapy. Oncology, 2006. p. 1363–400.
16. Singhal S. Infections in immunocompromised host. In: Handbook of HIC. 1st ed. CBS Publishers & Distributors; 2013.
17. Bhat S, Muthunatarajan S, Mulki SS, Archana Bhat K, Kotian KH. Bacterial infection among cancer patients: analysis of isolates and antibiotic sensitivity pattern. Int J Microbiol. 2021;2021:8883700.
18. Martin GS, Mannino DM, Eaton S, Moss M. The epidemiology of sepsis in the United States from 1979 through 2000. N Engl J Med. 2003;348:1546–54.
19. Carvalho AS, Lagana D, Catford J, Shaw D, Bak N. Blood stream infection in neutropenic patients with haematological malignancies. Infect Dis Health. 2020;25(1):P22–9.
20. Wong JL, Evans SE. Bacterial pneumonia in patients with cancer: novel risk factors and management. Clin Chest Med. 2017;38(2):263–77.
21. Huoi C, Vanhems P, Nicolle M-C, Michallet M, Bénet T. Incidence of hospital-acquired pneumonia, bacteraemia and urinary tract infections in patients with haematological malignancies, 2004–2010: a surveillance-based study. PLoS One. 2013;8:e58121.
22. Guidance on diagnosis & management of carbapenem resistant gram-negative infections. New Delhi: Division of Epidemiology & Communicable Diseases Indian Council of Medical Research; 2022.
23. Kumar A, et al. Intestinal colonization due to Carbapenem-resistant *Enterobacteriaceae* among hematological malignancy patients in India: prevalence and molecular characterisation. Indian J Hematol Blood Transfus. 2022;38(1):1–7.
24. Tackling drug-resistant infections globally: final report and recommendations. The Review on Antimicrobial Resistance, Chaired by Jim O'Neill, May 2016.
25. Bhagawati G, Paul S, Jaiswal SR, Bhardwaj A, Kumar RS, Mansi, Bhatia A, Chakrabarti S. Microbiological evaluation of patients admitted with acute respiratory illness during first wave of COVID-19 pandemic in New Delhi, India. J Clin Diagn Res. 2022;16(3):DC01–5.
26. https://www.cdc.gov/oralhealth/infectioncontrol/summary-infection-prevention-practices/standard-precautions.html. Accessed 13 May 22.
27. Sastry AS, Bhat S. Hospital infection control. In: Essentials of medical microbiology. 3rd ed. Jaypee Brothers Medical Publishers; 2021. p. 229–6.
28. Ekwere TA, Okafor IP. Hand hygiene knowledge and practices among health care providers in a tertiary hospital, south west, Nigeria. Int J Infect Control. 2013;34:1–10.
29. Kampf G, Löffler H, Gastmeier P. Hand hygiene for the prevention of nosocomial infections. Dtsch Arztebl Int. 2009;106(40):649–55.
30. WHO guidelines on hand hygiene in health care first global patient safety challenge clean care is safer care. WHO Patient Safety. 2009. https://www.who.int/publications-detailredirect/9789241597906. Accessed 13 May 22.
31. https://www.cdc.gov/infectioncontrol/pdf/strive/PPE103-508.pdf. Accessed 13 May 22.
32. Climo MW, Sepkowitz KA, Zuccotti G, et al. The effect of daily bathing with chlorhexidine on the acquisition of methicillin-resistant Staphylococcus aureus, vancomycin-resistant enterococcus, and healthcare-associated bloodstream infections: results of a quasi-experimental multicenter trial. Crit Care Med. 2009;37:1858–65.
33. Climo MW, Yokoe DS, Warren DK, et al. Effect of daily chlorhexidine bathing on hospital-acquired infection. N Engl J Med. 2013;368:533–42.

34. WHO guideline to prevent surgical site infections. 2016. https://www.who.int/teams/integrated-health-services/infection-prevention-control/surgical-site-infection. Accessed 13 May 22.
35. Epstein JB, Stevenson-Moore P. Periodontal disease and periodontal management in patients with cancer. Oral Oncol. 2001;37:613–9.
36. Guideline for disinfection and sterilization in healthcare facilities. 2017. https://www.cdc.gov/infectioncontrol/guidelines/disinfection/index.html. Accessed 13 May 22.
37. Bhagawati G, Jaiswal SR, Bhardwaj A, Sood N, Kumar RS, Lincy TP, Paul S, Mansi, Chakrabarti S. Species level identification of yeast and yeast like fungus for prompt infection control measures in prevention of outbreaks: with special reference to Candida auris in pre-covid era. Acta Sci Microbiol. 2021;4(8):19–25.
38. Micozzi A, Gentile G, Minotti C, Cartoni C, Capria S, Ballaro D, Santilli S, Pacetti E, Grammatico S, Bucaneve G, et al. Carbapenem-resistant Klebsiella pneumoniae in high-risk haematological patients: factors favouring spread, risk factors and outcome of carbapenem-resistant Klebsiella pneumoniae bacteremias. BMC Infect Dis. 2017;17(1):203.
39. Jaiswal SR, Gupta S, Kumar RS, Sherawat A, Rajoreya A, Dash SK, Bhagwati G, Chakrabarti S. Gut colonization with Carbapenem-resistant Enterobacteriaceae adversely impacts the outcome in patients with hematological malignancies: results of a prospective surveillance study. Mediterr J Hematol Infect Dis. 2018;10(1):e2018025.
40. Suleyman G, Alangaden G, Bardossy AC. The role of environmental contamination in the transmission of nosocomial pathogens and healthcare-associated infections. Curr Infect Dis Rep. 2018;20(6):12.
41. Dancer SJ. Controlling hospital-acquired infection: focus on the role of the environment and new technologies for decontamination. Clin Microbiol Rev. 2014;27(4):665–90.
42. Hobson RP, MacKenzie FM, Gould IM. An outbreak of multiply-resistant Klebsiella pneumoniae in the Grampian region of Scotland. J Hosp Infect. 1996;33:249–62.
43. Starlander G, Melhus A. Minor outbreak of extended-spectrum β-lactamase-producing Klebsiella pneumoniae in an intensive care unit due to a contaminated sink. J Hosp Infect. 2012;82:122–4.

Prevention and Management of Complications During Treatment of Childhood Tumors

46

Megha Saroha

There are many advancements that have been done in pediatric oncology with respect to early and better detection, improvement in survival and at the same time minimizing long term adverse effects in cancer survivors. Ameliorating the complications occurring during the treatment of childhood cancers can provide better outcomes and quality of life. Complications include febrile neutropenia (FN), nausea and vomiting, other gastrointestinal complications like colitis, diarrhea, constipation, extravasation of chemotherapy, pain as a result of tumor or treatment, etc. Few important ones are being covered in detail in this chapter and rest have been discussed elsewhere in the book.

46.1 Febrile Neutropenia

46.1.1 Definition

Febrile neutropenia is the occurrence of fever during a neutropenic episode. *Neutropenia* is defined as *absolute neutrophil count (ANC) of <500 cells/mm^3*, or an ANC expected to decrease to <500 cells/mm3 during the next 48 h. Fever is defined as a single oral temperature measurement of >38.3 °C (101 °F) or a temperature of >38.0 °C (100.4 °F) sustained over a 1-h period according to the *Infectious Diseases Society of America (IDSA)* Clinical Practice Guideline [1]. Fever is defined as an oral temperature of >38.5 °C or two consecutive readings of >38.0 °C for 2 h according to *European Society of Medical Oncology (ESMO)* Clinical Practice Guidelines

M. Saroha (✉)
Pediatric Oncology, Dharamshila Narayana Superspeciality Hospital, Delhi, New Delhi, India

Narayana Superspeciality Hospital, Gurugram, Gurugram, India

K. Sood Sharma et al. (eds.), *Complications of Cancer Therapy: Best Practices in Prevention and Management*, https://doi.org/10.1007/978-981-99-0984-1_46

[2]. The use of rectal temperature which is preferred in some centers should be avoided in children with neutropenic fever.

46.1.2 Incidence

In a prospective study, Castagnola et al. showed that the highest proportions of neutropenic periods with primary febrile episodes were observed after autologous HSCT (58%), aggressive treatment for acute leukemia (AL) or non-Hodgkin lymphoma (NHL, 48%), and allogeneic HSCT (44%); the lowest proportion (9%) was observed during maintenance chemotherapy for AL [3]. Mortality associated with FN in these patients ranges from 2% to 6% [4]. Studies from our India suggest that significant mortality is attributed to drug resistant Gram negative bacilli, early initiation of appropriate antibiotics are required to cover for drug resistance.

46.1.3 Management (Flowchart 46.1)

Time to the initial dose of antibiotics should be within 1 h from the onset of fever (*golden hour*). Delay in treatment can lead to worse outcomes as the progress from bacteremia to septicemia to septic shock in immune compromised children is rapid. Signs of inflammation like redness and swelling may be absent and a thorough examination or previous cultures can guide the antibiotic therapy. Presence of indwelling catheters or venous access devices needs to be noted and site examined for signs of infection.

Following are the recommendations from the *Guideline for the Management of Fever and Neutropenia in Children with Cancer and Hematopoietic Stem-Cell Transplantation Recipients: 2017 Update* [5].

Initial assessment and investigations:

1. Adopt a validated risk stratification strategy according to your hospital setting and available facilities and incorporate it into routine clinical management.
2. Obtain blood cultures at the onset of FN from all lumens of central venous catheters. Consider obtaining peripheral blood cultures concurrent with central venous catheter cultures. Consider urinalysis and urine culture in patients in whom a clean-catch, midstream specimen is readily available. Obtain chest radiography (CXR) only in patients with respiratory signs or symptoms

Antibiotic policy in high risk and low risk FN:

1. In high-risk FN: Use monotherapy with an antipseudomonal b-lactam, a fourth-generation cephalosporin, or a carbapenem as empirical therapy in pediatric high-risk FN. Reserve the addition of a second gram-negative agent or a glycopeptide for patients who are clinically unstable, when a resistant infection is suspected, or for centers with a high rate of resistant pathogens

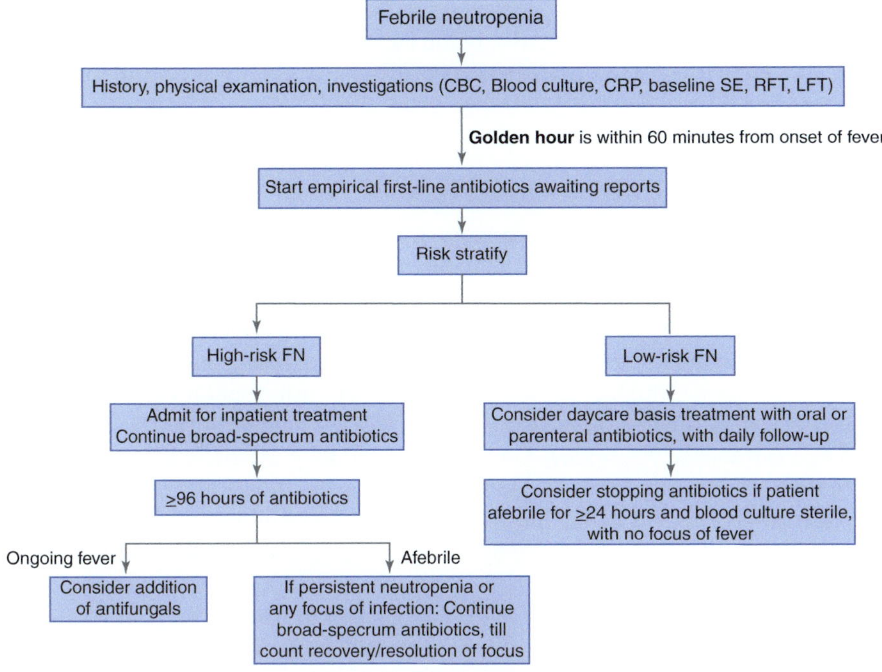

Flowchart 46.1 Management of febrile neutropenia (FN). (Adapted from standard treatment guidelines 2022 IAP. https://iapindia.org/pdf/ch-028.febrileneutropenia.pdf)

2. In low-risk FN: Consider initial or step-down outpatient management if the infrastructure is in place to ensure careful monitoring and follow-up. Consider oral antibiotic administration if the child is able to tolerate this route of administration reliably.

Modification of ongoing treatment:

1. In patients who are responding to initial empirical antibiotic therapy, discontinue double coverage for gram-negative infection or empirical glycopeptide (if initiated) after 24–72 h if there is no specific microbiologic indication to continue combination therapy.
2. Do not modify the initial empirical antibacterial regimen based solely on persistent fever in children who are clinically stable. In children with persistent fever who become clinically unstable, escalate the initial empirical antibacterial regimen to include coverage for resistant gram negative, gram-positive, and anaerobic bacteria.
3. In all patients, discontinue empirical antibiotics in patients who have negative blood cultures at 48 h, who have been afebrile for at least 24 h, and who have evidence of marrow recovery.

4. In patients with low-risk FN, consider discontinuation of empirical antibiotics at 72 h in patients who have negative blood cultures and who have been afebrile for at least 24 h, irrespective of marrow recovery status, as long as careful follow-up is ensured.

Antifungal policy:

1. Patients at high risk of IFD are those with AML, high-risk ALL, or relapsed acute leukemia, and children undergoing allogeneic HSCT. Children with prolonged neutropenia and children receiving high dose corticosteroids are also at high risk of IFD. All others should be categorized as IFD low risk.
2. In terms of biomarkers to guide empirical antifungal management for prolonged (96 h) FN in IFD high-risk patients: consider not using serum GM. Do not use b-D-glucan. Strong recommendation. Poor positive predictive values and limited data in prolonged FN setting. Do not use fungal PCR testing in blood.
3. In terms of imaging for the evaluation of prolonged (96 h) FN in IFD high-risk patients: perform CT of the lungs. Optimal timing of initial and repeated imaging not known. Consider imaging of abdomen in patients without localizing signs or symptoms.
4. Consider not routinely performing CT of sinuses in patients without localizing signs or symptoms In IFD high-risk patients with prolonged (96 h) FN unresponsive to broad spectrum antibacterial agents, initiate caspofungin or liposomal amphotericin B for empirical antifungal therapy.
5. In IFD low-risk patients with prolonged (96 h) FN, consider withholding empirical antifungal therapy.

46.2 Extravasation

46.2.1 Definition

Extravasation in chemotherapy refers to the inadvertent infiltration of chemotherapy into the subcutaneous or subdermal tissues surrounding the intravenous or intra-arterial administration site. Prior knowledge about the extravasation potential of each drug helps in cautious administration and prevention of extravasation. Given the higher chances of extravasation in children, preemptively putting central venous access device (CVAD) also decrease the chances. Though the extravasation can occur from CVAD also but he data is limited. Newly started units or with staff not trained to deal with children or chemotherapy adds to the chances of extravasation.

46.2.2 Classification

Extravasated drugs are classified according to their potential for causing damage as ‘vesicant’, ‘irritant’ and ‘nonvesicant’.

46.2.3 Incidence

Incidence varies highly due to variable reporting across the institutes. Estimates between 0.01% and 7% are noted in various publications [6].

46.2.4 Risk Factors

1. Patient related
    - Small and fragile veins
    - Hard and/or sclerosed veins as a consequence of multiple previous chemotherapy courses
    - Predisposition to bleeding, increased vascular permeability or those with coagulation abnormalities
    - Obesity in which peripheral venous access is more difficult
    - Communication difficulties or young children, which hinder the early reporting of the signs and symptoms allowing the identification of extravasation
    - Prolonged infusion
2. Cannulation and infusion procedure-related (peripheral or port)
    - Untrained or inexperienced staff
    - Multiple attempts at cannulation
    - Unfavorable cannulation site
    - Bolus injections
    - High flow pressure
    - Choice of equipment (peripheral catheter choice, size, steel 'Butterfly' needle)
    - Inadequate dressings or poor cannula fixation or irritable child in which cannula is expected to misplace
    - Poorly implanted CVAD (too deep for cannula, difficult to secure cannula)

46.2.5 Prevention

1. Site of insertion: Large veins in the forearm are recommended for administration of chemotherapy. Avoid putting cannula over the joints, inner wrist, lower extremities, anticubital fossa.
2. Cannula: Flexible large cannula are preferred.
3. For infusion of vesicant drugs of longer duration (e.g. 12–24 h) CVAD is highly recommended.
4. Bolus of vesicant drugs like vincristine should be administered after checking backflow, with a concurrent fast running infusion of iv fluid. Also flush with 5–10 mL saline after giving the drug. Continue monitoring of the cannula insertion site and check regularly for the appearance of symptoms such as swelling, pain or redness sluggish infusion rate.

46.2.6 Management of Extravasation

Comparative studies checking benefit of one antidote over other have not been done due to ethical reasons. Photographic documentation of the extravasation should be kept to allow a comparison at follow visits (Figs. 46.1 and 46.2). Stepwise approach has been shown in Fig. 46.3 [7].

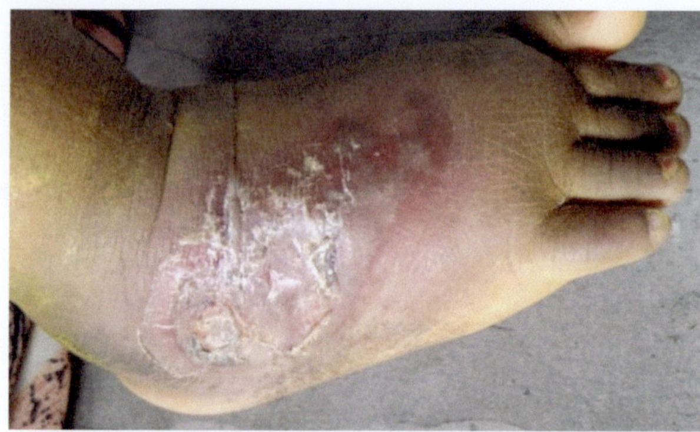

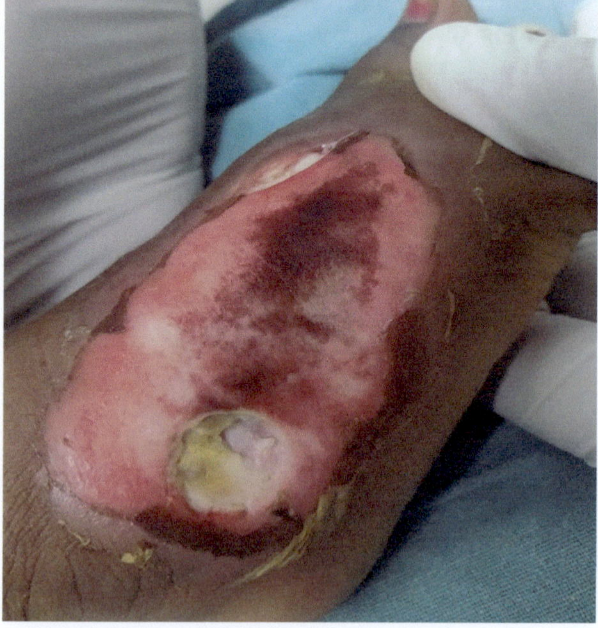

Figs. 46.1 and 46.2 Extravasation in a child post vincristine administration (day 1 and day 6)

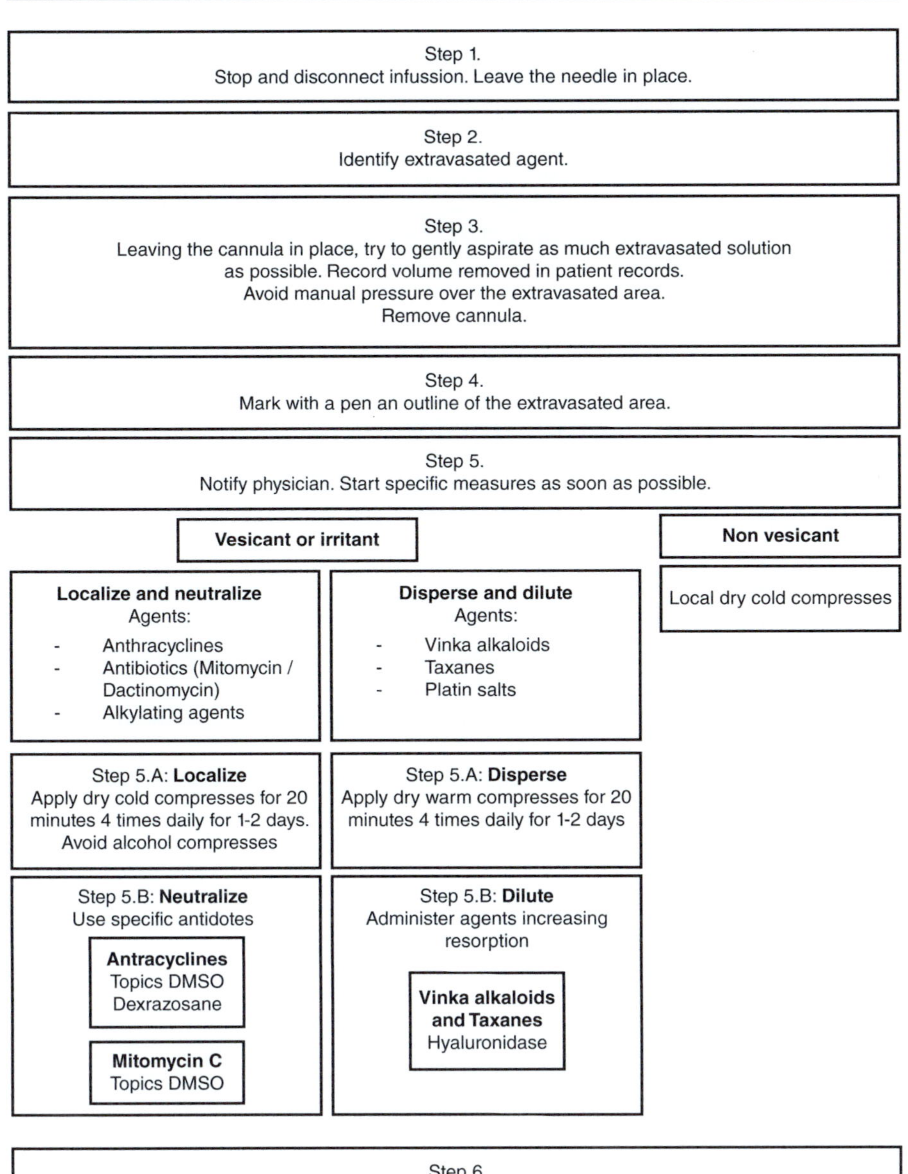

Fig. 46.3 Stepwise approach to management of extravasation

46.3 Pain

46.3.1 Definition

Pain is an unpleasant sensory and emotional experience associated with actual or potential tissue damage or described in terms of such damage. Pain in children is managed on extrapolation from adult data and is generally poorly controlled due to inadequate knowledge.

46.3.2 Incidence

Around 70% of children with cancer experience severe pain during their illness [8].

46.3.3 Cause of Pain

1. Disease itself CNS tumors with raised ICP, spinal cord compression, bone tumors, visceral invasion, leukemia with bony pains
2. Pain arising after treatment like chemotherapy induced neuropathy or mucositis, radiation induced dermatitis or mucositis, post operative pain
3. Procedures like repeated iv cannualation, lumbar puncture, bone marrow aspiration, biopsy
4. Also incidental, non cancerous pain occurring in general pediatric population

46.3.4 Pathophysiology

Nociception is a complex process whereby actual (or potential) tissue damage is perceived as pain by an individual. It may occur on three levels: peripheral, spinal or supraspinal. Through transduction, the primary afferent nociceptorsm which are thinly myelinated A delta and unmyelinated C fibres, transmit biochemical changes at the sensory nerve endings that are generated by painful (chemical, thermal, or mechanical)stimuli into electrical signals. This stimulation may be increased or decreased by molecules such as prostaglandins, leukotrienes, bradykinin and histamine. From the dorsal horn, second order neurons convey signals via ascending tracts (anterolateral spinothalamic tracts to supraspinal sites (brainstem, thalamus, cortex).

46.3.5 Pain Assessment

1. History and physical examination: To elicit factors contributing to pain, quality, location, onset and severity of pain.
2. Measurement of pain scales and validated tools. Common ones include:

(REVISED) FLACC Scale SCORING			
Categories	**0**	**1**	**2**
Face	No particular expression or smile.	Occasional grimace or frown, withdrawn, disinterested, **Sad, appears worried.**	Frequent to constant quivering chin, clenched jaw, **distressed looking face, expression of fright/ panic.**
Legs	Normal position or relaxed; **usual tone and motion to limbs.**	Uneasy, restless, tense, **occasional tremors.**	Kicking, or legs drawn up, **marked increase in spasticity, constant tremors, jerking.**
Activity	Lying quietly, normal position, moves easily, **regular, rhythmic respirations.**	Squirming, shifting back and forth, tense. **tense/guarded movements, mildly agitated, shallow/ splinting respirations, intermittent sighs**	Arched, rigid or jerking, **severe agitation, head banging, shivering, breath holding, gasping, severe splinting.**
Cry	No cry (awake or asleep)	Moans or whimpers: occasional complaint, **occasional verbal outbursts, constant grunting**	Crying steadily, screams or sobs, frequent complaints, **repeated outbursts, constant grunting.**
Consolability	Content, relaxed	Reassured by occasional touching, hugging, or being talked to: distractible	Difficult to console or comfort, **pushing caregiver away, resisting care or comfort measures.**
Each of the five categories (**F**) Face; (**L**) Legs; (**A**) Activity; (**C**) Cry; (**C**) Consolability is scored from 0-2, which results in a total score between zero and ten.			
References: Merkel, S. et al. The FLACC: A Behavioural Scale for Scoring Postoperative Pain in Young Children, Pediatric Nurse 23(3): 293-297, 1997. Copyright: Jannetti Co. University of Michigan Medical Centre. **Malviya, S., Vopel-Lewis, T. Burke, Merkal, S., Tait, A.R. (2006). The revised FLACC Observational Pain Tool: Improved Reliability and Validity for Pain Assessment in Children with Cognitive Impairment. (Pediatric Anesthesia 16: 258-265).**			

Fig. 46.4 FLACC scale

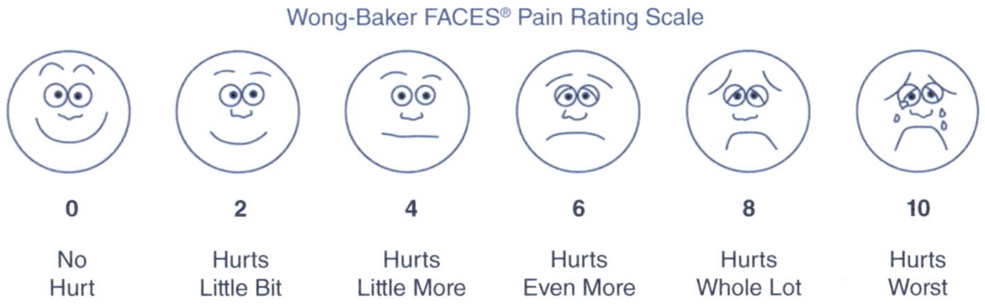

Wong-Baker FACES® Pain Rating Scale

0	2	4	6	8	10
No Hurt	Hurts Little Bit	Hurts Little More	Hurts Even More	Hurts Whole Lot	Hurts Worst

Fig. 46.5 The Wong-Baker FACES pain rating scale

(a) FLACC (Face, Legs, Activity, Cry, Consolability) scale, recommended for use in children younger than 3 years. Each of the five categories is scored from 0 to 2, which results in total score between 0 and 10 (Fig. 46.4).

(b) The Wong-Baker FACES pain rating scale, recommended for children 3 years and older. Child is asked to point to face that describes his pain best (Fig. 46.5).

The Numeric Pain Rating Scale Instructions

General Information:

- The patients is asked to make three pain ratings, corresponding to current, best and worst pain experienced over the past 24 hours.
- The average of the 3 ratings was used to represent the patient's level of pain over the previous 24 hours.

Patient Instructions (adopted from (Mccaffery, Beebe et al. 1989):
"Please indicate the intensity of current, best, and worst pain levels over the past 24 hours on a scale of 0 (no pain) to 10 (worst pain imaginable)"

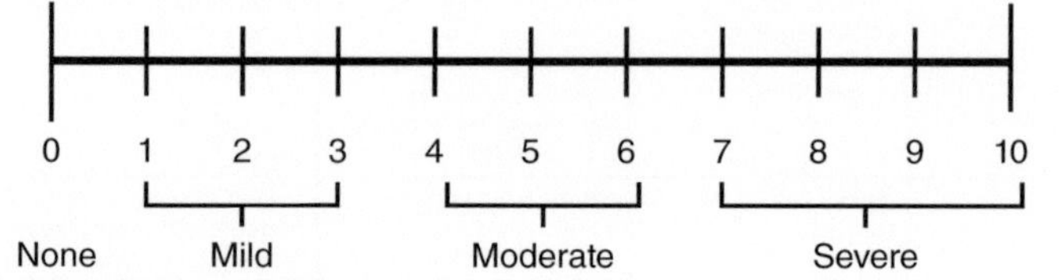

Fig. 46.6 Numerical pain rating scale

(c) Numerical pain rating scale, recommended for children 8 years and older (Fig. 46.6).

46.3.6 Management of Pain in Children

Anticipation and prevention of pain is the most important aspect of dealing with pain in children with cancer. Both pharmacologic and non pharmacologic approaches should be included. WHO recommends adequate pain control "By the ladder, by the clock, by the appropriate route, by the child". Previously used WHO 3 step ladder approach to pain provided effective approach to pain control for adults but was not found to be useful for patients with advanced disease. Two step ladder in which treatment passes from step 1 (non opioids) to step 3 (opioids) for mild to moderate pain provides superior pain relief. Following are the recommendations and salient features from WHO 2012 guidelines on the pharmacological treatment of persisting pain in children with medical illnesses [9].

Recommendations regarding use of NSAIDS:

(a) Paracetamol and ibuprofen are the medicines of choice in the first step (mild pain). In children above 3 months of age who can take oral medication and whose pain is assessed as being mild, paracetamol and ibuprofen are the medicines of choice. For children below 3 months of age, the only option is paracetamol

(b) Both paracetamol and ibuprofen have potential toxicity: there are concerns about potential renal and gastrointestinal toxicity, and bleeding with ibuprofen and other NSAIDs; and there are risks of hepatotoxicity and acute overdose associated with paracetamol. Hence both the drugs have maximum doses (Table 46.1).

Table 46.1 Non opioid analgesics for the relief of pain in neonates, infants and children (dose, oral route)

Medicine	Neonates form 0 to 29 days	Infants from 30 days to 3 months	Infants from 3 to 12 months or child from 1 to 12 years	Maximum dose
Paracetamol	5–10 mg/kg every 6–8 hourly[a]	10 mg/kg every 4–6 h[a]	10–15 mg/kg every 4–6 h[a,b]	Neonates, infants and children: 4 doses/day
Ibuprofen	–	–	5–10 mg/kg every 6–8 h	Child 40 mg/kg/day

Adapted from WHO 2012 guidelines on the pharmacological treatment of persisting pain in children with medical illnesses [9]

[a] Children who are malnourished or in a poor nutritional state are more likely to be susceptible to toxicity at standard dose regimens due to reduced natural detoxifying glutathione enzyme

[b] Maximum of 1 g at a time

Recommendations regarding use of opioids:

(a) If pain severity associated with a medical illness is assessed as moderate or severe, the administration of a strong opioid is necessary. Morphine is the medicine of choice for the second step, although other strong opioids should be considered and made available to ensure an alternative to morphine in case of intolerable side-effects.

(b) Medication should be administered on a regular schedule for persisting pain, rather than on an "as required basis", unless pain episodes are truly intermittent and unpredictable.

(c) To obtain a dose that provides adequate relief of pain with an acceptable degree of side-effects the

- Doses of morphine or other strong opioids need to be gradually increased until effective.
- Unlike paracetamol and NSAIDs, there is no upper dosage limit for opioid analgesics because there is no "ceiling" analgesic effect.
- The appropriate dose is the dose that produces pain relief for the individual child (with no maximum dose, unless further increase is not possible because of untreatable side-effects).
- The maximum dosage increase is 50% per 24 h in outpatient settings. Experienced prescribers can increase up to 100% while monitoring the patient carefully

(d) Long-term opioid use is usually associated with constipation and patients should also receive a combination of a stimulant laxative and a stool softener prophylactically

Recommendations regarding change of opioids:

(a) Selection of alternative opioid analgesics to morphine should be guided by considerations of safety, availability, cost and suitability including patient-related factors.

(b) Switching opioids and/or route of administration in children is strongly recommended in the presence of inadequate analgesic effect with intolerable side-effects. Routine rotation of opioids is not recommended.

Table 46.2 Formulations of morphine listed in the *WHO model list of essential medicines for children*, 2010 [9]

- *Injection*: 10 mg in 1 mL ampoule (morphine hydrochloride or morphine sulfate)
- *Granules (prolonged-release) (to mix with water)*: 20, 30, 60, 100, 200 mg (morphine sulfate)
- *Oral liquid*: 10 mg/5 mL (morphine hydrochloride or morphine sulfate)
- *Tablet (immediate-release)*: 10 mg (morphine sulfate)
- *Tablet (prolonged-release)*: 10, 30, 60, 100, 200 mg (morphine sulfate)

Table 46.3 Starting dosages for opioid analgesics in opioid-naive children (1–12 years) [9]

Medicine	Route of administration	Starting dose
Morphine	Oral (immediate release)	1–2 years: 200–400 mcg/kg every 4 h 2–12 years: 200–500 mcg/kg every 4 h (max 5 mg)
	Oral (prolonged release)	200–800 mcg/kg every 12 h
	IV injection[a]	1–2 years: 100 mcg/kg every 4 h 2–12 years: 100–200 mcg/kg every 4 h (max 2.5 mg)
	SC injection	
	IV infusion	Initial IV dose: 100–200 mcg/kg[a], then 20–30 mcg/kg/h
	SC infusion	20 mcg/kg/h
Fentanyl	IV injection	1–2 mcg/kg[b], repeated every 30–60 min
	IV infusion	Initial IV dose 1–2 mcg/kg[b], then 1 mcg/kg/h
Hydromorphone[c]	Oral (immediate release)	30–80 mcg/kg every 3–4 h (max 2 mg/dose)
	IV injection[d] or SC injection	15 mcg/kg every 3–6 h
Methadone[e]	Oral (immediate release)	100–200 mcg/kg every 4 h for the first 2–3 doses, then every 6–12 h (max 5 mg/dose initially)[f]
	IV injection[g] and SC injection	
Oxycodone	Oral (immediate release)	125–200 mcg/kg every 4 h (max 5 mg/dose)
	Oral (prolonged release)	5 mg every 12 h

Adapted from WHO 2012 guidelines on the pharmacological treatment of persisting pain in children with medical illnesses

[a] Administer IV morphine slowly over at least 5 min

[b] Administer IV fentanyl slowly over 3–5 min

[c] Hydromorphone is a potent opioid and significant differences exist between oral and intravenous dosing. Use extreme caution when converting from one route to another. In converting from parenteral hydromorphone to oral hydromorphone, doses may need to be titrated up to five times the IV dose

[d] Administer IV hydromorphone slowly over 2–3 min

[e] Due to the complex nature and wide inter-individual variation in the pharmacokinetics of methadone, methadone should only be commenced by practitioners experienced with its use

[f] Methadone should initially be titrated like other strong opioids. The dosage may need to be reduced by 50% 2–3 days after the effective dose has been found to prevent adverse effects due to methadone accumulation. From then on dosage increases should be performed at intervals of one week or over and with a maximum increase of 50%

[g] Administer IV methadone slowly over 3–5 min

Recommendations regarding opioids formulation:

(a) When selecting morphine formulations for the management of moderate to severe pain in children, priority should be given to the selection and procurement of immediate-release formulations (tablets and liquids).

(b) Liquid preparations allow for easier dose administration than tablets in infants and small children, although they may be more expensive and present challenges related to stability, portability and storage (Tables 46.2 and 46.3).

(c) Patient-controlled analgesia (PCA) is an approach to intravenous or subcutaneous administration of medicines. It allows children from approximately the age of seven to self administer "rescue" doses of analgesics for breakthrough pain. A pre-set dose is delivered into an infusion line by a computer-driven pump. For safety, there is a limited lock-out period after each dose so that additional doses cannot be delivered before a specified time has elapsed.

Non pharmacological treatment modalities like books, music, games, toys, relaxation techniques are equally important for holistic care of pain. Details regarding non pharmacological interventions, interventional techniques such as nerve blocks, epidural analgesia, intrathecal therapies, radiofrequency ablation and management of procedural pain are beyond the scope of this chapter.

46.4 CINV (Chemotherapy Induced Nausea and Vomiting)

Nausea and vomiting are important side effects associated with various modalities of cancer treatment especially chemotherapy and even with radiotherapy and surgery. CINV in children has been discussed in this section.

46.4.1 Pathophysiology

Chemotherapy can cause nausea and vomiting due to various mechanisms.

1. Stimulation of CTZ (lies in area postrema). It contains chemoreceptors outside the BBB that can detect emetogenic agents present in circulation as well as in spinal fluid.
2. Chemotherapy can also stimulate the gut leading to release of serotonin, which in turn stimulates the vagus nerve, which activates the vomiting center.
3. Central cortex may also be involved in CINV by mediating emotions such as anxiety that play a role in genesis of nausea.
4. Neurotransmitters important in CINV are serotonin, dopamine and substance P.

46.4.2 Classification

CINV is classified into acute, delayed or anticipatory type depending upon the time period of vomiting [2].

1. Vomiting occurring in the first 24 h of administering chemotherapy is labeled as acute CINV and in the absence of effective prophylaxis; it most commonly begins within 1–2 h of chemotherapy and usually peaks in the first 4–6 h.
2. Vomiting occurring later is called delayed CINV. Especially associated with cisplatin.
3. Anticipatory emetic episodes are triggered by taste, odor, sight, thoughts, or anxiety secondary to a history of poor response to antiemetic agents or inadequate antiemetic prophylaxis in the previous cycle of chemotherapy. It usually starts 1–4 h before chemotherapy but can sometimes occur days before chemotherapy

46.4.3 Predisposing Factors

The American Society of Clinical Oncology has classified the cancer chemotherapeutic drugs in four categories of high, moderate, low, and minimal emetogenecity, depending on their emetogenic potential (mentioned elsewhere in the book).

46.4.4 Management

The key to effective control of nausea and vomiting is to prevent it before it occurs whenever possible. Choice of antiemetic drug to be used in a chemotherapy regimen should include not only the chemotherapeutic drug being used but also the possible patient characteristics and etiology of emesis. Antiemetic drugs may be used alone or in combination (Table 46.4). The traditional drugs for management of CINV have been the dopamine antagonists (metoclopramide); steroids (dexamethasone), the 5-HT3 antagonists (ondansetron). Only some newer antiemetics have established efficacy and safety data. Neurokinin-1 antagonists aprepitant is not being used in children >6 months (3 mg/kg on day 1 up to 125 mg, 2 mg/kg on days 2–3 up to 80 mg). Palonosetron is a newer 5HT3 antagonist with a longer half-life than ondansetron which has been shown to be effective in preventing CINV in adults and now is recommended for children of all age groups (dose 0.2 mg/kg).

Table 46.4 Recommendations for antiemetic combinations according to emetogenic potential [10]

Emetogenic potential	Antiemetic regimen				
High	*>6 months of age, chemotherapy NOT known to interact with aprepitant* **Granisetron, ondansetron, or palonosetron + dexamethasone + aprepitant**	*>6 months of age, chemotherapy KNOWN to interact with aprepitant* **Granisetron, ondansetron, or palonosetron + dexamethasone**	*>6 months of age, chemotherapy NOT known to interact with aprepitant and who cannot receive dexamethasone* **Palonosetron + aprepitant**	*<6 months old* **Granisetron, ondansetron or palonosetron + dexamethasone**	*<6 months old who cannot receive dexamethasone% OR >6 months old and cannot receive aprepitant or dexamethasone* **Palonosetron**
Moderate	*No restrictions* **Granisetron, ondansetron, or palonosetron + dexamethasone**	*>6 months of age, who cannot receive dexamethasone* **Granisetron, ondansetron or, palonosetron + aprepitant**	*>6 months of age, chemotherapy KNOWN to interact with aprepitant and cannot receive dexamethasone%* **Palonosetron**		*<6 months old who cannot receive dexamethasone* **Palonosetron**
Low	**Ondansetron or granisetron**				
Minimal	No routine prophylaxis				

Key Points

1. Ameliorating the complications occurring during the treatment of childhood cancers can provide better outcomes and quality of life.
2. Time to the initial dose of antibiotics should be within 1 h from the onset of fever (*golden hour*).
3. Use monotherapy with an antipseudomonal b-lactam, a fourth-generation cephalosporin, or a carbapenem as empirical therapy in pediatric high-risk FN.
4. A second gram-negative agent or a glycopeptide for patients who are clinically unstable, when a resistant infection is suspected, or for centers with a high rate of resistant pathogens.
5. Extravasation can be prevented by choosing the right site for the right patient for iv cannulation. Large veins in the forearm are recommended for administration of chemotherapy.
6. Central venous access device is highly recommended for longer infusions, for smaller children and for vesicant chemotherapy drugs.
7. WHO recommends adequate pain control "By the ladder, by the clock, by the appropriate route, by the child".
8. Two step ladder in which treatment passes from step 1 (non opioids) to step 3 (opioids) for mild to moderate pain provides superior pain relief in children.
9. The key to effective control of nausea and vomiting is to prevent it before it occurs whenever possible.
10. Choice of antiemetic drug to be used in a chemotherapy regimen should include not only the chemotherapeutic drug being used but also the possible patient characteristics and etiology of emesis. Newer antiemetics like aprepitant and palonesetron are also efficacious and safe in children.

References

1. Freifeld AG, Bow EJ, Kent A, et al. Clinical practice guideline for the use of antimicrobial agents in neutropenic patients with cancer: 2010 update by the Infectious Diseases Society of America. Clin Infect Dis. 2011;52(4):56–93.
2. Naurois J. On behalf of the ESMO guidelines working group, management of febrile neutropenia: ESMO clinical practice guidelines. Ann Oncol. 2010;21(5):252–6.
3. Castagnola E, Fontana V, Caviglia I, Caruso S, Faraci M, Fioredda F, Garrè ML, Moroni C, Conte M, Losurdo G, et al. A prospective study on the epidemiology of febrile episodes during chemotherapy-induced neutropenia in children with cancer or after hemopoietic stem cell transplantation. Clin Infect Dis. 2007;45:1296–304.
4. Basu SK, Fernandez ID, Fisher SG, Asselin BL, Lyman GH. Length of stay and mortality associated with febrile neutropenia among children with cancer. J Clin Oncol. 2005;23:7958–66.
5. Lehrnbecher T, Robinson P, Fisher B, Alexander S, Ammann RA, Beauchemin M, et al. Guideline for the management of fever and neutropenia in children with cancer and hematopoietic stem-cell transplantation recipients: 2017 update. J Clin Oncol. 2017;35(18):2082–94.
6. Schulmeister L. Extravasation management: clinical update. Semin Oncol Nurs. 2011;27(1):82–90.
7. Perez Fidalgo JA, Garcia Fabregat L, Cervantes A, Margulies A, Vidall C, Roila F, ESMO Guidelines Working Group. Management of chemotherapy extravasation: ESMO–EONS

clinical practice guidelines. Eur J Oncol Nurs. 2012;16:528–34. https://doi.org/10.1016/j.ejon.2012.09.004.

8. Schulte FSM, Patton M, Alberts NM, Kunin-Batson A, Olson-Bullis BA, Forbes C, Russell KB, Neville A, Heathcote LC, Karlson CW, et al. Pain in long-term survivors of childhood cancer: a systematic review of the current state of knowledge and a call to action from the Children's Oncology Group. Cancer. 2020;127:35–44.
9. World Health Organization. WHO guidelines on pharmacological treatment of persisting pain in children with medical illnesses. Geneva: World Health Organization; 2012.
10. Sherani F, Boston C, Mba N. Latest update on prevention of acute chemotherapy-induced nausea and vomiting in pediatric cancer patients. Curr Oncol Rep. 2019;21:89.

Anaesthesia Related Implications and Complications in Cancer Patients

47

Neha Agrawal

47.1 Introduction

Three common modalities of cancer treatment chemotherapy, radiotherapy (RT) and surgery have certain associated risks besides being curative/palliative in nature. Various local and systemic involvement are well known in all cancer patients because of the type and extent of the disease per se and because of the side effects associated with chemotherapy drugs, radiotherapy and surgical procedures.

Almost 80% of cancer patients undergo anaesthesia administration [1] during their course of disease for surgical resection and others as a part of chemotherapy and/or radiotherapy associated interventional procedures. Due consideration needs to be given in perioperative period for all cancer patients during preoperative/pre-procedural anaesthesia evaluation, peroperative anaesthetic management in order to reduce peroperative and postoperative anaesthesia related risks and complications in view of side effects associated with different treatment modalities, the disease itself and augmentation/deterioration of such effects under anaesthesia.

Besides local and systemic complications, acute and long-term complications of tumour recurrence and metastasis are also being implicated in relation with anaesthesia agents/techniques and drugs used in perioperative period including blood transfusion [1–6].

Hence, it is imperative for the anaesthetist and oncology team to be aware of cancer therapy related complications and its further implications during anaesthesia. A careful preoperative anaesthesia evaluation, peroperative anaesthetic

N. Agrawal (✉)
Department of Anaesthesiology and Critical Care, Dharamshila Narayana Superspeciality Hospital, Delhi, New Delhi, India

Administration, Dharamshila Rahat Medical Centre, New Delhi, India

Healthcare Safety, Healthcare Integrals, Ghaziabad, India

K. Sood Sharma et al. (eds.), *Complications of Cancer Therapy: Best Practices in Prevention and Management*, https://doi.org/10.1007/978-981-99-0984-1_47

management, implementation of preventive measures is mandatory and any occurrence of actionable complications require timely and appropriate intervention to reduce associated morbidities and mortality.

47.2 Risks and Complications

Most cancer patients with advanced stage disease may be cachectic and pose significant challenge to anaesthesiologists because of disturbed homeostasis [7]. Various other risks or complications are associated with disease itself or cancer therapies which have implications in perioperative period and may further predispose patients for enhanced risk during anaesthesia.

47.2.1 Airway/Respiratory Risks

1. Difficult intubation and failure to intubate/ventilate: Airway compromise is commonly encountered in cancer patients because of the disease per se, e.g., head and neck cancers or because of cancer therapy (post radiation [8, 9] or prior surgical treatment). Literature review predicts 15.7–27.17% incidence of difficult intubation because of limited mouth opening, poor tissue mobility and airway distortion in such patients [10, 11] which may further be associated with failure to intubate and a need for surgical access for airway management. Postoperatively laryngeal oedema may further compromise airway and there may be need of mechanical ventilation [7]. Radiotherapy to head and neck is also known to cause airway narrowing due to tissue fibrosis and glottic/subglottic oedema (Figs. 47.1 and 47.2) [8]. Critical mediastinal mass syndrome is a well-known entity in mediastinal cancer patients resultant from airway obstruction [12]. These mediastinal tumours pose the risk of complete/exacerbation of airway obstruction, inability to ventilate with resultant hypoxaemia and hypotension any time during anaesthesia including preinduction, induction, positioning, surgery, emergence, extubation and in recovery area [13].
2. Pulmonary toxicity: Various chemotherapy drugs are known to result in pulmonary toxicity in the form of pulmonary oedema (methotrexate) or pulmonary fibrosis (bleomycin most commonly, carmustine, ifosfamide, panitumumab). Radiotherapy by way of production of oxygen free radical cause tissue damage with resultant pneumonitis and pulmonary fibrosis. High inspired concentration of oxygen even for a short period during anaesthesia or postoperatively can lead to faster progression of pulmonary toxicity with worsening of clinical signs and symptoms [5, 14].
3. Decrease in pulmonary compliance: In 2020, Marguerite Mulin in literature review "Anaesthetic Implications of Intraarterial Chemotherapy (IAC) for Retinoblastoma: A Literature Review" has reported sudden decrease in pulmonary compliance due to trigemino cardiac reflex during intraarterial chemotherapy under general anaesthesia in retinoblastoma paediatric patients followed by

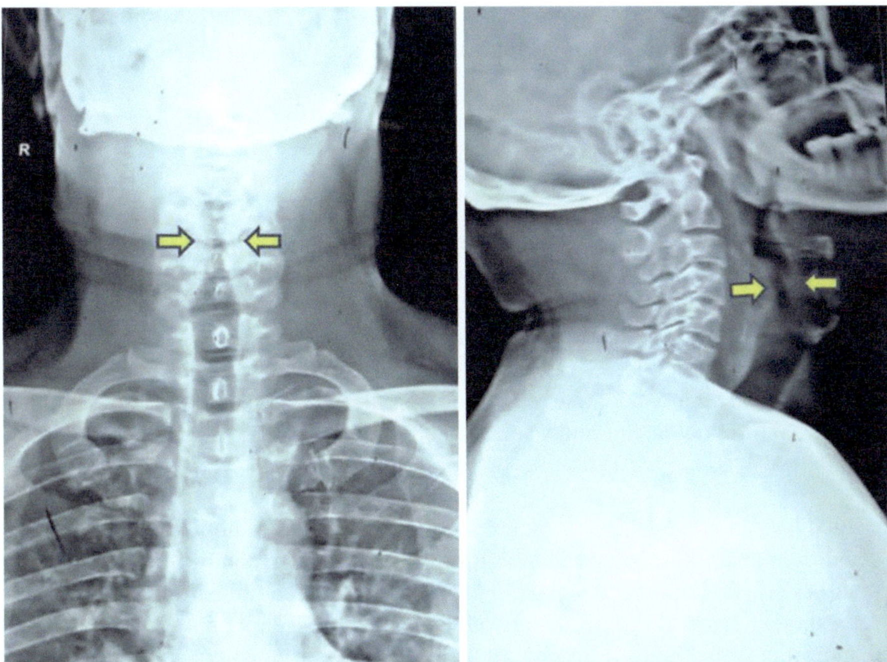

Fig. 47.1 Anteroposterior and lateral X-ray of the neck showing a narrowing in the airway (arrow marked) [8]. (Under open licence: CC BY-NC 4.0)

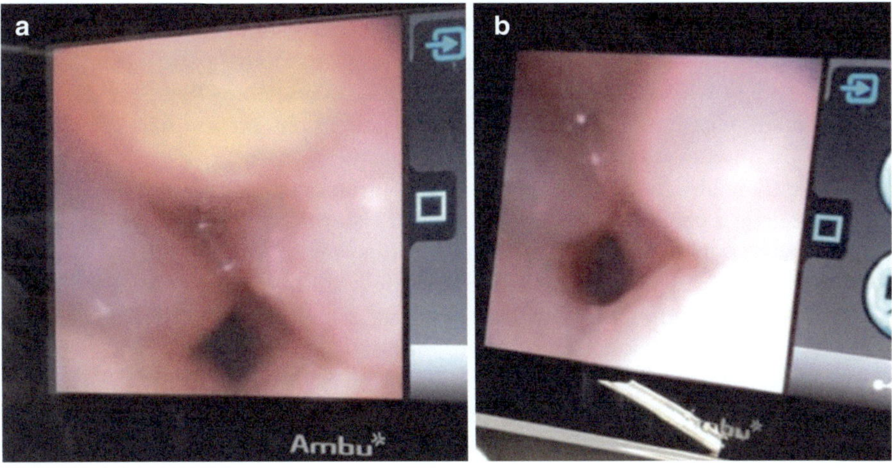

Fig. 47.2 Fibreoptic view: oedema in the glottic (**a**) and subglottic areas (**b**) [8]. (Under open licence: CC BY-NC 4.0)

associated hypoxemia, hypotension, bradycardia and cardiovascular collapse [15]. This cardiopulmonary event is reported in 29% cases of IAC in retinoblastoma cases.

47.2.2 Cardiovascular Risks

Multiple chemotherapy drugs have cardiovascular concerns in the perioperative period as anaesthesia administration can further compromise the cardiac reserve of the patients by way of anaesthetic agents' myocardial depressant effects and resultant decreased cardiac output and hypotension. Radiotherapy is also known for causing myocarditis. Besides the therapy side effects, tumours can cause anatomical effects (cardiac tamponade) due to metastasis to pericardium or as a primary tumour with resultant hypotension under anaesthesia. Following are the associated cardiovascular risks [5, 14, 16, 17]:

1. Tachycardia, bradycardia or other cardiac arrythmias: Radiotherapy to heart and multiple chemotherapy drugs are implicated in rhythm abnormalities, e.g., procarbazine, fludarabine, docetaxel etc. with resultant complications under anaesthesia. QT interval prolongation with drugs like crizotinib, dasatinib, sorafenib, sunitinib, lenvatinib are at risk of potentially fatal arrythmia like torsades de pointes with concurrent use of QT prolongation drugs or electrolyte abnormalities.
2. Hypotension or hypertension: Drugs like vincristine, vinblastine, sorafenib, bevacizumab are implicated. Tamponade effects by tumour encasing pericardium (mesotheliomas and sarcomas) or pericardial effusion with resultant pericarditis can result in hypotension during anaesthesia. Constrictive pericarditis or effusions with or without tamponade is known post-radiotherapy to the mediastinum with its implication under anaesthesia and patients can present with pericarditis even after months to years post radiation treatment.
3. Cardiomyopathy: Drugs like doxorubicin, epirubicin, trastuzumab, sunitinib are implicated in cardiotoxicity. Patients are at risk for heart failure which further can lead to hypotension and respiratory distress under anaesthesia.
4. Coronary and valvular heart disease: Patients with history of thoracic radiation have been known to have premature coronary artery disease. Valvular heart disease, especially aortic or mitral valve, is also reported post thoracic radiation therapy [17]. Pre anaesthesia evaluation must be done with due diligence in younger patients to prevent untoward cardiac events in perioperative period.

47.2.3 Nephrotoxicity

Nephrotoxic chemotherapeutic agents (platinum based, e.g., cisplatin, carboplatin and oxaliplatin) can cause acute or chronic renal failure. Anaesthesia administration if associated with dehydration and inadvertent use of non-steroidal anti-inflammatory drugs can augment the nephrotoxic process [5, 14].

47.2.4 Gastrointestinal and Hepatic System Toxicity

1. Nausea, vomiting, diarrhoea: Gastrointestinal (GI) toxicity is common in the form of nausea, vomiting, diarrhoea and mucositis after chemotherapy administration. Grade 3 [common terminology criteria for adverse events (CTCAE)] diarrhoea occurs in 30% of patients receiving chemotherapy which can lead to dehydration and electrolyte imbalance [18].
2. Typhlitis and neutropenic enterocolitis: Typhlitis and neutropenic enterocolitis is seen as a consequence of chemotherapy induced neutropenia where patient may present with signs and symptoms of perforation and multiorgan failure [18].
3. Colitis: Immunotherapy have diarrhoea as an adverse effect with 2% of the patients developing colitis where patients with severe colitis are at risk of developing bowel necrosis, perforation and toxic megacolon.
4. Hepatitis: Hepatitis incidents in the range of 5–10% is commonly seen in patients on immunotherapy, onset occurring 4–12 weeks after initiation of the therapy and deranged liver function is seen in grade 2–4 hepatitis [18] which warrants checking of liver function tests. Impaired liver function can lead to coagulopathy with regional anaesthesia being a contraindication [14]. Radiation induced acute hepatitis is known to occur within 2–6 weeks of therapy initiation and may lead to hepatic enlargement and portal hypertension with abnormal liver function. Chronic form of hepatic injury leading to cirrhosis occurs after 6 months of radiotherapy [7]. Anaesthesia drug dosage need precaution as in any other hepatic disease.
5. Mucositis: Bleeding can occur due to mucositis during direct laryngoscopy which can obstruct the airway [5, 14].
6. Radiotherapy induced enteritis [7]: This is seen within 1 month of the radiotherapy and ulceration can lead to abscess, perforation and fistulae. With healing of ulcers, fibrosis of the tissues and stricture formation occurs. Patient can present with signs and symptoms of intestinal obstruction and perforation [18] many years after treatment. Patient may complain of pain abdomen at the time of pre anaesthetic evaluation because of above complications. Anaesthesiologists need to order relevant referrals and investigations for appropriate perioperative optimisation of the patients.

47.2.5 Nervous System/Neurotoxicity

Neurological risks and complications are associated with variety of tumours as well as with radiotherapy and various chemotherapeutic agents [7, 13, 14, 17, 19, 20].

1. Vincristine and cisplatin are most common agents implicated for neurological side effects. Peripheral neuropathy (vincristine, paclitaxel and oxaliplatin), muscle pain, cranial neuropathy and seizures are common.
2. High dose methotrexate besides causing hemiparesis can cause encephalopathy which is also associated with ifosfamide which may complicate anaesthesia outcome.

3. Involvement of autonomic nervous system can lead to orthostatic hypotension and rarely vocal cord palsy which further complicates anaesthesia administration with vocal cord palsy increasing risk of aspiration in perioperative period.
4. Regional anaesthesia, being a relative contraindication, if attempted in such patients need careful perioperative monitoring.
5. Certain cancers (small cell carcinoma lung) are associated with paraneoplastic syndrome and anaesthetic agent can exacerbate neuromuscular dysfunction which can lead to respiratory failure or delayed extubation [7].
6. Stroke risk is associated with patients undergoing neck irradiation [21] and high suspicion should be kept for patients receiving neck radiotherapy and chemotherapy for head and neck cancers with its obvious implications for patients undergoing anaesthesia administration.

47.2.6 Endocrinology and Electrolyte Imbalance Risk

1. Suppression of the hypothalamic pituitary adrenal (HPA) axis: Various chemotherapeutic protocols include glucocorticoids as a therapeutic or supportive treatment component. Suppression of HPA axis may exist in patients taking 5 mg/day of prednisone or its equivalent for more than 3 weeks [17]. The resultant adrenal insufficiency places patients at risk of insufficient adrenal response to surgical stress and resultant unresponsive hypotension in perioperative period. The careful work up and management is vital in such patients [22] (Flowchart 47.1).
2. Hyponatremia: Hyponatremia in cancer patients due to paraneoplastic effects of tumour or because of treatment may occur with its resultant complications under anaesthesia and increased post-operative 30-day morbidity and mortality [23]. Exacerbation of hyponatremia is to be avoided by administering non-hypotonic fluids during anaesthesia for surgery and in post-operative period besides careful monitoring and other standard treatment measures [17, 24].
3. Hypercalcaemia: Hypercalcaemia occurs in up to 30% of cancer patients during their course of disease which further complicates the patient care [25]. This is most common in patients with squamous cell cancers of head and neck, breast cancer, non-small cell lung cancer, urothelial carcinomas, ovarian cancer or multiple myeloma [25]. Cardiac arrhythmias and ECG abnormalities like short QT interval and widened T wave are known with hypercalcaemia. Whereas mild to moderate hypercalcaemia is often asymptomatic, symptoms are usually seen with severe hypercalcaemia more than 3 mmol/L and coma or cardiac arrest may occur if the calcium concentration is more than 3.75 mmol/L [26]. Patient may present with fatigue, depression, confusion, anorexia, nausea, vomiting, constipation, peptic ulceration or pancreatitis signs and symptoms. Patients with muscle weakness may have enhanced response to neuromuscular blocking agents.
4. Hypothyroidism: Literature review shows incidence of radiation induced hypothyroidism in head and neck cancer patients in the range of 23–53% [9]. Hypothyroidism may be overt (clinical hypothyroidism, low free T4 and high TSH) or sub clinical (compensated normal free T4 and high TSH) and in most

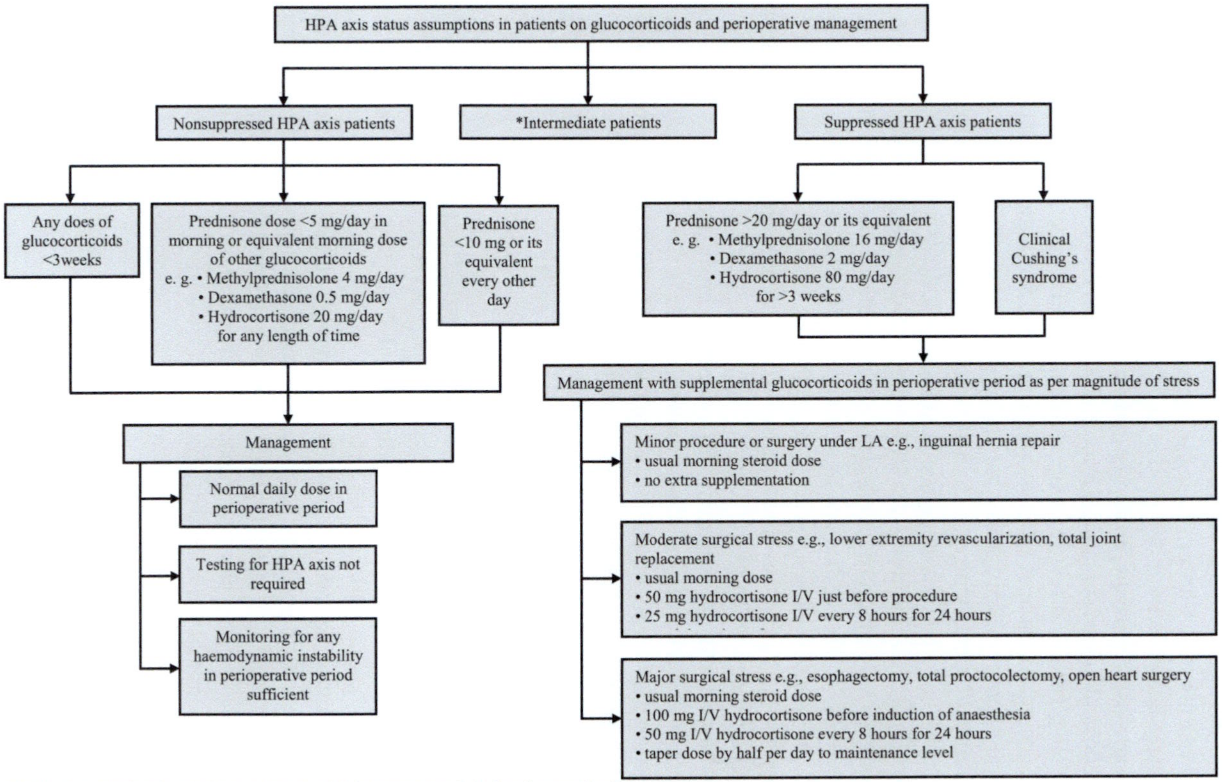

HPA axis status assumptions in patients on glucocorticoids and perioperative management

Nonsuppressed HPA axis patients

*Intermediate patients

Suppressed HPA axis patients

Any does of glucocorticoids <3weeks

Prednisone dose <5 mg/day in morning or equivalent morning dose of other glucocorticoids
e. g. • Methylprednisolone 4 mg/day
• Dexamethasone 0.5 mg/day
• Hydrocortisone 20 mg/day
for any length of time

Prednisone <10 mg or its equivalent every other day

Management

- Normal daily dose in perioperative period
- Testing for HPA axis not required
- Monitoring for any haemodynamic instability in perioperative period sufficient

Prednisone >20 mg/day or its equivalent
e. g. • Methylprednisolone 16 mg/day
• Dexamethasone 2 mg/day
• Hydrocortisone 80 mg/day
for >3 weeks

Clinical Cushing's syndrome

Management with supplemental glucocorticoids in perioperative period as per magnitude of stress

Minor procedure or surgery under LA e.g., inguinal hernia repair
• usual morning steroid dose
• no extra supplementation

Moderate surgical stress e.g., lower extremity revascularization, total joint replacement
• usual morning dose
• 50 mg hydrocortisone I/V just before procedure
• 25 mg hydrocortisone I/V every 8 hours for 24 hours

Major surgical stress e.g., esophagectomy, total proctocolectomy, open heart surgery
• usual morning steroid dose
• 100 mg I/V hydrocortisone before induction of anaesthesia
• 50 mg I/V hydrocortisone every 8 hours for 24 hours
• taper dose by half per day to maintenance level

(HPA: hypothalamic-pituitary-adrenal; I/V: intravenous; LA: local anaesthesia)
* Prednisone dose 5-20 mg or equivalent. Preoperative evaluation of HPA axis status required

Flowchart 47.1 HPA axis status in patients on glucocorticoids and perioperative management [17, 22]. *HPA* hypothalamic-pituitary-adrenal, *I/V* intravenous, *LA* local anaesthesia. *Prednisone dose 5–20 mg or equivalent. Preoperative evaluation of HPA axis status required

cases sub clinical hypothyroidism progresses to clinical hypothyroidism at the rate of 5–20% per year [9]. Study by Lechner et al. has shown the development of hypothyroidism in 40% of patients after tyrosine kinase inhibitor (TKI) therapy in non-thyroid cancer patients [27]. Chemotherapy with agents like sorafenib, sunitinib has also been known to cause hypothyroidism. A careful anaesthetic management becomes more imperative as atherosclerotic disease, cardiac dysfunction and cardiovascular mortality and progression to clinical hypothyroidism as a consequence of subclinical hypothyroidism is known [28–30]. Moreover, intraoperative cardiac arrest in cancer patient with undetected hypothyroidism [28] and increased chances of post-operative atrial fibrillation in patients with subclinical hypothyroidism who have undergone aortic valve surgery [31] have been reported. Patients with sub clinical hypothyroidism show improvement in cardiac function with eltroxin replacement therapy [32].

5. Carcinoid crisis: Carcinoid crisis is a life-threatening condition which develops in patient with serotonin producing well differentiated neuroendocrine tumour, e.g., tumour of GI tract at the time of tumour manipulation during surgery or by induction of anaesthesia. Tachycardia, arrhythmias, bronchospasm are some of the symptoms [17] and wide blood pressure fluctuations with the predominance of hypotension are known [33].
6. Phaeochromocytoma and hypertensive/hypotensive crisis: Because of excessive circulating catecholamines in adrenal tumours, there is risk of hypertensive crisis and arrythmias during intubation, change of position of the patient or manipulation of the tumour during surgery. Post excision of the tumour, there is sudden fall in blood pressure with resultant complications under anaesthesia and in post-operative period [34].

47.2.7 Myelosuppression and Haematological Effects

Most chemotherapy drugs and radiotherapy affect bone marrow and peripheral blood cells. Neutropenic patients carry risk of developing life-threatening sepsis and rapid deterioration following infection. Emergency surgeries and anaesthesia administration in such patients may be a cause of increased morbidity and mortality. Anaesthesia and surgery in pancytopenic patients can have serious implications because of reduced oxygen carrying capacity, increased risk of bleeding and any opportunistic infection [14, 19, 20].

1. Neutropenia: Absolute neutrophil count or ANC less than 1500/μL or less than $1.5 \times 10^9/L$ has been defined as neutropenia with following gradings [35, 36]:
   Mild: 1000–1500/μL or $1.5 \times 10^9/L$
   Moderate: 500–999/μL or $0.5–0.999 \times 10^9/L$
   Severe: 200–499/μL or $0.2–0.499 \times 10^9/L$
   Very severe: <200/μL or less than $0.2 \times 10^9/L$

ANC below 500/μL carries risk of life-threatening infection. Although Joshua et al. in their article on “Timing and Outcome of Abdominal Surgery in Neutropenia Patients” [37] have advocated for early consideration of operations on neutropenic patients with obvious surgical pathology with suggestion for lower threshold of ANC less than 350 cells/μL. This has been recommended in view of multiple literature evidence between non operative medical management and adverse outcomes in neutropenic cancer patients with surgical pathology [37].

2. Thrombocytopenia: Thrombocytopenia is associated with increased risk of bleeding depending upon grades of thrombocytopenia and type of procedure or surgery being performed in the patient and pose patient for consequent risk under anaesthesia and perioperative period. US National Cancer Institute have classified thrombocytopenia (platelet level <150,000/μL) in four grades [38]:
   Grade 1—platelet greater than 75,000
   Grade 2—platelet 50,000–75,000
   Grade 3—platelet 10,000–50,000
   Grade 4—platelet less than 10,000

Indications of platelet transfusion in actively bleeding patients and as preparation for some common procedures are enumerated in Table 47.1 [39].

Table 47.1 Indications of platelet transfusion [39]

Platelet transfusion		
S. no.	Indication	Platelet level/μL
1	• Actively bleeding patient (including DIC)	• To keep platelet count above 50,000/μL
	• Central nervous bleeding	• To keep platelet count above 100,000/μL
2	Preparation for an invasive procedure:	
	• Neurosurgery or ocular surgery	<100,000
	• Most other major surgery	<50,000
	• Endoscopic procedure	
	– Therapeutic	<50,000
	– low risk diagnostic procedure	<20,000
	• Bronchoscopy with bronchoalveolar lavage (BAL)	<20,000–30,000
	• Central line placement	<20,000
	• Lumbar puncture	
	– Hematologic malignancy	<10,000–20,000
	– Without hematologic malignancy	<40,000–50,000
	– Immune thrombocytopenia (ITP)	Lower thresholds may be used
	• Neuraxial analgesia/anaesthesia	<80,000
	• Bone marrow aspiration or biopsy	<20,000
3	Prevention of spontaneous bleeding (can vary depending on patient and clinical scenario):	
	• Afibrile patient and low platelets due to myelosuppression	<10,000
	• Fibrile or septic patients	<20,000–30,000
	• Acute promyelocytic leukemia (APC) with coagulopathy	<30,000–50,000

3. Anaemia: Anaemia is seen in more than 50% of cancer patients undergoing anti-cancer therapy [40]. Anaemia correction with perioperative blood transfusion has been implicated for immunosuppression, increased role of cancer recurrence and worse overall oncological prognosis [41].

47.2.8 Other Risks or Complications

1. Venous thromboembolism (VTE): Cancer patients are known to have increased risk of venous thromboembolism with an associated increased morbidity and mortality in comparison to general population. Mulder et al. have reported a 12-month cumulative incidence of VTE around 3% after cancer diagnosis which is nine-fold higher than in general population [42]. This risk of VTE in cancer patients may be further enhanced with duration of anaesthesia more than 2 h and immobilisation during surgery [43] and an incidence of 45–69% post-operative VTE in cancer patients without prophylaxis is known [7]. Moreover, patients on VTE treatment or prophylaxis have risk of epidural haematoma formation at the time of epidural catheter insertion or removal and it is prudent that time of insertion and removal of epidural catheter as per standard guidelines is followed [44].
2. Tumour lysis syndrome: Tumour lysis syndrome is seen with cytotoxic chemotherapy agents and presents with multiple metabolic derangements causing hypocalcaemia, hyperuricaemia, hyperkalaemia and uraemia [7, 45, 46] with its obvious implications and challenges for anaesthesiologist in perioperative period. This syndrome has been seen in Burkitt's lymphoma, acute lymphoblastic leukaemia being treated with chemotherapeutic agents. Anaesthesia, fever, radiotherapy or corticosteroid administration are other known triggering factors for manifestation of tumour lysis syndrome [46].
3. Risk of hypothermia: Most of cancer patients are prone for hypothermia in intraoperative and postoperative period because of their poor nutrition status and disturbed homeostasis. Use of forced convective air warming device is indicated to maintain normothermia and to prevent perioperative complications [7].
4. Inability to get intravenous (I/V) access: Inability to get peripheral I/V access in cancer patients as a result of chemotherapy, radiotherapy or prior surgical procedures is known. A healthcare professionals' estimated incidence of 31% of peripheral vein sclerosis has been reported in breast cancer patients [47]. Even jugular venous (peripheral or central) or subclavian venous access may be difficult in head and neck cancer patients post radiotherapy, due to previous surgery or because of tumour mass effect. Vein visualisation tool (near infrared light/US as per availability) to aid peripheral IV access is being used and recommended [48].
5. Risk of tumour recurrence: Literature review suggest role of anaesthesia agents or techniques and drugs used in perioperative period including blood transfusion in tumour recurrence [1–6, 36, 49, 50]
   (a) Volatile anaesthetics and opioids impair natural killer cell function which is primary host defence against cancer [4].

(b) Few studies have reported shorter time of diagnosis of new cancer and of cancer free survival with higher concentration of oxygen usage and fraction of inspired oxygen (FIO_2) of 0.3–0.4 is being suggested during anaesthesia and post anaesthesia period [49].
(c) Dexmedetomidine (alpha 2 adrenoceptor) used in perioperative period may play a role in development of breast cancer [49].

47.3 Preoperative Anaesthesia Evaluation

A careful detailed history, general and systemic examination are the main stay for better outcome in cancer patients with relevant investigations and optimisation preoperatively as well as for appropriate management per and postoperatively. Besides routine pre anaesthesia workup specific evaluations are stressed upon depending upon type of tumour, its local and systemic effects and associated ongoing anticancer therapies.

47.3.1 Airway and Respiratory System Evaluation

1. Airway assessment:
   (a) Various predictors for difficult airway and intubation and its management have been used preoperatively in head and neck cancer patients. Hazariwalla et al. in their observational study in 2020 [11] have used Modified Mallampatti (MMT) classification, jaw protrusion (Calder's test), thyromental distance (TMD), mobility of cervical spine, Atlanto occipital joint extension, Cormack and Lehane grading as predictors and have suggested combination of MMT and jaw protrusion to be a better predictor of difficult airway.
   (b) Side to side mobility of thyroid cartilage: Radiotherapy in head and neck cancers leads to tissue fibrosis and fixity of thyroid cartilage leading to inability of lifting up of epiglottis during direct laryngoscopy and is a common cause of failed intubation in such patients.
   (c) X-Ray neck: Antero posterior and lateral view in case of head and neck cancer patients to assess for airway deviation or compression (Fig. 47.1).
   (d) Computed tomography (CT) neck: May be required in relatively asymptomatic large or symptomatic neck tumours as fibreoptic intubation may not be feasible and even tracheostomy tube may not bypass tumour.
2. Assessment for signs and symptoms of airway obstruction especially in mediastinal tumour patients:
   (a) History for episodes of dyspnoea, stridor/wheezing and/or orthopnoea
   (b) Raised jugular venous pressure (JVP)
   (c) CT scan chest
   (d) Pulmonary function test (PFT) to differentiate between dyspnoea of chronic obstructive pulmonary disease (COPD) and mediastinal tumour (Table 47.2)

Table 47.2 Classification and anaesthesia management of patients with anterior mediastinal mass [52]

S. no.	Category of patient	Symptoms	Radiological evidence	Anesthesia management	Monitoring standard
1	Low risk	Asymptomatic or mildly symptomatic without postural symptoms	No radiological evidence of significant compression of structures	GA with positive pressure ventilation	Routine anaesthesia monitoring
2	Intermediate risk	Mild to moderate	Tracheal compression <50% of normal CSA	• Awake fibreoptic intubation with LA • Spontaneous ventilation during GA I/V anesthetic agent, dexmedetomidine, ketamine • Use of "rescue" position, if required • Consider post op ventilation in case of: – Tracheomalacia – In long standing large mass – Long operative period – Significant blood loss and fluid shifts	• Routine anaesthesia monitoring • Invasive arterial monitoring mandatory • Large bore I/V access in lower extremity if preoperative evidence of SVC syndrome exists
3	High risk	Severe postural symptoms, stridor cyanosis	Tracheal compression >50% of normal CSA + associated tracheal compression, pericardial effusion or SVC syndrome	• Awake fibreoptic intubation with LA • Spontaneous ventilation during GA, I/V anaesthetic agent, dexmedetomidine, ketamine • Use of "rescue" position, if required • Consider post op ventilation in case of: – Tracheomalacia – In long standing large mass – Long operative period – Significant blood loss and fluid shifts • Cardiopulmonary bypass in highest risk patients. Cannulation should occur prior to induction of anesthesia. Post op ventilation required	• Routine anaesthesia monitoring • Invasive arterial monitoring mandatory • Large bore I/V access in lower extremity if preoperative evidence of SVC syndrome exists

CSA cross sectional area, *GA* general anaesthesia, *I/V* intravenous, *LA* local anaesthesia, *SVC* superior vena cava syndrome

3. Assessment for signs and symptoms of pulmonary fibrosis
   (a) Pulmonary function test
   (b) Arterial blood gas (ABG)
   (c) Carbon monoxide diffusion capacity

47.3.2 Cardiovascular Assessment

1. Younger patients with history of thoracic radiation: ECG, careful chest auscultation for heart sounds and murmur in view of associated coronary and valvular heart disease is required.
2. Signs and symptoms of arrythmia post chemotherapy need to be assessed.
3. Signs and symptoms of cardiomyopathy and reduced ejection fraction: breathlessness, raised JVP.
4. Signs and symptoms of cardiac tamponade (pericardial effusion or mass effect).
   (a) Progressive dyspnoea
   (b) Retrosternal chest pain
   (c) Abdominal discomfort from hepatic enlargement
   (d) Raised JVP
   (e) Diminished heart sound
   (f) Narrow pulse pressure
   (g) Pulsus paradoxus
   (h) Hepatic engorgement
5. Investigations required for tamponade:
   (a) ECG: ECG shows decreased voltage
   (b) Echocardiography
   (c) Chest X-ray: Chest X-ray shows cardiomegaly, pulmonary oedema, pleural effusion (may be the cause).
6. Investigations for chemotherapy dependent cardiotoxicity
   (a) ECG: Non-specific ST and T wave changes, premature atrial and ventricular contractions, sinus tachycardia or low voltage QRS complex may be seen. Torsedes de Pointes may be seen in chemotherapeutic agents causing QT prolongation.
   (b) Echocardiography: Cardiomyopathy may have reduced left ventricular ejection fraction.

47.3.3 Gastrointestinal and Hepatic System Evaluation

1. Patients with radiotherapy in abdominal region may have long term effects (months after completion of therapy) in the form of strictures, bowel obstruction, perforation, bleeding or fistula formation and may complain of pain in abdomen during pre-anaesthesia evaluation.

2. Investigations required:
   (a) Biochemical tests: Liver function test (LFT), serum electrolytes, coagulation profile, serum albumin.
   (b) Ultrasound abdomen: for grade of hepatitis when indicated.

47.3.4 Renal System Evaluation

1. All relevant renal panel investigations.

47.3.5 Nervous System Evaluation

1. Neurological assessment as per history and examination.
2. Assessment for involvement of autonomic nervous system: Check for postural hypotension.
3. Carotid ultrasound: Required in case of head and neck radiotherapy in view of risk of ischaemic stroke [21]. Review and documentation are must before anaesthesia.

47.3.6 Endocrinological and Electrolyte Imbalance Evaluation

1. Serum electrolytes: sodium, chloride, calcium.
2. Thyroid function test (TFT): Free T3, Free T4, TSH in case of history of radiotherapy to head and neck region and patients on chemotherapeutic agents causing hypothyroidism, e.g., TKI group of drugs. Thyroid function test measurement is being recommended prior to initiating treatment with TKI and then periodically afterwards for at least 6 months and especially in female patients [27].
3. HPA axis status assessment when indicated (Flowchart 47.1): Morning serum cortisol, ACTH stimulation test. Suggested reading is an article by Hamrahian et al. [22].
4. Other relevant investigations suggesting endocrinal tumours, e.g.
   (a) Phaeochromocytoma: (triad of headache, palpitation and sweating) Urinary and plasma metanephrine [34] and urinary vanillylmandelic acid.
   (b) Carcinoid syndrome: 24-hour urinary excretion of 5-hdroxyindoleaceticacid (5-HIAA). Suggested reading is an article by Jonathan R. Strosberg [51].

47.3.7 Myelosuppression Assessment

1. Complete blood count and absolute neutrophil count is indicated to look for neutropenia, thrombocytopenia, anaemia or pancytopenia. Timing of investigation is of paramount importance as the nadir of myelosuppression is known to occur between 7 and 14 days of chemotherapy or radiotherapy [38].

47.4 Management of Risk and/or Complications

47.4.1 Airway/Respiratory

1. Difficult airway management mandates careful planning and availability of difficult airway drill trolley including fibreoptic endoscope for awake intubations, intubating LMA, I gel and tracheostomy trays along with the surgical team. In case of mediastinal mass anaesthesia plan has to be formulated for each patient. Blank et all have enumerated use of risk stratification strategies and further anaesthetic management [52]. Table 47.2 elucidates the classification of patients with anterior mediastinal mass and anaesthesia management.
2. In large head and neck or mediastinal tumour with tracheal compression at the caudal end tracheostomy may need to be planned with smaller size endo tracheal tube as tracheostomy tube may not bypass the obstruction.
3. Administration of injection dexamethasone 8 mg IV in adults to prevent laryngeal oedema which facilitates safer extubation postoperatively.
4. Careful administration of oxygen concentration to maintain oxygen saturation between 88% and 92% in case of pulmonary fibrosis patients to prevent exacerbation of pulmonary toxicity. Use of PEEP as ventilatory strategy is mandated in such patients [5].

47.4.2 Cardiovascular

1. For management of cardiovascular risks and complications continuous five lead ECG monitoring peroperatively along with intra-arterial blood pressure monitoring and CVP monitoring is required wherever needed. Readiness with vasopressors, antiarrhythmic and antihypertensive agents is required for timely administration.
2. Certain anaesthesia drugs, e.g., propofol (moderate risk), dexmedetomidine (low risk) or opioids, e.g., methadone (moderate risk) and buprenorphine (low risk) have QT prolongation properties and are to be avoided or to be used cautiously under anaesthesia in patients having QT prolongation [17], e.g., post chemotherapy with crizotinib, sorafenib, sunitinib, etc.

47.4.3 Renal and GI System Considerations

1. Appropriate hydration needs to be maintained in perioperative period in patients in risk associated with renal or gastrointestinal function as indicated.
2. Anaesthesia drug dosage need precaution as in any other renal or hepatic disease.

47.4.4 Neurological/Nervous System

1. Regional anaesthesia is to be used cautiously in patients with ANS dysfunction and with coagulopathy.
2. It is recommended to maintain intraoperative mean arterial blood pressure of >70 mmHg and avoid hypocarbia [53] in patients with risk of stroke as in post radiotherapy of head and neck tumours.

47.4.5 Endocrinological and Electrolyte Imbalance

1. Patients on glucocorticoids:
   (a) Management in perioperative period to be done as per HPA axis status [22] to prevent unresponsive hypotension in perioperative period (Flowchart 47.1).
   (b) Intermediate category patients requiring urgent or emergency surgery should receive empiric perioperative glucocorticoid coverage [22] as per Flowchart 47.1 depending upon the type of surgery without waiting for tests for HPA axis status.
   (c) Etomidate is best avoided as it inhibits steroid synthesis and precipitates acute adrenal insufficiency. In case it is to be used the perioperative glucocorticoid coverage or close monitoring of the patient is required [22].
2. Hypercalcaemia:
   (a) Hydration, calcitonin, bisphosphonates, denosumab, corticosteroids and cinacalcet are treatment modalities depending upon the cause of hypercalcemia [54, 55]. Anaesthetic management involves the maintenance of euvolemia with sodium containing fluid.
   (b) Continuous ECG monitoring is mandatory to detect PR interval and QT interval shortening.
   (c) Reduced doses of non-depolarising neuromuscular blocking agents are to be used in patients with muscle weakness.
3. Phaeochromocytoma hypertensive/hypotensive crisis: Alpha receptor and beta receptor blockade and intravascular volume expansion in preoperative preparation and serial haematocrit estimation are the mainstay of management [17, 34, 56]. Intraoperatively invasive monitoring of blood pressure and central venous pressure is imperative even in pre-operative normotensive patients [34]. Immediately post excision of tumour and in post-operative period fluid loading and vasopressors are required as incidence of hypotension in the range of 20–70% has been reported. Severe hypoglycaemia is also known because of rebound hyperinsulinemia [34] and requires management.
4. Carcinoid crisis: It's been recommended to have ready availability of octreotide intraoperatively and to be used when needed. The prophylactic preoperative use of octreotide is optional in patients with carcinoid syndrome especially in patients who are already on long-acting somatostatin analogues [33]. Recommended dose of injection octreotide is 50–200 mcg/h.

47.4.6 Myelosuppression and Haematologic Status

1. Anaemia: Restrictive transfusion strategies (haemoglobin threshold of 7–8 g/dL) are being indicated in cancer patients for surgery [57] although associated comorbidities, clinical signs and symptoms and the age factor play a major role in final decision of blood transfusion. Haemoglobin value of 10–11 g/dL is being suggested for patients with significant risk factors [7].
2. Neutropenia: Management of neutropenia patients for surgery involves multidisciplinary approach by involving oncologists and surgical team. Use of antibiotic is prudent and granulocyte stimulating factor (G-CSF) is being used by oncologists as per NCCN guidelines [58].
3. Thrombocytopenia: Some of platelet transfusion indications are enumerated in Table 47.1 and dosage in Fig. 47.3.

47.4.7 Patients on VTE Prophylaxis

1. As per International Initiative on Thrombosis and Cancer (ITAC) guidelines 2022 [59] anticoagulation prophylaxis should be started between 12 and 2 h preoperatively. It is recommended to continue the prophylaxis for at least 7–10 days post operatively and once daily low dose low molecular weight heparin (LMWH) or low dose unfractionated heparin thrice a day. In patients undergoing major cancer abdominal or pelvic surgery (laparotomy or laparoscopy) and without a high bleeding risk, grade 1A recommendation is for extended duration low molecular weight heparin prophylaxis for 4 weeks [59]. Mechanical prophylaxis as monotherapy is indicated only when pharmacological methods are contraindicated. An intermittent pneumatic compression plus low molecular weight heparin has been shown to be the best VTE prevention method in patients with

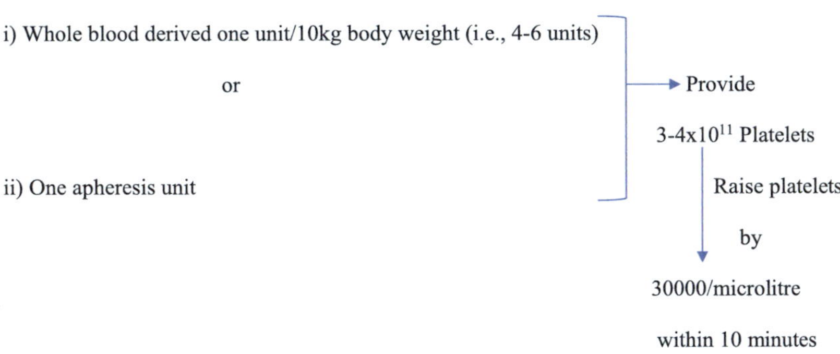

Fig. 47.3 Dosage of platelets [39]

gynaecological cancer undergoing major abdominopelvic surgery [60]. Inferior vena cava filters are not recommended for routine prophylaxis (grade 1A recommendation) in cancer patients undergoing surgery as per 2022 ITAC guidelines for thromboprophylaxis [59].

2. Guidelines for epidural catheter insertion or removal: Fonseca et al. in 2020 have reviewed various aspects of VTE prevention drugs and epidural anaesthesia need and have made recommendations [44]. The interval between last dosage of LMWH and neuraxial blockade as well as epidural catheter removal has been recommended from >12 h (prophylactic dosage) to >24 h (patients on therapeutic dosage). The interval between catheter removal and next dose (prophylactic or therapeutic) has been recommended to be more than 4 h. The article reading is suggested for complete guidelines in case of usage of other thromboprophylactic agents. Other suggested reading is an article on regional anaesthesia in patients on anti-thrombotic drugs where joint European Society of Anaesthesiology and Intensive Care (SAIC) and European Society of Regional Anaesthesia (ESRA) guidelines are published in 2022 [61].

47.4.8 Tumour Recurrence

There are multiple contradictory reports of beneficial or detrimental effects of one or another anaesthetic techniques for tumour recurrence or progression.

1. As of now local anaesthetic lidocaine and propofol intravenous anaesthetic agents are being implicated to improve host immunity and potentially reduce cancer recurrence [50].
2. Although various previous studies have implicated regional anaesthesia as beneficial effect on cancer recurrence versus general anaesthesia, one of the latest randomised trial has shown 30% recurrence free survival in patients who received volatile anaesthetics based general anaesthesia with opioid based patient control analgesia (PCA) versus 24% among patient who had received epidural anaesthesia analgesia technique [50].
3. In view of implication of role of blood transfusion in tumour recurrence and poor prognosis of cancer patients especially in abdominopelvic surgery, restrictive blood transfusion strategies as stated above are to be implemented. Other measures like use of antifibrinolytics may be considered [62].
4. No change in any current anaesthesia practice is recommended as more prospective trials are needed for any definitive technique recommendation in view of various contradictory reports.

47.5 Conclusion

Cancer patients by way of tumour's local or systemic effects or because of anticancer treatment pose multiple challenges for anaesthesiologists, surgeons and oncologists in perioperative period. Flowchart 47.2 depicts overview of associated major

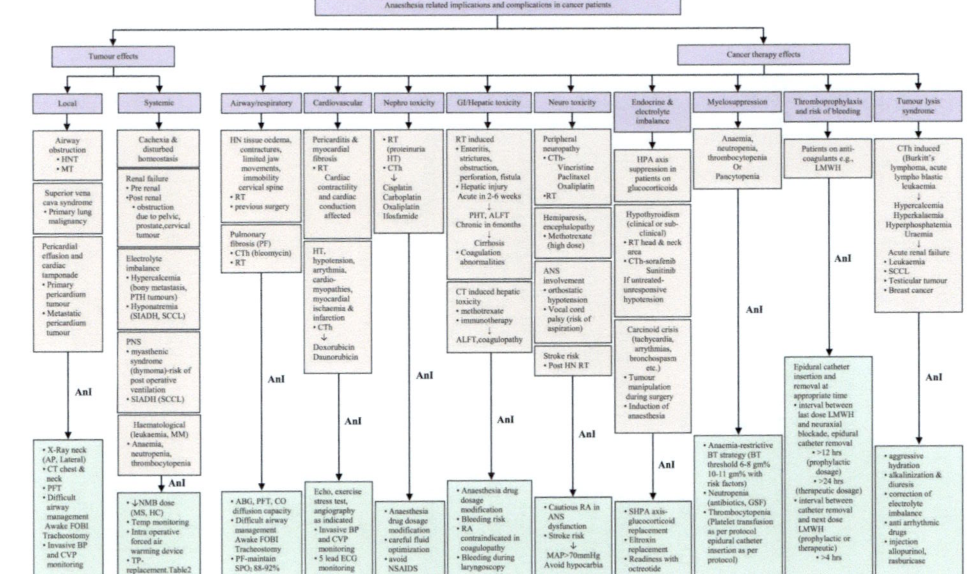

ABG: arterial blood gas; ALFT: abnormal liver function test; AnI: anaesthesia plan/implications; ANS: autonomic nervous system; AP: antero posterior; BP: blood pressure; BT: blood transfusion; CO: carbon monoxide; CT: computed tomography; CTh: chemotherapy; CVP: central venous pressure; Echo: echocardiogram; GI: gastrointestinal; GSF: granulocyte stimulating factor; HC: hypercalcemia; HN: head & neck; HNT: head & neck tumour; HPA: hypothalamic-pituitary-adrenal; HT: hypertension; LMWH: low molecular weight heparin; MAP: mean arterial pressure; MM: multiple myeloma; MS: myasthenic syndrome; MT: mediastinal tumour; NMB: neuro muscular blocker; NSAIDS: non-steroidal anti-inflammatory drugs; PFT: pulmonary function test; PHT: pulmonary hypertension; PNS: para neoplastic syndrome; PTH: parathyroid hormone; RA: regional anaesthesia; RT: radiotherapy; SCCL: small cell carcinoma lung; SHPA: suppressed hypothalamic-pituitary-adrenal; SIADH: syndrome of inappropriate antidiuretic hormone; Temp: temperature; TP: thrombocytopenia

Flowchart 47.2 Anaesthesia related implications and complications in cancer patients: an overview [5, 7, 14, 17, 45, 46]. *ABG* arterial blood gas, *ALFT* abnormal liver function test, *AnI* anaesthesia plan/implications, *ANS* autonomic nervous system, *AP* antero posterior, *BP* blood pressure, *BT* blood transfusion, *CO* carbon monoxide, *CT* computed tomography, *CTh* chemotherapy, *CVP* central venous pressure, *Echo* echocardiogram, *GI* gastrointestinal, *GSF* granulocyte stimulating factor, *HC* hypercalcemia, *HN* head & neck, *HNT* head & neck tumour, *HPA* hypothalamic-pituitary-adrenal, *HT* hypertension, *LMWH* low molecular weight heparin, *MAP* mean arterial pressure, *MM* multiple myeloma, *MS* myasthenic syndrome, *MT* mediastinal tumour, *NMB* neuro muscular blocker, *NSAIDS* non-steroidal anti-inflammatory drugs, *PFT* pulmonary function test, *PHT* pulmonary hypertension, *PNS* para neoplastic syndrome, *PTH* parathyroid hormone, *RA* regional anaesthesia, *RT* radiotherapy, *SCCL* small cell carcinoma lung, *SHPA* suppressed hypothalamic-pituitary-adrenal, *SIADH* syndrome of inappropriate antidiuretic hormone, *Temp* temperature, *TP* thrombocytopenia

risks and complications in patients with malignancy along with important anaesthesia related implications/action points which need a collaborative and multidisciplinary approach. In depth knowledge of cancer therapies and it's side effects, careful history and examination, further evaluation and optimization in preoperative period by the anaesthesiologist, and management per and postoperatively along with the team lead to safer and better outcome in these patients.

Key Points

1. Airway obstruction by head and neck and mediastinal tumours mandates careful preoperative assessment and planning for intubation and extubation to prevent adverse respiratory events in perioperative period. Large head and neck tumours with caudal tracheal extension or compression may require tracheostomy with small size endotracheal tube instead of tracheostomy tube.
2. Careful administration of oxygen concentration to maintain oxygen saturation between 88% and 92% in case of pulmonary fibrosis patients to prevent exacerbation of pulmonary toxicity is required. Use of PEEP as ventilatory strategy is recommended in such patients.
3. Cardiac complications as a tumour mass effect, post radiotherapy or chemotherapy in the form of pericarditis, cardiac tamponade or cardiac myopathies require echocardiography to evaluate left ventricular ejection fraction and pericardiocentesis in compromising pericardial effusion in preoperative period. Intraoperatively invasive blood pressure, central venous pressure and cardiac output monitoring may be required.
4. Cautious use of anaesthetic drugs having propensity for QT prolongation, e.g., propofol, dexmedetomidine, methadone, buprenorphine is warranted in patients receiving chemotherapy associated with QT interval prolongation, e.g., crizotinib, sorafenib, sunitinib etc. in order to prevent dangerous arrythmias like torsades de pointes.
5. Chemotherapy induced (4–12 weeks post immunotherapy) and radiation induced hepatic injury (acute within 2–6 weeks and chronic after 6 months) with portal hypertension, deranged liver function and coagulopathy requires appropriate pre anaesthetic evaluation, optimization and anaesthesia drug modification as in any other hepatic disease. Regional anaesthesia is contraindicated in patients with coagulopathy.
6. Stroke risk is associated with patients undergoing neck irradiation and carotid ultrasound review and documentation is must before anaesthesia. Peroperatively maintenance of mean arterial blood pressure >70 mmHg and avoidance of hypocarbia is recommended.
7. Patients receiving glucocorticoid therapy may have suppressed HPA axis and may require perioperative glucocorticoid replacement to prevent hypotensive haemodynamic complications.
8. Hypothyroidism post radiotherapy (23–53% incidence) in head and neck cancer patients, post TKI inhibitor therapy (40% incidence) and with other chemotherapy agents like sorafenib, sunitinib is known in patients with malignancy. As literature review has shown cardiac complications like atrial fibrillation,

unresponsive hypotension in perioperative period in patients with undetected and untreated subclinical hypothyroidism, cautious perioperative management with eltroxin replacement therapy may be required in such patients as a preventive measure as per defined institutional protocol.

9. Hypercalcaemia is a common manifestation occurring in 30% of cancer patients with its resultant cardiac complications in the form of short QT interval on ECG, arrythmias and even cardiac arrest with calcium concentration of more than 3.75 mmol/L. Anaesthesia management involves continuous ECG monitoring, maintenance of euvolemia with isotonic saline, reduced doses of non-depolarising neuromuscular blocking agents in patients presenting with muscle weakness along with other standard treatment modalities in perioperative period.
10. Myelosuppression and resultant thrombocytopenia need platelet transfusion in perioperative period as per thrombocytopenia grade and type of invasive procedure or surgery being performed.
11. Patients on VTE treatment or prophylaxis have risk of epidural haematoma formation at the time of epidural catheter insertion or removal and it is prudent that time of insertion and removal of epidural catheter as per standard guidelines is followed.
12. Tumour lysis syndrome with its manifestations of hyperkalaemia, hyperuricemia, hyperphosphatemia with resultant hypocalcaemia may be triggered by chemotherapeutic agents, corticosteroids, radiotherapy, fever and anaesthesia itself and aggressive management is required by attending anaesthesiologist.
13. Various anaesthesia agents or technique chosen for surgical intervention have the potential to harm or benefit the patient in relation to tumour progression or recurrence. Although numerous studies have been performed, currently the data available is insufficient to recommend a definitive anaesthetic choice.

Acknowledgement The author acknowledges the artwork and assistance of Mr. Yash Agarwal in composing the manuscript.

References

1. Montejano J, Jevtovic-Todorovic V. Anesthesia and cancer, friend or foe? A narrative review. Front Oncol. 2021;11:1–7.
2. Liu Q, Sheng Z, Cheng C, Zheng H, Lanuti M, Liu R, Wang P, Shen Y, Xie Z. Anesthetic propofol promotes tumor metastasis in lungs via GABAA R-dependent TRIM21 modulation of Src expression. Adv Sci (Weinh). 2021;8(18):e2102079.
3. Raigon Ponferrada A, Guerrero Orriach J, Malo Manso A, Sepúlveda Haro E, Romero Molina S, Fontaneda Heredia A, et al. Anaesthesia and cancer: can anaesthetic drugs modify gene expression? Ecancermedicalscience. 2020;14:1–13.
4. Wall T, Sherwin A, Ma D, Buggy D. Influence of perioperative anaesthetic and analgesic interventions on oncological outcomes: a narrative review. Br J Anaesth. 2019;123(2):135–50.
5. Gudaitytė J, Dvylys D, Šimeliūnaitė I. Anaesthetic challenges in cancer patients: current therapies and pain management. Acta Med Litu. 2017;24(2):121–7.

6. Kim R. Effects of surgery and anesthetic choice on immunosuppression and cancer recurrence. J Transl Med. 2018;16(1):1–13.
7. Bajwa S, Kulshrestha A. Anaesthesia considerations and implications during oncologic and non-oncologic surgery in cancer patients. Apollo Med. 2014;11(3):191–6.
8. Sriramka B, Karan D, Parida M. Post-radiation airway management—an anesthesiologist's challenge. J Dent Anesth Pain Med. 2019;19(1):73–5.
9. Khan Joad S, Jain D. Head and neck radiotherapy—a risk factor for anaesthesia? Indian J Anaesth. 2020;64:488–94.
10. Shamim F, Khan A, Khan F. First-pass success of tracheal intubation with videolaryngoscopy in head and neck cancer patients: a registry-based retrospective cohort study. Cureus. 2021;13(12):1–8.
11. Hajariwala V, Pathak B. Predicting difficult intubation in head and neck cancer patients using clinical predictors: an observational study. Int J Anesthesiol. 2020;13(3):191–5.
12. Jilani TN, Killeen RB, Siddiqui AH. Mediastinal cancer [Updated 2022 Apr 9]. In: StatPearls. Treasure Island, FL: StatPearls Publishing; 2022.
13. Ku CM. Anesthesia for patients with mediastinal masses. In: Slinger P, editor. Principles and practice of anesthesia for thoracic surgery. Springer; 2011. p. 201–10.
14. Allan N, Siller C, Breen A. Anaesthetic implications of chemotherapy. Contin Educ Anaesth Crit Care Pain. 2012;12(2):52–6.
15. Mullin M. Anesthetic implications of Intraarterial chemotherapy for retinoblastoma: a literature review. Nurse Anesthesia Capstones. 2020, p. 35. https://dune.une.edu/na_capstones/35.
16. Gómez-Henao P, Carreño-Dueñas J. Cardiovascular pre-anesthesia evaluation in oncological surgery. Colomb J Anesthesiol. 2016;44(1):17–22.
17. UpToDate. Uptodate.com. Preoperative evaluation and management of patients with cancer [reviewed 2022 Jun; cited 2022 Jul 21]. Available from: https://www.uptodate.com/contents/preoperative-evaluation-and-management-of-patients-with-cancer.
18. O'Reilly M, Mellotte G, Ryan B, O'Connor A. Gastrointestinal side effects of cancer treatments. Ther Adv Chronic Dis. 2020;11:1–7.
19. Huitink JM, Teoh WHL. Current cancer therapies—a guide for perioperative physicians. Best Pract Res Clin Anaesthesiol. 2013;27(4):481–92.
20. Sahai SK. Perioperative assessment of the cancer patient. Best Pract Res Clin Anaesthesiol. 2013;27(4):465–80.
21. Plummer C, Henderson R, O'Sullivan J, Read S. Ischemic stroke and transient ischemic attack after head and neck radiotherapy. Stroke. 2011;42(9):2410–8.
22. UpToDate. Uptodate.com. The management of the surgical patient taking glucocorticoids [reviewed 2022 Jun; cited 2022 Jul 22]. Available from: https://www.uptodate.com/contents/the-management-of-the-surgical-patient-taking-glucocorticoids.
23. Leung A, McAlister F, Rogers S, Pazo V, Wright A, Bates D. Preoperative hyponatremia and perioperative complications. Arch Intern Med. 2012;172(19):1474–81.
24. Vassalotti JA, Dupree E. Preoperative hyponatremia. An opportunity for intervention? Arch Intern Med. 2012;172(19):1482–3.
25. Guise T, Wysolmerski J. Cancer-associated hypercalcemia. N Engl J Med. 2022;386(15):1443–51.
26. Parikh M, Webb S. Cations: potassium, calcium, and magnesium. Contin Educ Anaesth Crit Care Pain. 2012;12(4):195–8.
27. Lechner M, Vyas C, Hamnvik O, Alexander E, Larsen P, Choueiri T, et al. Hypothyroidism during tyrosine kinase inhibitor therapy is associated with longer survival in patients with advanced nonthyroidal cancers. Thyroid. 2018;28(4):445–53.
28. Sudha P, Koshy R, Pillai V. Undetected hypothyroidism and unexpected anesthetic complications. J Anaesthesiol Clin Pharmacol. 2012;28(2):276–7.
29. Garcia-Serra A, Amdur RJ, Morris CG, Mazzaferri E, Mendenhall WM. Thyroid function should be monitored following radiotherapy to the low neck. Am J Clin Oncol. 2005;28:255–8.

30. Rodondi N, Newman AB, Vittinghoff E, de Rekeneire N, Satterfield S, Harris TB, et al. Subclinical hypothyroidism and the risk of heart failure, other cardiovascular events and death. Arch Intern Med. 2005;165:2460–6.
31. Martinez-comendador J, Marcos-Vidal JM, Gualis J, Martin CE, Martin E, Otero J, et al. Subclinical hypothyroidism might increase the risk of postoperative atrial fibrillation after aortic valve replacement. Thorac Cardiovasc Surg. 2016;64:427–33.
32. Garber J, Cobin R, Gharib H, Hennessey J, Klein I, Mechanick J, et al. Clinical practice guidelines for hypothyroidism in adults: cosponsored by the American Association of Clinical Endocrinologists and the American Thyroid Association. Thyroid. 2012;22(12):1200–35.
33. UpToDate. Uptodate.com. Treatment of the carcinoid syndrome [reviewed 2022 Jun; cited 2022 Jul 22]. Available from: https://www.uptodate.com/contents/treatment-of-the-carcinoid-syndrome.
34. Ramachandran R, Rewari V. Current perioperative management of pheochromocytomas. Indian J Urol. 2016;33(1):19–25.
35. BMJ best practices. Bmj.com. Assessment of neutropenia [reviewed 2022 Jun; cited 2022 Jul 23]. Available from: https://bestpractice.bmj.com/topics/en-gb/893.
36. Cata J, Gottumukkala V. Blood transfusion practices in cancer surgery. Indian J Anaesth. 2014;58(5):637–42.
37. Jolissaint J, Harary M, Saadat L, Madenci A, Dieffenbach B, Al Natour R, et al. Timing and outcomes of abdominal surgery in neutropenic patients. J Gastrointest Surg. 2019;23(4):643–50.
38. Hospital Pharmacy Europe. Hospitalpharmacyeurope.com. Management of myelosuppression in cancer patients. 2010 [cited 2010 Jun 9]. Available from: https://hospitalpharmacyeurope.com/news/editorspick/management-of-myelosuppression-in-cancer-patients.
39. UpToDate. Uptodate.com. Platelet transfusion: indications, ordering, and associated risks [reviewed 2022 Jun; cited 2022 Jul 20]. Available from: https://www.uptodate.com/contents/platelet-transfusion-indications-ordering-and-associated-risks.
40. Radziwon P, Krzakowski M, Kalinka E, Zaucha R, Wysocki P, Kowalski D, et al. Anemia in cancer patients—expert group recommendations. Revision 2020. Oncol Clin Pract. 2020;16(5):261–9.
41. Odell D, Bilimoria K. Evaluating appropriate blood transfusion in cancer surgery. JAMA Surg. 2016;151(6):525.
42. Mulder FI, Horvath-Puho E, Van Es N, Van Laarhoven HWM, Pedersen L, Moik F, et al. Venous thromboembolism in cancer patients: a population-based cohort study. Blood. 2021;137(14):1959–69.
43. Agnelli G, Bolis G, Capussotti L, Scarpa R, Tonelli F, Bonizzoni E, et al. A clinical outcome-based prospective study on venous thromboembolism after cancer surgery. Ann Surg. 2006;243(1):89–95.
44. Fonseca N, Pontes J, Perez M, Alves R, Fonseca G. SBA 2020: regional anesthesia guideline for using anticoagulants update. Braz J Anesthesiol (Eng Ed). 2020;70(4):364–87.
45. Mayet S. A practical approach to the patient receiving chemotherapy and anaesthesia. S Afr J Anaesth Analg. 2018;24(3 Suppl 1):38–42.
46. Verma A, Mathur R, Chauhan M, Ranjan P. Tumor lysis syndrome developing intraoperatively. J Anaesthesiol Clin Pharmacol. 2011;27(4):561–3.
47. LeVasseur N, Stober C, Daigle K, Robinson A, McDiarmid S, Mazzarello S, et al. Optimizing vascular access for patients receiving intravenous systemic therapy for early-stage breast cancer—a survey of oncology nurses and physicians. Curr Oncol. 2018;25(4):298–304.
48. Bertoglio S, van Boxtel T, Goossens G, Dougherty L, Furtwangler R, Lennan E, et al. Improving outcomes of short peripheral vascular access in oncology and chemotherapy administration. J Vasc Access. 2017;18(2):89–96.
49. UpToDate. Uptodate.com. Anesthesia and cancer recurrence [reviewed 2022 Jun; cited 2022 Jun 20]. Available from: https://www.uptodate.com/contents/anesthesia-and-cancer-recurrence.
50. Buggy D, Riedel B, Sessler D. Can anaesthetic technique influence cancer outcome? The next steps…. Br J Anaesth. 2021;127(1):5–7.

51. UpToDate. Uptodate.com. Diagnosis of carcinoid syndrome and tumor localization [reviewed 2022 Jun; cited 2022 Jul 29]. Available from: https://www.uptodate.com/contents/diagnosis-of-carcinoid-syndrome-and-tumor-localization.
52. Blank R, de Souza D. Anesthetic management of patients with an anterior mediastinal mass: continuing professional development. Can J Anaesth. 2011;58(9):853–67.
53. Benesch C, Glance L, Derdeyn C, Fleisher L, Holloway R, Messé S, et al. Perioperative neurological evaluation and management to lower the risk of acute stroke in patients undergoing noncardiac, nonneurological surgery: a scientific statement from the American Heart Association/American Stroke Association. Circulation. 2021;143(19):923–46.
54. Asonitis N, Angelousi A, Zafeiris C, Lambrou G, Dontas I, Kassi E. Diagnosis, pathophysiology and management of hypercalcemia in malignancy: a review of the literature. Horm Metab Res. 2019;51(12):770–8.
55. Bassatne A, Rahme M, Piggott T, Murad M, Hneiny L, El-Hajj Fuleihan G. Values and other decisional factors regarding treatment of hypercalcaemia of malignancy: a systematic review protocol. BMJ Open. 2021;11(10):e051141.
56. Connor D, Boumphrey S. Perioperative care of phaeochromocytoma. BJA Educ. 2016;16(5):153–8.
57. Wu H, Tai Y, Lin S, Chan M, Chen H, Chang K. The impact of blood transfusion on recurrence and mortality following colorectal cancer resection: a propensity score analysis of 4,030 patients. Sci Rep. 2018;8(1):1–8.
58. Neutropenia. Medscape.com. 2021 [cited 2022 Jul 29]. Available from: https://emedicine.medscape.com/article/204821-overview.
59. Farge D, Frere C, Connors JM, Khorana AA, Kakkar A, Ay C, Muñoz A, Brenner B, Prata PH, Brilhante D, Antic D, Casais P, Guillermo Esposito MC, Ikezoe T, Abutalib SA, Meillon-García LA, Bounameaux H, Pabinger I, Douketis J, International Initiative on Thrombosis and Cancer (ITAC) Advisory Panel. 2022 International clinical practice guidelines for the treatment and prophylaxis of venous thromboembolism in patients with cancer, including patients with COVID-19. Lancet Oncol. 2022;23(7):e334–47.
60. Insin P, Vitoopinyoparb K, Thadanipon K, Charakorn C, Attia J, McKay G, et al. Prevention of venous thromboembolism in gynecological cancer patients undergoing major abdominopelvic surgery: a systematic review and network meta-analysis. Gynecol Oncol. 2021;161(1):304–13.
61. Kietaibl S, Ferrandis R, Godier A, Llau J, Lobo C, Macfarlane A, et al. Regional anaesthesia in patients on antithrombotic drugs. Eur J Anaesthesiol. 2022;39(2):100–32.
62. Sampaio AM, Guimarães GMN, Medeiros GP, Damasceno GMM, Silva RMA, Nunes RR, Rocha HAL, Nascimento JCR. Efficacy and safety of antifibrinolytics in oncological surgery: a systematic review and meta-analysis. Braz J Anesthesiol. 2019;69(5):484–92.

MIX
Papier aus verantwortungsvollen Quellen
Paper from responsible sources
FSC® C105338

If you have any concerns about our products,
you can contact us on
ProductSafety@springernature.com

In case Publisher is established outside the EU,
the EU authorized representative is:
Springer Nature Customer Service Center GmbH
Europaplatz 3, 69115 Heidelberg, Germany

Printed by Libri Plureos GmbH
in Hamburg, Germany